New Concepts in Immunodeficiency Diseases

New Concepts in Immunodeficiency Diseases

Edited by

SUDHIR GUPTA

Division of Basic and Clinical Immunology, University of California, Irvine,
California, USA

and

CLAUDE GRISCELLI

Immunology and Haematology Unit, Department of Paediatrics,
Groupe Hospitalier Necker Enfants Malades, Paris, France

JOHN WILEY & SONS
Chichester · New York · Brisbane · Toronto · Singapore

Other Wiley Editorial Offices

John Wiley & Sons, Inc., 605 Third Avenue,
New York, NY 10158-0012, USA

Jacaranda Wiley Ltd, G.P.O. Box 859, Brisbane,
Queensland 4001, Australia

John Wiley & Sons (Canada) Ltd, 22 Worcester Road,
Rexdale, Ontario M9W 1L1, Canada

John Wiley & Sons (SEA) Pte Ltd, 37 Jalan Pemimpin #05-04,
Block B, Union Industrial Building, Singapore 2057

Library of Congress Cataloging-in-Publication Data

New concepts in immunodeficiency diseases / edited by Sudhir Gupta and
   Claude Griscelli.
      p.   cm.
   Includes bibliographical references and index.
   ISBN 0 471 93880 7
   1. Immunological deficiency syndromes.   I. Gupta, Sudhir.
II. Griscelli, Claude.
   [DNLM: 1. Immunologic Deficiency Syndromes—genetics.
2. Immunologic Deficiency Syndromes—immunology.   3. Immunologic
Deficiency Syndromes—therapy.   WD 308 N53125]
RC606.N48   1993
616.97'9—dc20
DNLM/DLC
for Library of Congress   92-48950
                                                                      CIP

British Library Cataloguing in Publication Data

A catalogue record for this book is available from the British Library

ISBN 0 93880 7

Typeset in Palatino 10/12pt by Inforum, Rowlands Castle, Hants
Printed and bound in Great Britain by Biddles Ltd, Guildford & King's Lynn

Contents

Contributors

M. AMIN ARNAOUT — *Department of Medicine, Renal Unit, 8th Floor, Massachusetts General Hospital, East 149 13th Street, Charlestown, Massachusetts 02129, USA*

BARBARA E. BIERER — *Division of Pediatric Oncology, Dana-Farber Cancer Institute, 44 Binney Street, Boston, Massachusetts 02115, USA*

R. MICHAEL BLAESE — *Cellular Immunology Section, Metabolism Branch, National Cancer Institute, National Institutes of Health, Building 10, Room 6B05, Bethesda, Maryland 20892, USA*

STEVEN J. BURAKOFF — *Division of Pediatric Oncology, Dana-Farber Cancer Institute, 44 Binney Street, Boston, Massachusetts 02115, USA*

HELEN M. CHAPEL — *Department of Immunology, Nuffield Department of Medicine, John Radcliffe Hospital, Headington, Oxford OX3 9UD, UK*

MARY ELLEN CONLEY — *Department of Pediatrics, University of Tennessee College of Medicine, 332 N Lauderdale, Memphis, Tennessee TN 38101, USA*

MAX D. COOPER — *Department of Immunology, Howard Hughes Medical Institute, University of Alabama at Birmingham, T263, Birmingham, Alabama 35294, USA*

KENNETH W. CULVER — *Cellular Immunology Section, Metabolism Branch, National Cancer Institute, National Institutes of Health, Bethesda, Maryland 20892, USA*

CHARLOTTE CUNNINGHAM-RUNDLES — *Departments of Medicine and Pediatrics, Mount Sinai Medical Center, 1 Gustave L. Levy Place, Box 1089, New York, New York 10029, USA*

JOHN I. GALLIN — *Laboratory of Host Defenses, National Institute of Allergy and Infectious Diseases, National Institutes of Health, Building 10, Room 11C103, Bethesda, Maryland 20892, USA*

RICHARD A. GATTI — *Department of Pathology, UCLA School of Medicine, Center for the Health Sciences, 10883 Le Conte Avenue, Los Angeles, California 90024-1732, USA*

ERWIN W. GELFAND — *Division of Basic Sciences, Department of Pediatrics, National Jewish Center for Immunology and Respiratory Medicine, 1400 Jackson Street, Denver, Colorado 80206, USA*

JOHN GORDON — *Department of Immunology, The Medical School, University of Birmingham, Edgbaston, Birmingham B15 2TT, UK*

CLAUDE GRISCELLI — *Unite d'Immunologie et d'Hematologie, Departement de Pediatrie, Hôpital des Enfants Malades, 149 Rue de Sèvres, 75743 Paris Cedex 15, France*

SUDHIR GUPTA — *Division of Basic and Clinical Immunology, Department of Medicine, University of California, Irvine, California 92717, USA*

MICHAEL S. HERSHFIELD — *Division of Rheumatology and Immunology, Box 3049, Room 418, Sands Building, Duke University Medical Center, Durham, North Carolina 27710, USA*

CARL H. JUNE — *Immune Cell Biology Program, Naval Medical Research Institute, 8901 Wisconsin Avenue, Bethesda, Maryland 20889-5055, USA*

ANNE KESSINGER — *Section of Oncology/Hematology, University of Nebraska Medical Center, 600 South 42nd Street, Omaha, Nebraska 68198-3330, USA*

TAKASHI KEI KISHIMOTO — *Department of Immunology, Boehringer-Ingelheim Pharmaceuticals Inc., 90 East Ridge, PO Box 368, Ridgefield, Connecticut 06877, USA*

JACOV LEVY — *Department of Pediatrics, Soroka Medical Center, PO Box 151, Beer-Sheva, Israel 84101*

BARBARA LISOWSKA-GROSPIERRE — *Unite d'Immunologie et d'Hematologie, Departement de Pediatrie, Hôpital des Enfants Malades, 149 Rue de Sèvres, 75743 Paris Cedex 15, France*

ELWYN LOH

Division of Hematology and Oncology, Department of Medicine, School of Medicine, Hospital of the University of Pennsylvania, 3400 Spruce Street, Philadelphia, Pennsylvania 19104-4283 USA

BERNARD MACH

Department of Microbiology, University of Geneva, Geneva, Switzerland

MASAHIRO MICHISHITA

Department of Medicine, Renal Unit, 8th Floor, Massachusetts General Hospital, East 149 13th Street, Charlestown, Massachusetts 02129, USA

JOHN K. PARK

Division of Pediatric Oncology, Dana-Farber Cancer Institute, 44 Binney Street, Boston, Massachusetts 02115, USA

ROGER M. PERLMUTTER

Department of Immunology, 1264 Health Sciences Building—SL-05, University of Washington, Seattle, Washington 98195, USA

ALFRED REITER

Paediatric Haematology and Oncology, Medical School Hannover, D-3000-Hannover-61, Germany

HANSJÖRG RIEHM

Paediatric Haematology and Oncology, Medical School Hannover, D-3000-Hannover-61, Germany

DIRK ROOS

c/o Publication Secretariat, Central Laboratory of The Netherlands Red Cross Blood Transfusion Service, PO Box 9190, 1006 AD Amsterdam, The Netherlands

YVONNE ROSENSTEIN

Division of Pediatric Oncology, Dana-Farber Cancer Institute, 44 Binney Street, Boston, Massachusetts 02115, USA

ROBERT ROTHLEIN

Department of Immunology, Boehringer-Ingelheim Pharmaceuticals Inc., 90 East Ridge, PO Box 368, Ridgefield, Connecticut 06877, USA

MENAHEM SCHLESINGER

Barzilai Hospital, Ashkelon, Israel

HARRY W. SCHROEDER

Division of Developmental and Clinical Immunology, University of Alabama at Birmingham, Birmingham, Alabama 35294-3300, USA

JEFFREY N. SIEGEL

Immune Cell Biology Program, Naval Medical Research Institute, Bethesda, Maryland 20814, USA

JOHN E. VOLANAKIS   *Division of Clinical Immunology and Rheumatology, Department of Medicine, Howard Hughes Medical Institute, University of Alabama at Birmingham, T263, Birmingham, Alabama 35294, USA*

KARL WELTE   *Paediatric Haematology and Oncology, Medical School Hannover, D-3000-Hannover-61, Germany*

CORNELIA ZEIDLER   *Paediatric Haematology and Oncology, Medical School Hannover, D-3000-Hannover-61, Germany*

Preface

The primary immunodeficiency disorders have been known for the past seven decades; however, immunological defects were described at the cellular level and the therapies were limited to the use of γ-globulin, antibiotics, and bone marrow transplantation. During the past decade, rapid progress has been made in the understanding of the basic concepts of immune response at the biochemical and molecular levels. This new information has been instrumental in understanding the defects of many primary immunodeficiency disorders at the molecular level. As a result, innovative techniques are now available to diagnose them at a very early stage and to detect their carrier states. Novel therapeutic approaches, including gene therapy and use of biological response modifiers, have emerged. This book reviews these rapidly developing concepts in primary immunodeficiency disorders.

The book is divided into three major sections. Part A addresses basic mechanisms in the immune response. This includes development of the human antibody repertoire, pathways of human B cell growth and differentiation, development of the T cell repertoire, signalling mechanisms in T cell activation and T cell tolerance, and the role of adhesion molecules in neutrophil–endothelial cell interactions. Also included is a review on substituted guanine ribonucleoside compounds as B cell activators and their potential future use in the therapy of antibody deficiency syndromes. Part B deals with the genetic and molecular basis of primary immunodeficiency disorders. The genetic and molecular basis of Leu-CAM (adhesion molecules) deficiency is reviewed. The biochemistry and function of the CD43 molecule as co-receptor in signal transduction in lymphocytes and monocytes, and its role in the pathophysiology of Wiskott–Aldrich syndrome, are discussed. The nature of the genetic defects, detection of carrier state by various techniques to delineate X chromosome inactivation, and linkage analyses in severe combined immunodeficiency are reviewed. A chapter is devoted to combined immunodeficiency with defective expression of MHC class II antigen. The molecular and genetic basis of chronic granulomatous disease and detection of carrier state is detailed. A role for MHC class II and class III antigens in selective IgA deficiency and common variable immunodeficiency and genetic defects in ataxia–telangiectasis are discussed. Included in Part C are the advances in the area of therapy for primary immunodeficiency disorders. The current status of peripheral stem cell transplantation, PEG–ADA, and gene therapy in severe combined immunodeficiency have been reviewed. The use of biological response modifiers, including interferons in chronic granulomatous disease and IL-2 in common variable immunodeficiency, has been discussed. A chapter is devoted to the use of colony-stimulating factor and its haematological and clinical effects in congential neutropenia, cyclic neutropenia, and acquired idiopathic neutropenia. The uses, guidelines, and mechanisms of action of intravenous immunoglobulin are reviewed.

This book should be of interest to academic paediatricians, internists, basic and clinical immunologists, and transplantation biologists.

We wish to thank Miss Nancy Doman for excellent secretarial assistance.

Sudhir Gupta
Claude Griscelli

Part A
BASIC MECHANISMS

Chapter 1

Development of the Human Antibody Repertoire

HARRY W. SCHROEDER JR

Division of Developmental and Clinical Immunology, University of Alabama at Birmingham, Birmingham, Alabama, USA

ROGER M. PERLMUTTER

Department of Immunology, and Howard Hughes Medical Institute, University of Washington, Seattle, Washington, USA

INTRODUCTION

Immunoglobulins are heterodimeric proteins composed of two heavy and two light chains (1–5). Each chain can be divided into a variable domain that contributes to antigen specificity and a constant domain that mediates effector functions and permits stabilization of the H_2L_2 complex. These variable domains are the products of an ordered series of gene-splicing events that occur in fetal liver and in fetal and adult bone marrow. Assembly begins with the joining of D_H to a J_H gene segment in the next gene locus. Due to promoter-like elements positioned 5' to D_H gene segments, these initial products of heavy chain rearrangement can be transcribed and even translated into protein products (6, 7). After DJ joining has occurred on both homologous chromosomes, V to DJ rearrangements occur. The splice points between V and DJ may vary, hence on average in only one out of three cases will this rearrangement result in the formation of a product wherein the V is in the same reading frame as the J. In those cases where an in-frame join occurs, heavy chain rearrangement ceases and the homologous chromosome retains its D→J join. Should an out-of-frame join between V and DJ occur, the cell can undergo a second V→DJ rearrangement on the homologous chromosome. In this latter case, although both VDJ genes can be transcribed

New Concepts in Immunodeficiency Diseases. Edited by S. Gupta and C. Griscelli
© 1993 John Wiley & Sons Ltd

and produce mRNA, in general only one generates a functional product. Following successful rearrangement of a functional heavy chain, light chain splicing begins. After both heavy and light chain loci have produced functional products, the lymphocyte expresses its antigen receptor on the cell surface and thus becomes susceptible to selection based on the specificity of that receptor.

Each heavy and light chain variable domain contains three intervals of sequence hypervariability (termed complementarity-determining regions or CDRs) that are separated from each other by four intervals of relatively constant sequence (termed frameworks or FRs) (Figure 1.1, reviewed in ref. 5). Solution of the crystal structure of immunoglobulins has documented that the CDRs of the heavy and light chains contribute significantly to the formation of the antigen binding site. CDRs 1 and 2 of the heavy and light chains are completely encoded by their respective V gene segments, whereas the CDR 3 regions are the direct product of VDJ and VJ joining, respectively. CDRs 1 and 2 form the outside border of the binding site, while the CDR 3 regions are positioned at the boundary between the heavy and light chains and create the center of the antigen binding pocket. Hence the sequences of the CDR 3 regions greatly influence the specificity of the mature antigen receptor.

Several mechanisms contribute to the diversity of the heavy chain CDR 3 (1–4). During the splicing process, nucleotides can be lost from the 3' end of the V_H, from either the 5' or 3' end of the D_H, or from the 5' end of the J_H gene segments. Unlike V_H and J_H gene segments that have only one reading frame, D_H gene segments can potentially encode peptide sequence in six reading frames since they can rearrange by either deletion or inversion. D_H gene segments can also rearrange to each other, creating D–D products and thus doubling the extent of diversity. Finally, non-germ line encoded nucleotides can be inserted at the gene segment splice site during rearrangement. Two types of nucleotide addition exist: random and templated. Templated additions, termed "P" junctions, can be detected adjacent to the terminus of a coding sequence that has not undergone base loss (8). These nucleotide additions, typically only 1 or 2 bp in length, are palindromic copies of the terminal nucleotides of the gene segment. Random addition of nucleotides, termed "N" nucleotides or regions, is associated with the activity of terminal deoxynucleotidyl transferase (TdT), a non template-dependent DNA polymerase (9). Because non-templated nucleotides are inserted at random, each codon added by N regions increases the potential diversity of the repertoire 20-fold. Hence, even though individual B cells may rearrange the same V, D, and J gene segments, the CDR 3 sequences of their expressed heavy chain variable domains may differ, generating dramatically different antigen specificities.

5

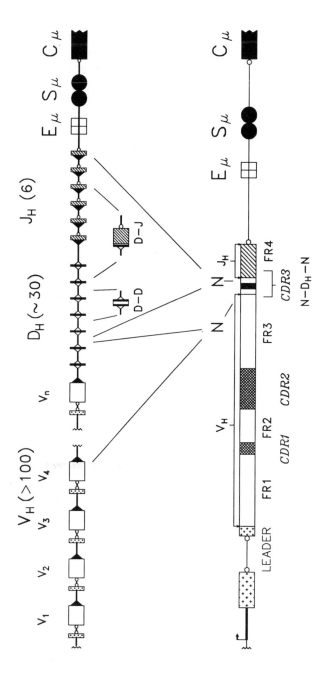

Figure 1.1. The V domain of an H chain is the product of a series of gene rearrangement events. Rearrangement in the human H chain locus is illustrated here. See text for further details (E = enhancer, S = switch region, C = constant domain(s), CDR = complementarity-determining regions, FR = framework regions)

DEVELOPMENT OF THE HEAVY CHAIN REPERTOIRE IN THE MOUSE

Although the adult repertoire of antigen specificities appears to be the product of random gene rearrangement and N region addition, the ability to respond to specific antigens develops in a programmatic fashion during fetal and neonatal life (10–13). This phenomenon has been studied in greatest detail in the mouse, using adoptive transfer methods (12). Antibody-forming cell precursors reactive with some antigens, notably dinitrophenyl (DNP) haptens, are detectable by day 14 of fetal life (14), while precursors reactive with many other antigens, e.g. phosphorylcholine (PC) (15) or $\alpha{\rightarrow}1,3$-dextran, do not appear until late in the first neonatal week. The existence of this strict developmental program is paradoxical given the stochastic nature of mechanisms underlying antibody diversification.

Analysis of the fetal and neonatal immune response in the mouse has demonstrated an association between the step-wise acquisition of antigen responsiveness and an ordered developmental program of heavy chain V_H utilization, as well as control of the extent of diversity available at the VDJ join that encodes CDR 3 (16, 17). In both mouse and man, V_H gene segments have been grouped into families of elements of high relative sequence homology (i.e. >80% sequence identity (18–21)). Thus it is possible to assess the representation of each V_H family in populations of developing B cells by measuring the abundance of cross-hybridizing mRNA using a standard set of V_H probes. With this technique, we demonstrated that about 80% of murine fetal pre-B cell hybridomas utilize a member of the V_H7183 family, but that this family contributes only 20% of rearrangements in neonatal hybridomas (22). More detailed analysis of fetal rearrangements by Yancopoulos and colleagues (23) revealed that more than 50% of heavy chain rearrangements in Abelson virus-transformed BALB/c fetal pre-B cell lines utilized a single member of the V_H7183 family, V_H81X (23). A similar preference for V_H81X and the V_H7183 family has been demonstrated in B lineage cells from adult bone marrow (17, 24). These findings suggest that there may be a preference for the V_H7183 family in general, and for the V_H81X gene segment in particular, that is intrinsic and common to pre-B cells at all stages of development. This extraordinary restriction in V_H repertoire at the earliest stages of B cell differentiation may well explain the developmentally programmed acquisition of antibody specificities, but in addition raises the possibility that the preferential rearrangement of certain V_H gene segments early in life provides some advantage to the developing organism (25).

(For lack of better terms, we have chosen to label B lineage cells enriched for a heavy chain repertoire characteristic of fetal liver-derived mononuclear cells as "fetal" in type, in contrast to "mature" B lineage cells that express a repertoire more characteristic of peripheral blood lymphocytes.)

Although a consistent preference for V_H7183 and for V_H81X appears to exist among murine fetal B lineage cells and pre-B cells at all stages of development, emerging B cells from mature bone marrow already have a diminished frequency of V_H7183-containing cells (26) and rarely express functional V_H81X-containing transcripts (27). These observations suggest that there has been a selection against V_H7183-expressing B cells during the progression from the pre-B to the circulating B cell stage in the mature organism. Similarly, although neonatal splenic B cell lines continue to express 7183-family gene segments more frequently than expected by random chance alone (17), V family expression in adult splenic B cells appears most compatible with random utilization of the various families (17, 22, 23, 28). These studies do not allow us to distinguish between the possibility that the antigen specificities expressed by the fetal repertoire become disadvantageous to the mature organism, or that exposure to a diverse array of antigens—either endogenous, exogenous, or antigen in the form of anti-idiotypic antibodies—has led to diversification of the repertoire (26, 29).

Taken as a whole, these V_H utilization studies could be interpreted to suggest that the pre-B cell heavy chain antibody repertoire remains the same throughout life, and that the differences in the repertoires expressed in newly emergent and splenic B cells are the product of antigen receptor-mediated selection. However, analysis of V_H family utilization does not completely address the actual diversity of the repertoire. Variability in heavy chains is also dependent on the extent of N region addition and D and J utilization. It is thus remarkable that sequence analysis of CDR 3 regions from pre-B cells at different stages of gestation demonstrate striking differences in repertoire diversity (16).

Mouse fetal and neonatal heavy chain rearrangements typically lack N regions (16, 30). When present, non-germ line encoded nucleotides are often templated "P" junctions rather than random base additions. Further restrictions in the extent of repertoire diversity are induced by the preferential use of only one of the six possible D_H reading frames: reading frame one. Thus, the heavy chain fetal repertoire is primarily germ line encoded. In contrast, adult heavy chains contain numerous N regions that enhance CDR 3 variability. These developmental differences in CDR 3 diversity can be detected at the DJ rearrangement step, prior to the formation of a VDJ product capable of encoding a functional antigen receptor. Thus, there appears to be a fundamental difference in the nature of gene segment rearrangement in "fetal" pre-B cells versus "mature" pre-B cells, even though these populations appear identical by morphological analysis.

The controlled diversification of the heavy chain repertoire probably results from intrinsic differences in the B-lineage progenitors found in fetal liver versus adult bone marrow, as reflected by differences in VDJ splicing and N region addition, and external selection of B cells by antigen, which occurs following generation of functional VDJ products. This selection may

8

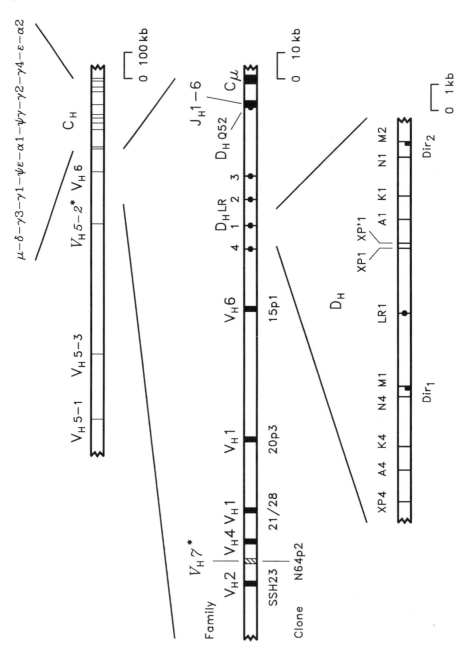

reflect deletion or silencing of B cells expressing self-reactive antibodies, modulation of the repertoire by idiotypic network interactions, or positive selection by foreign antigen.

THE HUMAN IMMUNOGLOBULIN HEAVY CHAIN LOCUS

The extraordinary restriction in H chain repertoire diversification during murine fetal life may well explain the developmentally programmed acquisition of antibody specificities, but in addition raises the possibility that the preferential rearrangement of certain V_H elements early in life provides some advantage to the developing organism. With these thoughts in mind, we have focused our efforts on direct examination of the heavy chain repertoire expressed by human fetal and neonatal B lineage cells. We found that V_H expression in man appears to follow a developmental program that is strikingly similar to that previously documented in the mouse.

The immunoglobulin heavy or H chain locus encodes both the receptor and effector functions of the antibody, and its germ line locus on chromosome 14 is complex (2–4, 31). More than 100 V_H gene segments, which can be grouped into at least seven families (20, 32), are positioned 5' to six J_H gene segments (33). Located in a 70 kb block of DNA 20 kb 5' of the J_H locus is the D_H (D for diversity) locus (Figure 1.2). There are eight families of D_H gene segments (33–41). Each D locus contains one or more repeats of a 9 kb block of DNA that contains one or more members of seven of the eight D_H families. The single exception to this rule is the D_HQ52 gene segment that is positioned immediately adjacent to the J_H locus.

Unlike the mouse, D–D rearrangements occur quite frequently in man (42–44). D–D rearrangement and the potential for additional N region addition, coupled to the increase in the number of D_H gene segments, yields an extraordinarily diverse human H chain-variable domain repertoire. Random

---

Figure 1.2. (*opposite*) Map of IGH locus on chromosome 14q32 (from refs 34, 35, 41, 46, 50, 51, 55, 56, 88–90). Shown at the top is a representation of the 1500 kb block of DNA that contains the C_H, J_H and major D_H loci, as well as the majority of the functional V_H repertoire. The three gene segments that comprise the V_H5 family and the single member of the V_H6 family serve as useful markers delimiting the major V_H locus. Unlike the mouse, members of the different V_H families in man are interspersed. Shown in the middle panel are the five most J_H-proximal functional V_H gene segments in the human genome. Family designation is noted above the gene position and known clones that contain these V_H gene segments are depicted below the gene. Clones 15p1 and 20p3 were isolated from a 130-day fetal liver library (58), clone 21/28 is an anti-DNA binding antibody (72), clone N64p2 was isolated from a cord blood mononuclear cell library (44), and clone SSH23 is a rheumatoid factor (75). Asterisks identify genes that are absent in some haploid genomes. The bottom panel contains an expanded view of the repeating structure of the major D_H locus. See text for further details

combinatorial rearrangement of the germ line V_H, D_H and J_H repertoire can theoretically generate $100 \times 30 \times 6$, or 1.8×10^4 different variable domains. Every codon added by N region addition increases the potential diversity of the repertoire 20 times, and N regions can be inserted both between the V and the D, between Ds, and between the D and the J. In total, potentially more than 10^9 different H chain VDJ junctions, or CDR 3-encoding intervals, can be generated at the time of the gene segment rearrangement. Because any L chain can theoretically associate with any H chain, random combination of the H and L chain partners yields a potential pre-immune antibody repertoire of greater than 10^{14} different immunoglobulins.

DEVELOPMENT OF THE HUMAN H CHAIN REPERTOIRE

A timetable for B cell development in humans can be extrapolated from murine data on the basis of age equivalence between fetal mouse and man. Pre-B cell development in the mouse is first apparent at days 12–13 and corresponds to a human fetal gestational age of 5–6 weeks (45). B cell development also begins at day 17 corresponding to a human gestational age of 9–12 weeks (45). Experimentally, immunofluorescent staining of fetal liver has shown the presence of cytoplasmic C_μ+/surface IgM– (pre-B cells) by the 7th to 8th week of gestation, immature B lymphocytes (sIgM+,sIgD–) by the 9th week of gestation, and mature B lymphocytes (sIgM+,sIgD+) by the 12th week of gestation (45).

Although some gene segments, such as V_H6 (32, 46, 47), are highly conserved in the human population, a number of polymorphisms in the H chain locus have been recently described (42, 48–56). Polymorphisms can be divided into two general classes: alleles and insertions/deletions. In many cases, single base-pair changes can be detected in V_H or J_H gene segments that occupy the same relative physical location in the germ line. These variants are true allelic forms of the same V_H or J_H gene segment. Likely as a result of the near-identity of related immunoglobulin gene segments and their surrounding DNA, the H chain locus has undergone many insertions, deletions and gene duplications as well as gene conversion events (57). Thus, in addition to allelic forms of the same V_H gene segment, individuals may have multiple copies of highly similar gene segments or lack other gene segments entirely.

By generating cDNA libraries from human fetal liver and cord blood mononuclear cells, we hoped to sample in a relatively unbiased way the early fetal antibody repertoire. Because of the considerable polymorphism in the human heavy chain locus, we elected to generate libraries using individual fetal and cord blood samples. Mononuclear cells were isolated from fetal liver, and their RNA was used to independently generate oligo(dT)-primed cDNA libraries from samples derived from two unrelated fetuses of 104 and

130 days gestation, respectively ((25, 48, 58); Bertrand and Schroeder, unpublished observations). These stages were chosen because early second trimester fetal liver is of sufficient quantity to allow generation of a cDNA library by traditional means.

Heavy chain transcripts were identified purely on the basis of their hybridization to a $C_\mu+$ probe. A third of these transcripts contained identical 5' non-variable sequences with numerous stop codons in all three reading frames. The presence of these "sterile" transcripts is common in early lymphoid cells (59). Unlike the mouse, these sterile transcripts initiated immediately upstream of the C_H1 exon and were transcribed without an intervening intronic sequence (Figure 1.3). The complete nucleotide sequences of three $D_H–J_H–$ and 30 $V_H–D_H–J_H–C_\mu+$ transcripts, selected solely on the basis of hybridization with a C_μ probe, were determined. Examination of these sequences revealed that each derived from an independent $D_H–J_H$ and $V_H–D_H–J_H$ joining event, hence our libraries were not biased by the presence of a few clones expressing large amounts of particular mRNAs. Nevertheless, only 12 different V_H gene segments were used to generate the 30 V_H-containing sequences, five of which belong to the V_H3 family. Three of these sequences contained out-of-frame $V_H–DJ$ joins, hence 10% of these cDNAs represented non-translatable transcripts that could not influence the antigen specificity of their parent B cells. As shown graphically in Figure 1.4, all but three of the 30 V_H gene segments were used more than once, with similar representation in both libraries. None of the three single representatives contained out-of-frame joins. Representation of the same limited population of V_H gene segments in both translatable and non-translatable

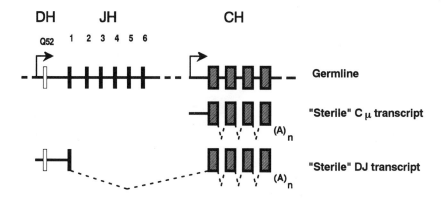

Figure 1.3. Unrearranged transcripts from the Ig H locus in fetal liver B lineage cells. The majority of non-translatable or "sterile" transcripts include germ line sequences immediately 5' to the C_H1 domain (48, 58, 91). Also depicted are $D_HQ52–J_H1$-containing $C_\mu+$ transcripts that include the intervening DNA between D_H and J_H (48)

12

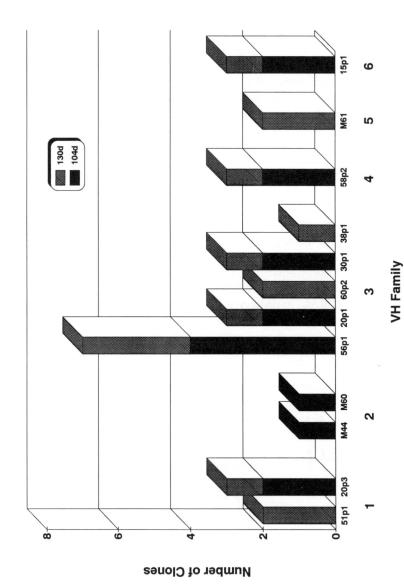

Figure 1.4. Thirty randomly isolated C_μ+ VDJ-containing transcripts have been cloned and sequenced from two unrelated fetuses of 104 and 130 days of gestation. The limited set of 12 V_H elements that contributed to these rearrangments are grouped by family and identified by a representative cDNA clone (refs 48, 58, and Bertrand and Schroeder, unpublished observations)

transcripts indicates that the preference for these V_H gene segments reflects B cell events prior to antigen selection.

Due to technical considerations related to tissue quantity, random analysis of the heavy chain repertoire expressed at the earliest stages of B cell development has been difficult. Initial hybridization analyses with V_H family-specific probes of RNA isolated from 7-week fetal liver revealed apparent preferential expression of members of the V_H5 and V_H6 families (60). However, the slot blot technique used could not differentiate between sterile transcripts of unrearranged V_H genes (61) and functional VDJ joins. In five separate polymerase chain reaction (PCR) amplifications of C_μ+ transcripts from fetal liver samples of 8–10 weeks gestation, we have isolated transcripts derived from the same set of V_H gene segments identified in our second trimester libraries (Mortari and Schroeder, unpublished observations). Similar results have been obtained by other investigators (62, 63). A statistical treatment of these data suggests that the preferred V_H repertoire of these two unrelated fetal samples is most probably encoded by fewer than 14 elements. The similarities in the V_H repertoires expressed by unrelated human fetuses of 2–5 months gestation indicate the existence of a conserved B cell developmental program of heavy chain variable element expression.

Non-random representation of H chain variable gene segments extends to the D_H and J_H loci. Preference was shown for D_HQ52, the most J_H-proximal D_H, and for J_H3 and J_H4 (Figure 1.4). Although this pattern of V, D and J utilization was first described in two individual samples of 104-day and 130-day fetal liver-derived mononuclear cells, this same preference has also been seen in five separate PCR amplifications of C_μ+ transcripts from fetal liver samples of 8–10 weeks gestation (Mortari and Schroeder, unpublished observations), as well as in studies by other investigators (43, 62). The three D_H–J_H-containing transcripts from the second trimester libraries all contained D_HQ52 in association with J_H1, 2 and 3, respectively. Intriguingly, one of these transcripts contained unrearranged D_HQ52 and J_H1 gene segments, complete with the intervening intron (Figure 1.3) (48). This transcript may represent the initial activation product of the D_H–J_H locus. A preference for D_HQ52 in association with V_H-proximal J_H gene segments has also been found in fetal Epstein–Barr virus (EBV)-transformed cell lines (64). The preferential use of D_HQ52 in the incomplete products of H chain rearrangement as well as in mature VDJ transcripts again indicates that non-random gene segment expression reflects a regulatory process intrinsic to the B cell itself.

In order to determine if the antibody repertoire expressed at birth differed from that expressed in the fetus, we performed sequence analysis of VDJ-containing C_μ cDNA transcripts from unselected cord blood mononuclear cells (65). Of the 13 V_H-containing cord blood C_μ+ transcripts sequenced, only one of the V_H gene segments had been previously observed in fetal transcripts. In contrast, three of these transcripts contained gene segments belonging to the newly described V_H7 family. To our knowledge, members of this family have not been detected in fetal liver. The V_H7 and V_H1 families are likely derived from a common progenitor (20). They share 90% nucleotide identity in FR 1, CDR 1, and FR 2; but only 64% identity in CDR 2 and FR 3. The FR 3 and CDR 2 regions contribute significantly to the structure and sequence of the antigen binding site (5, 20, 66).

In addition to differences in V_H utilization, there were significant differences in the gene segment composition, sequence and length distribution of the cord blood C_μ^+ CDR 3 intervals in comparison to the fetus (Figure 1.4). Cord blood C_μ^+ transcripts were enriched for use of J_H4, 5 and 6; whereas the fetal repertoire had been enriched for J_H3 and 4 (Figure 1.5). The cord blood transcripts used a number of different D_H gene segments, whereas fetal transcripts were enriched for D_HQ52. Cord blood C_μ^+ CDR 3 sequences contained an average of 17 codons, ranging between six and 24 codons in length. In contrast, the fetal liver-derived CDR 3 sequences averaged 11 codons in size and were all less than 18 codons long ((43, 48, 58); Mortari and Schroeder, unpublished data). Of the fetal transcripts where D_H identity could be assigned with certainty, all of the VD junctions, but only 57% of the DJ junctions, contained N regions.

As summarized in the Introduction, each codon added by N region addition expands the potential diversity of the H chain repertoire by as much as 20-fold. Thus, the increase in the length of the CDR 3 region generated by N region addition and changes in D_H and J_H utilization expands the potential diversity of the cord blood repertoire by 20^7 or 10^9 in different sequences. As the number of amino acids in the loops increases, the size of the binding loop is likely to expand, generating new binding structures not seen in the fetal repertoire.

In the mouse, diversity in fetal CDR 3 regions was limited by absence of N region addition, use of ''P'' junctions, use of D_H reading frame 1, and preferential sites fo VDJ splicing (16, 30, 43). In man, fetal DJ joins contain fewer N regions, although non-germ line encoded nucleotides are present in a substantial minority of the splice sites. However, P junctions are rare, N regions are common at the VD join, D_H reading frame appears random, and a preferred splice site has not been detected. Unlike the mouse, limitations in the length and potential diversity of fetal sequences are the result of preferential use of the smallest D_H gene segment, D_HQ52; preferential use of the shortest J_H gene segments, J_H3 and 4; and an absence of D–D joining. In contrast, D–D joining, enhanced N region addition at the DJ junction, and use of the J_H5 and 6 gene segments, which are one and five codons longer than both J_H 3 and 4, respectively, loosen these restrictions in more mature repertoires. Therefore, although the specific mechanisms differ, control of CDR 3 diversity in man, as in the mouse, likely plays a key role in the stepwise acquisition of the ability to respond to specific antigens.

15

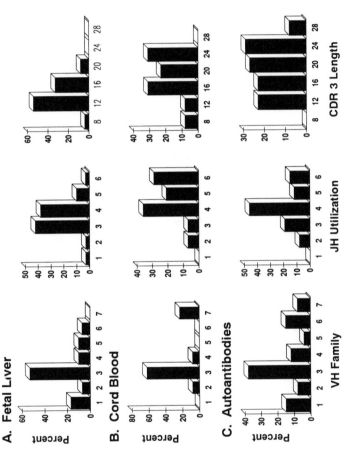

Figure 1.5. Graphic comparison of the patterns of V_H and J_H utilization in (A) 30 fetal liver Cμ+ transcripts (refs 48, 58, and Bertrand and Schroeder, unpublished observations), (B) 14 cord mononuclear cell C$_\mu$+ transcripts (65) and (C) 26 self-reactive antibodies derived from B cell lines (69–75). Shown on the left are the percentage of transcripts that utilize members of the designated V_H families and in the middle are the percentage of transcripts that utilize the designated J_H gene segment. Shown on the right is the distribution of the lengths of the CDR 3 intervals of these transcripts, divided into four residue intervals (e.g. <8 amino acids (a.a.), 9–12 a.a., 13–16 a.a., 17–20 a.a., 21–24 a.a, and 25–28 a.a.)

HUMAN AUTOANTIBODIES FREQUENTLY CONTAIN "FETAL" V_H GENE SEGMENTS

The genetic composition of autoantibodies in man has been the focus of intense investigation for a number of years. In the mouse, V_H genes belonging to the families most frequently expressed during fetal life (e.g. V_H7183 and Q52) are frequent components of self-reactive antibodies (67). Over the past 5 years, a number of investigators have generated B cell lines that express antibodies with the self-reactive specificities typical of autoantibodies expressed in many major human autoimmune diseases (68), e.g. anti-DNA, rheumatoid factor, and anti-SM antibodies, among others. Of the 12 V_H gene segments that we have shown to be frequently expressed in fetal liver, seven (20p1, 30p1, M60, V_H6, 56p1, 51p1, and 58p2) have been described, in germ line or near-germ line form, as components of these types of autoantibodies (69–75). In light of our analysis of fetal and cord blood transcripts, we reviewed published nucleotide sequences of 26 self-reactive antibodies. These antibodies are expressed by cell lines that have been selected for their antigen reactivity and thus may not represent an entirely random sampling of peripheral B cells capable of self-reactivity. However, of these 26 autoantibodies, fully 16 share greatest sequence similarity with members of the fetal repertoire. These findings suggest that in man, as in the mouse, the fetal liver-derived antibody repertoire is enriched for use of potentially self-reactive gene segments. Moreover, it is possible that the early generation of self-reactive antibodies may represent a critical feature of immune repertoire development (76).

Two sets of sequences deserve special note. Like V_H81X, the single member V_H6 family is the most J_H proximal V_H gene segment in man (see Figure 1.2 (46)) and is more frequently represented in pre-B cells than expected by random chance (48, 58, 77). We are aware of the antigen reactivities of four functional antibodies from V_H6-expressing cell lines (69). All four express the same reactivity: anti-DNA. It is possible that the drop in V_H6 utilization from the pre-B to B cell stage, like the drop in V_H81X, reflects selection against a deleterious antibody. The V_H30p1 sequence is also frequently found in anti-DNA antibodies that express the common 16/6 idiotype (71, 72). V_H gene segments similar to 30p1 are recurrent components of anti-bacterial-polysaccharide antibodies (78). Thus, the frequency of use of 30p1 sequences may reflect a delicate balance between self-reactivity and protection from bacterial infection.

HUMAN AND MURINE FETAL V_H GENE SEGMENTS ARE EVOLUTIONARILY CONSERVED

Through pairwise comparisons of known germ line (as opposed to somatically generated) antibody V_H elements, we have shown that mammalian immunoglobulin V_H families can be grouped into three distinct clans based upon conserved nucleotide and peptide features common to all known sets of murine and human V_H gene segments (19). Mouse and human V_H elements probably derive from three distinct progenitor V_H elements whose descendants populate these three clans (20, 32, 79). Clan I includes the human $V_H 1$, $V_H 5$, and the $V_H 7$ families, and the murine J558 and Vgam3.8 ($V_H 9$) families (Figure 1.6). Primordial clan II split into two distinct sets of families before the divergence of mouse and man: the V_H II subclan (human $V_H 2$, mouse 3609), and the V_H IV subclan (human $V_H 4$, $V_H 6$, and mouse Q52, 36–60, $V_H 12$). Clan III consists of the human $V_H 3$ family and the murine 7183, T15, J606, X24, $V_H 10$, $V_H 11$, and $V_H 13$ families. Through replacement/silent site substitution analysis and molecular modeling of known immunoglobulin crystal structures, we have shown that this conservation reflects preservation of protein sequence and structure. The patterns of conservation observed suggest that these subdomains play an important role in antibody function. Each clan contains a characteristic FR 1 interval that is solvent exposed and structurally separated from the antigen binding site. Families within a clan contain their own unique FR 3 interval that is capable of either influencing the conformation of the antigen binding site or interacting directly with antigen.

Homologous proteins typically demonstrate a location-dependent tolerance to amino acid substitution in evolution. Due to degeneracy in the genetic code, codons undergoing random mutation are predicted to yield an amino acid replacement (R) to silent site (S) substitution ratio (R/S ratio) of

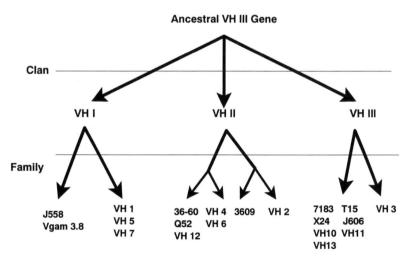

Figure 1.6. A scheme for the evolutionary relationships among the human and murine V_H families based upon analysis of conserved nucleotide and peptide sequences as well as studies of solved crystallographic structures (19, 20)

2.9 (80, 81). Peptide conservation due to positive selection yields R/S ratios of less than 2.9, whereas ratios significantly greater than 2.9 can only be achieved through selection for diversity. For example, the catalytic site of a soluble enzyme will exhibit the lowest R/S ratios, followed by the hydrophobic interior which stabilizes the structure, while the hydrophilic exterior often demonstrates R/S ratios typical of random mutation. Similarly, the enhanced affinity for antigen demonstrated by antibodies of the secondary response which have undergone somatic hypermutation is associated with R/S ratios significantly greater than 2.9, indicating positive selection for high-affinity antigen binding sites (81).

The 12 V_H gene segments that are preferentially expressed in the human fetal repertoire derive from six of the seven known human V_H families. However, five are members of the V_H3 family whose closest mouse counterpart is the V_H7183 family, which is also preferentially expressed during fetal life. Indeed, the V_H gene segments that exhibit the highest sequence identity between man and mouse, V_H30p1 (58) and V_HE415 (23) (Figure 1.7), are both components of the fetal repertoire. Depicted in Figure 1.7 are the location of the residues that have diverged between these two fetal sequences, as well as the R/S ratios of each of the functional domains (5). The average R/S ratio for the coding portion of the sequence is only 0.95, indicating strong evolutionary conservation of sequence. If evolutionary pressure was being exerted on fetal V_H gene segments in order to maintain the sequence and structure of a specific antigen binding site, we would predict that the CDR regions would evidence the greatest conservation. However, examination of the actual location and number of peptide changes reveals that sequence conservation is centered on the sequence intervals that define clan and family. Within these two regions, these fetal gene segments are 90% identical in nucleotide sequence.

The extensive diversity of the germ line repertoire of V_H gene segments makes it difficult to interpret the significance of the similarity or differences between two gene segments drawn at random from the germ line pool. Because V_H gene segments undergo gene conversion within a family (57), we reasoned that the confounding effects of individual gene segment variation could be minimized by treating each family as a group. Family-specific consensus sequences for the FR 1 and 3 intervals of the known human and mouse families were generated by identifying the most commonly utilized nucleotide at each base pair position for all the germ line elements available to us. These consensus sequences comprise the group norm for each family. Remarkably, the human fetal repertoire is enriched for sequences identical (e.g. the V_H3 30p1 and the V_H4 58p2) or nearly identical (e.g. the V_H1 20p3 gene segment) to their family consensus sequence (20). These findings suggest that the fetal repertoire contains a set of prototypical, phylogenetically conserved gene segments. These gene segments might provide a plastic,

19

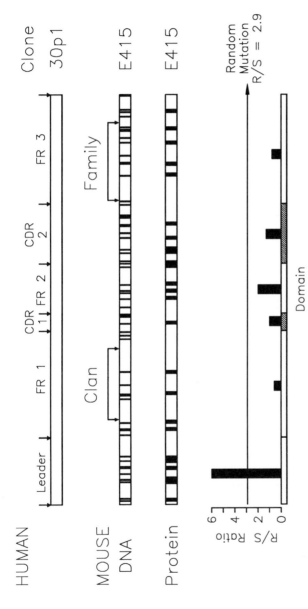

Figure 1.7. The murine and human fetal V_H repertoires include many similar sequences. Shown is a representation of the extensive nucleotide and peptide identity of the human 30p1 sequence (58) to a V_H7183 gene segment that is also a frequent component of the murine BALB/c fetal repertoire, V_HE415 (23). The different domains that characterize each V_H gene segment are marked above the human sequence. Each bar reflects a nucleotide or peptide difference between the murine sequence and the human one. In the bottom panel, we present a graphic depiction of the ratio between replacement and silent mutations (R/S ratio) in each of these domains (leader R/S ratio = 6.0, FR 1 = 0.6, CDR 1 = 1.0, FR 2 = 2.0, CDR 2 = 1.3, FR 3 = 0.8). An arrow marks the predicted R/S ratio for random mutation, 2.9. Superimposed upon the mouse sequence are the locations of the conserved intervals that define clan (residues 6–24) and family (residues 67–85). See text for further details

polyreactive natural antibody repertoire capable of delivering a low-affinity defense against a wide array of antigens (82). In this context, it is provocative that the highest conservation of sequence throughout the vertebrate radiation has been exerted on the FR 3 sequence of Clan III members, whose descendants can be detected in the primitive shark *Heterodontus*, as well as *Xenopus*, chicken, man and mouse (20, 83–86).

SUMMARY

In man as in mouse, diversification of the H chain repertoire appears to follow a developmental program. Control is exerted on V, D and J utilization, on N region addition, and thus on the potential diversity of the available repertoire of antigen binding sites. The fetal repertoire appears biased towards low-affinity, multi-specific antibodies containing highly conserved structures (20, 87). We may speculate that this repertoire is the product of evolutionary pressure to express a plastic set of antibodies that enable an immunologically naive individual to respond to a wide range of antigenic challenge. The cost of maintaining a multi-reactive repertoire appears to include the risk of generating potentially deleterious self-reactive antibodies. Preliminary data from a number of laboratories, including our own, suggest that alterations or abnormal regulation of the components of the fetal repertoire may contribute to diseases of immune function in man.

REFERENCES

1. Leder, P. (1982) The genetics of antibody diversity. *Sci. Am.*, **246** (5), 102–115.
2. Tonegawa, S. (1983) Somatic generation of antibody diversity. *Nature*, **302**, 575–581.
3. Honjo, T. (1983) Immunoglobulin genes. *Annu. Rev. Immunol.*, **1**, 499.
4. Yancopoulos, G.D. and Alt, F.W. (1986) Regulation of the assembly and expression of variable region genes. *Annu. Rev. Immunol.*, **4**, 339–368.
5. Kabat, E.A., Wu, T.T., Reid-Miller, M., Perry, H.M. and Gottesman, K.S. (1987) *Sequences of Proteins of Immunological Interest*, 4th edn. US Department of Health and Human Services, Bethesda, pp. vii–804.
6. Reth, M. and Alt, F.W. (1984) Novel immunoglobulin heavy chains are produced from DJH gene segment rearrangements in lymphoid cells. *Nature*, **312**, 418–423.
7. Gu, H., Kitamura, D. and Rajewsky, K. (1991) B cell development regulated by gene rearrangement: Arrest of maturation by membrane-bound Dµ protein and selection of DH element reading frames. *Cell*, **65**, 47–54.
8. Lafaille, J.J., DeCloux, A., Bonneville, M., Takagaki, Y. and Tonegawa, S. (1989) Junctional sequences of T cell receptor γδ genes: Implications for γδ T cell lineages and for a novel intermediate of V-(D)-J joining. *Cell*, **59**, 859–870.
9. Desiderio, S.V., Yancopoulos, G.D., Paskind, M., Thomas, E., Boss, M.A., Landau, N., Alt, F.W. and Baltimore, D. (1984) Insertion of N regions into heavy-chain genes is correlated with expression of terminal deoxytransferase in B cells. *Nature*, **311**, 752–755.

10. Silverstein, A.M., Uhur, J.W., Kraner, K.L. and Lukes, R.J. (1963) Fetal response to antigenic stimulus. II. Antibody production by the fetal lamb. *J. Exp. Med.*, **117**, 799–812.
11. Sherwin, W.K. and Rowlands, D.T., Jr (1974) Development of humoral immunity in lethally irradiated mice reconstituted with fetal liver. *J. Immunol.*, **113**, 1353–1360.
12. Klinman, N.R. and Press, J.L. (1975) The B cell specificity repertoire: Its relationship to definable subpopulations. *Transplant. Rev.*, **24**, 41–75.
13. Denis, K.A. and Klinman, N.R. (1983) Genetic and temporal control of neonatal antibody expression. *J. Exp. Med.*, **157**, 1170.
14. Klinman, N.R. and Press, J.L. (1975) The characterization of the B-cell repertoire specific for the 2,4-dinitrophenyl and 2,4,6-trinitrophenyl determinants in neonatal BALB/c mice. *J. Exp. Med.*, **141**, 1133–1146.
15. Kamps, W.A. and Cooper, M.D. (1982) Microenvironmental studies of pre-B and B cell development in human and mouse fetuses. *J. Immunol.*, **129**, 526–531.
16. Gu, H., Forster, I. and Rajewsky, K. (1990) Sequence homologies, N sequence insertion and J_H gene utilization in $V_H D J_H$ joining: Implications for the joining mechanism and the ontogenetic timing of Ly1 B cell and B-CLL progenitor generation. *EMBO J.*, **9**, 2133–2140.
17. Malynn, B.A., Yancopoulos, G.D., Barth, J.E., Bona, C.A. and Alt, F.W. (1990) Biased expression of J_H-proximal V_H genes occurs in the newly generated repertoire of neonatal and adult mice. *J. Exp. Med.*, **171**, 843–859.
18. Brodeur, P.H. and Riblet, R.J. (1984) The immunoglobulin heavy chain variable region (Igh-V) locus in the mouse. I. One hundred Igh-V genes comprise seven families of homologous genes. *Eur. J. Immunol.*, **14**, 922–930.
19. Schroeder, H.W., Jr, Hillson, J.L. and Perlmutter, R.M. (1990) Evolution of mammalian V_H families. *Int. Immunol.*, **20**, 41–50.
20. Kirkham, P.M., Mortari, F., Newton, J.A. and Schroeder, H.W., Jr (1992) Immunoglobulin V_H clan and family identity predicts variable domain structure and may influence antigen binding. *EMBO J.*, **11**, 603–609.
21. Kodaira, M., Kinashi, T., Umemura, I., Matsuda, F., Noma, T., Ono, Y. and Honjo, T. (1986) Organization and evolution of variable region genes of the human immunoglobulin heavy chain. *J. Mol. Biol.*, **190**, 529–541.
22. Perlmutter, R.M., Kearney, J.F., Chang, S.P. and Hood, L.E. (1985) Developmentally controlled expression of immunoglobulin V_H genes. *Science*, **227**, 1597.
23. Yancopoulos, G.D., Desiderio, S.V., Paskind, M., Kearney, J.F., Baltimore, D. and Alt, F.W. (1984) Preferential utilization of the most J_H-proximal V_H gene segments in pre-B cell lines. *Nature*, **311**, 727–733.
24. Lawler, A.M., Lin, P.S. and Gearhart, P.J. (1987) Adult B-cell repertoire is biased toward two heavy-chain variable region genes that rearrange frequently in fetal pre-B cells. *Proc. Nat. Acad. Sci. USA*, **84**, 2454–2458.
25. Perlmutter, R.M., Schroeder, H.W., Jr and Hillson, J.L. (1988) Diversification of the human fetal antibody repertoire. In Witte, O., Howard, M. and Klinman, N. (eds) *UCLA Symposia on Molecular and Cellular Biology, New Series, Vol. 85: B Cell Development*. Liss, New York, pp. 91–104.
26. Freitas, A.A., Burlen, O. and Coutinho, A.A. (1988) Selection of antibody repertoires by anti-idiotypes can occur at multiple steps of B cell differentiation. *J. Immunol.*, **140**, 4097–4102.
27. Decker, D.J., Boyle, N.E., Koziol, J.A. and Klinman, N.R. (1991) The expression of the IgH chain repertoire in developing bone marrow B lineage cells. *J. Immunol.*, **146**, 350–361.

28. Dildrop, R., Krawinkel, U., Winter, E. and Rajewsky, K. (1985) V_H gene expression in murine lipopolysaccharide blasts distributes over the nine known V_H-gene groups and may be random. *Eur. J. Immunol.*, **15**, 1154–1156.

29. Vakil, M., Sauter, H., Paige, C.J. and Kearney, J.F. (1986) *In vivo* suppression of perinatal multispecific B cells results in a distortion of the adult B cell repertoire. *Eur. J. Immunol.*, **16**, 1159–1165.

30. Feeney, A.J. (1990) Lack of N regions in fetal and neonatal mouse immunoglobulin V-D-J junctional sequences. *J Exp. Med.*, **172**, 1377–1390.

31. Geiger, M.J., Gorski, J. and Eckels, D.D. (1991) T cell receptor gene segment utilization by HLA-DR1-alloreactive T cell clones. *J. Immunol.*, **147**, 2082–2087.

32. Berman, J.E., Mellis, S.J., Pollock, R., Smith, C.L., Suh, H., Heinke, B., Kowal, C., Surti, U., Chess, L., Cantor, C.R. and Alt, F.W. (1988) Content and organization of the human Ig V_H locus: Definition of three new V_H families and linkage to the Ig C_H locus. *EMBO J.*, **7**, 727–738.

33. Ravetch, J.V., Siebenlist, U., Korsmeyer, S., Waldmann, T. and Leder, P. (1981) Structure of human immunoglobulin μ locus: Characterization of embryonic and rearranged J and D genes. *Cell*, **27**, 583–591.

34. Ichihara, Y., Abe, M., Yasui, H., Matsuoka, H. and Kurosawa, Y. (1988) At least five D_H genes of human immunoglobulin heavy chains are encoded in 9-kilobase DNA fragments. *Eur. J. Immunol.*, **18**, 649–652.

35. Matsuda, F., Lee, K.H., Nakai, S., Sato, T., Kodaira, M., Zong, S.Q., Ohno, H., Fukuhara, S. and Honjo, T. (1988) Dispersed localization of D segments in the human immunoglobulin heavy-chain locus. *EMBO J.*, **7**, 1047–1051.

36. Siebenlist, U., Ravetch, J.V., Korsmeyer, S., Waldmann, T. and Leder, P. (1981) Human immunoglobulin D segments encoded in tandem multigenic families. *Nature*, **294**, 631–635.

37. Buluwela, L., Albertson, D.G., Sherrington, P., Rabbitts, P.H., Spurr, N. and Rabbitts, T.H. (1988) The use of chromosomal translocations to study human immunoglobulin gene organization: Mapping D_H segments within 35 kb of the Cμ gene and identification of a new D_H locus. *EMBO J.*, **7**, 2003–2010.

38. Zong, S.Q., Nakai, S., Matsuda, F., Lee, K.H. and Honjo, T. (1988) Human immunoglobulin D segments: Isolation of a new D segment and polymorphic deletion of the D1 segment. *Immunol. Lett.*, **17**, 329–334.

39. Kurosawa, Y. and Tonegawa, S. (1982) Organization, structure, and assembly of immunoglobulin heavy chain diversity DNA segments. *J. Exp. Med.*, **155**, 201–218.

40. Matsuda, F., Shin, E.K., Hirabayashi, Y., Nagaoka, H., Yoshida, M.C., Zong, S.Q. and Honjo, T. (1990) Organization of variable region segments of the human immunoglobulin heavy chain: Duplication of the D5 cluster within the locus and interchromosomal translocation of variable region segments. *EMBO J.*, **9**, 2501–2506.

41. Ichihara, Y., Matsuoka, H. and Kurosawa, Y. (1988) Organization of human immunogobulin heavy chain diversity gene loci. *EMBO J.*, **7**, 4141–4150.

42. Yamada, M., Wasserman, R., Reichard, B.A., Shane, S., Caton, A.H. and Rovera, G. (1991) Preferential utilization of specific immunoglobulin heavy chain diversity and joining segments in adult human peripheral blood B lymphocytes. *J. Exp. Med.*, **173**, 395–407.

43. Sanz, I. (1991) Multiple mechanisms participate in the generation of diversity of human H chain CDR3 regions. *J. Immunol.*, **147**, 1720–1729.

44. Mortari, F., Newton, J.A., Wang, J.Y. and Schroeder, H.W. Jr (1992) the human cord blood antibody repertoire: Frequent use of the V_H7 gene family. *Eur. J. Immunol.*, **22**, 241–245.
45. Owen, J.J.T., Raff, M.C. and Cooper, M.D. (1975) Studies on the generation of B lymphocytes in the mouse embryo. *Eur. J. Immunol.*, **5**, 468–473.
46. Schroeder, H.W., Jr, Walter, M.A., Hosker, M.H., Ebens, A., Willems van Dijk, K., Lau, L., Cox, D.W., Milner, E.C.B. and Perlmutter, R.M. (1988) Physical linkage of a unique human immunoglobulin vh gene segment (VH6) to D_H and J_H gene segments. *Proc. Nat. Acad. Sci. USA*, **85**, 8196–8200.
47. Sanz, I., Kelly, P., Williams, C., Scholl, S., Tucker, P.W. and Capra, J.D. (1989) The smaller human VH gene families display remarkably little polymorphism. *EMBO J.*, **8**, 3741–3748.
48. Schroeder, H.W., Jr and Wang, J.Y. (1990) Preferential utilization of conserved immunoglobulin heavy chain variable gene segments during human fetal life. *Proc. Nat. Acad. Sci. USA*, **87**, 6146–6150.
49. Willems van Dijk, K., Schroeder, H.W., Jr, Perlmutter, R.M. and Milner, E.C.B. (1989) Heterogeneity in the human Ig V_H locus. *J. Immunol.*, **142**, 2547–2554.
50. Shin, E.K., Matsuda, F., Nagaoka, H., Fukita, Y., Imai, T., Yokoyama, K., Soeda, E. and Honjo, T. (1991) Physical map of the 3' region of the human immunoglobulin heavy chain locus: Clustering of the autoantibody-related variable segments in one haplotype. *EMBO J.*, **10**, 3641–3645.
51. Walter, M.A., Surti, U., Hofker, M.H. and Cox, D.W. (1990) The physical organization of the human immunoglobulin heavy chain gene complex. *EMBO J.*, **9**, 3303–3313.
52. Benger, J.C. and Cox, D.W. (1989) Polymorphisms of the immunoglobulin heavy-chain delta gene and association with other constant-region genes. *Am. J. Hum. Genet.*, **45**, 606–614.
53. van Dijk, K.W., Sasso, E.H. and Milner, E.C.B. (1991) Polymorphism of the human Ig V_H4 gene family. *J. Immunol.*, **146**, 3646–3651.
54. Sasso, E.H., Willems van Dijk, K. and Milner, E.C.B. (1990) Prevalence and polymorphism of human V_H3 genes. *J. Immunol.*, **145**, 2751–2757.
55. Walter, M.A. and Cox, D.W. (1991) Nonuniform linkage disequilibrium within a 1,500-kb region of the human immunoglobulin heavy-chain complex. *Am. J. Hum. Genet.*, **49**, 917–931.
56. Bottaro, A., Cariota, U., DeMarchi, M. and Carbonara, A.O. (1991) Pulsed-field electrophoresis screening for immunoglobulin heavy-chain constant-region multigene deletions and duplications. *Am. J. Hum. Genet.*, **48**, 745–756.
57. Perlmutter, R.M., Berson, B., Griffin, J.A. and Hood, L.E. (1985) Diversity in the germline antibody repertoire: Molecular evolution of the T15 V_H gene family. *J. Exp. Med.*, **162**, 1988.
58. Schroeder, H.W., Jr, Hillson, J.L. and Perlmutter, R.M. (1987) Early restriction of the human antibody repertoire. *Science*, **238**, 791–793.
59. Kelley, D.E. and Perry, R.P. (1986) Transcriptional and posttranscriptional control of immunoglobulin mRNA production during B lymphocyte development. *Nucleic Acids Res.*, **14**, 5431–5447.
60. Cuisinier, A.-M., Guigou, V., Boubli, L., Fougereau, M. and Tonnelle, C. (1989) Preferential expression of V_H5 and V_H6 immunoglobulin genes in early human B-cell ontogeny. *Scand. J. Immunol.*, **30**, 493–497.
61. Berman, J.E., Humphries, C.G., Barth, J., Alt, F.W. and Tucker, P.W. (1991) Structure and expression of human germline V_H transcripts. *J. Exp. Med.*, **173**, 1529–1535.

62. Berman, J.E., Nickerson, K.G., Pollock, R.R., Barth, J.E., Schuurman, R.K.B., Knowles, D.M., Chess, L. and Alt, F.W. (1991) *Eur. J. Immunol.*, **21**, 1311–1314.

63. Raaphorst, F.M., Timmers, E., Kenter, M., Van To, M., Vossen, J.M. and Schuurman, R.K. (1992) Restricted utilization of germ-line V_H3 genes and short diverse third complementarity-determining regions (CDR3) in human fetal B lymphocyte immunoglobulin heavy chain rearrangements. *Eur. J. Immunol.*, **22**, 247–251.

64. Nickerson, K.G., Berman, J.E., Glickman, E., Chess, L. and Alt, F.W. (1989) Early human IgH gene assembly in Epstein–Barr virus-transformed fetal B cell lines. *J. Exp. Med.*, **169**, 1391–1403.

65. Mortari, F., Newton, J.A., Wang, J.-Y. and Schroeder, H.W., Jr (1992) The human cord blood antibody repertoire: Frequent use of the V_H7 gene family. *Europ. J. Immunol.*, **22**, 241–245.

66. Tramontano, A., Chothia, C. and Lesk, A.M. (1990) Framework residue 71 is a major determinant of the position and conformation of the second hypervariable region in the VH domains of immunoglobulins. *J. Mol. Biol.*, **215**, 175–182.

67. Kofler, R., Dixon, F.J. and Theofilopoulos, A.N. (1987) The genetic origin of autoantibodies. *Immunol. Today*, **8**, 374–376.

68. Carson, D.A., Chen, P.P. and Kipps, T.J. (1991) New roles for rheumatoid factor. *J. Clin. Invest.*, **87**, 379–383.

69. Logtenberg, T., Young, F.M., Van Es., J.H., Gmelig-Meyling, F.H.J. and Alt, F.W. (1989) Autoantibodies encoded by the most J_H-proximal human immunoglobulin heavy chain variable region gene. *J. Exp. Med.*, **170**, 1347–1355.

70. Sanz, I., Dang, H., Takei, M., Talal, N. and Capra, J.D. (1989) V_H sequence of a human anti-SM autoantibody. *J. Immunol.*, **142**, 883–887.

71. Sanz, I., Casali, P., Thomas, J.W., Notkins, A.L. and Capra, J.D. (1989) Nucleotide sequences of eight human natural autoantibody V_H regions reveals apparent restricted use of V_H families. *J. Immunol.*, **142**, 4054–4061.

72. Dersimonian, H., Schwartz, R.S., Barrett, K.J. and Stollar, B.D. (1987) Relationship of human variable region heavy chain germ-line genes to genes encoding anti-DNA autoantibodies. *J. Immunol.*, **139**, 2496–2501.

73. Pascual, V., Randen, I., Thompson, K., Sioud, M., Forre, O., Natvig, J. and Capra, J.D. (1990) The complete nucleotide sequences of the heavy chain variable regions of six monospecific rheumatoid factors derived from Epstein–Barr virus-transformed B cells isolated from the synovial tissue of patients with rheumatoid arthritis. Further evidence that some autoantibodies are unmutated copies of germ line genes. *J. Clin. Invest.*, **86**, 1320–1328.

74. Dersimonian, H., McAdam, K.P.W.J., Mackworth-Young, C. and Stollar, B.D. (1989) The recurrent expression of variable region segments in human IgM anti-DNA autoantibodies. *J. Immunol.*, **142**, 4027–4033.

75. Stuber, F., Lee, S.K., Bridges, S.L. Jr, Koopman, W.J., Schroeder, H.W. Jr, Gaskin, F. and Fu, S.M. (1992) A rheumatoid factor from a normal individual encoded by V_H2 and V_κ II gene segments. *Arthritis Rheum.*, **35**, 900–904.

76. Vakil, M. and Kearney, J.F. (1988) Regulatory influences of neonatal multispecific antibodies on the developing B cell repertoire. *Int. Rev. Immunol.*, **3**, 117–131.

77. Berman, J.E., Nickerson, K.G., Pollock, R.R., Barth, J.E., Schuurman, R.K., Knowles, D.M., Chess, L. and Alt, F.W. (1991) V_H gene usage in humans: Biased usage of the V_H6 gene in immature B lymphoid cells. *Eur. J Immunol.*, **21**, 1311–1314.

78. Silverman, G.J. and Lucas, A.H. (1991) Variable region diversity in human circulating antibodies specific for the capsular polysaccharide of *Haemophilus influ-*

enzae type b: Preferential usage of two types of V_H3 heavy chains. *J. Clin. Invest.*, **88**, 911–920.

79. Tutter, A. and Riblet, R. (1989) Conservation of an immunoglobulin variable-region gene family indicates a specific, noncoding function. *Proc. Nat. Acad. Sci. USA*, **86**, 7460–7464.
80. Jukes, T.H. and King, J.L. (1979) Evolutionary nucleotide replacements in DNA. *Nature*, **281**, 605–606.
81. Shlomchik, M.J., Nemazee, D.A., Sato, V.L., van Snick, J., Carson, D.A. and Weigert, M.G. (1986) Variable region sequences of murine IgM anti-IgG monoclonal autoantibodies (rheumatoid factors): A structural explanation for the high frequency of IgM anti-IgG B cells. *J. Exp. Med.*, **164**, 407–427.
82. Dighiero, G., Lymberi, P., Mazie, J.-C., Rouyre, S., Butler-Browne, G.S., Whalen, R.G. and Avrameas, S. (1983) Murine hybridomas secreting natural monoclonal antibodies reacting with self antigens. *J. Immunol.*, **131**, 2267–2276.
83. Litman, G.W., Berger, L., Murphy, K., Litman, R., Hinds, K. and Erickson, B.W. (1985) Immunoglobulin V_H gene structure and diversity in *Heterodontus*, a phylogenetically primitive shark. *Proc. Nat. Acad. Sci. USA*, **82**, 2082–2086.
84. Yamawaki-Kataoka, Y. and Honjo, T. (1987) Nucleotide sequences of variable region segments of the immunoglobulin heavy chain of *Xenopus laevis*. *Nucleic Acids Res.*, **15**, 5888.
85. Reynaud, C.-A., Dahan, A., Anques, V. and Weill, J.-C. (1989) Somatic hyperconversion diversifies the single V heavy gene of the chicken with a high incidence in the D region. *Cell*, **59**, 171–183.
86. Kirkham, P.M. and Schroeder, H.W., Jr (1991) Peptide sequence analysis of *Xenopus laevis* V_H gene families reveals homology to mammalian VH clans. *FASEB J.*, **5** (6), A1775 (Abstract).
87. Digheiro, G., Lymberi, P., Holmberg, D., Lundquist, I., Coutinho, A. and Avrameas, S. (1985) High frequency of natural autoantibodies in normal newborn mice. *J. Immunol.*, **134**. 765–771.
88. Olsson, P.G., Marten, H.H., Walter, M.A., Smith, S., Hammarstrom, L., Smith, C.I.E. and Cox, D. (1991) Ig H chain variable and C region genes in common variable immunodeficiency. *J. Immunol.*, **147**, 2540–2546.
89. Hofker, M.H., Walter, M.A. and Cox, D.W. (1989) Complete physical map of the human immunoglobulin heavy chain constant region gene complex. *Proc. Nat. Acad. Sci. USA*, **86**, 5567–5571.
90. Matsuda, F., Shin, E.K., Hirabayashi, Y., Nagaoka, H., Yoshida, M.C., Zong, A.Q. and Honjo, T. (1990) Organization of variable region segments of the human immunoglobulin heavy chain: Duplication of the D5 cluster within the locus and interchromosomal translocation of variable region segments. *EMBO J.*, **9**, 2501–2506.
91. Milili, M., Fougereau, M., Guglielmi, P. and Schiff, C. (1991) Early occurrence of immunoglobulin isotype switching in human fetal liver. *Mol. Immunol.*, **28**, 753–761.

Chapter 2

Pathways of Human B Cell Growth and Differentiation

JOHN GORDON

Department of Immunology, The Medical School, University of Birmingham, UK

INTRODUCTION

Someone once said (and with apologies, I cannot remember who) that "to understand the normal first study the abnormal". The contrary, however, must equally hold true. Thus, the intended aim of this contribution is to "set the scene" for chapters in this volume which concern themselves with a description of those immune deficiencies that impinge—either directly or indirectly—upon B cell function. As such, it does not attempt a comprehensive review of human B cell differentiation, but rather stresses recent information obtained on the role of cell surface molecules and soluble factors which are likely to be central to the control of the diverse and complex processes involved in persuading a small primary B cell to undergo rapid clonal expansion and terminal differentiation toward plasma cells secreting specific antibody with high affinity for the antigen which initiated the process. While unashamedly focusing on information obtained from *in vitro* models, the final section will nevertheless deal with some of the issues relating to the anatomical microenvironments where such events will be occurring *in vivo*. The heterogenity of B cells found at different sites within secondary tissues will be examined and their varying potential for maturation in response to defined signals discussed.

New Concepts in Immunodeficiency Diseases. Edited by S. Gupta and C. Griscelli
© 1993 John Wiley & Sons Ltd

ACTIVATION OF RESTING B CELLS

Resting B Cells

Newly formed virgin B cells leaving the bone marrow are initially immuno-globulin M (IgM) positive and, from studies in the rat, only some 10% are believed to be incorporated into the peripheral B cell pool. Some will be deleted by virtue of expressing antigen receptors encoding autoreactivities, while an element of positive recruitment may also be operative. A cell "counting system" could additionally be in force to ensure the maintenance of homeostasis outside of the previously mentioned mechanisms (1). What-ever the precise details, successfully recruited B cells soon begin to co-express antigen receptors of IgM and IgD classes at their surfaces, and this phenotype marks the immunocompetent primary B cell which dominates peripheral blood and can be found in the follicular mantle zones of second-ary lymphoid tissues. These B cells are quiescent and remain so unless they receive a positive signal for activation. The majority of studies on human B cells *in vitro* have focused on this population, obtained either directly from blood or isolated as high-density B lymphocytes from solid lymphoid tissues and particularly from tonsils.

Primary peripheral B cells can be stimulated through a number of surface receptors, each taking the cell to a distinct stage of activation (2). The major driving signal is assumed to be via antigen receptor, while other factors may be considered as being more instrumental in programming the direction of the response or modifying that delivered through surface Ig (2). Many of the receptors which receive signals impinging directly upon resting B cells appear to be T cell derived: these may be received as soluble factors or via direct contact with corresponding counterstructures on the T cell surface. Some of these will now be considered in detail, while signalling of resting B cells through smIg is covered adequately in chapter 11 of this volume.

Interleukin 4

Interleukin 4 (IL-4) is a product of TH cells that encourages a number of phenotypic changes on the resting B cell and may be intimately involved in its programming along a defined route of subsequent development. Dense resting B cells cultured with IL-4 increase in size, up-regulate surface expres-sion of IgM, CD40, CD72 and major histocompatibility complex (MHC) class II antigen, and begin to express high levels of CD23 (3–5). There is no evidence for human B cells, in contrast to the mouse, that exposure to IL-4 prepares B cells for heightened responses to signals delivered through anti-gen receptors, although the up-regulation of IgM expression would suggest a function of this type (4). Interestingly, the amount of IL-4 required to provoke this latter change is 10- to 100-fold less than that needed for some of the other alterations in B cell phenotype (5).

The signal transduction pathway through which IL-4 triggers phenotypic change in resting B cells is currently controversial, primarily because what has been observed in human B cells is apparently quite different from that previously established for mouse. Moreover, studies on human B cell lines provide data that also seem at odds with that generated from the study of primary resting B cells. Nevertheless, there is compelling evidence that—at least for the induction of CD23 expression—IL-4 activates a novel second messenger cascade in resting B cells (6). This comprises transient phosphatidyl inositol (PI) hydrolysis with a corresponding rise in intracellular free Ca^{2+}, which peaks at 15 seconds and is over by 1 minute: this is followed, with a delay of around 10 minutes, by a sustained increase in levels of intracellular cAMP. When compared to signals triggered through surface membrane immunoglobulin (smIg) activation via IL-4 generates similar amounts of Ca^{2+}-mobilizing inositol trisphosphate (IP3) but little inositol tetrakisphosphate (IP4): the latter appears to facilitate the ability of IP3 to mediate release of Ca^{2+} from intracellular stores. Phenotypic change other than CD23 induction (or triggering for cell cycle progression which appears to be similar) may utilize different pathways of activation: thus, concentrations of IL-4 sufficient for up-regulation of smIgM do not generate significant increases in either intracellular Ca^{2+} or cAMP (6). These observations may explain, in part, the apparent differences between human and murine B cells in the second messengers generated on binding of IL-4 to its receptors. Another consideration, however, is the different way in which human and mouse B cells are isolated for study. This has been discussed in detail elsewhere (6).

There is now good reason to believe that IL-4 will both strengthen and direct interaction of the primary B cell with activated T cells. Increase in MHC class II antigen expression would clearly encourage cognate interactions, while recent evidence implicates CD23, CD40 and CD72 as accessory molecules in this process. Counterstructures for CD40 and CD72 have now been identified on T cell surfaces, while an involvement for CD23 in T–B conjugation has been described (7, 8). Recent data now implicate CD21 as a ligand for CD23 in such interaction (9). There is compelling reason to speculate that these changes may be instrumental in directing B cell responses to IgE production. IL-4 is essential to IgE production both *in vitro* and *in vivo*, while the only major B cell impairment reported for IL-4 gene-deleted mice was the inability to produce IgE (10, 11). CD23 is the low-affinity receptor for IgE on B cells, while its cleaved fragments constitute earlier-described IgE regulants (12). Resting B cells can be driven directly to IgE synthesis by a combination of IL-4 and mAb binding to CD40, which would mimic interaction of CD40 with its ligand on activated TH cells (10).

CD40

The binding between 48 kDa CD40 and its recently identified ligand (CD40-L) may be a major signal involved in driving the cognate activation of resting B cells (7). As will be discussed in later sections, it is undoubtedly central to the maintenance of B cell expansion and survival, at least as indicated from experiments *in vitro*. Current efforts to produce CD40-"knockout" mice will answer whether this is also the case *in vivo*. Regarding the activation of resting, primary B cells, ligation of CD40 (by monoclonal antibody) brings about an increase in size but, as yet, no dramatic change in the expression of other functional molecules on the B cell surface has been observed from this mode of activation (4). Nevertheless, resting B cells triggered in this fashion are modified functionally. Whereas control (or IL-4) cultured B cells rapidly wane in their ability to respond to polyclonal stimuli, those engaged through CD40 via mAb remain "alert" to such signalling (4). This observation provided the first indication that CD40 might somehow be involved in enhancing B cell survival—a concept that, as we shall see later, became reinforced by studies on germinal centre B cells (13).

The most dramatic phenotypic change engendered in resting B cells on engaging CD40 is the induction of rapid and extensive homotypic adhesions (4). This process is energy and temperature dependent, and also requires Ca^{2+}. LFA-1 is involved but LFA-1-independent mechanisms of binding also appear to be operative: aggregation can be blocked partially by mAb to either CD18 or CD54. Expression of ICAM-1 (CD54) appears to increase on activating resting B cells through CD40 (14). The signal transduction mechanism whereby CD40 activates this, or other phenotypic change, is, at the time of writing, unknown. Inositol lipid hydrolysis does not appear to be involved, nor increases in intracellular Ca^{2+} levels. At least in resting B cells, no tyrosine kinase activity has been observed on engaging CD40. Phosphorylation of proteins on serines and threonines has been reported (14). An intriguing finding was that in the murine B lymphoma cell line, M12, introduction of DNA encoding human CD40 conferred responsiveness (by growth inhibition) of the cells to human IL-6. There is no evidence to suggest that CD40 binds IL-6 directly, so the explanation seems to be that indirect transmodulation between CD40 and IL-6R must be occurring (14).

Whatever the mechanism is by which CD40 delivers its signal, it seems to engage in particularly intimate cross-talk with the IL-4R. Signals through CD40 synergize strongly with IL-4 for the induction of CD23. The production and turnover of soluble CD23 is especially enhanced (15). It was recently shown that normal inhibitors of IL-4-induced change on this phenotype—including interferons (IFNs), transforming growth factor-β (TGF$_\beta$) and anti-CD19—no longer exert their influence if CD40 is simultaneously engaged (16).

The intimacy of the cross-talk involved in these two receptors is underscored by the recent finding that CD40 signalling is even able to overcome the potent inhibition of IL-4 induction of CD23 observed with either glucocorticoids or the broad kinase inhibitor, staurosporine. Interestingly, staurosporine significantly enhances the amount of CD23 induced, both on the B cell surface and as soluble fragments, on co-ligation of CD40 and IL-4R (Gordon and Katira, manuscript in preparation).

CD19

This member of the Ig superfamily is expressed throughout B cell differentiation from the very earliest "pro-B cell", and only becomes diminished in expression on terminal maturation to plasma cells. Its counterstructure is, at the time of writing, unknown. Nevertheless, there is a relatively large body of data available on functional properties of CD19 engagement as gleaned from presumed mimetic mAb. Reports of direct effects on resting B cells are limited and its main function may be to co-modulate via signals delivered through smIg (14). CD19 and smIgM have been found to co-cap on individual B cells, although there is no other direct evidence that the two glycoproteins are physically associated (17). Rather, CD19 is now known to be part of a macromolecular complex of several proteins which include CD21, the C3d/EBV-R (18). No change in MHC class II expression, adhesion molecules, or other markers of phenotypic change are obvious on engaging CD19. CD19 does, however, deliver signals for strong homotypic aggregation of B cells (14).

The mode of direct signalling through CD19 to the resting B cell has been controversial. Initial reports suggested a behaviour similar to that of smIg, with an increase in intracellular Ca^{2+} and the translocation of protein kinase C (PKC) to membranes. These changes were, however, dependent upon cross-linking with a second antibody (19). Simple exposure of B cells to CD19 mAb is known to be sufficient for the initiation of functional change, and this proceeds without any detectable change in $[Ca^{2+}]$.

CD20

The 35/37 kDa phosphoprotein, originally termed B1, has been considered as a surface molecule capable of invoking an alternative pathway of B cell activation in a manner somewhat analogous to that of CD2 on the T cell. This concept has evolved primarily because CD20 appears to prime resting B cells for subsequent responses to cell cycle progression factors completely independently of a need to engage smIg (14). CD20 parallels smIg in its ability to stimulate increases in c-myc expression and in up-regulating MHC class II and CD18 expression. Divergence in the two pathways is also evident, however, inasmuch as CD20 does not signal for increases in either CD54 or in the expression of the CD28 ligand, B7/BBI (14).

The predicted topology of CD20 is that of multiple (four) transmembrane domains, with both the amino- and carboxy-terminus being cytoplasmic. This overall pattern is reminiscent of several typical transmembrane ion channels. Using classical patch-clamp techniques, it has been shown that CD20 may indeed serve as a Ca^{2+} ion channel. Separate studies indicate multiple phosphorylation sites on CD20 itself and it is tempting to speculate that, depending on the activation signals being received, differential phosphorylation may serve to effectively open or close the ion channel function of this B cell surface protein (20). This would be in keeping with the observed dichotomous behaviour of CD20 mAb on resting and activated B cells, being in turn stimulatory or inhibitory.

A recent report indicates a relationship between the actions of CD40 and IL-4 and the conformation—and hence the potential functional status—of CD20. Dancescu and co-workers found that exposure of B cells to IL-4 extinguished the expression of an epitope on CD20 defined by the Leu-16 antibody, while leaving the binding capacity of seven other CD20 mAbs unchanged (21). The steady-state level of CD20 mRNA similarly remained unchanged. Joint exposure of the B cells to CD40 antibody antagonized the ability of IL-4 to influence this apparent conformational change. The full functional consequences of these interesting observations remain to be determined. They do, nevertheless, highlight once again the intimate relationship existing between IL-4 and CD40 in modifying B cell behaviour.

CD22

This heavily glycosylated surface protein of mature B cells has been found to share close homology with myelin-associated glycoprotein (22). A recent report claimed to have identified two counterstructures for CD22, namely CD45RO and CD75. The latter may be an artefact, however (23). The ability of B cell-associated CD22 to couple with T cell CD45RO—a marker of memory or activated T cells—suggests that this pairing may assume particular significance at specific stages of a B cell response to TD antigen. The finding of CD45RO on a minority population of peripheral blood B cells raises the possibility of cross-talk between B cells at different stages of activation through CD22 (14).

Although cytoplasmic CD22 is a characteristic marker of pre-B cells, its surface expression is closely linked to that of CD21. Engagement of CD22 on resting B cells promotes no obvious direct change but it does modify the outcome of triggering through smIg. Indeed, certain mAbs to CD22 enhances the level of Ca^{2+} flux mediated through smIg and alters the threshold at which anti-Ig induces stimulation of resting B cells into S phase (14).

Interestingly, CD22 expression appears to be a prerequisite for smIg to activate resting B cells (14).

CD72

CD72, a member of the C-type family of animal lectins, is the human counterpart of the murine B cell differentiation antigen Lyb-2 (24). Both are expressed constitutively on mature B cells and each is capable of delivering activation signals when using appropriate antibodies (3). CD72/Lyb-2 represents one of those rare surface glycoproteins where univalent binding by Fab fragments of antibody is sufficient for stimulation of the receptor—cross-linking is not required to elicit a response (25). In both human and murine systems, the consequence of occupying CD72/Lyb-2 shares features in common with that of signalling B cells via IL-4. Thus the expression of MHC class II antigen is increased, and cells enlarge and enter the early G1 phase of the cell cycle (26).

At one stage there was speculation that Lyb-2 might represent the IL-4R on mouse B cells. This is clearly not the case although a functional relationship between IL-4R and CD72/Lyb-2 may exist (26). Although in many ways similar, signalling through CD72 differs from that initiated via IL-4R by the ability of the latter but not the former to induce expression of CD23. Nevertheless, it was recently demonstrated that mAb to CD72 significantly enhances IL-4-dependent up-regulation of CD23 on small resting B cells (25). Moreover, and perhaps more importantly, engagement of CD72 reduced the threshold requirement for IL-4 to induce such phenotypic change.

The discovery that CD5 is a counterstructure to CD72 was unexpected, as the ability to trigger on univalent binding was considered to favour a soluble factor as its natural ligand (3, 8). Nevertheless, the changes observed on activating CD72 sit comfortably within the context of T–B collaboration via CD5–CD72 pairing. It is of note that B cell-associated CD5 is down-regulated on exposure to IL-4, suggesting a reprogramming of cells along a CD23-directed pathway enhanced by the ability of the B cell now to interact with T cell-expressed CD5 (27). The presence of a CD23 counterstructure (CD21) on a subset of CD4+ T cells increases further the level of interplay available in such a scenario.

CD5-positive B Cells

The debate surrounding the exact nature of CD5+ B cells is too extensive to address fully within the confines of this chapter. Nevertheless, certain aspects of this important phenotype needs to be covered as there are clear repercussions for the understanding of B cell behaviour in general. In the mouse, there appears little doubt that, particularly during fetal development, the Ly-1/CD5 B cell dominates and represents a lineage that is quite distinct from the majority "conventional" population encountered in adulthood. These cells—recently classified as "B1"—are bright for smIgM and dull for smIgD and the B220 antigen. A key distinction between CD5+ and conventional (or "B2" cells) is the capacity for self-renewal, being apparent for the former but not for the latter population (28).

The cytokine IL-10 may be intimately involved in the regulation of B1 cells. O'Garra and colleagues have shown that production of IL-10 by B cells is restricted to the CD5+ subset, whereas the laboratory of Howard has presented experiments arguing that IL-10 is necessary for the development of this population (29, 30). Thus mice treated from birth with anti-IL-10 possess normal total B cell numbers but are void of B1 cells. Although IL-10-"knockout" mice do not reveal this disturbed pattern of B cell subsets, such experiments do not discount the important role of IL-10 in normal development, as other elements may take over when an animal is genetically deficient for a given component from the outset of its development.

Perhaps the most important feature of B1 cells is their bias toward early V gene usage, which results in the expression of autoreactive and polyspecific antigen receptors (28). The precise role of such autoreactive clones is not clear, although a function in general "housekeeping", in autoregulation, and in maintenance of B cell memory have each been mooted. It is of interest that the malignant populations expanded in B-CLL are universally CD5+ and show a high frequency of V gene usage encoding polyspecific and autoreactive antibodies. Whether this contributes to the longevity of the leukaemic cells remains to be established.

Much of the controversy relating to CD5+ B cells has arisen from the observation that, in the adult human, CD5 seems to be more a marker of activation status than of lineage. It was already discussed above that IL-4 can down-regulate pre-existing levels of CD5 on adult B cells (27). Moreover, the expression of CD5 on B cells from activated tissues, such as tonsil, appears disproportionately high in human, while this number can be further increased on activation (particularly with phorbol esters) *in vitro* (Holder and Gordon, unpublished observations). The possibility that CD5 might also represent a "movable marker" even in the mouse was raised by a study from Wortis and colleagues. Here it was shown that anti-Ig plus IL-6, but not lipopolysaccharide (LPS), was able to stimulate a large number of conventional adult B cells to CD5 positivity (31). This group has argued that the CD5 phenotype is primarily a consequence of extensive cross-linking of smIgM by antigen with highly repetitive epitopes as would be encountered with thymus-independent type 2 (TI-2) antigens (28). As is often the case in such immunological controversies, it would not be surprising if each school of thought was correct, in that CD5 can be *both* a lineage-specific marker and a functional surface glycoprotein which is induced on conventional B cells under appropriate circumstances. A rationale for the latter is presented next.

A Role for CD5–CD72 Interactions in TI-2 Responses?

The first report to detail the role of CD72 in stimulating human B cells noted that mAb to CD72 was unable to provide a direct proliferative signal, nor did it co-stimulate particularly well with a wide variety of co-factors. The one exception to this was provided by immobilized—but not by soluble—anti-IgM (3). Such a clear-cut dichotomy in the ability to co-stimulate with soluble versus immobilized ligand for sIg has not been observed with any other mode of B cell signalling. It was concluded that CD72 may have a special role to play in activation of B cells via TI antigens. More recently, the same group has demonstrated that antibody to CD5 selectively inhibits stimulations of purified B cells mediated by immobilized anti-Ig (Kamal and Gordon, manuscript in preparation).

It becomes tempting to speculate that the autonomous nature of stimulations via TI-2 antigens is due partly to signalling through CD72 achieved by inducing CD5 on neighbouring B cells. Given that B-CLL cells carry both CD5 and CD72 and that the polyspecific nature of their antigen receptors might result in continuous low-level signalling through this route, then all the requirements for self-maintenance in the absence of exogenous antigen seem to be in place.

GROWTH SIGNALS FOR HUMAN B CELLS

Soluble Factors

Of the plethora of soluble activities which have been described as influencing B cell growth, very few have so far gained respectability by being molecularly cloned and sequenced. An attempt to survey these disparate activities is essentially fruitless in the absence of any recognized standard. Instead, this section will limit itself to a discussion of factors which are available in recombinant form and investigated sufficiently that some consensus can be reached on their influence on B cell growth.

"Growth factors" operationally fall into two categories: those that promote the progression of the activated B cell from early G1 through to S phase of the cell cycle; and those that elicit cell division (2). Clearly, these are not mutually exclusive activities. A third category may be included when considering the perhaps equally important negative regulators, or inhibitors, of growth (2).

Among the interleukins, IL-1, IL-2, IL-3, IL-4, IL-6, IL-7 and IL-10 may each have a role to play in B cell growth, while IFNs, tumour necrosis factors

(TNFs) and TGF_β have also been implicated as B lymphotropic regulators. Studies on IL-7 indicate that its influence may be restricted to early B cell development. Indeed, IL-7 together with appropriate stromal support may be *the* growth factor for pre-B cells (32). Denial of either of these components appears to result in death of the developing B cell, probably through self-destruction by apoptosis. By contrast, IL-6 comes into its own during late B cell development. Early synonyms for this interleukin included "hybridoma growth factor" and "plasmacytoma growth factor". IL-6, together with IL-3, may be particularly important for the replication of plasmablasts isolated from peripheral blood (Hardie and MacLennan, personal communication). Inappropriate response to IL-6 may be contributory to the longevity of the neoplastic clones comprising multiple myeloma (33). Whether IL-3 is an important B cell regulator in its own right is unclear, although a recent study indicates that it may be at selective stages of activation (34).

IL-5 has not been included for discussion as its proposed role in the stimulation of murine B cells has not been substantiated by studies on human B cells, despite extensive and diverse efforts in that direction. Whether this represents a true species difference remains to be determined. The role of IL-1 is considered as being modulatory rather than the monokine being a major player in deciding the fate of a B cell response: it can probably best be viewed as a general enhancer of the action of other B lymphotropic factors.

There is now little doubt that, at least *in vitro*, IL-2 has the capacity to promote B cell growth and replication. This conclusion can be reached from studies made on both neoplastic and normal B cell populations. Moreover, B cells can be encouraged to express both chains of the high-affinity IL-2R. The reported actions of IL-2 make it compatible with its being a relatively late-acting B cell growth factor, most likely exerting its influence at the late G1 or G2/M phase of the cell cycle (35). Unpublished studies have revealed that IL-2 is a major growth factor for IgM plasmablasts found in the germinal centres of secondary lymphoid tissues. Such cells actively multiply and differentiate to IgM-secreting plasma cells in the presence of low concentrations of IL-2 and without the need for any filler cell support (Holder and Gordon, manuscript in preparation).

The first fully characterized "B cell growth factor" ("BCGF") was what is now termed IL-4. This TH2-derived factor exerts diverse influence on mature B cells at almost every stage of the cell cycle and is central to isotype regulation. Its actions on resting B cells were outlined earlier. Several studies have detailed the potent cell cycle progression activity of IL-4 on B cells which have been pre-stimulated via a variety of activation regimens (2). Paradoxically, B cell stimulations dependent upon IL-2, a product of TH1 cells, are generally antagonized by IL-4 (36).

One of the central features of IL-4 action is its ability to synergize with signals delivered through CD40 for long-term B cell proliferation. This striking synergy was first noted in a study reported in 1987, where a combination of IL-4 and mAb to CD40 provided an optimal signal for maintaining the cell cycle of B cells which had been driven into proliferation by phorbol ester and calcium ionophore (37). A later study was able to improve on this dual action of IL-4 and mAb to CD40 by incorporating a feeder layer of L cells which had been transfected with CDw32, an FcR which was able to capture the antibody and present it to the B cell in a particularly efficacious manner (38). It is likely that the transformed fibroblasts also provide signals which facilitate B cell growth and survival in this powerful system (39).

A more recently identified player in the game is IL-10. Originally cloned as CSIF (cytokine synthesis inhibition factor of T cells) a potential importance in B cell regulation soon emerged from the identification of a striking homology to BCRF1, an open reading frame in the Epstein–Barr virus (EBV) genome (40). In the mature protein-coding sequences, the homology between hIL-10 and BCRF1 is 84% identical (40). No direct influence of IL-10 on resting B cells has been recorded but it is capable of enhancing DNA synthesis in B cells activated with immobilized anti-Ig, although the degree of stimulation was small by comparison with that achieved by either IL-4 or IL-2 (40). IL-10 was, however, found to be particularly potent when used in the system described above of CDw32-transfected L cells carrying mAb to CD40. Indeed, over a 2-week period its efficacy was equal to that of IL-4, promoting a 10- to 25-fold increase in B cell numbers. Moreover, IL-4 and IL-10 were found to cooperate with one another in that a 60- to 100-fold increase in B cells was now registered with the two factors working together (40).

IFNs have been described as having both positive and negative effects on B cell growth. The precise role of TNF remains obscure, although lymphotoxin has been claimed to contribute up to 70% of the activity contained within a commercial source of "BCGF" (41). TGF$_\beta$ can clearly be a potent inhibitor of B cell growth and may have a major role to play in the regulation of apoptosis at susceptible stages of B cell development (42, 43).

Cell Surface Molecules

Several of the cell surface molecules regulating B cell growth have already been discussed: CD5, CD19, CD20, CD22, CD40 and CD72. The studies using the CDw32–L cell transfectants exemplify the importance of CD40 signalling in B cell proliferation—an event that would be encountered physiologically during cognate B–T interactions. Using the same system, it was recently found that co-ligation of CD19 and smIg greatly reduced the threshold at which B cells can be triggered to growth through antigen receptor (44). CD19 therefore appears to be a critical accessory molecule for smIg signalling, and identification of its natural counterstructure will be particularly rewarding.

An important surface molecule so far not mentioned in detail is CD21, or CR2, which in the human serves not only to bind C3d but also provides the route of entry for EBV into the B cell (45). CD21 belongs to a family of complement proteins, and its major function on B cells may involve interaction with C3d-containing immune complexes. Signalling through CD21 appears not to be PI linked, although ligation of CD21 has been reported to enhance increases in [Ca^{2+}] provoked by anti-Ig (46). Certain mAbs to CD21 have been shown to supply a T cell-dependent signal for B cell growth and differentiation (47). The physical association noted between CD21 and CD19 on B cells is clearly of interest (18).

While the previously discussed glycoproteins are expressed constitutively on the B cell surface already at significant levels, the 45 kDa C-type lectin family member CD23 needs to be actively induced before it can be readily detected. Expression is super-induced on EBV infection and following exposure to phorbol esters (26). Physiologically, IL-4 appears to be the major regulator of CD23 expression; IL-4-dependent expression is dramatically up-regulated on engagement of CD40 by mAb or by cognate and non-cognate interaction with TH cells. Selected mAbs to CD23 binding to a restricted epitope within the lectin homology domain trigger cell cycle progression in activated B cells while others appear to block B cell stimulations (26). Whether the stimulating mAbs map to the epitope on CD23 utilized in binding to CD21—a recently identified counterstructure— remains to be determined. A full account of the behaviour and functional properties of membrane-bound CD23 has been given in a number of recent reviews (26, 48).

DIFFERENTIATION PATHWAYS

Events in Secondary Lymphoid Tissues

Most of our understanding of human B cell behaviour has, by necessity, been gleaned from the study of immune cells *in vitro*. The reductionist approach afforded by such analysis clearly provides important information but, nevertheless, can only hope at best to approximate the complex array of interactions occurring *in vivo*. Such analysis can, however, be supplemented with knowledge obtained by immunohistological examination of human B cells *in situ* and by following the fate of *in vivo* antigen-specific responses using appropriate animal models. The type of synthesis that can emerge by such a combined approach has been fully illustrated in a recent review (49). The conclusions reached will not be reiterated in detail here but some of the more salient points relating to later stages of B cell development will be covered briefly.

Activation of B Cells by TD antigen

The focus for initial B cell responses to TD antigens is the interdigitating cell (IDC) found in the T cell-rich paracortex of secondary lymphoid tissues. It is of interest that IDCs express CD40, heavily suggesting the possibility of an amplification loop being created between IDCs, T cells and B cells congregating at this site. The first wave of B cell proliferation occurs outside of follicles and culminates in the production of IgM plasma cells, the product of which characterizes the primary response. The second wave is established by B cells entering follicles and giving rise to germinal centres, the outcome of which is the generation of memory and affinity maturation of the antibody response. It is currently a matter of debate as to whether separate subsets, or even lineages, of B cells give rise independently to primary and memory responses.

Signal, Driving Germinal Centre Cell Responses

Once a primary follicle has become fully occupied with the progeny of the antigen-specific B cell blast, differentiation occurs to provide: (a) *centroblasts*, which comprise the dark zone of germinal centres and are a self-renewing population that also give rise to (b) *centrocytes*—non-dividing cells occupying the light zone. The evidence for these cells being, respectively, the targets for somatic hyper-mutation and selection of high-affinity antigen-binding clones has been adequately reviewed elsewhere (49).

Once centrocytes have been selected on their ability to bind antigen, a bifurcation occurs which will allow: the production of plasma cells producing antibody with high affinity for the antigen which initiated the response; and the establishment of a memory pool for creating a rapid and effective response on subsequent antigen rechallenge. From studies on isolated germinal centre cells *in vitro*, two sets of signals have been identified as potential mediators of these separate pathways.

Culture of germinal centre B cells with mAb to CD40 appears to promote development toward a possible memory phenotype (49). These cells can be restimulated by IL-4, particularly when they are placed on a stromal support. Encounter with CD40-L may naturally occur in the germinal centre light zone where CD57+/CD69+ TH cells are located. Simultaneous or proximal interaction with antigen held as immune complexes on FDC and CD40-L presented by T cells—perhaps also participating in response to the same antigen which is driving the B cell response—may be a necessary component for long-term B cell survival: this would provide a mechanism to militate against the selection of autoreactive clones which could arise by random somatic mutation on Ig V genes. Encounter with (self) antigen in the absence of TH-expressed CD40-L would be insufficient for the establishment of memory and may even provide a direct trigger for apoptosis. It should be noted that Burkitt lymphoma lines—which appear to represent neoplastic counterparts of germinal centre B cells—can be activated to undergo apoptosis by anti-Ig, a process which, in turn, is arrested on engaging CD40 (50).

Development of antigen-selected germinal centre B cells along a plasmacytoid pathway of differentiation may be promoted by their exposure to soluble CD23. A role for CD23 in germinal centre cell processes was initially suggested by the high-level expression of this C-type lectin in a discrete subset of follicular dendritic cells located within the light zone (12). Germinal centre B cells are, themselves, negative for CD23 expression. It was found that culture with soluble CD23 and IL-1 *in vitro* not only provided rescue of germinal centre cells from apoptosis but also encouraged their differentiation toward a plasmacytoid phenotype. Such cells showed an increased content of cytoplasmic IgG but high-rate Ig secretion was not evident (49). Clearly other signals are required for their terminal differentiation to mature plasma cells.

B Cell Differentiation Factors

Soluble factors can influence B cell differentiation both by directing isotype commitment and by driving terminal maturation of pre-committed cells. In order to discriminate between these two possibilities, studies must be performed using cells sorted on the basis of Ig isotype expression and plated at limiting number. Such an approach has revealed that IL-4 is highly efficient at promoting switching of uncommitted IgM+/IgD+ cells to IgE and IgG4 production. Engagement of CD40 also appears to provide a necessary co-factor, at least for IgE production, which can be provided by mAb to CD40 or by activated TH membranes presumably carrying the CD40-L. The inability of IL4-"knockout" mice to mount IgE responses supports the observations made *in vitro*. Both IFNs (types I and II) and TGF$_\beta$ have been shown to antagonize the ability of IL4 to promote IgE production. At least with IFN, engagement of CD40 overcomes its inhibitory action on IL-4-promoted IgE synthesis (10).

IL-4 can also promote general Ig production in *in vitro* culture of pre-activated B cells, but this might simply reflect an effect on already isotype-committed populations. Similarly, IL-10 has a potent and broad influence on B cells when placed with anti-CD40 on CDw32-transfected L cells: large amounts of IgM, IgG and IgA are secreted under these conditions (40). It was also noted that *Staphylococcus aureus* Cowan I (SAC)-activated B cells respond particularly well to IL-10 by Ig secretion. Again, it is not clear whether this factor is driving isotype commitment or promoting terminal differentiation of pre-committed cells.

Another factor shown to drive high-rate Ig production is IL-2. In a recent study using T cells or their membranes as a support, it was shown that large amounts of IgM, IgG and IgA were produced in response to IL-2 (51). In this case, there was no evidence in favour of isotype switching; rather, that IL-2 induced a selective expansion of committed B cells. IL-4 was found to block selectively the IL-2-driven production of IgA. In contrast, TGF$_\beta$ in the same system has been found to promote IgA production, this time by directing IgA switching in B cells (52).

CLOSING COMMENT

The range of recently developed *in vitro* systems available for assessing B cell responses to growth and differentiation factors has been reviewed elsewhere (53). It is clear that these high-efficiency systems are providing, and will continue to provide, important insights into the possibilities open to human B cells in their progress to antibody-producing cells following their initial encounter with antigen. It will be of special interest to apply these systems to the study of perturbed B cells as encountered in immunodeficiencies and other immune disorders.

ACKNOWLEDGEMENTS

The work of the author is supported by a Programme Grant from the Medical Research Council (UK), by the Leukaemia Research Fund, the Wellcome Trust, and the Arthritis and Rheumatism Council. This chapter was written in May to June of 1992 during a leave of absence at DNAX, Palo Alto. I wish to thank Maureen Howard and her group for providing a stimulating atmosphere in which to prepare this work: special thanks to my "twin brother" Andy Heath for his British humour and converting me to the use of the MAC; Leopoldo Santos-Argumedo is acknowledged for his continual nagging; Christopher Grimaldi for *excellent* company; Debbie Cockayne, for being a "knock-out".

REFERENCES

1. MacLennan, I.C.M. and Gray, D. (1986) Antigen-driven selection of virgin and memory B cells. *Immunol. Rev.*, **91**, 61–85.
2. Gordon, J. and Guy, G.R. (1987) The molecules controlling B lymphocytes. *Immunol. Today*, **8**, 339–344.
3. Kamal, M., Katira, A. and Gordon, J. (1991) Stimulation of B lymphocytes via CD72 (Human Lyb-2). *Eur. J. Immunol.*, **21**, 1419–1424.
4. Gordon, J., Millsum, M.J., Guy, G.R. and Ledbetter, J.A. (1988) Resting B lymphocytes can be triggered directly through the CDw40 (Bp50) antigen. *J. Immunol.*, **140**, 1425–1430.
5. Rigley, K.P., Thurstan, S.M. and Callard, R.E. (1991) Independent regulation of IL4 induced human B cell surface CD23 or IgM: Functional evidence for two IL4-receptors. *Int. Immunol.*, **3**, 197–204.
6. Finney, M., Guy, G.R., Michell, R.H., Gordon, J., Dugas, B., Rigley, K.P. and Callard, R.E. (1990) Interleukin-4 activates human B lymphocytes via transient

inositol lipid hydrolysis and transient cAMP generation. *Eur. J. Immunol.,* **20,** 541–548.

7. Armitage, R.J., Fanslow, W.C., Strockbine, L., Sato, T.A. *et al.* (1992) Molecular and biological characterization of a murine ligand for CD40. *Nature,* **357,** 80–82.

8. van de Velde, H., von Hoegen, I., Luo, W., Parnes, J.R. and Thielemans, K. (1991) The B cell surface protein CD72/Lyb-2 is the ligand for CD5. *Nature,* **351,** 662–664.

9. Aubry, J-P., Pochon, S., Grabere, P., Jansen, K. and Bonnefoy, J-Y. (1992) CD_{21} is a ligand for CD_{23} and regulates IgE production. *Nature,* **358,** 505–508.

10. de Vries, J.E., Gauchat, J.-F., Aversa, G.G., Punnonen, J., Gascan, H. and Yssel, H. (1991) Regulation of IgE synthesis by cytokines. *Curr. Opinion Immunol.,* **3,** 851–858.

11. Kuhn, R., Rajewsky, K. and Miller, W. (1991) Generation and analysis of inter-leukin 4-deficient mice. *Science,* **254,** 707–710.

12. Gordon, J., Flores-Romo, L., Cairns, J.A., Millsum, M., Lane, P.J.L., Johnson, G.D. and MacLennan, I.C.M. (1989) CD23: A novel multifunctional receptor/lymphokine. *Immunol. Today,* **10,** 153–159.

13. Liu, Y.-J., Joshua, D.E., Williams, G.T., Smith, C.A., Gordon, J. and MacLennan, I.C.M. (1989) Mechanism of antigen-driven selection in germinal centers. *Nature,* **342,** 929–931.

14. Clark, E.A. and Lane, P.J. (1991) Regulation of human B cell activation and adhesion. *Annu. Rev. Immunol.,* **9,** 97–127.

15. Cairns, J.A., Flores-Romo, L., Millsum, M.J., Guy, G.R., Gillis, S., Ledbetter, J.A. and Gordon, J. (1988) Soluble CD23 is released by B lymphocytes cycling in response to interleukin 4 and anti-Bp50 (CDw40). *Eur. J. Immunol.,* **18,** 349–354.

16. Gordon, J., Katira, A., Strain, A.J. and Gillis, S. (1991) Inhibition of interleukin-4-promoted CD23 production in human B lymphocytes by TGFB, interferons, or anti-CD19 is overridden on engaging CD40. *Eur. J. Immunol.,* **21,** 1917–1922.

17. Pesando, J.M., Bouchard, L.S. and McMaster, B.E. (1989) CD19 is functionally and physically associated with surface immunoglobulin. *J. Exp. Med.,* **170,** 2159–2164.

18. Matsumoto, A.K., Kopicky-Burd, J., Carter, R.H., Tuveson, D.A., Tedder, T.F. and Fearon, D.T. (1991) Intersection of the complement and immune systems: A signal transduction complex of the B-lymphocyte containing CR2 and CD19. *J. Exp. Med.,* **175,** 55–64.

19. Ledbetter, J.A., Rabinovitch, P.S., June, C.H., Song, C.W., Clark, E.A. and Uckun, F.M. (1988) Antigen-independent regulation of cytoplasmic calcium in B cells with a 12-kDa B-cell growth factor and anti-CD19. *Proc. Nat. Acad. Sci. USA,* **85,** 1897–1901.

20. Tedder, T.F., Zhou, L.J., Bell, P.D., Frizzell, R.A. and Bubien, J.K. (1990) The CD20 surface molecule of B lymphocytes functions as a calcium channel. *J. Cell Biochem.,* **140,** 195–201.

21. Dancescu, M., Wu, C., Rubio, M., Delespesse, G. and Sarfati, M. (1992) IL4 induces conformational change of CD20 antigen via a protein kinase C-independent pathway: Antagonistic effect of anti-CD40 monoclonal antibody. *J. Immunol.,* **148,** 2411–2416.

22. Stamenkovic, I. and Seed, B. (1990) The B lymphocyte antigen CD22 mediates monocyte and erythrocyte adhesion. *Nature,* **345,** 74–77.

23. Munro, S., Bast, B.J.E.G., Colley, K.J. and Tedder, T.F. (1992) The B lymphocyte surface antigen CD75 is not an α-2,6-sialyltransferase but is a carbohydrate antigen, the production of which requires the enzyme. *Cell,* **68,** 1003–1004.

24. von Hoegen, I., Hsieh, C.-L., Shwarting, R., Francke, U. and Parnes, J.R. (1991) Identity of human CD72 and Lyb-2 and localization of the gene to chromosome 9. *Eur. J. Immunol.*, **21**, 1425–1432.

25. Katira, A., Kamal, M. and Gordon, J. (1992) Occupancy of CD72 (the CD5 counterstructure) enhances IL4-dependent CD23 induction. *Immunology*, **76**, 422–426.

26. Gordon, J. (1993) CD23 and CD72: C-type lectins and B lymphocyte regulation. *Adv. Cell. Mol. Immunol.*, **1** (in press).

27. Defrance, T., Vanberlivet, B., Durand, I. and Banchereau, J. (1989) Human interleukin 4 down-regulates the surface expression of CD5 on normal and leukemic B cells. *Eur. J. Immunol.*, **19**, 293–300.

28. Kantor, A.B. (1991) The development and repertoire of B-1 cells (CD5 B cells). *Immunol. Today*, **14**, 389–392.

29. O'Garra, A., Chang, R., Go, N., Hastings, R., Haughton, G. and Howard, M. (1992) Ly-1 B cells are the main source of B-cell derived Il-10. *Eur. J. Immunol.*, **22**, 711–718.

30. Ishida, H., Hastings, R., Kearney, J. and Howard, M. (1992) Continuous anti-interleukin 10 antibody administration depletes mice of Ly-1 B cells but not conventional B cells. *J. Exp. Med.*, **175**, 1213–1220.

31. Cong, Y., Rabin, E. and Wortis, H.H. (1991) Treatment of murine CD5– B cells with anti-Ig, but not LPS, includes surface CD5: Two B cell activation pathways. *Int. Immunol.*, **5**, 467–476.

32. Rolink, A. and Melchers, F. (1991) Molecular and cellular origins of B lymphocyte diversity. *Cell*, **66**, 1081–1094.

33. Kishimoto, T. and Hirano, T. (1988) Molecular regulation of B lymphocyte response. *Annu. Rev. Immunol.*, **6**, 485–512.

34. Xia, X., Li, L. and Choi, Y.S. (1992) Human recombinant IL3 is a growth factor for normal B cells. *J. Immunol.*, **148**, 491–497.

35. Kishimoto, T. (1985) Factors affecting B cell growth and differentiation. *Annu. Rev. Immunol.*, **3**, 133–157.

36. Karray, S., Defrance, T., Merle-Beral, H., Banchereau, J., Debre, P. and Galanaud, P. (1988) Interleukin 4 counteracts interleukin 2-induced proliferation of monoclonal B cells. *J. Exp. Med.*, **168**, 85–94.

37. Gordon, J., Millsum, M.J., Guy, G.R. and Ledbetter, J.A. (1987) Synergistic interaction between interleukin-4 and anti-Bp50 (CDw40) revealed in a novel B cell restimulation assay. *Eur. J. Immunol.*, **17**, 1535–1538.

38. Banchereau, J., de Paoli, P., Valle, A., Garcia, E. and Rousset, F. (1991) Long term human B cell lines dependent on interleukin-4 and antibody to CD40. *Science*, **251**, 70–73.

39. Holder, M., Liu, Y.-J., Defrance, T., Flores-Romo, L., MacLennan, I.C.M. and Gordon, J. (1991). Growth factor requirements for the stimulation of germinal center B cells: Evidence for an IL2-dependent pathway of development. *Int. Immunol.*, **3**, 1243–1252.

40. Moore, K.W., Rousset, F. and Banchereau, J. (1991) Evolving principles in immunopathology: Interleukin 10 and its relationship to Epstein–Barr virus protein BCRF1. *Springer Semin. Immunopathol.*, **13**, 157–166.

41. Paul, N.L. and Ruddle, N.H. (1988) Lymphotoxin. *Annu. Rev. Immunol.*, **6**, 407–438.

42. Warner, G.L., Ludlow, J.W., Nelson, D.A., Gaur, A. and Scott, D.W. (1992) Anti-immunoglobulin treatment of murine B cell lymphomas induces active TGFB but pRB hypophosphorylation is TGFB independent. *Cell Growth Differ.*, **5**, 175–181.

43. Holder, M.J., Knox, K.A. and Gordon, J. (1992) Factors regulating survival in germinal center B cells: Glucocorticoids and TGFB, but not cyclosporin A or anti-CD19, block smIg-dependent rescue from apoptosis. *Eur. J. Immunol.*, **22**, 2725–2728.

44. Carter, R.H. and Fearon, D.T. (1992) CD19: Lowering the threshold for antigen receptor stimulation of B lymphocytes. *Science,* **256**, 105–107.

45. Cooper, N.R., Moore, M.D. and Nemerow, G.R. (1988) Immunobiology of CR2, the B lymphocyte receptor for Epstein–Barr virus and C3d complement component. *Annu. Rev. Immunol.*, **6**, 85–113.

46. Carter, R.H., Spycher, M.O., Ng, Y.C., Hoffman, R. and Fearon, D.T. (1988) Synergistic interaction between complement receptor type 2 and membrane IgM on B lymphocytes. *J. Immunol.*, **141**, 457–463.

47. Bohnsack, J.F. and Cooper, N.R. (1988) CR2 ligands modulate human B cell activation. *J. Immunol.*, **141**, 2569–2576.

48. Delespesse, G.T., Sarfati, M., Wu, C.Y., Fournier, S. and Letellier, M. (1992) The low affinity receptor for IgE. *Immunol. Rev.*, **125**, 156–172.

49. Liu, Y.-J., Johnson, G.D., Gordon, J. and MacLennan, I.C.M. (1992) Germinal centres in T-cell-dependent antibody responses. *Immunol. Today,* **15**, 17–22.

50. Gregory, C.D., Dive, C., Henderson, S., Smith, C.A., Williams, G.T., Gordon, J. and Rickinson, A.B. (1991) Activation of Epstein–Barr virus latent genes protects human B cells from death by apoptosis. *Nature,* **349**, 612–615.

51. Vlasselaer, P.V., Gascan, H., de Waal Malefyt, R. and de Vries, J.E. (1992) IL-2 and a contact-mediated signal provided by CD4+ T cells induce polyclonal Ig production by committed human B cells: Enhancement by IL-5, specific inhibition of IgA synthesis by IL-4. *J. Immunol.*, **148**, 1674–1684.

52. Vlasselaer, P.V., Punnonen, J. and de Vries, J.E. (1992) Transforming growth factor-B directs IgA switching in human B cells. *J. Immunol.*, **148**, 2062–2067.

53. Gordon, J. (1991) Human B lymphocytes mature. *Clin. Exp. Immunol.*, **84**, 373–375.

Chapter 3

Substituted Guanine Ribonucleosides as B Cell Stimulators: Their Potential Clinical Application

SUDHIR GUPTA*

Division of Basic and Clinical Immunology, University of California, Irvine, California, USA

INTRODUCTION

The role of cyclic nucleotides as "second messengers" in lymphocyte activation differentiation has been controversial. However, during the course of their studies aiming to probe the role of cyclic GMP as "second messenger" in B cell activation, Goodman and Weigle (1) observed a family of substituted guanine ribonucleosides that exhibited enhancing activities for T cells and B cells. Further investigations revealed that these compounds also activate macrophages and natural killer (NK) cells. The critical determinant of biological activity is the substitution with an inductive electron-withdrawing group at the C-8 position (2, 3). The potency of the substituted compounds could be further enhanced by an additional substitution at the N-7 position (4). Substituted guanine ribonucleoside compounds are low-molecular-weight analogs of the fundamental building blocks of cellular nucleic acid. These analogs are taken up by a carrier-facilitated transport mechanism and act intracellularly by bypassing the biochemical steps of membrane signal transduction. In this chapter, I will review the effects of

---

*Address for correspondence: Department of Medicine, Medical Sciences I, C–240, University of California, Irvine, CA 92717, USA.

New Concepts in Immunodeficiency Diseases. Edited by S. Gupta and C. Griscelli
© 1993 John Wiley & Sons Ltd

mono- and disubstituted guanine ribonucleoside compounds on various immune responses, both in animals and humans, and their potential clinical uses in human diseases, with a particular reference to antibody deficiency syndromes.

EFFECTS ON T CELL-MEDIATED IMMUNITY

Substituted guanine ribonucleoside compounds alone do not induce T cell proliferation but influence certain T cell functions (2, 4). In mice, 8-mercaptoguanosine (8MGuo) enhances proliferation of T cells to alloantigens and soluble recall antigens (5). Feldbush and Ballas (6) have shown that 8MGuo induces generation of cytotoxic T lymphocyte (CTL) activity in allogeneic mixed lymphocyte culture reaction without any effect on T cell proliferation in rats. This effect is observed when suboptimal conditions are used for the generation of CTL activity. Therefore, in rats 8MGuo induces T cell differentiation without concomitant T cell proliferation. These compounds also enhance the education of T helper cells *in vivo* to provide increased help to primary B cells in mice (5). Scheuer *et al.* (7) demonstrated that 8-bromoguanosine (8BrGuo) is a potent adjuvant for the primary IgG antibody response *in vivo* to a highly T cell-dependent antigen-deaggregated human γ-globulin (DHGG) in A/J mice, suggesting that 8BrGuo can transform a tolerogenic signal by DHGG into an immunogenic signal that apparently involves both T helper cells and B cells. Weigle *et al.* (8) have shown that the induction of tolerance by 8BrGuo *in vivo* is mediated by interleukin 1 (IL-1). Approximately at day 60, T cells remain tolerant to HGG; however, B cells regain responsiveness. Therefore 8BrGuo acts as an alternate T cell signal, bypassing tolerant T cells and terminating the overall tolerant state. Goodman (9) demonstrated that 7-allyl-8-oxoguanosine (7a8OGuo) induces significant production of interferon-γ (IFNγ) from CBA/CaJ spleen cells. The peak response was observed on day 3 and at 30 μM concentration. Although 8MGuo alone had no effect on IL-2 production, however, 8MGuo enhanced IL-2 production in mixed lymphocyte culture reaction in mice and enhanced concanavalin A (Con A)-induced IL-2 production by human mononuclear cells. The response on IL-2 production was less dramatic as compared to its effect on IFNγ production. Gupta *et al.* (10) also demonstrated an enhancing effect of 7a8OGuo on antibody response to a T cell-dependent antigen (tetanus toxoid) in human peripheral blood. 7a8OGuo alone had no effect on the transition of naive CD4+ T cells to memory CD4+ T cells in humans. 7a8OGuo depolarized the plasma membrane potential of peripheral blood mononuclear cells; however, it is unclear whether the effect on plasma membrane potential is on T cells, B cells, NK cells and macrophages or selective to one of these populations. The mechanism of 7a8OGuo-induced depolarization of plasma membrane remains to be determined.

These data suggest that substituted guanine ribonucleosides by themselves have little effect on T cells (except IFNγ production), but significantly enhance T cell functions induced by other antigens in suboptimal conditions.

EFFECT ON NATURAL KILLER CELLS, LYMPHOKINE-ACTIVATED KILLER CELLS AND MACROPHAGES

NK cells play an important role in defenses against viruses and tumors. NK cell activity is potentiated by interferons (11). Koo *et al.* (12) demonstrated that 8BrGuo enhances murine NK cell activity that was blocked by anti-interferon (IFN) antibodies, indirectly suggesting that 8BrGuo activates NK cells via production of IFN. Recently Jin *et al.* (13) have reported *in vivo* enhancement of activity of NK cells by 7-thia-8-oxoguanosine (7T8OGuo). This enhanced activity appears to be due to an induction of interferon (14). In addition, Smee *et al.* (15) demonstrated that 7T8OGuo induces *in vivo* antiviral activity against Semiliki forest virus infection in mice. This antiviral activity appears to be due to increased interferon production and enhanced NK activity. Sharma *et al.* (16) have shown that 7T8OGuo inhibits pulmonary murine melanoma metastases in B16 melanoma model and these effects were associated with *in vivo* enhanced NK activity. Thompson and Ballas (17) reported that 8MGuo synergizes with extremely low concentrations of IL-2 *in vitro* to influence lymphokine-activated killer (LAK) cell (CD4–, CD8–, asialo-GMI+)-mediated activity. However, the role of IFN in potentiation of LAK activity was not explored.

Macrophages play an important role in antigen presentation and as effector cells in killing of tumor and virally infected target cells. Goodman (18) demonstrated that 8BrGuo and 8MGuo induce production of IL-1-like activity from irradiated splenic adherent cells and mouse macrophage P388D cell line. We also reported induction of IL-1 production from human peripheral blood adherent cells by 7a8OGuo (10). 7T8OGuo also appears to induce Ia on murine macrophages (19). Koo *et al.* (12) reported that 8BrGuo enhances peptone-elicited peritoneal macrophage cytolytic activity to P815 cells. This induction of cytolytic activity was blocked by anti-IFNα, β and γ antibodies, indicating that these cells possibly produce IFN. Sharma *et al.* (16) also reported enhanced *in vivo* effect of 7T8OGuo on cytolytic activity of macrophages, resulting in successful treatment of murine melanoma metastasis. They entertained the possibility of the involvement of cytokines.

In summary, substituted guanine ribonucleosides appear to activate NK cells and macrophages, via production of interferons and perhaps other cytokines as well. The biochemical and molecular events involved in NK cell and macrophage activation remains to be determined. A role of substituted guanosine compounds in antigen processing/presentation also remains to be evaluated.

EFFECT ON B CELL ACTIVATION, PROLIFERATION AND
DIFFERENTIATION

B lymphocytes, the precursors of antibody-forming cells, undergo a process of activation, proliferation and differentiation following stimulation with anti-immunoglobulin and B cell mitogens (20, 21). Substituted guanosine compounds have been shown to increase the expression of Ia antigen on murine B lymphocytes (20, 21). Wicker *et al.* (20), using fractionated B cells, based on cell size, demonstrated that 8BrGuo and 8MGuo increased Ia expression on small resting B cells but failed to induce proliferation and differentiation, whereas both compounds increased Ia expression and induced proliferation and differentiation of large B cells. The proliferation of resting B cells (in the presence of these compounds) was Mac-1+ adherent cell dependent, whereas the proliferation of large B cells was Mac-1+ adherent cell independent. Adherent cells failed to induce differentiation of resting B cells. 7T8OGuo also induces Ia antigen on murine B cells and further increases Ia density on pre-activated B cells (19). Goodman and Weigle (1, 22–25) observed that compounds that have bromination or thiolation of guanosine at the C-8 position confer the capacity of these compounds to induce B cell proliferation and increased antibody production when given along with antigen. They also demonstrated that 8MGuo, when added to highly purified B cells, resulted in an antigen-specific, antigen-dependent immune response, presumably attributable to the nucleosides serving as an alternate T cell-like signal (22, 23). Goodman (26) suggested that T cell-like signal transmitted to B cells by 8MGuo differs qualitatively from that provided by T cells, most probably in their ability to activate a particular B cell subset to responsiveness. The predominant B cell population that responds by proliferation bears surface δ chain, Ia antigens, complement receptors, and Lyb-5 antigen (27). Goodman and Hennen (4) compared the B cell proliferative potential of 8MGuo to disubstituted 7m8OGuo. 7m8OGuo appears to have greater mitogenic activity and has greater adjuvant property in antibody response (requiring ten times less concentration to achieve a similar degree of immuno-enhancing activity as 8MGuo). Adjuvant activity appears early and persists late (4). The adjuvant effect of 8MGuo on B cell response is both T cell dependent and T cell independent (26). The majority of the increased numbers of antibody-producing cells contributing to the adjuvant effect are recruited from cells primarily participating in the immune response, with clonal expansion accounting for a minor contribution. In contrast, Feldbush and Ballas (6) reported that 8MGuo does not cause proliferation of rat B lymphocytes and does not have B cell growth factor-like activity. However, 8MGuo causes a marked increase in IgM and a modest increase in IgG by mitogen-stimulated B cells. They showed that 8MGuo along with condition medium act synergistically to stimulate secretion of both immunoglobulin isotypes. This would suggest that 8MGuo has both B cell differentiation factor-μ (BCDF-μ) and BCDF-γ activities. In mice, Mond *et al.* (28) demonstrated that 8MGuo *in vivo* enhances anti-trinitrophenol (anti-TNP)–Ficoll IgG1, IgG2, and IgG3 response but had no effect on specific IgM antibody response. Furthermore, 8MGuo enhanced the antibody response to weak antigen, pneumococcal polysaccharide. Ahmed and Mond (3) examined a number of C-8-substituted guanine ribonucleosides for their role in murine B cell activation. They observed that 8-hydroxyguanosine (8OHGuo) stimulates both B cell proliferation and differentiation of murine B cells, while 8-methoxyguanosine (8MeGuo) stimulates only differentiation, and 8-aminoguanosine (8aGuo) had no significant effect on B cell activation. 8OHGuo and 8MeGuo increase the magnitude of primary antibody response to the type 2 antigen TNP–Ficoll. 8MGuo, 8BrGuo, 8OHGuo, 8MeGuo and 8aGuo also increase polyclonal immunoglobulin secretion and increase anti-TNP response when incubated with the antigen. These observations would suggest the requirement for C-8 substitution for guanosine analogs to activate B lymphocytes. Furthermore, substitution of the thio and bromo groups at the C-8 position of guanosine is not an absolute requirement for potentiating B cell differentiation. Goodman (29) demonstrated that a large subset of potentially reactive B cells remains unresponsive to antigen even in the presence of signals provided by guanosine nucleosides, except when this signal is provided by a soluble factor present in the mixed lymphocyte culture reaction supernatants. IL-1, IL-2, IL-3, IL-4, IL-5, granulocyte–macrophage colony-stimulating factor (GM–CSF) and IFNγ have no synergism, whereas IFNα and IFNβ synergize with guanosine compounds. In human peripheral blood mononuclear cells, 7m8OGuo markedly augments antibody response to sheep red blood cells (SRBC) if B cells are supplemented with IL-2 (30). Gupta *et al.* (10) showed an enhancing effect of 7a8OGuo on tetanus-specific antibody response in human peripheral blood mononuclear cells *in vitro*.

EFFECT IN IMMUNODEFICIENT/IMMUNODYSFUNCTION STATES

The potential clinical use of these compounds is evident by their remarkable effects in reconstituting/correcting the immune dysfunction in experimental models and human immunodeficiency states.

Activity in SJL Mice

SJL mice express a number of immunological abnormalities and increased susceptibility to autoimmunity (31) and malignancies (32). Goodman and

Weigle (33) showed that SJL mice are hyporesponsive to the inductive or antigen-independent signals delivered by the C-8-substituted guanine ribonucleosides, although they respond normally to antigen-non-specific signals delivered by other B cell activators. These substituted compounds, however, restore antigen-dependent response. There appear to be two distinct mechanisms that are involved in the adjuvant activity of 8MGuo: one whereby pre-existing antigen-specific B cells undergo clonal expansion, and the other in which cells not normally participating in the response are recruited in the absence of clonal expansion. Goodman (34) showed that B cells from SJL mice exhibit a K_d value of low-affinity nucleoside binding sites 10- to 20-fold lower than that of normal CBA mice.

Aging Mice

Aging mice serve as a good model for combined T and B cell immunodeficiency. B cells from these animals are unresponsive to antigen. 8MGuo induces polyclonal immunoglobulin production in both young and old mice, whereas lipopolysaccharide induces in young mice alone (35). Furthermore, 8MGuo provides effective T cell-like signal to produce antibody response to T-dependent type 1 antigen (SRBC) in aged mice. Similar results were observed *in vivo* (36). Aged mice injected with aggregated human γ-globulin (HGG) made only a feeble anti-HGG response. Injection of 7m8OGuo resulted in enhanced response in aging mice to the levels in young mice injected with aggregated HGG alone. In neonates, which are entirely unresponsive to antigen, 8MGuo restored the antigen-specific antibody response to the level observed in young adult animals (26).

Xid Mice and Congenitally Athymic Mice

The CBA/N ([CBA/N × CBA/CAJ]F1) mice bear the *xid* B cell defect in the Lyb-5+ subpopulation of B cells (37). Goodman and Weigle (24) reported that 8MGuo *in vitro* restored the antibody response to SRBC of F1 male animals to the levels generated by normal F1 female. Goodman and Weigle (38) demonstrated that substituted guanosine compounds exert powerful *in vivo* adjuvant activity in CBA/N mice. The adjuvant activity was not observed with non-substituted guanosine compounds. Guanosine compounds reconstituted antibody response in CBA/N (NCF1 male) mice to the level of NCF1 female. The effect of these compounds was due to a recruitment of Lyb-5–, G-10 non-adherent B cells to respond to antigen. Ahmad and Mond (21) reported reconstitution of anti-TNP–Ficoll response in CBA/N mice by guanosine compound. They suggested that the defect in CBA/N mice is not in the inability of TNP–Ficoll to stimulate *xid* B cells from G0 to G1 phase, but rather inability of antigen-activated cells to respond to a second signal that can be substituted by 8MGuo. Similar results were obtained *in vivo* (28). They demonstrated that 8MGuo enhanced IgG1, IgG2 and IgG3 response to polysaccharide antigen and restored anti-TNP response to TNP–Ficoll in CBA/N *xid* male mice.

Goodman and Weigle (23) successfully restored the T cell-dependent antigen response in Nu/Nu mice with 8MGuo. This underscores the ability of these compounds to act in a T cell-independent manner.

Common Variable Immunodeficiency

Common variable immunodeficiency (CVI) is the second commonest primary immunodeficiency disorder, characterized by decreased serum IgG, IgA and/or IgM. The basic defect in the majority of cases appears to be a primary B cell defect (although circulating B cells are often present in normal numbers). Increased suppressor and/or decreased T cell help has also been documented. We have performed an *in vitro* study in nine patients with CVI with primary defect in B cells, suppressor and/or helper T cells. 7m8OGuo restored antibody response to SRBC in eight of nine subjects to a level observed in normal subjects stimulated with antigen (39). This effect was independent of membrane signal pathway via protein kinase C activation. In this study specific antibody response of IgG and IgA isotypes were not measured. Dosch *et al.* (40) showed that 8MGuo could reconstitute polyclonal IgA response *in vitro* in patients with selective IgA deficiency. In contrast, patients with congenital agammaglobulinemia failed to show any response to nucleosides. This would suggest that substituted nucleosides lack the property of differentiation of pre-B cells to B cells as the latter patients appear to have a defect in the differentiation of pre-B cells to mature B cells. In a recent phase I *in vivo* study with 7a8OGuo in patients with advanced malignancy, no significant serious side effects were noted (41). Phase I/II clinical trial in patients with CVI is about to begin.

MECHANISM OF ACTION OF SUBSTITUTED GUANINE RIBONUCLEOSIDES

Several cellular studies with substituted guanosine compounds have led to the identification of at least three subsets of B lymphocytes that contribute to specific antibody responses in experimental systems. These include the mature antigen-reactive B cells that do not require nucleosides for specific antibody response, nucleoside-dependent B cells that require the signal provided by the nucleosides to be responsive to antigen, and a large pool of B cell subset that requires antigen, and signal provided by cytokine(s) and nucleoside. The nature of cytokine remains to be defined. In the murine systems, it appears that 8MGuo does not synergize with IL-1 through IL-5,

Basic Mechanisms

GM-CSF or IFNγ; however, it synergizes with IFNα and IFNβ (29). In human B cell response, IL-2 appears to synergize with 7m8OGuo for antibody response to SRBC (30).

The regulatory role of macrophages and their soluble products has also been explored. Wicker *et al.* (42) reported that small resting B cell proliferation in the presence of 8BrGuo and 8MGuo was dependent on Mac-1+ adherent cells, whereas proliferation of large B cells was independent of Mac-1+ adherent cells and could occur in the presence of Mac-1– adherent cells. The oxidative metabolites of arachidonic acid (AA) appear to have distinct immunoregulatory effects on B cell proliferation induced by membrane-directed ligands as compared to substituted guanosine compounds (43). The metabolites of the cyclooxygenase pathway (PGE_2, PGE_1 and $PGF_{2\alpha}$) amplify anti-Ig-mediated B cell proliferation, whereas products of the lipoxygenase pathway (HETEs and/or HPETEs) inhibit Ig-mediated B cell proliferation. In contrast, murine B cell proliferation induced by 8MGuo is inhibited by the products of the cyclooxygenase pathway, whereas products of the lipoxygenase pathway enhance 8MGuo-induced B cell proliferation.

Substituted guanine ribonucleosides are taken up into B cells by a process of carrier-mediated diffusion (44) similar to that by naturally occurring nucleosides. In contrast, however, substituted nucleosides are not a substrate for salvage by purine nucleoside phosphorylase (45). There is a short initial period of unidirectional flux of nucleoside into the cell, followed by bidirectional flux resulting in a state of equilibrium. The period of rapid efflux is followed by a much slower phase. The intracellular compartment would contain both free and bound pools of nucleoside. Incubation of murine B cells with variable concentrations of radiolabeled nucleoside demonstrates the presence of two binding interactions: the high affinity interaction with a K_d of 4–10 µM, and 700 µM for the lower-affinity interaction (34, 46). Studies in SJL mice suggest that low-affinity binding sites play a role in antigen-independent differentiative events, whereas high-affinity binding sites play a role in antigen-dependent differentiation events mediated by substituted guanosine nucleosides (46). Furthermore, experiments with radiolabeled nucleosides show that they do not incorporate into cellular nucleic acid. This would suggest that unmetabolized nucleosides are active regulatory molecules. Substituted guanine ribonucleosides do not act via a classical transmembrane signaling pathway. They do not modulate the binding of GTP to G proteins, elevate inositol phosphates, increase free intracellular calcium, or translocate protein kinase C from cytosol to the plasma membrane (47).

POTENTIAL CLINICAL USES OF GUANINE RIBONUCLEOSIDES

Because of their role in the reconstitution of immune responses both *in vitro* and *in vivo* in immunodeficient animals and *in vitro* in patients with CVI, substituted guanine ribonucleosides are promising candidates for clinical use in a variety of clinical disorders. First, they could be used in the correction of specific antibody response. This would include patients with primary hypogammaglobulinemias (exclusive of X-linked agammaglobulinemia and severe combined immunodeficiency disorders) without mature B cells, because of the lack of activity of guanosine compounds on pre-B or immature B cells). Promising results have already been observed *in vitro* in patients with CVI (39). Secondary immunodeficiencies would include patients with chronic lymphocytic leukemia, multiple myeloma, and Waldenstrom's macroglobulinemia, and children with HIV infection. In addition, studies of substituted guanosine compounds with neonates and aged subjects suggest that they could be used in boosting the response of infants to vaccine against *Hemophilus influenzae* and *Streptococcus pneumoniae* in newborns and infants, and to *S. pneumoniae* in aged subjects.

The second potential use of substituted guanine ribonucleosides would be in patients with malignancies. Because guanosine compounds potentiate macrophage, NK, LAK and CTL activities, and production of antibodies (all effector mechanisms against tumors), they are promising candidates (as an adjuvant) for the treatment of a variety of malignancies. Sharma *et al.* (48) have shown promising results in murine metastatic melanoma model. They have also shown that substituted guanosine compound increases the immunogenicity of leukemic cells and improves the survival of experimental animals. Therefore, substituted guanine ribonucleosides have a promising future as an adjuvant to vaccine therapy.

ABBREVIATIONS USED

8aGuo	= 8-aminoguanosine
7a8OGuo	= 7-allyl-8-oxoguanosine
8BrGuo	= 8-bromoguanosine
8MGuo	= 8-mertcaptoguanosine
7m8OGuo	= 7-methyl-8-oxoguanosine
8MeGuo	= 8-methoxyguanosine
8OHGuo	= 8-hydroxyguanosine
7T8OGuo	= 7-thia-8-oxoguanosine

REFERENCES

1. Goodman, M.G. and Weigle, W.O. (1981) Activation of lymphocytes by brominated nucleoside analogues: Implication for the "second messenger" function of cyclic GMP. *Proc. Nat. Acad. Sci. USA*, **78**, 7604–7608.
2. Goodman, M.G. and Weigle, W.O. (1983) Activation of lymphocytes by a thiol-derivatized nucleoside: Characterization of cellular parameters and responsive subpopulations. *J. Immunol.*, **130**, 551–558.

3. Ahmad, A. and Mond, J.J. (1985) 8-Hydroxyguanosine and 8-methoxyguanosine possess immunostimulating activity for B lymphocytes. *Cell. Immunol.*, **94**, 276–280.

4. Goodman, M.G. and Hennen, W.J. (1986) Distinct effect of dual substitution on inductive and differentiative activities of C8-substituted guanine ribonucleosides. *Cell. Immunol.*, **102**, 395–402.

5. Goodman, M.G. and Weigle, W.O. (1986) Enhancement of T cell proliferation and differentiation by 8 mercaptoguanosine. In Nyhan, W.L., Thompson, L.F. and Watts, R.W.E. (eds) *Purine and Pyrimidine Metabolism in Man.* Plenum Press, New York, pp. 443–449.

6. Feldbush, T.L. and Ballas, Z.K. (1985) Lymphokine-like activity of 8-mercaptoguanosine: Induction of T and B cell differentiation. *J. Immunol.*, **134**, 3204–3211.

7. Scheuer, W.V., Goodman, M.G., Parks, D.E. and Weigle, W.O. (1985) Enhancement of the *in vivo* antibody response by an 8-derivatized guanine nucleoside. *Cell. Immunol.*, **91**, 294–300.

8. Weigle, W.O., Gahring, L.C., Romball, C.G. and Goodman, M.G. (1989) The effect of lipopolysaccharide desensitization on the regulation of *in vivo* induction of immunological tolerance and antibody production and *in vitro* release of IL-1. *J. Immunol.*, **142**, 1107–1113.

9. Goodman, M.G. (1991) Cellular and biochemical studies of substituted guanine ribonucleoside immunostimulants. *Immunopharmacology*, **21**, 51–68.

10. Gupta, S., Vayuvegula, B. and Gollapudi, S. (1991) Substituted guanine ribonucleosides as B cell activators. *Clin. Immunol. Immunopathol.*, **61**, S21–S27.

11. Djeu, J.Y., Heinbaugh, J.A., Holden, H.J. and Herberman, R.B. (1979) Augmentation of mouse natural killer cells activity by interferon and interferon inducers. *J. Immunol.*, **122**, 175–181.

12. Koo, G.C., Jewell, M.E., Manyak, C.L., Sigal, N.H. and Wicker, L.S. (1988) Activation of murine natural killer cells and macrophages by 8-bromoguanosine. *J. Immunol.*, **140**, 3249–3252.

13. Jin, A., Sharma, B., Mhaskar, S., Balazs, L., Siaw, M. and Jolley, W. (1989) Potentiation of mouse natural killer cell activity by a novel nucleoside, 7-thia-8-oxoguanosine. *FASEB J.*, **3**, 490 (Abstract).

14. Smee, D.F., Alaghamandan, H.A., Cottam, H.B., Sharma, B., Jolley, W.B. and Robins, R.K. (1989) Broad spectrum *in vivo* antiviral activity of 7-thia-8-oxoguanosine, a novel immunopotentiating agent. *Antimicrob. Agents Chemother.*, **33**, 1487–1492.

15. Smee, D.F., Alaghamanadan, H.A., Jin, A., Sharma, B. and Jolley, W.B. (1990) Role of interferon and natural killer cells in the antiviral activity of 7-thia-8-oxoguanosine against Semiliki forest virus in mice. *Antiviral Res.*, **13**, 91–102.

16. Sharma, B., Balazs, L., Jin, A., Jolley, W.B. and Robins, R.K. (1991) Successful immunotherapy of murine melanoma metastases with 7-thia-8-oxoguanosine. *Clin. Exp. Metastasis*, **9**, 429–439.

17. Thompson, R.A. and Ballas, Z.K. (1989) 8-Mercaptoguanosine (8MG) synergizes with minimal doses of IL-2 in the generation of lymphokine activated killer (LAK) *in vitro. FASEB J.*, **3**, A490 (Abstract).

18. Goodman, M.G. (1988) Induction of interleukin 1 activity from macrophages by direct interaction with C8-substituted guanine ribonucleosides. *Int. J. Immunopharmacol.*, **10**, 579–586.

19. Lee, V., Sharma, B. and Jolley, W.B. (1989) 7-Thia-8-oxoguanosine induces *de novo* expression of surface Ia antigens and Ig. *FASEB J.*, **3**, 794 (Abstract).

20. Wicker, L.S., Boltz, R.C., Nichols, E.A., Miller, B.J., Sigal, N.H. and Peterson, L.B. (1987) Large, activated B cells are the primary B-cell target of 8-bromoguanosine and 8-mercaptoguanosine. *Cell. Immunol.*, **106**, 318–329.

21. Ahmad, A. and Mond, J.J. (1986) Restoration of *in vitro* responsiveness of *xid* B cells to TNP–Ficoll by 8-mercaptoguanosine. *J. Immunol.*, **136**, 1223–1226.

22. Goodman, M.G. and Weigle, W.O. (1984) Mechanism of 8-mercaptoguanosine-mediated adjuvanticity: Roles of clonal expansion and cellular recruitment. *J. Immunol.*, **133**, 2910–2914.

23. Goodman, M.G. and Weigle, W.O. (1983) T cell-replacing activity of C8-derivatized guanine ribonucleosides. *J. Immunol.*, **130**, 2042–2045.

24. Goodman, M.G. and Weigle, W.O. (1983) Derivatized guanine nucleosides: A new class of adjuvant for *in vitro* antibody responses. *J. Immunol.*, **130**, 2580–2585.

25. Goodman, M.G. and Weigle, W.O. (1982) Induction of immunoglobulin secretion by a simple nucleoside derivative. *J. Immunol.*, **128**, 2399–2404.

26. Goodman, M.G. (1985) Demonstration of T-cell-dependent and T-cell-independent components of 8-mercaptoguanosine-mediated adjuvanticity (42126). *Proc. Soc. Exp. Biol. Med.*, **179**, 479–486.

27. Goodman, M.G. and Weigle, W.O. (1981) Activation of lymphocytes by a thiol-derivatized nucleoside: Characterization of cellular parameters and responsive subpopulations. *J. Immunol.*, **130**, 551–557.

28. Mond, J.J., Hunter, K., Kenny, J.J., Finkelman, F. and Witherspoon, K. (1989) 8-Mercaptoguanosine-mediated enhancement of *in vivo* IgG1, IgG2 and IgG3 antibody responses to polysaccharide antigens in normal and *xid* mice. *Immunopharmacology*, **18**, 205–212.

29. Goodman, M.G. (1987) Interaction between cytokines and 8-mercaptoguanosine in human immunity: Synergy with interferon. *J. Immunol.*, **139**, 142–146.

30. Goodman, M.G. and Weigle, W.O. (1985) Enhancement of the human antibody response by C8-substituted guanine ribonucleosides in synergy with interleukin 2. *J. Immunol.*, **135**, 3284–3288.

31. Pettinelli, C.B. and McFarlin, D.E. (1981) Adoptive transfer of experimental allergic encephalomyelitis in SJL-J mice after *in vitro* activation of lymph node cells by myelin basic protein: Requirement for Lyt 1+ 2– T lymphocytes. *J. Immunol.*, **127**, 1420–1423.

32. Bonavida, B. (1983) The SJL-J spontaneous reticulum cell sarcoma: New insights in the field of neoantigens, host tumor interactions, and regulation of tumor growth. *Adv. Cancer Res.*, **38**, 1–21.

33. Goodman, M.G. and Weigle, W.O. (1985) Dissociation of inductive from differentiative signals transmitted by C8-substituted guanine ribonucleosides to B cells from SJL mice. *J. Immunol.*, **134**, 91–94.

34. Goodman, M.G. (1990) B lymphocytes from hyporesponsive SJL mice contain aberrant nucleoside binding sites. *Cell. Immunol.*, **129**, 377–384.

35. Goodman, M.G. and Weigle, W.O. (1985) Restoration of humoral immunity *in vitro* in immunodeficient aging mice by C8-derivatized guanine ribonucleosides. *J. Immunol.*, **134**, 3808–3811.

36. Weigle, W.O., Thoman, M.L. and Goodman, M.G. (1987) Augmentation of the antibody response in aged mice with an 8-derivatized guanosine nucleoside and its effect of immunological memory. *Cell. Immunol.*, **109**, 332–337.

37. Shultz, L.D. and Sidman, C.L. (1987) Genetically determined murine models of immunodeficiency. *Annu. Rev. Immunol.*, **5**, 367–403.

38. Goodman, M.G. and Weigle, W.O. (1985) Manifold amplification of *in vivo* immunity in normal and immunodeficient mice by ribonucleosides derivatized at C8 of guanine. *Proc. Nat. Acad. Sci. USA*, **80**, 3452–3455.
39. Goodman, M.G., Gupta, S., Rosenthale, M.K., Capetola, R.J., Bell, S.C. and Weigle, W.O. (1991) C-kinase independent restoration of specific immune responsiveness in common variable immunodeficiency. *Clin. Immunol. Immunopathol.*, **59**, 26–36.
40. Dosch, H.-M., Osundwa, V. and Lam, P. (1988) Activation of human B lymphocytes by 8' substituted guanosine derivatives. *Immunol. Lett.*, **17**, 125–131.
41. Agarwala, S., Kirkwood, S., Bryant, J.M., Abels, R. and Troetschel, M. (1992) A double-blind, Phase I, placebo-controlled study of the safety, pharmacokinetics, and immunological effect of single, ascending doses of 7-allyl-8-oxoguanosine in patients with advanced cancer. *Proc. Am. Assoc. Cancer Res.*, **33**, 263 (Abstract).
42. Wicker, L.S., Ashton, W.T., Boltz, R.C., Jr, Meurer, L.C., Miller, B.J., Nichols, E.A., Sigal, N.H., Tolman, R.L. and Peterson, L.B. (1988) 5 halo-6-phenyl by rimidinones and 8-substituted guanosines. Biological response modifiers with similar effects on B cells. *Cell. Immunol.*, **112**, 156–165.
43. Goodman, M.G. and Weigle, W.O. (1984) Regulation of B-lymphocyte proliferative responses by arachidonate metabolites: Effects on membrane-directed versus intracellular activators. *J. Allergy Clin. Immunol.*, **74**, 418–425.
44. Goodman, M.G. and Weigle, W.O. (1984) Intracellular lymphocyte activation and carrier-mediated transport of C8-substituted guanine ribonucleosides. *Proc. Nat. Acad. Sci. USA*, **81**, 862–866.
45. Goodman, M.G. (1988) Role of salvage and phosphorylation in the immunostimulatory activity of C8-substituted guanine ribonucleosides. *J. Immunol.*, **141**, 2394–2399.
46. Goodman, M.G. and Cherry, D.M. (1989) Ligand binding sites for a synthetic B cell growth and differentiation factor. *Cell. Immunol.*, **123**, 417–426.
47. Goodman, M.G., Speizer, L., Bokoch, G., Kanter, J. and Brunton, L.L. (1990) Activity of an intracellular stimulator is independent of G-protein interactions, $[Ca^{2+}]_i$ elevation, phosphoinositide hydrolysis, and protein kinase C translocation. *J. Biol. Chem.*, **265**, 12248–12252.
48. Sharma, B., Balazs, L., Jin, A., Wnag, J.C.-J., Jolley, W.B. and Robins, R.K. (1991) Potentiation of the efficacy of murine L1210 leukemia vaccine by a novel immunostimulator 7-thia-8-oxoguanosine: Increased survival after immunization with vaccine plus 7-thia-8-oxoguanosine. *Cancer Immunol. Immunother.*, **33**, 109–114.

Chapter 4

Development of the Human T Cell Repertoire

ELWYN LOH

Division of Hematology and Oncology, Department of Medicine, University of
Pennsylvania, Philadelphia, USA

The specific genetic defects that cause inherited immunodeficiencies are gradually being discovered. While none of those described for human diseases is a mutation of a gene specifically expressed in T cells, immunodeficiency diseases invariably involve alterations in T cell function and diversity that arise from the primary defect. This chapter describes the normal genetics and development of the T cell receptor.

ROLE OF T CELL ANTIGEN RECEPTOR IN ACTIVATION OF T CELLS

T cells play a central role in the decision-making process of the immune system. In the vernacular of information science, the T cell serves multiple functions in the storage and processing of analog information (Figure 4.1). The input information that the T cell receives comes through many routes: receptors specific for protein or peptide molecules, receptors for other messengers such as glucocorticoids, and possibly other changes in the environment not related to specific receptors. The past information that the T cell has received is stored as the number, localization, and differentiation state of the T cell. Each T cell operates as a parallel processor for information such that the output of the entire immune system is the sum of the outputs of each individual cell. Thus, eventually, it will be necessary to understand not only how individual cells work but also how the entire system operates as an integrated entity.

The T cell receptor for antigen (TCR) is one of many surface glycoproteins of the T cell that transfers information to the T cell. The uniqueness of its role is not

New Concepts in Immunodeficiency Diseases. Edited by S. Gupta and C. Griscelli
© 1993 John Wiley & Sons Ltd

58

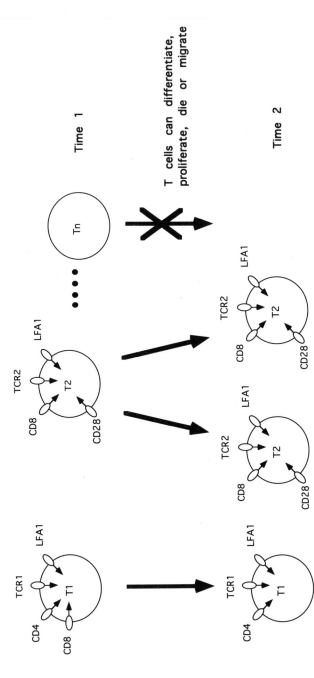

Figure 4.1. T cells serve as parallel processors of information. Each T cell has a unique set of input devices, including many cell surface receptors, of which the TCR, LFA1, CD2, and CD4 are examples. Each T cell also has a set of output mechanisms which are not shown, including secretion of interleukins and alterations of adhesion receptors, morphology and mobility functions. In a continual process of change, the cell integrates the input information and can differentiate, replicate, die, or migrate

that a signal through the TCR is always necessary for activation or that the strength of that signal is greater or different from that of other inputs; rather that only the TCR can differentiate one antigen from another. Thus the discrimination between self and non-self must be performed by the T cell through the TCR. The ability of the TCR to recognize a vast universe of foreign antigens requires that itself be equally complex, and the description and understanding of that complexity will be the challenge of this chapter. One fundamental generalization that can be made is that, just as each B cell expresses only one species of immunoglobulin receptor, each T cell expresses only one species of TCR (with roughly 2×10^4 to 10^5 identical copies (1)), thus allowing the decision to respond or not to respond to a specific antigen to be made at the cellular level of a T cell. It is also a receptor that for most purposes defines a T cell, in that its expression is necessary and sufficient for a cell to be called a T cell, including some cells which are not thymically derived, which is the older use of the term. Because of this unique role, the nature of the TCR, and how and what it recognizes, plays a central role in immunology. The other general point to emphasize about the role of the TCR in T cell activation is the dynamic state of the T cell. What happens when antigen is presented to the T cell depends not only on what the T cell is simultaneously seeing through all of its other receptors, but also on the history of the T cell in terms of what differentiation state it is in. This chapter will not discuss the events that occur after the antigen receptor interaction has taken place; instead, we will summarize the current state of knowledge about the functional protein structure and genetics of the T cell receptor. In the context of medical applications of this knowledge, there are several possible implications: (a) mutations or polymorphisms in the genes that code for the structural genes or regulatory genes of the TCR may alter susceptibility of persons to autoimmune or infectious diseases; and (b) steps in the pathophysiology of a disease that requires T cells may be manipulable in a therapeutic way through the TCR. While neither of these situations has been proven in man, animal models exist which hold promise for the application of this knowledge.

BIOCHEMICAL CHARACTERIZATION OF THE ANTIGEN RECOGNITION COMPLEX OF THE T CELL

The T cell receptor for antigen is a complex of at least six different proteins. This is shown schematically in Figure 4.2. The antigen specificity of the receptor is determined by an $\alpha\beta$ or $\gamma\delta$ heterodimer, referred to in this chapter as the TCR, as contrasted with the T cell receptor complex which includes the other polypeptide chains. (An alternative nomenclature refers to the heterodimer as Ti, and the entire complex as the TCR.) The determination of the antigen specificity by the $\alpha\beta$ heteroduplex has been demonstrated by several lines of evidence, including the transfer of specificity for a major histocompatability complex (MHC) peptide by the molecular transfer of the TCR (2). In those experiments, the TCR from a T cell that recognizes a specific peptide MHC molecule was molecularly cloned and transfected into a recipient cell. It was then shown that the recipient cell could now respond to the peptide MHC. In general, an individual T cell has either αβ or γδ receptors. There may rarely be other combinations of the heterodimer such as a δβ, but whether these combinations are biologically significant is not known. Physically and functionally associated with the TCR are the CD3 molecules that are involved in the signaling process of transferring the information of antigen recognition into the cell. The tight physical association between TCR and CD3 is shown by the observation that antibodies that precipitate the TCR in non-ionic detergents also precipitate the CD3 complex. Conversely, antibodies that precipitate the CD3 molecules generally precipitate the TCR. Not only are the TCR and the CD3 molecules physically associated, but in most circumstances one cannot appear on the cell surface without the other. When mutations are introduced in the TCR that abrogate their expression, the CD3 molecule is not expressed on the cell surface. Similarly, in cases where mutants of CD3 are made that effect CD3 expression, the TCR cannot get to the cell surface. The stoichiometry of the associated complex is not precisely known but is likely to occur in several forms, possibly even within a single cell. These possible combinations include TCR–αβ CD3δεγεζ2 and TCR–αβ CD3δεγεζη in the mouse, while the situation in man is less clear (3). The proteins that are included in the entire complex may differ depending

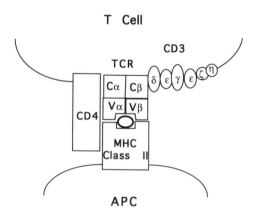

Figure 4.2. Schematic diagram of the T cell receptor complex. The complex includes molecules that are physically associated, namely TCR α (shown as a C region and V region domain), TCR β, CD3-γ, CD3-δ, CD3-ε, CD3-ζ, CD3-η, as well as other molecules functionally and possibly physically associated, including CD4 or CD8. The two cell types involved are the T cell and the antigen-presenting cell (APC)

on the type of T cell. For example, some large granular lymphocytes have an FcεRIγ as part of the complex, instead of CD3ζη (4).

Also contributing to the recognition specificity of the complex is either a CD4 or CD8 molecule. In general, the CD4 molecule will recognize MHC class II molecules, while CD8 recognizes MHC class I molecules. Some experiments of the αβ chains recognizing an antigen have been unsuccessful without the concomitant expression of a CD4 or CD8 molecule on the T cell (5, 6). The association between the TCR and the CD4 and CD8 molecules is not covalent or physically tight since even in gentle dissociation conditions antibodies directed against the TCR do not precipitate the CD4 or CD8 molecules. Thus the association of the TCR with the CD4 or CD8 molecule is a functional one that may require the presence of the antigen molecule. The role of the CD3, CD4 and CD8 molecules and their role in activation are not discussed in detail. We will focus on the structure of the antigen receptor that comprises either an αβ or γδ heterodimer.

The function of the TCR has been studied in detail only in the presence of the entire complex on the surface of a cell. Many attempts have been made to produce soluble TCR which could be used to specifically recognize antigen, just as the immunoglobulin molecule recognizes its antigen (7, 8). While significant amounts of soluble receptor have been produced through molecular manipulations, the function of those molecules to recognize peptide MHC has been difficult to demonstrate convincingly, possibly because the affinity of the receptor for antigen is too low. A recent paper has described a soluble TCR–immunoglobulin chimeric molecule that could be used to block specifically peptide–T cell interactions (9). This may be an unusual TCR with high affinity. It is possible that only with the increased avidity of many cell surface receptors can specific recognition take place. It is of potential interest that there have been reports of soluble TCR that occur naturally, associated with biologically important functions such as suppression and delayed type hypersensitivity. What the molecular form of the soluble receptors may be and what their role is in immunology remains to be demonstrated.

The TCR is a protein which can be divided into regions of functional importance. Based on its primary protein structure, the TCR is a member of the immunoglobulin super-family, with close homology to immunoglobulins. All of the TCR chains can be divided into presumptive functional domains consisting of a leader peptide that is cleaved off during synthesis, two immunoglobulin-like domains, V region and a C region domain, each of approximately 90 amino acids, followed by a connecting peptide (CP), a transmembrane region (TM) and a short cytoplasmic tail (CY) (Figure 4.3). The V region domain interacts with antigen and can be subdivided into functional regions based on patterns of diversity similar to the hypervariable regions described for immunoglobulins. The four regions of increased variability are designated CDR 1, 2, and 3, representing the complementarity-

determining regions 1, 2, and 3, as well as HV4 for hypervariable region 4
(10). The functional implications for these regions are described in the next
paragraph and the genetic relationship between the domains and the structure will be discussed later. One set of V regions, the Vγl family of γ chains,
illustrates the diversity patterns in Figure 4.3B (11). As one can see, the rest
of the V region which can be termed framework regions is remarkably
conserved, with the diversity within this family being found predominantly
within the CDRs and HV4. When more sequences are compared, the cluster-

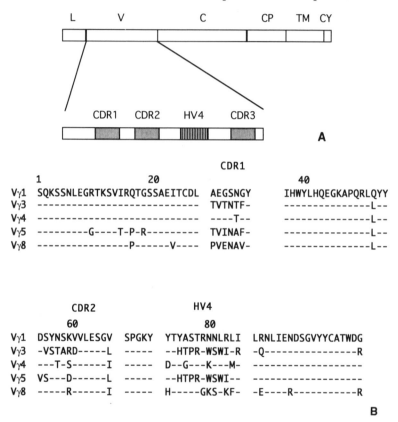

Figure 4.3. Structure of the TCR protein. (A) Schematic illustration of the division of
the primary structure of the TCR into functional domains. The leader sequence (L) is
cleaved off during protein synthesis. The V region domain recognizes antigen and
can be subdivided into complementarity-determining regions (CDR) and HV4
(hypervariable region 4). The C region contains the first domain which interacts with
the other chain of the heterodimer, followed by the connecting peptide (CP), the
transmembrane domain (TM) and the cytoplasmic tail (CY). (B) Hypervariable regions in the TCR γ chain family (Vγl). Five V regions are included. The single-letter
code is used for the amino acids and dashes indicate identity with the sequences
above. CDR 3 is not included because it is not coded by germ line genes

ing of the differences into CDR becomes obscured because the framework regions vary. Only the first two CDRs and the HV4 are shown because CDR 3 is coded for by a separate genetic region with far greater diversity.

A hypothetical model exists that describes the structural relationship of the TCR to antigen. After the description of MHC restriction of antigens, the key question was raised whether the TCR was two molecular structures: one interacting with the antigen and one interacting with the presenting molecule. After the characterization of the TCR, experiments proved that the TCR was responsible both for peptide and MHC recognition. After the first crystal structure of an MHC molecule was determined, a model was proposed that united what was known about the structure of MHC and peptide with what was known about the TCR (12). The assumptions of the model were that the three-dimensional structure of the TCR was essentially that of the immunoglobulin molecule and, therefore, the surface of the TCR that interacts with peptide MHC is composed of the CDR 1, CDR 2, and CDR 3 of the two polypeptide chains (Figure 4.4 upper panels). It was further proposed that the linear pocket of the MHC molecule in which the peptide resides could orient beneath the linear structure of the CDR 3s of TCR as in models A and D in the figure. Since the model has been published, it has become widely used in the conceptualization of the ternary structure of peptide MHC–TCR structure. A more general application of the model would allow the rotation of the structure at other angles such as 90° in models B and C. Even more general would be the possibility of an infinite number of other rotations and translations. One set of TCRs that recognize cytochrome c peptides has been experimentally examined to try to test the model. While the details of the approach are complex, the idea was to mutate the peptide and see where adaptive changes in the TCR would occur. By lining up the changes, it was interpreted that the α chain of the TCR was oriented above the α helix of the polymorphic β chain of the MHC molecule, model D (13). It is important to note that even if one TCR is oriented in a particular fashion over the MHC molecule, other TCR–MHC combinations may be oriented in very different ways. No known general constraints exist that dictate that all TCR have the same alignment with respect to the MHC molecule. The theoretical model of the three-dimensional structure of the TCR–MHC–peptide complex will be replaced in the near future by the actual structure as determined by crystal structure.

The binding affinity of the interaction between the TCR and peptide antigen has been measured by two approaches. One measured the amount of soluble MHC peptide required to block the binding of an antibody to TCR; and the other measured the amount of soluble TCR required to block T cell responses (1, 9). Both gave values of approximately 10^{-4} to 10^{-5} M. That level of affinity can be viewed in the context of antibody affinities which are in a much higher range.

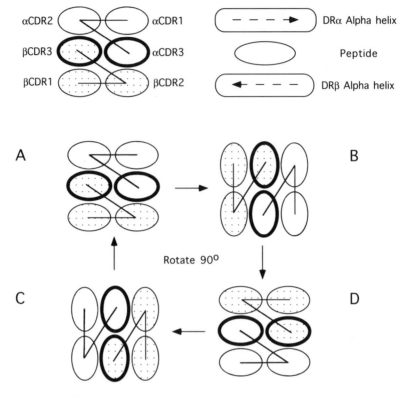

Figure 4.4. Model of the interaction between the TCR and the MHC peptide. The upper panel shows a schematic diagram of the domains of the surface of the TCR and MHC. The lines connecting the domains in the TCR show the three domains that belong to the same polypeptide chain. The CDR 3 are in bold and are in the middle of the TCR surface. The orientation of the TCR domains is actually from the back, so that to see the interaction of the domains with MHC one need only place the TCR over the MHC. The four simplest possible orientations of the TCR to the MHC are illustrated in the bottom panel (A–D). In reality, the TCR could be rotated to any angle and translated laterally or vertically. Experiments are in progress to see if the simplest models may be generally true

   TCRs can recognize a second class of molecules that has been loosely termed super-antigens (14). These differ from conventional peptide antigens in several remarkable ways: (a) the antigens do not require processing but instead stimulate T cells if they are intact; (b) presentation by class II molecules is necessary but there is not a strict MHC restriction. This is interpreted to mean that superantigens are bound to class II molecules when they stimulate T cells but they can associate with a wide range of class II molecules, unlike peptides which can fit into a narrow choice of MHC grooves; (c) recognition of superantigens is determined predominantly by their interaction with the β chain of the TCR. The data have shown that when one assays a complex mixture of T cells for stimulation by a superantigen, T cells with certain Vβs will respond and others will not, suggesting that recognition is a function of the Vβ. More recent data suggest that the α chain contributes as well to the recognition of superantigens; (d) the region of the TCR that interacts with superantigen has been examined in two mouse models (15, 16) and one human example (17). For example, the observation was made that in a strain of mouse with a polymorphism of Vβ8, the T cells expressing that Vβ were no longer recognizing the mouse Mls-1[a] molecule, a known superantigen. Replacement of some of those residues that were different in the polymorphic form restored recognition of the superantigen. This work and the other examples have suggested that the region around HV4 could be important for the interaction with superantigen.

THE GERM LINE GENES CODING FOR THE TCR

The general description of the germ line genes that code for the TCR has been a major success of molecular immunology. Eventually with research related to the human genome project, the complete sequence of the loci, involving several megabases, will be completed. The following description is therefore incomplete but includes the major features. Beyond the completion of one genomic individual sequence, which actually will be a compilation of several individuals' genes, the description of the polymorphic nature of the loci is unfolding. The clinical significance of such polymorphisms may be important, as we discuss later. It is important to emphasize that we describe the human genes and that other species will be different.

The Structure of the β Locus

Essential features of the β locus are illustrated in the central structure of Figure 4.5 (adapted from multiple sources, including refs 18, 19). The locus is at band q35–36 of chromosome 7. The figure also illustrates the rearrangements which will be discussed in the next section.

1. A cluster of V regions lies centromeric to the C regions. Various attempts have been made to estimate the number of V regions that are present in the genome. The straightforward approach has been partially accomplished, that is, to isolate and sequence the entire region. Because this region covers approximately a megabase, the final results of this effort have not been published, although it has been partially mapped with genetic and physical techniques (20). A second approach has been to sequence randomly selected cDNAs from the peripheral blood of a given individual. Using that approach, four recent papers have analyzed more

66

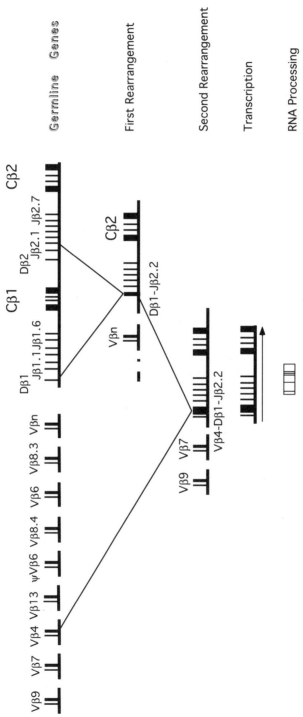

Figure 4.5. TCR β locus. At the top are shown the germ line configuration of the locus. Note the set of V regions on one side and two J–C clusters on the other. Each V region consists of two exons: one corresponding to the leader peptide and one to the V region. Each rearrangement deletes the region of the chromosome between the two pieces. After two rearrangements, transcription creates an mRNA containing the intronic sequences that are spliced out during RNA processing

than 700 β chain cDNA sequences (21–24). Interpretation of these data has led to the conclusion that there exist 24 families of V regions and a total of approximately 60 functional V region genes. [This interpretation involves some problems of nomenclature and ambiguity. Repetitions of identical V region sequences are interpreted to represent repeat sequences of one V region. Sequences that differ by only a few bases can be due to separate V regions, sequencing errors, or polymorphisms. Sequences that differ by up to 25% are felt to be different genes but have been grouped within a family (some have called these subfamilies). The V gene family concept developed because of historical and technical reasons. Workers used individual V region probes for hybridization studies, and sequences that differed by less than 25% generally could cross-hybridize. Thus by probing Southern digests of unrearranged DNA, one could estimate the number of members of a given family. Using this criterion of defining families, a total of 24 β families have been described.] The number of members within each family is usually greater than one, ranging up to six or more. A second approach to the characterization of V regions has been cloning the germ line copies of all of the members of a family, using an individual member as a probe. This has been done for the Vβ8 and Vβ6 as well as partially for the Vβ12 subfamily (25, 26). It is remarkable that in these cases multiple pseudogenes for the TCR were found. (Pseudogenes are homologous sequences to the functional TCR genes but appear to have mutations that render them nonfunctional, such as internal stop codons.) This suggests that like other clusters of homologous genes, the Vβs are undergoing homologous but unequal cross-overs that can expand and contract the set during evolution, with gradual divergence of related genes. The related members of a family have not been found grouped together, suggesting that these homologous but unequal cross-overs can occur throughout the region. The orientation of the V regions that have been examined are all in the same translational direction, a finding that may have unknown functional importance. One exception is a V region, Vβ17 (mouse), which has been identified in the mouse to be found 3' to the C region cluster and oriented in the opposite direction (27). A human counterpart may exist as well. While the rearrangement of that V region necessarily needs to occur by an inversional rather than a deletional mechanism, the significance of the position is unknown. For immunoglobulin heavy chain genes there is the suggestion that V regions proximal to the C region rearrange first. No such data have been found for the human β locus.

2. Centromeric of the V region cluster are the genes coding for the D–J–C region of the molecule. The sequence of nearly the entire region has been published (18). Two homologous clusters exist; each has one D region followed by either six J regions and one C region for the first cluster, or

seven J regions and one C region for the second cluster. The formal possibility remains that other D regions may exist but they have not been described. The two C regions are closely related and have no known functional differences.

3. Numerous polymorphisms of the β locus are certain to exist, and a few have been described (28, 29).

The Structure of the γ Locus

The overall structure of the γ locus, on chromosome band 7p15, resembles that of the β locus, with multiple V regions and two clusters of J–C genes (Figure 4.6) (30, 31). While the β V region locus has not been described in detail, the γ chain locus has been characterized and the following description is likely to be complete, although again the entire region has not been sequenced.

1. A cluster of V regions precedes the rest of the locus, with the V regions oriented in one direction. Unlike the β locus, there is a structural organization of the V regions in that the nine most closely related sequences come first, while the more divergent sequences follow. This suggests that homologous but unequal cross-over events have not occurred recently between the first set and the others. The first set of nine V regions contains several pseudogenes that may not code for functional genes. Five can clearly code for functional proteins and are designated Vγ2, Vγ3, Vγ4, Vγ5, and Vγ8; these are closely related and have been given a family name of VγI (Figure 4.3B). Five other γ chain V regions follow, including two more pseudogenes. Three functional V regions not in the VγI family are widely divergent from each other and have been designated Vγ9 (VγII), Vγ10 (VγIII), and Vγ11 (VγIV).

2. Centromeric to the V regions are two clusters of J regions, each with a C region following the J regions. The first cluster of J regions has three members, while the second has two members which closely resemble the first and third of the first set, explaining the notation of not having a Jγ2.2. The two C regions have a marked difference, in that Cγ1 has one second exon, which codes for the connecting peptide of the constant region, while Cγ2 has a duplication of the second exon. Even more remarkable is that the second exons of Cγ2 have lost the cysteine that forms the disulfide bond between the C regions of the γ and δ chains. There is probably a functional difference between Cγ1 and Cγ2 because of the observation that most of the γδ cells in the peripheral blood are Cγ1 while those of the thymus are Cγ2. The possibility exists, however, that J region or V region differences may account for the presence of Cγ1 or Cγ2 in certain populations of cells, since specific V or J regions are associated with the C regions.

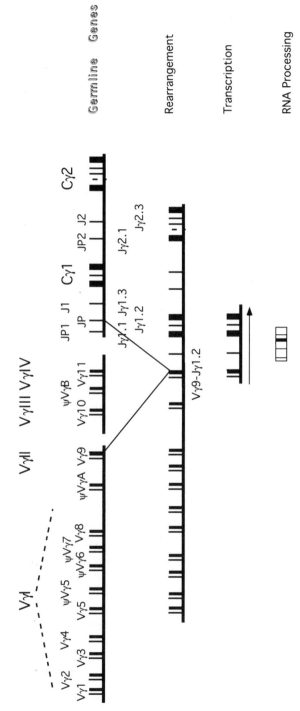

Figure 4.6. TCR γ locus. At the top are the germ line genes for the γ locus. The two notations for the V regions are shown. Pseudogenes are indicated by a ψ. An example of a rearrangement is shown, followed by transcription and splicing

3. Polymorphisms of the γ chain: the most striking polymorphism of the γ chain is the presence of either two or three second exons. The form with three tandem second exons occurs in up to 68% of the Black African population but only in 16% of the French and 13% of the Chinese population (32, 33). This polymorphism leads to a significant measurable difference in the molecular weight of the γ chain, in part because of the asparagine-linked carbohydrate on the connecting peptide. No functional difference or disease association is known, but no systematic attempts have been made to find a functional difference. For example, it has not been determined if the distribution of the genotypes in a population is in Hardy–Weinberg equilibrium. Two polymorphic forms of the VγI set of genes have been described. One haplotype has seven instead of nine genes with the loss of Vγ4 and Vγ5; this occurs in approximately 21% of the French population. Another haplotype has ten VγI genes with the addition of a pseudo-Vγ3 gene. A functional difference has not been appreciated for these polymorphisms either.

The Structure of the α–δ Locus

The most complex TCR locus is the α–δ locus at band 14q11 (Figure 4.7) (34, 35). The overall structure of the locus resembles the γ and β locus in having a cluster of V regions, followed by two J–C clusters. A major difference is that the two J–C regions are very divergent genetically and functionally. Related to the wide divergence of α and δ constant regions, some V regions are rearranged and expressed with the δ J and C region and others are consistently found as α chains. The mechanism for that separation is not known. It may be due simply to the physical clustering of Vδ since they are found mostly near the J–C region. It may also relate to unknown regulation of rearrangements and/or transcription.

1. The V regions of the cluster have again been divided into families based on criteria similar to those used for the β chains. The most extensive characterization of a population of T cells has recently been published, where sequences of 300 α chains were determined. A total of 29 families were defined (21). Most of the families had small numbers of members such that the current estimates of the number of V region families is 30, with a total number of V regions being 50. This does not include the three V region subfamilies that have been associated primarily with δ chains. The order of the V regions has only been partially determined and the orientation is exclusively in one direction, with the exception of one Vδ which lies 3' of the δ constant region in an inverted orientation (36).
2. The δ chain cluster consists of three D regions, three J regions and the constant region (36).

3. No polymorphisms have been described for the δ chains, while some have been described for the α chain (37–39).
4. The α chain cluster consists of a large domain of J regions that number approximately 100, covering 75 kb between the inverted Vδ3 and the α C region (40). A single α chain C region exists.
5. While many polymorphisms are likely to exist in the α J regions, they have yet to be described.

T CELL RECEPTOR REPERTOIRE DEVELOPMENT

Every fully functional T cell must necessarily have undergone a developmental process that includes multiple steps and decision points. A major goal of modern immunology has been the delineation of that process. As a part of the early developmental pathways of the T cell, every fully functional TCR on the surface of a T cell must have similarly undergone a series of developmental steps that are described in a general way in Figure 4.8 within the overall development of the T cell. The details of the process with respect to the TCR are described for each of the TCR families following a general discussion of repertoire development.

In the germ line and in early T committed cells, the TCR genes are unrearranged, with separate V, D, J and C region segments as described earlier. The number of V genes in the germ line defines the "germ line diversity" of a locus. If all of the germ line genes that are functional can rearrange randomly, those rearrangements constitute the "potential diversity" or potential repertoire of a receptor family, which is shown in Table 4.1. The potential diversity of the TCR loci is an enormous number which is well beyond the number of cells in the body. Thus the repertoire that is actually expressed as a functional receptor is a tiny fraction of the potential repertoire. Early in the commitment process to T cells, a rearrangement of one of the TCR loci occurs, usually either in the α or δ locus. The rearrangement process has been described in the earlier chapter on immunoglobulin genes. The enzymology of the rearrangements is probably generally the same in B and T cells in that the types of joints produced appear to be the same, the SCID mutation of the mouse affects immunoglobulin and TCR gene rearrangement equally (41), and the RAG1 and RAG2 gene "knockout" mice generate animals incapable of rearranging either TCR or Ig genes. What is clearly different between the B and T cells is the process of choosing what loci to rearrange. Thus the cell with the rearrangement machinery turned on must selectively rearrange the TCR loci and not the immunoglobulin loci and, more precisely, it must select correctly a specific TCR locus and not others. The details of how that selection is made remains an important unanswered question but it may be related to transcriptional regulation, i.e. the same mechanisms that open up a locus to transcription may open it up for rearrangement.

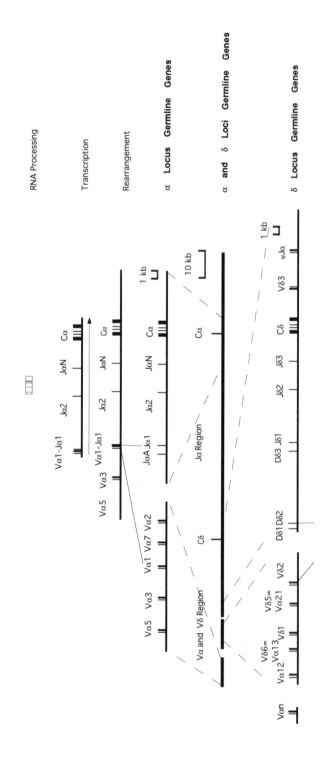

73

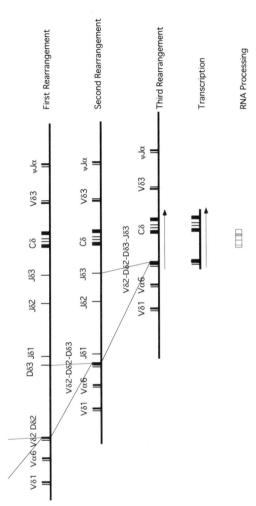

Figure 4.7. TCR α–δ locus. The middle three lines show germ line genes. Because the two sets of genes are imbedded, two separate lines show the expanded α and δ loci. One rearrangement can create a functional α gene, but up to four rearrangements are necessary to make a δ gene

74

State of the TCR and T cells	Developmental process	Regulatory decision affecting TCR repertoire
Germ line receptor genes	All unrearranged genes prior to commitment to T cell lineage	
One receptor gene rearranged	First rearrangement of either α or δ locus. For δ two rearrangements are necessary	Selection of V, D, J
Both receptors rearranged	A second rearrangement of either γ or β locus	Selection of V, D, J
A cell surface receptor is expressed	The cells that successfully rearrange an in-frame receptor that can associate with each other can express a cell surface TCR	Elimination of cells that do not express a functional receptor. Termination of the recombinase activity
T cells that recognize self-MHC are selected	Positive selection	Cells recognizing self-MHC differentiate and proliferate
T cells that recognize self-peptide MHC are eliminated	Negative selection	Cells recognizing self-peptide MHC die
Cells leave the thymus and migrate to peripheral organs or stay in the blood	Expression of cell surface molecules dictate migratory pathway	Different lineages of cells express different cell surface molecules
T cells that recognize antigen increase in number	Antigen stimulation through TCR	Cells specific for antigen proliferate

Figure 4.8. Developmental steps involved in TCR repertoire differentiation. On the left are the progressive states of the genes of the TCR or T cells during development of a mature immune system. The second column describes the developmental process that changes the previous state to that level. The right-hand column describes the decision the cell makes during that developmental process

Table 4.1 Sequence diversity in T cell receptor and immunoglobulin genes*

Gene locus:	H	κ	α	β	γ	δ
	IG		α:β TCR		γ:δ TCR	
Variable segments	250–1000	250	50	60	9	6
Diversity segments	10(?)	0	0	2	0	3
Ds read in all frames	Rarely	None	None	Often	None	Often
N-region addition	V–D, D–J	None	V–J	V–D, D–J	V–J	V–D1, D1–D2, D2–D3, D3–J
Joining segments	6	5	90	13	5	3
Variable region combinations	62 500–250 000		3000		54	
Junctional combinations	$\sim 10^{11}$		$\sim 10^{15}$		$\sim 10^{20}$	

* Adapted from ref. 12

The first locus in a potential T cell to rearrange is probably either the β or δ locus. Following the rearrangement of one locus, a second locus must rearrange: the α for the αβ lineage and a γ for the γδ lineage. All of the possible rearrangements that occur within a lineage generate the *potential* repertoire. In other words, if in αβ T cells the γδ loci do not rearrange, then the potential repertoire of the αβ cell does not include any receptors of the γδ type. These events are not mutually exclusive. In many, if not most, αβ T cells there are rearrangements of the γ locus and sometimes of the δ locus; α or β rearrangements have not been commonly found in γδ T cells.

Many rearrangements do not generate the possibility of a functional molecule. Many such defective rearrangements have been described: (a) a pseudogene is rearranged; (b) the junction between the segments does not preserve the translational frame of the sequence; (c) the addition of N region sequences introduces a stop codon; (d) the exonuclease activity deletes an essential part of the V region or J region such as the cysteine residue. By far the most frequent event is the generation of out-of-frame products which have been found in approximately two-thirds of the junctions which are taken from cells that have not been selected for function. If the first allele of the locus produces an aberrant rearrangement, the second allele may rearrange. If the first rearranges correctly, a second rearrangement of the same locus on the other allele may be prohibited. This may be an explanation for the phenomenon of allelic exclusion, originally described for B cells where a given B lymphocyte expresses only one allele of a polymorphic locus (such as *Inv* for the Ig κ chain) while having two ostensible alleles coding for each of the chains involved. Multiple mechanisms probably exist for the phenomenon, which has been studied to a limited extent for T cells. No general studies have been done because no allele-specific C region antibodies have been available. On a cellular level, no T cell clones have been described that express two different β chains, two δ chains or two γ chains. Multiple instances have been described where two α chain cDNAs are expressed in the same cell (42). The general rule, which is probably not absolute, is that allelic exclusion does not exist for α chains while it does exist for β chains, with the story for γ and δ being less clear.

A further barrier to the successful development of a functional TCR is the association between the two chains. For example, certain combinations of γ and δ TCRs have not been observed. One explanation of that phenomenon is that structural constraints exist between the two chains of a heterodimer that prevents certain combinations existing as a stable heterodimer. Such a phenomenon has been observed for the two chains of an immunoglobulin molecule. Thus the next level of repertoire of T cells is the *expressed* repertoire which would include all receptors that can actually appear on the surface of T cells.

When a functional TCR appears on the surface of the cell, functional selection of the T cell can now occur on at least four levels: thymic-positive selection for self-MHC, thymic-negative selection against self-peptide MHC; positive or negative stimulation with super-antigens in the periphery; and positive or negative stimulation by peptide antigens in the periphery. Thus the *selected* repertoire of T cells will shrink further.

While each T cell has only one receptor, the biological effect of a T cell response is dictated by a population of T cells with a heterogeneous array of antigen receptors. Attempts to describe and measure the diversity of the receptors have been described as the T cell receptor repertoire question. Because the measurements are incomplete, the repertoire is a complex issue that combines theory and data. Aspects of the repertoire can be discussed on the level of a species, an individual, a population of cells, or by an individual specificity.

ORDERED AND REGULATED REARRANGEMENTS IN T CELL DEVELOPMENT

Lineages of T cells may express limited repertoires of TCR. Examples in the mouse and to a more limited extent in man have provided a model where certain lineages of T cells with specialized function express TCR with limited diversity. This model implies that some diseases may be associated with the over- or under-expression of these subsets of cells, and more importantly that the lineages may recognize different antigens that presumably have an etiological role in the growth of these lineages. An analogy is with the CD5+ B cells which have unique immunoglobulin receptors and are expressed on B cell lymphomas and CLL. The existence of a lineage of cells implies that the cells can be distinguished from another lineage by a set of important functional and molecular criteria. The CD4+ and CD8+ lineages are examples where it is known that the MHC molecules that stimulate the two sets of cells are different. Recently, evidence suggests that the α chain repertoire may differ between those two populations of cells. An example of a lineage of cells with a unique receptor comes from studies of dendritic epithelial cells (DEC) of the mouse, which were found to be γδ T cells with a nearly homogeneous TCR with very limited junctional diversity (43). Remarkably, these γδ cells were found to be one of the first to develop in mouse embryo genesis in the thymus, leaving the thymus to populate the skin prior to the appearance of other T cells. Following those cells, other waves of γδ T cells, each with its own set of receptors, appear in the thymus (44).

Regulation of rearrangements may determine the TCR repertoire of separate lineages of T cells. Data have been presented that T cells make an early commitment to either an αβ or a γδ lineage (45). One suggestion has been that the decision to rearrange the δ or α locus is also made very early. The alternative theory would be that the cells can rearrange both loci, but the cells that successfully make an αβ receptor become αβ T cells and those that make a successful γδ receptor become γδ cells. Because the rearrangements are not reversible, one can obtain evidence of a cell's developmental history by examining the rearranged products in mature T cells. One study found, in mature cells of the αβ lineage, no evidence that the δ locus had also rearranged, as one might expect if the decision to commit to a lineage is made after the rearrangement step. (Some conflicting data have also been described such that the relationship of the lineage determination to the rearrangement process remains not entirely clear.) In man, when the early fetal rearrangements were examined it was found that Vδ2–Dδ3 rearrangements appeared first, with other rearrangements Vδ1–Dδ2 appearing later (46, 47). These early rearrangements have not yet been associated with any adult lineage of T cells. They may have a special role in fetal immunity and disappear, or they may be in a compartment of the adult immune system that has not been carefully examined.

TCR REPERTOIRE AND DISEASE ASSOCIATIONS

There have been many reports where differences in the TCR genes or repertoire have been associated with human diseases. The reports have fallen into two categories. First are reports of diseases that appear to be associated with TCR locus polymorphisms. Prominent among these diseases are autoimmune disorders such as multiple sclerosis (48, 49). These studies find increased frequency of certain TCR alleles in groups of unrelated patients when compared to control groups. These suggest that structural or regulatory polymorphisms in the TCR genes may play a role in the susceptibility to immunological diseases analogous to MHC associations. Precedent for these studies was established by the use of the approach in finding disease associations between HLA polymorphisms and diseases of the immune system. To date, none of these associations with the TCR has been documented in multiple studies from different laboratories. It is unclear whether those associations are not real or if technical problems and disease heterogeneity have obscured real biologically important effects (50). Family or twin studies of disease associations would be more convincing but are not yet available. Importantly, this type of study makes no direct link between a gene and a disease. It could be any genetic locus that is linked to the polymorphism studied that is really associated mechanistically to the disease.

The second category comprises reports of diseases that have an altered TCR repertoire. A strong impetus to those studies was the finding in rodents that the TCRs that recognized myelin basic protein, an immunogen that could cause experimental allergic encephalomyelitis (EAE), a demyelinating disease, were of a very limited heterogeneity (51–53). For example, TCR sequences were obtained from T cell clones that react to an MBP (myelin basic protein) peptide in PL/J mice. All of the clones used the same Vα; many used the same Vβ. Not only were the V regions of limited heterogeneity but also the junctional sequences were closely related in terms of the amino acid structure, suggesting that the disease process that produces anti-MBP T cells, which were shown to cause the symptoms of the demyelination, expanded out T cells of a very narrow spectrum. Furthermore, it has been possible to treat the clinical disease with antibodies against the disease-associated T cell receptors (54). If human syndromes could be found with similar pathophysiology, the prospects for treatment are exciting.

Since the early reports of altered repertoire in animal models of autoimmune diseases, many attempts have been made to ask if human diseases were similar. Reports of that type have been common in many diseases, most prominently multiple sclerosis (55), but also sarcoidosis, rheumatoid arthritis (56, 57), inflammatory bowel disease, HIV infection, autoimmune thyroiditis (58), and many others. These studies have not been repeated in large well-controlled patient populations, and it is too early to know if any of them will be found to mean that the TCR repertoire has any fundamental role in the evolution of a disease. The key to the interpretation of those studies is the understanding that basic immunological knowledge is not available to do the studies correctly or to interpret them. It is known that the T cell repertoire can be very different depending on where and how one looks. Superantigens can expand *in vitro* populations of T cells with certain Vβ. The TCR repertoire after other antigen stimulation in the mouse can be very homogeneous, as with the MBP example, or fairly diverse, as with a peptide from myoglobin. Different tissues can have a limited TCR repertoire, as with the increase in Vα12 in the human intestine (59). Thus when one finds that the repertoire is altered in a disease one may be looking at tissue or developmental differences rather than disease-associated changes. Furthermore, technical difficulties in measuring TCR repertoire may have a great impact on the observations. In the mouse, most studies of V region use of β chains were made possible through the use of monoclonal antibodies against specific V regions. In man those antibodies have not been widely available. Polymerase chain reaction (PCR) techniques have largely replaced Southern blot as a molecular method to examine TCR repertoire. The quantitative PCR with specific primers has become the predominant technology, even though the reproducibility, accuracy, and specificity of the techniques remain to be clearly demonstrated.

In conclusion, the role of the T cell in a range of human disease is unquestioned. It remains a fascinating possibility that alterations in the T cell receptor repertoire caused by genetic polymorphisms, by altered developmental steps or by interactions with the environment could be causal in human disease. If that proves to be true, it could have very important implications both diagnostically and therapeutically.

REFERENCES

1. Matsui, K., Boniface, J.J., Reay, P.A., Schild, H., Fazekas de St. Groth, B. and Davis, M.M. (1991) Low affinity interaction of peptide–MHC complexes with T cell receptors. *Science*, **254**, 1788.

2. Saito, T. and Germain, R.N. (1988) The molecular basis of MHC-restricted antigen recognition by T cells. *Int. Rev. Immunol.*, **3**, 147.

3. Jensen, J.P., Hou, D., Ramsburg, M., Taylor, A., Dean, M. and Weissman, A.M. (1992) Organization of the human T cell receptor zeta/eta gene and its genetic linkage to the FcgammaRII-FcgammaRIII gene cluster. *J. Immunol.*, **148**, 2563.

4. Koyasu, S., D'Adamio, L., Arulanandam, A.R., Abraham, S., Clayton, L.K. and Reinherz, E.L. (1992) T cell receptor complexes containing Fc epsilon RI gamma homodimers in lieu of CD3 zeta and CD3 eta components: A novel isoform expressed on large granular lymphocytes. *J. Exp. Med.*, **175**, 203.

5. Gabert, J., Langlet, C., Zamoyska, R., Parnes, J.R., Schmitt-Verhulst, A.M. and Malissen, B. (1987) Reconstitution of MHC class I specificity by transfer of the T cell receptor and Lyt-2 genes. *Cell*, **50**, 545.

6. Ballhausen, W.G., Reske-Kunz, A.B., Tourvieille, B., Ohashi, P.S., Parnes, J.R. and Mak, T.W. (1988) Acquisition of an additional antigen specificity after mouse CD4 gene transfer into a T helper hybridoma. *J. Exp. Med.*, **167**, 1493.

7. Grégoire, C., Rebaï, N., Schweisguth, F., Necker, A., Mazza, G., Auphan, N., Millward, A., Schmitt-Verhulst, A.–M. and Malissen, B. (1991) Engineered secreted T-cell receptor αβ heterodimers. *Proc. Nat. Acad. Sci. USA*, **88**, 8077.

8. Devaux, B., Bjorkman, P.J., Stevenson, C., Greif, W., Elliott, J.F., Sagerstrom, C., Clayberger, C., Krensky, A.M. and Davis, M.M. (1991) Generation of monoclonal antibodies against soluble human T cell receptor polypeptides. *Eur. J. Immunol.*, **21**, 2111.

9. Weber, S., Traunecker, A., Oliveri, F., Gerhard, W. and Karjalainen, K. (1992) Specific low-affinity recognition of major histocompatibility complex plus peptide by soluble T-cell receptor. *Nature*, **356**, 793.

10. Jores, R., Alzari, P.M. and Meo, T. (1990) Resolution of hypervariable regions in T-cell receptor beta chains by a modified Wu-Kabat index of amino acid diversity. *Proc. Nat. Acad. Sci USA*, **87**, 9138.

11. Huck, S., Dariavach, P. and Lefranc, M.P. (1988) Variable region genes in the human T-cell rearranging gamma (TRG) locus: V–J junction and homology with the mouse genes. *EMBO J.*, **7**, 719.

12. Davis, M.M. and Bjorkman, P.J. (1988) T-cell antigen receptor genes and T-cell recognition [published erratum appears in *Nature* (1988) **335**, 744]. *Nature*, **334**, 395.

13. Jorgensen, J.L., Reay, P.A., Ehrich, E.W. and Davis, M.M. (1992) Molecular components of T-cell recognition. *Annu. Rev. Immunol.*, **10**, 835.

14. Marrack, P. and Kappler, J. (1990) The staphylococcal enterotoxins and their relatives [published erratum appears in *Science* (1990) **248**, 1066]. *Science*, **248**, 705.

15. Pullen, A.M., Bill, J., Kubo, R.T., Marrack, P. and Kappler, J.W. (1991) Analysis of the interaction site for the self superantigen Mls-1a on T cell receptor V beta. *J. Exp. Med.*, **173**, 1183.

16. Dellabona, P., Peccoud, J., Kappler, J., Marrack, P., Benoist, C. and Mathis, D. (1990) Superantigens interact with MHC class II molecules outside of the antigen groove. *Cell*, **62**, 1115.

17. Choi, Y.W., Kotzin, B., Herron, L., Callahan, J., Marrack, P. and Kappler, J. (1989) Interaction of *Staphylococcus aureus* toxin "superantigens with human T cells". *Proc. Nat. Acad. Sci. USA*, **86**, 8941.
18. Toyonaga, B. and Mak, T.W. (1987) Genes of the T-cell antigen receptor in normal and malignant T cells. *Annu. Rev. Immunol.*, **5**, 585.
19. Klein, M.H., Concannon, P., Everett, M., Kim, L.D., Hunkapiller, T. and Hood, L. (1987) Diversity and structure of human T-cell receptor alpha-chain variable region genes. *Proc. Nat. Acad. Sci. USA*, **84**, 6884.
20. Lai, E., Wilson, R.K. and Hood, L.E. (1989) Physical maps of the mouse and human immunoglobulin-like loci. *Adv. Immunol.*, **46**, 1.
21. Roman-Roman, S., Ferradini, L., Azocar, J., Genevee, C., Hercend, T. and Triebel, F. (1991) Studies on the human T cell receptor alpha/beta variable region genes. I. Identification of 7 additional V alpha subfamilies and 14 J alpha gene segments. *Eur. J. Immunol.*, **21**, 927.
22. Rosenberg, W.M.C., Moss, P.A.H. and Bell, J.I. (1992) Variation in human T cell receptor V_b and J_b repertoire: Analysis using anchor polymerase chain reaction. *Eur. J. Immunol.*, **22**, 541.
23. Robinson, M.A. (1991) The human T cell receptor beta-chain gene complex contains at least 57 variable gene segments: Identification of six V beta genes in four new gene families. *J. Immunol.*, **146**, 4392.
24. Plaza, A., Kono, D.H. and Theofilopoulos, A.N. (1991) New human V beta genes and polymorphic variants. *J. Immunol.*, **147**, 4360.
25. Siu, G., Strauss, E.C., Lai, E. and Hood, L.E. (1986) Analysis of a human V beta gene subfamily. *J. Exp. Med.*, **164**, 1600.
26. Li, Y., Szabo, P. and Posnett, D.N. (1991) The genomic structure of human Vb6 T cell antigen receptor genes. *J. Exp. Med.*, **174**, 1537.
27. Malissen, M., McCoy, C., Blanc, D., Trucy, J., Devaux, C., Schmitt-Verhulst, A.M., Fitch, F., Hood, L. and Malissen, B. (1986) Direct evidence for chromosomal inversion during T-cell receptor beta-gene rearrangements. *Nature*, **319**, 28.
28. Li, Y., Szabo, P. and Posnett, D.N. (1991) The genomic structure of human Vb6 T cell antigen receptor genes. *J. Exp. Med.*, **174**, 1537.
29. Charmley, P., Chao, A., Concannon, P., Hood, L. and Gatti, R.A. (1990) Haplotyping the human T-cell receptor beta-chain gene complex by use of restriction fragment length polymorphisms. *Proc. Nat. Acad. Sci. USA*, **87**, 4823.
30. Lefranc, M.P. and Rabbitts, T.H. (1989) The human T-cell receptor gamma (TRG) genes. *Trends Biochem. Sci.*, **14**, 214.
31. Lefranc, M.P., Chuchana, P., Dariavach, P., Nguyen, C., Huck, S., Brockly, F., Jordan, B. and Lefranc, G. (1989) Molecular mapping of the human T cell receptor gamma (TRG) genes and linkage of the variable and constant regions. *Eur. J. Immunol.*, **19**, 989.
32. Ghanem, N., Buresi, C., Moisan, J.P., Bensmana, M., Chuchana, P., Huck, S. Lefranc, G. and Lefranc, M.P. (1989) Deletion, insertion, and restriction site polymorphism of the T-cell receptor gamma variable locus in French, Lebanese, Tunisian, and black African populations. *Immunogenetics*, **30**, 350.
33. Buresi, C., Ghanem, N., Huck, S., Lefranc, G. and Lefranc, M.P. (1989) Exon duplication and triplication in the human T-cell receptor gamma constant region genes and RFLP in French, Lebanese, Tunisian, and black African populations [published erratum appears in *Immunogenetics* (1989), **30**, 148]. *Immunogenetics*, **29**, 161.
34. Griesser, H., Champagne, E., Tkachuk, D., Takihara, Y., Lalande, M., Baillie, E., Minden, M. and Mak, T.W. (1988) The human T cell receptor alpha–delta locus: A

physical map of the variable, joining and constant region genes. *Eur. J. Immunol.*, **18**, 641.

35. Satyanarayana, K., Hata, S., Devlin, P., Roncarolo, M.G., De Vries, J.E., Spits, H., Strominger, J.L. and Krangel, M.S. (1988) Genomic organization of the human T-cell antigen-receptor alpha/delta locus. *Proc. Nat. Acad. Sci. USA*, **85**, 8166.

36. Loh, E.Y., Cwirla, S., Serafini, A.T., Phillips, J.H. and Lanier, L.L. (1988) Human T-cell-receptor delta chain: Genomic organization, diversity, and expression in populations of cells. *Proc. Nat. Acad. Sci. USA*, **85**, 9714.

37. Chan, A., Du, R.P., Reis, M., Baillie, E., Meske, L.M., Sheehy, M. and Mak, T.W. (1989) Polymorphism of the human T cell receptor alpha chain variable genes: Identification of a highly polymorphic V gene probe. *Int. Immunol.*, **1**, 267.

38. Chan, A., Du, R.P., Reis, M., Meske, L.M., Sheehy, M., Baillie, E. and Mak, T.W. (1990) Human T cell receptor V alpha gene polymorphism. *Exp. Clin. Immunogenet.*, **7**, 26.

39. Posnett, D.N. (1990) Allelic variations of human TCR V gene products. *Immunol. Today*, **11**, 368.

40. Champagne, E., Sagman, U., Biondi, A., Lewis, W.H., Mak, T.W. and Minden, M.D. (1988) Structure and rearrangement of the T cell receptor J alpha locus in T cells and leukemic T cell lines. *Eur. J. Immunol.*, **18**, 1033.

41. Carroll, A.M. and Bosma, M.J. (1991) T-lymphocyte development in scid mice is arrested shortly after the initiation of T-cell receptor δ gene recombination. *Genes Dev.*, **5**, 1357.

42. Malissen, M., Trucy, J. Letourneur, F., Rebai, N., Dunn, D.E., Fitch, F.W., Hood, L. and Malissen, B. (1988) A T cell clone expresses two T cell receptor alpha genes but uses one alpha beta heterodimer for allorecognition and self MHC-restricted antigen recognition. *Cell*, **55**, 49.

43. Allison, J.P., Asarnow, D.M., Bonyhadi, M., Carbone, A., Havran, W.L., Nandi, D. and Noble, J. (1991) γδ T cells in murine epithelia: Origin, repertoire, and function. *Adv. Exp. Med. Biol.*, **292**, 63.

44. Haas, W. and Tonegawa, S. (1992) Development and selection of γδ T cells. *Curr. Opinion Immunol.*, **4**, 147.

45. Winoto, A. and Baltimore, D. (1989) Separate lineages of T cells expressing the alpha beta and gamma delta receptors. *Nature*, **338**, 430.

46. Spits, H., Yssel, H., Brockelhurst, C. and Krangel, M. (1991) Evidence for controlled gene rearrangements and cytokine production during development of human TCR γδ+ lymphocytes. *Curr. Top. Microbiol. Immunol.*, **173**, 47.

47. Krangel, M.S., Yssel, H., Brocklehurst, C. and Spits, H. (1990) A distinct wave of human T cell receptor gamma/delta lymphocytes in the early fetal thymus: Evidence for controlled gene rearrangement and cytokine production. *J. Exp. Med.*, **172**, 847.

48. Charmley, P., Beall, S.S., Concannon, P., Hood, L. and Gatti, R.A. (1991) Further localization of a multiple sclerosis susceptibility gene on chromosome 7q using a new T cell receptor beta-chain DNA polymorphism. *J. Neuroimmunol.*, **32**, 231.

49. Kumar, V., Kono, D.H., Urban, J.L. and Hood, L. (1989) The T-cell receptor repertoire and autoimmune diseases. *Annu. Rev. Immunol.*, **7**, 657.

50. Hillert, J. and Olerup, O. (1992) Debate: Do TCR genes influence susceptibility to autoimmune disease in humans? Germ-line polymorphism of TCR genes and disease susceptibility—Fact or hypothesis? *Immunol. Today*, **13**, 47.

51. Acha-Orbea, H. (1991) Limited heterogeneity of autoantigens and T cells in autoimmune diseases? *Res. Immunol.*, **142**, 487.

52. Esch, T., Clark, L., Zhang, X.-M., Goldman, S. and Heber-Katz, E. (1992). Observations, legends, and conjectures concerning restricted T-cell receptor usage and autoimmune disease. *Crit. Rev. Immunol.*, **11**, 249.

53. Acha Orbea, H., Mitchell, D.J., Timmermann, L., Wraith, D.C., Tausch, G.S., Waldor, M.K., Zamvil, S.S., McDevitt, H.O. and Steinman, L. (1988) Limited heterogeneity of T cell receptors from lymphocytes mediating autoimmune encephalomyelitis allows specific immune intervention. *Cell*, **54**, 263.

54. Zaller, D.M., Osman, G., Kanagawa, O. and Hood, L. (1990) Prevention and treatment of murine experimental allergic encephalomyelitis with T cell receptor V beta-specific antibodies. *J. Exp. Med.*, **171**, 1943.

55. Hood, L., Kumar, V., Osman, G., Beall, S.S., Gomez, C., Funkhouser, W., Kono, D.H., Nickerson, D., Zaller, D.M. and Urban, J.L. (1989) Autoimmune disease and T-cell immunologic recognition. *Cold Spring. Harbor Symp. Quant. Biol.*, **54**, Pt 2, 859.

56. Pluschke, G., Ricken, G., Taube, H., Kroninger, S., Melchers, I., Peter, H.H., Eichmann, K. and Krawinkel, U. (1991) Biased T cell receptor V_a region repertoire in the synovial fluid of rheumatoid arthritis patients. *Eur. J. Immunol.*, **21**, 2749.

57. Paliard, X., West, S.G., Lafferty, J.A., Clements, J.R., Kappler, J.W., Marrack, P. and Kotzin, B.L. (1991) Evidence for the effects of a superantigen in rheumatoid arthritis. *Science*, **253**, 325.

58. Davies, T.F., Martin, A., Concepcion, E.S., Graves, P., Lahat, N., Cohen, W.L. and Ben Nun, A. (1992) Evidence for selective accumulation of intrathyroidal T lymphocytes in human autoimmune thyroid disease based on T cell receptor V gene usage. *J. Clin. Invest.*, **89**, 157.

59. DerSimonian, H., Band, H. and Brenner, M.B. (1991) Increased frequency of T cell receptor V alpha 12.1 expression on CD8+ T cells: Evidence that V alpha participates in shaping the peripheral T cell repertoire. *J. Exp. Med.*, **174**, 639.

Chapter 5

Signal Transduction in T Cell Activation and Tolerance

JEFFREY N. SIEGEL and CARL H. JUNE

Immune Cell Biology Program, Naval Medical Research Institute, Bethesda, Maryland, USA

SIGNAL TRANSDUCTION IN HUMAN T LYMPHOCYTES

T lymphocytes communicate with their environment through a large array of specialized cell surface receptors. These receptors provide signals which influence T cell ontogeny, activation by antigen, homing and many other aspects of T cell biology. Recent advances have provided a wealth of new information regarding the mechanism by which these surface receptors influence intracellular biochemical events. Transmembrane signaling is initiated by the binding of specific ligand to the extracellular portion of cell surface receptors. The signal is believed to be transmitted across the plasma membrane via either a conformational change in the receptor, by receptor dimerization (1) or by a change in its association with other proteins (2). This change in the receptor in turn induces changes in the level and activity of critical regulatory proteins and second messenger molecules. Then the signal is transmitted into the nucleus, where it induces changes in transcription-regulatory factors. Finally, changes in the activity of transcription factors induce changes in gene expression, leading to the functional and phenotypic markers associated with engagement of that receptor. In this chapter, we will review current knowledge of the molecular events which transpire between engagement of cell surface receptors and transmission of the signal into the nucleus. A summary of current knowledge of the subsequent transcriptional events is beyond the scope of this chapter but may be obtained from recent reviews (3, 4).

New Concepts in Immunodeficiency Diseases. Edited by S. Gupta and C. Griscelli
© 1993 John Wiley & Sons Ltd

How can an understanding of signal transduction aid in our understanding of T lymphocyte function? One way is to help to explain those instances where stimulation of different T cell populations in identical ways leads to markedly different outcomes. This situation has been observed repeatedly. First, T cells differ in their responsiveness at different stages of development. T cells at different stages of thymic ontogeny respond differently to binding of the T cell antigen receptor (TCR) by monoclonal antibodies. Only the more mature subset increases intracellular Ca^{2+} in response to antibodies directed against the antigen-binding chains (5). Human cord blood T cells respond in a markedly different way to pharmacological mitogens than adult T cells *in vitro* (6). Second, different clones and subsets of mature T cells have been defined which respond differently to engagement of the TCR. *In vitro* derived T helper cell clones differ markedly in the second messenger pathways activated in response to engagement of the TCR (7, 8). Another example concerns naive and memory T cells, which constitute two readily distinguishable subsets of mature T cells differing in their surface markers and prior exposure to antigen (9). Recent studies have demonstrated that in spite of their equivalent surface expression of TCR, the naive subset is markedly impaired in its ability to proliferate and secrete lymphokines in response to cross-linking of either TCR or CD2 (10, 11). Finally, certain cell populations rendered non-responsive by exposure to specific antigen either *in vivo* or *in vitro* are impaired in their ability to increase intracellular Ca^{2+} and produce lymphokines in response to TCR engagement (12, 13). In each of these examples, T lymphocytes which exhibit comparable levels of surface TCR differ markedly in their response to TCR engagement. Studies of the signal transduction events occurring in these cells can help to determine what accounts for the observed differences. Under different circumstances, differences in responsiveness might occur at the level of the receptor, the signals produced by receptor engagement, or the response of the gene transcription elements to the signals produced.

Another important contribution of signal transduction studies is in elucidating T cell responses to multiple stimuli. During a T cell response to antigen, multiple receptors besides the TCR are engaged. The accessory molecules CD4, CD8, CD45, adhesion molecules and others contribute in important ways to the final outcome. In many cases, accessory molecules play a dual role in immune responses both by promoting cell–cell adhesion upon engagement of their specific ligand on the antigen-presenting cell and by generating an intracellular biochemical signal. Only by defining the nature of the signals they produce and how these signals interact with others generated by the TCR can the role of accessory molecules be fully understood. Accessory molecules play a major role in thymic selection of T cells and in providing the co-stimulatory signals required for antigenic responses of mature T cells. Signal transduction studies can help to sort out how the cell integrates information entering simultaneously through multiple surface receptors.

T CELL RECEPTOR SIGNAL TRANSDUCTION

Structure and Function of the T Cell Receptor

The T cell receptor for antigen (TCR) is a multi-chain glycoprotein complex (Figure 5.1) which mediates recognition of peptide antigen in association with products of the major histocompatibility complex (MHC) (14, 15). It consists of three components: (a) the clonotypic heterodimeric Ti-α and -β chains which bind specific antigen; (b) the CD3 chains γ, δ and ε; and (c) a disulfide-linked dimer consisting of the ζ chain (16) or members of the ζ family of proteins (17, 18). Ti-α and -β chains are members of the immunoglobulin super-gene family. They have a long extracellular domain which binds specific antigen in association with MHC molecules, and a short intracellular domain which is probably not involved in signal transduction. In contrast, the CD3 chains and ζ chain have relatively short extracellular domains and long cytosolic tails which mediate signal transduction. The CD3 chains are members of the immunoglobulin super-family. The genes encoding these proteins are homologous and are clustered together on chromosome 11, indicating derivation from a common ancestral gene (19, 20). The ζ chain is a member of a small family of related proteins. It is not a member of the immunoglobulin gene family (21, 22). The gene encoding the ζ chain is on chromosome 1 and is not related to the CD3 chains. The other known members of the ζ family are the η chain and the γ subunit of the Fc receptor for IgE (18, 23). The η chain is an alternatively spliced product derived from the same gene as ζ but differing in the C-terminal region (17, 24).

There is evidence for considerable variability in the composition of the TCR. While the Ti-α and -β chains are the antigen-binding chains on most T cells, Ti-γ and Ti-δ are found on an important subpopulation (25, 26). The composition of CD3 chains in the receptor is complex. Evidence from several studies indicates that these chains are not found as a triad. Rather, the CD3-ε chain is associated in a pairwise manner with either CD3-δ or -γ, with two CD3-ε chains per receptor (27, 28). There are also indications that there may be heterogeneity in the composition of the CD3 complex in a single cell in that CD3-ε may be expressed with either CD3-δ or -γ but not both chains in the same complex (29). Finally, TCRs are found with variable composition of ζ family members. Commonly, there is a disulfide-linked ζ–ζ homodimer. However, in murine T cells and possibly in human as well, a fraction (~ 10%) of surface TCRs contain the ζ–η heterodimer (17). Finally, in certain cells, e.g. CTLL, ζ is found associated with the γ chain of the Fc receptor for IgE (18). All of these ζ family dimers are competent for signaling (30, 18). The

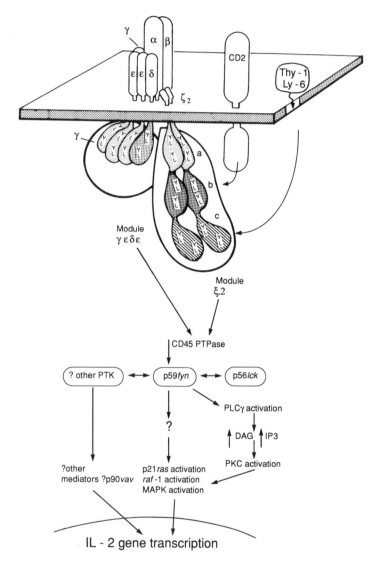

Figure 5.1. Initial events in T cell activation. Activation of either of two distinct modules can initiate signal transduction through the TCR, leading to IL-2 production. The first module consists of the CD3 chains γ, δ and ε, while the other consists of a dimer of chains of the TCR ζ family of proteins. The TCR initiates signal transduction by activating tyrosine kinase activity in a CD45 tyrosine phosphatase-dependent manner. As indicated, p21*ras*, *raf-1* and MAP kinase have all been implicated in mediating the subsequent transcriptional events. While PKC has been shown to activate each of these mediators, other activators may be involved as well. See text for details. A portion of this figure is modified from Wegener *et al.* (34), with permission

plasticity in the composition of the TCR components provides the potential for considerable variability in signal transduction through the receptor both in different stages of T cell ontogeny and in different subsets of mature T cells.

Which components of the TCR are responsible for signal transduction? As mentioned above, the antigen-binding α/β chains have short cytosolic tails, making them unlikely candidates. In contrast, both the CD3 chains and the ζ chain have long cytosolic tails which could serve to couple to intracellular signaling pathways. To study the signaling capabilities of these chains independent of the rest of the TCR, chimeric molecules have been constructed by several groups wherein the cytosolic tails have been expressed linked to the extracellular and transmembrane domain of an unrelated cell surface protein. These experiments have indicated that both the cytosolic tail of the ζ chain as well as that of CD3-ϵ are capable of generating a transmembrane signal alone, independent of the other TCR chains (31–33). Furthermore, the quality of the signal appears to be identical to that generated through the whole TCR. All components of signal transduction are seen, including tyrosine phosphorylation, increases in intracellular Ca^{2+}, phosphatidyl inositol (PI) turnover and interleukin 2 (IL-2) production. This finding demonstrates an unexpected redundancy in the structure of the TCR, with multiple components capable of generating a signal. However, there are indications from studies with murine T cells that CD3 chains and ζ chains may transduce different signals in intact T cells. These studies demonstrate that while ζ-deficient and ζ-containing TCR complexes can both signal in response to antigen, only TCR complexes containing ζ chains can support signaling through the accessory molecules Thy-1 and Ly-6 (34) (illustrated in Figure 5.1).

A major advance in understanding how the TCR transmits its intracellular signal came about when several groups determined the sequence motifs in the CD3 chains and the ζ chain which are responsible for signaling. Experiments dissecting the cytosolic tail of ζ have shown that there is an 18-amino acid stretch with two tyrosine residues capable of generating a signal when expressed linked to heterologous proteins (34, 35). This short stretch defines a consensus sequence which is found three times in the cytosolic tail of ζ. It is also found in the cytosolic tails of CD3-γ, -δ and -ϵ, as well in the immunoglobulin-associated mB-1 and B29 chains and the Fc-ϵ-associated β and γ chains. The broad distribution of the ζ consensus sequence suggests that it may represent a common mechanism used by a variety of immune system receptors to couple to signal transduction pathways (36).

T Cell Receptor Signaling Pathways

Engagement of the T cell receptor for antigen activates two intracellular signal transduction pathways (Figure 5.1) (37–40). A tyrosine kinase is activated which phosphorylates the ζ chain of the TCR as well as a large number of other cellular substrates. In addition, phospholipase C (PLC) is activated, which increases PI turnover, leading to increases in diacylglycerol (DAG) and inositil 1,4,5 trisphosphate (Ins(1,4,5)P3) (41). Ins(1,4,5)P3 in turn acts to increase intracellular Ca^{2+}, while DAG activates the serine/threonine kinase protein kinase C (PKC). Like the tyrosine kinase which is activated, PKC phosphorylates components of the TCR—in this case CD3-γ and -ε—as well as a number of other cellular substrates.

The existence of two signal transduction pathways activated through the TCR raises the question of the relationship between the two. Are these two pathways activated independently or is one pathway dependent on the other? Several lines of evidence indicate that they are not independent and that a tyrosine kinase is responsible for activation of the PLC pathway. First, tyrosine phosphorylation can be induced through the TCR in cells in which PKC has been down-regulated pharmacologically, indicating that tyrosine kinase activation is not dependent on PKC (37). Second, anti-phosphotyrosine immunoblotting studies show that tyrosine phosphorylation of substrates can be measured as early as 5–15 s after TCR engagement by monoclonal antibodies (42). This rapid kinetics is more rapid than the generation of Ins(1,4,5)P3 or increases in intracellular Ca^{2+}, suggesting that tyrosine kinase activation precedes PLC activation. Third, pharmacological studies using the selective tyrosine kinase inhibitor herbimycin A demonstrate that tyrosine phosphorylation is required for activation of PLC through the TCR (43). Furthermore, herbimycin A also prevented IL-2 production and expression of high-affinity IL-2 receptors on T cells stimulated through the TCR. Similar results have been obtained with the tyrosine kinase inhibitor genistein (43a). These studies indicate that tyrosine kinase activation is a necessary event for effective signaling through the TCR and that PLC activation is downstream.

Tyrosine Kinase Pathway

The induction of tyrosine phosphorylation following TCR stimulation can best be understood as the end result of two competing enzymatic processes. The level of tyrosine phosphorylation of cellular proteins at any point in time is determined by the rate of phosphorylation by tyrosine kinases, balanced by the rate of dephosphorylation by tyrosine phosphatases (44). Both of these processes appear to be important in regulating tyrosine phosphorylation in T lymphocytes.

What is the TCR-activated tyrosine kinase? While the specific kinase is not known with certainty, several candidates have been proposed which are likely to play an important role in TCR signaling. First of all, unlike the ligand-activated tyrosine kinase growth factor receptors like platelet-derived growth factor receptor (PDGF-R) or epidermal growth factor receptor (EGF-R), none of the chains of the TCR shares the consensus sequence characteristic of all of the known tyrosine kinases. For this reason, it is likely that the TCR-activated tyrosine kinase is a member of a different class of tyrosine kinase, possibly the p60^{src}-related family of cytosolic tyrosine kinases. Several p60^{src}-related tyrosine kinases are expressed in hematopoietic cells in general and T-lymphocytes in particular, including p62^{yes}, p56^{lck} and p59^{fyn} (45). There is evidence for the involvement of both p56^{lck} and p59^{fyn} in TCR signaling.

The cytosolic tyrosine kinase p56^{lck} is present in T cells in large part associated with the surface receptors of CD4 and CD8 (46–49). This association is mediated by short segments of the cytosolic tail of CD4 and CD8 which have several shared amino acid residues, including two conserved cysteines, a proline and a lysine. On the p56^{lck} molecule, the region responsible for the association is in the N-terminus and includes two critical cysteine residues. It has been postulated that the cysteine residues on CD4/CD8 and p56^{lck} may form a linkage via a metal ion, as has been found in the HIV-encoded tat protein (50). Several lines of evidence suggest a role for p56^{lck} in TCR-mediated signaling. The ligands for CD4 and CD8 are invariant regions of class II and class I MHC molecules, respectively. Thus, while CD4 and CD8 are not linked to the TCR complex in resting cells, they have the potential to become associated with the TCR when it is engaged by a complex of antigen and MHC on the surface of an antigen-presenting cell. Indeed the association of CD4 and p56^{lck} is essential for antigen-specific signal transduction in certain T cells (50a). In addition, a physical association between the TCR and CD4 has been demonstrated to occur in response to TCR engagement even in the absence of antigen-presenting cells (51–54). On cross-linking of either CD4 or CD8, it has been shown that p56^{lck} autophosphorylates and acquires tyrosine kinase activity toward exogenous substrates (47). Another potential mechanism by which the CD4/p56^{lck} and CD8/p56^{lck} complex may signal is suggested by the finding that it is specifically associated with a 32 kDa GTP-binding protein (54a). To determine what role p56^{lck} might play in TCR signalling if it is activated, Abraham *et al.* transfected T cell lines with a constitutively active form of p56^{lck} (55). They found that while active p56^{lck} induced little tyrosine phosphorylation by itself, in combination with TCR stimulation there was strong synergy in tyrosine phosphorylation of substrates and synergy in the resulting IL-2 production. A major role for p56^{lck} in signal transduction events involved in T cell development is indicated by the profound deficits in thymic maturation in mice where the endogenous p56^{lck} gene was knocked out by homologous recombination (56). While these studies indicate that p56^{lck} kinase activation undoubtedly plays a major role in TCR-mediated signaling, other studies indicate a role for other tyrosine kinases as well. In certain murine T cell lines, TCR is expressed in the absence of surface CD4 or CD8. Yet, in these cells, TCR cross-linking still activates tyrosine phosphorylation and IL-2 production. Furthermore, in the C8 T cell line, cross-linking of CD4 activates p56^{lck} but cross-linking the TCR does not (47). Thus p56^{lck} cannot be the sole tyrosine kinase involved in TCR signaling.

Samelson *et al.* demonstrated the existence of a tyrosine kinase interacting directly with the TCR by co-precipitating tyrosine kinase activity with the receptor (57). Using specific antibodies they determined that the cytosolic tyrosine kinase p59^{fyn} co-precipitated with the receptor, while p62^{yes} and p56^{lck} did not. They were unable to demonstrate an increase in p59^{fyn} kinase activity in response to TCR stimulation. However, the inability to detect a change in kinase activity may be technical in nature, possibly reflecting a detergent-induced activation of p59^{fyn} in the resting cells. An important role for p59^{fyn} in T cell function is further suggested by the fact that alternate splicing of one of the exons of p59^{fyn} gives rise to a unique form of this kinase in T cells compared to other tissues where it is expressed (58). Direct evidence for a potential role for p59^{fyn} in TCR-mediated signaling is provided by transgenic studies wherein p59^{fyn} is over-expressed in thymocytes (59). In normal mice, immature CD4+CD8+ thymocytes are characterized by ten-fold lower levels of p59^{fyn} compared to mature thymocytes, and depressed responsiveness to TCR stimulation as measured by Ca^{2+} mobilization. By contrast, in the transgenic mice, p59^{fyn} expression by the immature thymocytes and TCR-stimulated Ca^{2+} mobilization are both increased to the same levels seen in the mature population. While these studies suggest an important role for p59^{fyn} in TCR signaling, there are indications that it is not the only TCR-associated tyrosine kinase. Experiments in the Jurkat human T cell line have demonstrated a TCR-associated tyrosine kinase activity which is not p59^{fyn} (60). This kinase activity is observed specifically in stimulated cells and is selectively associated with the ζ chain of the TCR. Taken together, these studies show that while p59^{fyn} can clearly associate with the TCR, other tyrosine kinases can as well. Further experiments will be required to determine whether several different cytosolic tyrosine kinases including p59^{fyn} can serve as the TCR-stimulated tyrosine kinase or whether another as yet undefined tyrosine kinase acts as the common signal-transducing kinase.

Interest in the role of tyrosine phosphatases in TCR-mediated signaling was first kindled by the discovery that the highly expressed cell surface glycoprotein CD45 is a tyrosine phosphatase, as revealed by the presence of a tandemly repeated tyrosine phosphatase domain in its cytosolic tail (61). Since that time, it has been shown that CD45 is a member of a large family of transmembrane and cytosolic tyrosine phosphatases, several members of which are expressed in T lymphocytes (62). The importance of CD45 in T cell activation was shown by the finding that certain CD45– T cell lines are incapable of proliferating in response to antigenic stimulation or cross-linking of the antigen receptor (63). However, proliferation in response to exogenously added IL-2 was intact. Koretzky *et al.* demonstrated that early signaling events are also dependent on CD45 since CD45– HPB–ALL cells did not increase intracellular Ca^{2+}, PI turnover, tyrosine phosphorylation or IL-2 production in response to engagement of the TCR (64, 65). TCR-mediated tyrosine phosphorylation is also impaired by treatment of cells with the tyrosine phosphatase inhibitor phenyl arsine oxide (PAO) (66). These studies indicate that CD45 may be involved in the very earliest events in the TCR signal transduction cascade, perhaps by regulating events required for tyrosine kinase activation.

How does CD45 function in T cell activation? One approach to understanding its function is to identify tyrosine-phosphorylated substrates. Studies cross-linking CD45 with surface activation receptors have suggested some potential substrates for CD45. The physiological relevance of these substrates is suggested by the following studies. Cross-linking of CD2 or CD3 on T lymphocytes induces T cell activation. However, if these molecules are co-aggregated with CD45, activation is inhibited as measured by the failure to increase cytosolic Ca^{2+} or IP_3 levels (42, 67). Interestingly, this CD45-mediated inhibition is correlated selectively with impairment in tyrosine phosphorylation of a 100 kDa protein substrate on anti-phosphotyrosine blotting. This 100 kDa phosphoprotein may thus represent a substrate for CD45. Alternatively, CD45 co-aggregation may inhibit activation of a tyrosine kinase which phosphorylates this protein. The requirement for the expression of CD45 to induce tyrosine kinase activation may be explained by its ability to dephosphorylate an inhibitory tyrosine phosphorylation site on p56*lck* at residue 505 and possibly on other p56*lck*-related kinases such as p59*fyn* (68, 69). In one study of three independently derived pairs of CD45– and CD45+ murine T cell lymphomas, the CD45-expressing cells were consistently deficient in phosphorylation of p56*lck* at Tyr-505. Furthermore, co-cross-linking CD4 with CD45 induces dephosphorylation of p56*lck* at Tyr-505 (69). Clearly, CD45 is capable of influencing the state of phosphorylation and activity of p56*lck* *in vivo*. A determination of the other *in vivo* substrates of CD45 will help to further define the role of this key regulatory molecule.

Tyrosine Kinase Substrates

Defining the tyrosine phosphorylated substrates will be critical for understanding how tyrosine kinases mediate TCR signaling. Antiphosphotyrosine blotting demonstrates upwards of ten cellular proteins whose tyrosine phosphorylation is increased significantly in response to TCR cross-linking. Micro-sequencing of proteins identified by binding to antiphosphotyrosine antibodies is currently being used to determine the identity of these substrates (39). However, some substrates may be tyrosine phosphorylated at a level too low to detect in antiphosphotyrosine blots of whole cell lysates. Another approach which has been highly productive for defining substrates has been to look for tyrosine phosphorylation of enzymes and other proteins suspected to be involved in signal transduction. Fibroblasts stimulated through tyrosine kinase growth factor receptors has been a particularly fruitful system for discovering significant tyrosine-phosphorylated substrates. Some of these same substrates have been shown to be tyrosine phosphorylated in T cells as well. A list of the currently identified tyrosine-phosphorylated substrates is provided in Table 5.1.

Table 5.1   Identified tyrosine-phosphorylated substrates in T cell activation

Stimulus	Substrate	Potential function	Ref.
TCR stimulation	$PLC_\gamma 1$	Catalyzes PI hydrolysis	70–72
	p90*vav*	Mediates transcriptional activation	76, 77
	ezrin	?Mediates cytoskeletal rearrangement	39
	TCR_ζ	Activates signal transduction	16
	CD45	Modulates tyrosine dephosphorylation	79
IL-2 stimulation	PI-3K	?Promotes proliferation	212
	$IL-2R_\beta$	Activates signal transduction	210, 220
	p56*lck*	Activates tyrosine phosphorylation	222
	raf-1	Activates serine/threonine phosphorylation	213

One of the most important tyrosine-phosphorylated substrates following TCR stimulation is phospholipase C (70–72) (Table 5.1). Several isoforms of PLC exist in cells but only the γ isoforms have SH2 (*src*-homology region 2) and SH3 domains (see below). Following TCR engagement, the γ isoform of PLC is rapidly tyrosine phosphorylated in a time course which parallels activation of PLC activity *in vivo*. Tyrosine phosphorylation of PLC_γ has been demonstrated *in vitro* to activate its enzymatic activity (73–75). These observations complement the finding that tyrosine kinase activity is required for activation of the PLC pathway of TCR signaling and support the hypothesis that tyrosine kinase activation is indeed a primary event.

A newly defined tyrosine-phosphorylated substrate which may provide insight regarding transmission of signals into the nucleus is the proto-oncogene product p95*vav* (76, 77). This protein is expressed selectively in hematopoietic cells. On cross-linking of CD3 with CD4, T lymphocytes exhibit tyrosine phosphorylation of p95*vav* as rapidly as 30 s after stimulation. The predicted amino acid sequence of p95*vav* reveals several interesting properties. It has an SH2 domain and two SH3 domains (78). These sequences allow specific association with tyrosine-phosphorylated proteins and are found on many tyrosine-phosphorylated substrates, including PLC_γ. In addition, p95^{vav} has nuclear localization signals and sequences characteristic of transcription factors, including a leucine zipper domain and a helix–loop–helix domain. These features suggest that p95^{vav} may localize to the nucleus after TCR/CD4 stimulation, where it may modulate gene transcription.

Another protein which has been shown to be a possible tyrosine kinase substrate after TCR stimulation is CD45 (79). CD45 tyrosine phosphorylation was transient. If tyrosine phosphorylation of CD45 has effects on its function, this observation may demonstrate cross-talk between tyrosine kinase and tyrosine phosphatase components involved in early signal transduction. Several other important signaling molecules have been reported to be tyrosine phosphorylated in other cell types but not yet in T cells stimulated through the TCR, in particular a set of SH2-containing proteins which includes: c-*crk*; the 85 kDa subunit of phosphatidyl inositol 3-kinase; the p21^{ras}-GTPase activating protein (*ras*-GAP); and the 62 and 190 kDa GAP-associated proteins (80). In addition, a newly described protein tyrosine phosphatase (81) also has an SH2 domain, although it has not yet been shown to be tyrosine phosphorylated.

Phospholipase C Pathway

Activation of PLC is an early event following TCR stimulation. It acts to hydrolyze PIP2 (phosphatidyl-inositolbisphosphate) to IP3 and diacylglycerol. IP3 is a hydrophilic cytosolic mediator which binds to specific receptors located in the endoplasmic reticulum (82), opening channels which release stores of Ca^{2+} into the cytosol. Increases in cytosolic Ca^{2+} are also derived from the extracellular medium. The mechanism underlying this latter Ca^{2+} flux is still controversial. In combination with Ca^{2+}, diacylglycerol binds to and activates PKC. The events subsequent to PKC activation are not known in detail because few substrates of PKC have been defined with certainty. Further complexity is added by the fact that PKC is not a single enzyme but a family of related isoforms (83). Different isoforms of PKC are activated differently and have different subcellular localization (84). PKC is known to phosphorylate the CD3-γ and -ϵ chains of CD3 (85), but the effects of this phosphorylation are not known. It is known, however, that PKC activation induces the AP-1 transcription factor which consists of c-*fos* and c-*jun*. Binding sites for AP-1 are present in the promoter region of a variety of different genes, including the IL-2 gene (4). AP-1 is also a component of NFAT (nuclearfactor of activated T cells), a transcription factor present in activated T cells, which binds to the promoter region of the IL-2 gene (86). Thus activation of PKC by PLC has the potential to induce new gene expression, and is likely to contribute to IL-2 gene expression.

While much evidence supports the model that PKC activation is respons-ible for induction of IL-2 gene expression following TCR stimulation, there is evidence that other mechanisms may be involved. Supporting a role for PKC are experiments which have shown that pharmacological activation of PKC by phorbol ester in combination with calcium ionophores is a sufficient stimulus for IL-2 production (41). In addition, recent experiments have dem-onstrated that activation of the PLC pathway in Jurkat cells through a trans-fected G-protein-coupled receptor activates IL-2 production by itself without activation of tyrosine kinases (87). However, other experiments suggest that pathways not involving PKC may also induce IL-2 production. First, in certain cells, TCR engagement has been observed to induce IL-2 production without any evidence of PI hydrolysis or any increase in intra-cellular Ca^{2+}, therefore suggesting an absence of PLC activation (88). In addition, gene transfection experiments have suggested that tyrosine kinases may induce IL-2 production by themselves. Specifically, transfection of T cell hybridoma cells with an active cytosolic tyrosine kinase ($p60^{v-src}$) led to constitutive IL-2 production in a dose-dependent manner (89). None-theless, there was no evidence of PKC activation. These studies demonstrate that tyrosine phosphorylation may contribute to IL-2 production by path-ways which do not involve PKC.

Other Mediators

A variety of other signal transduction mediators have also been implicated in TCR signaling. Some of these—including the GTP-binding protein $p21^{ras}$ and the serine/threonine kinases *raf*-1, MAP kinase and $p90^{rsk}$ kinase—were first found to be involved in signaling through tyrosine kinase growth factor receptors and subsequently found to be activated in T cells as well.

The protooncogene product *ras* is a 21 kDa monomeric GTP-binding pro-tein which is found in mutated form in a large variety of transformed cells (90). It has been shown to have growth-promoting properties, as shown by its ability to transform cells *in vitro* when mutated forms are transfected in com-bination with other oncogenes. Inactive $p21^{ras}$, found in resting cells, is bound to GDP, while active $p21^{ras}$ binds GTP; $p21^{ras}$ has an intrinsic GTPase activity which hydrolyzes the bound GTP, rendering the protein inactive. To deter-mine whether $p21^{ras}$ was activated in response to TCR stimulation, Down-ward *et al.*, compared levels of GTP- and GDP-bound $p21^{ras}$ in resting and activated T cells (91). They found that TCR stimulation led to a substantial, rapid increase in the proportion of $p21^{ras}$ in the GTP-bound, active form. Increases in GTP-bound $p21^{ras}$ can occur by either of two mechanisms: there can be an increase in the guanine nucleotide exchange rate, thereby substitut-ing the more abundant GTP for GDP; alternatively, there can be a decrease in the intrinsic GTPase activity of $p21^{ras}$, leading to stabilization of the GTP-bound form. Cellular enzymes have been characterized which mediate both these activities: guanine nucleotide exchange factors (92) and GAP enzymatic activities, respectively. Downward *et al.* determined that increases in GTP-bound p21*ras* following TCR stimulation occurred because of a decrease in GAP activity in the cell with no change in the rate of nucleotide exchange. The proteins *ras*-GAP (93, 94) and NF1 (95–97) have both been shown to regulate the intrinsic GTPase activity of p21*ras*. However, it is not currently known what protein is responsible for regulating *ras* GTPase following TCR stimulation. Pharmacological activation of PKC also activates p21*ras* and decreases cellular activation, but it is not known whether this is the only mechanism responsible for the effects of TCR stimulation on *ras* activation (98).

The demonstration that p21*ras* is activated when the TCR is engaged suggests that it may serve to mediate some of the transcriptional effects of TCR stimulation. Support for this possibility is provided by studies of Baldari *et al.*, who introduced constitutively active p21*ras* into murine EL-4 T cells (99). Ordinarily these cells require calcium ionophore and phorbol ester for IL-2 production. While p21*ras* alone did not induce IL-2 gene expression, it did substitute for phorbol ester, allowing IL-2 gene expression with calcium ionophore alone. IL-2 production by these transfected cells in response to calcium ionophore was not inhibited by the PKC inhibitor H7. While the effects of H7 are not completely specific for PKC, these results suggest that p21*ras* activation is upstream of PKC in the sequence of events leading to new gene transcription.

The cytosolic protein *raf-1* (also known as c-*raf*) is a cytosolic serine/ threonine kinase which is activated within minutes of TCR stimulation (100). *raf-1* has been shown to occupy a key position in signal transduction through many different growth factor receptors (101–104). Down-regulation of *raf-1* protein by anti-sense mRNA expression prevents proliferation of fibro blasts in response to serum or purified growth factors (105). In addition, expression of constitutively active *raf-1* has been shown to induce expression of a variety of new genes, including c-fos (106) and a member of the jun gene family (107), showing that receptor-mediated activation of *raf-1* may influence transcriptional events. In murine T lymphocytes, TCR stimulation induces hyperphosphorylation of a majority of the *raf-1* present in the cell. The enzymatic activity of *raf-1* also increases with TCR stimulation as measured *in vitro* by phosphorylation of both endogenous and exogenous substrates. The pathway of activation of *raf-1* through the TCR has been shown to depend on the activation of PKC, as it is abolished in PKC-depleted cells. In this respect, the TCR behaves differently from growth factor receptors where *raf-1* activation is independent of PKC (108). In human T cells, *raf-1* activation occurs rapidly, reaching peak levels as early as 30 s after TCR cross-linking by anti-CD3 monoclo nal antibodies (39).

Nonetheless, it requires activation of both a tyrosine kinase and a tyrosine phosphatase, demonstrating that *raf-1* activation is downstream of these other signal transduction mediators. These observations suggest that the early events following TCR stimulation are coordinated in a highly efficient manner which allows coupling of the receptor to *raf-1* through a series of intermediate events with minimal delay. An important key to determining the role of *raf-1* will be to define its substrates *in vivo*. In view of the known effects of *raf-1* on gene transcription and the observed translocation of *raf-1* to the nucleus (109, 110), it is likely that *raf-1* activation mediates some of the transcription events following TCR stimulation, perhaps by phosphorylating nuclear factors involved in gene expression.

The study of signal transduction pathways activated following stimulation of tyrosine kinase growth factor receptors has revealed the existence of a protein kinase cascade wherein one protein kinase phosphorylates and activates another, thereby propagating the signal. Among the known growth factor-activated protein kinases are the serine/threonine kinases MAP kinase and p90^{rsk}. These kinases have also been shown to be activated in response to TCR stimulation (111). MAP kinase was first named for its ability to phosphorylate microtubule-associated protein-2 (112). MAP kinase is believed to phosphorylate and activate the serine/threonine kinase p90^{rsk} *in vivo*, supporting the likelihood of a protein kinase cascade. *In vitro* data suggests it may also phosphorylate a range of other substrates, including the transcription factors myc and jun; however, further experiments are required to assess whether it has the same effect *in vivo*. MAP kinase has been shown to be activated by phosphorylation on both tyrosine and threonine residues (113, 114). Enzyme activities capable of catalyzing these phosphorylation events have been isolated from activated cells, but the identity of the proteins involved has not yet been determined (112, 115, 116). In T lymphocytes, MAP kinase has been shown to be activated in response to cross-linking of both CD3 and CD2 (117, 118). Phorbol ester stimulation also activates MAP kinase, suggesting that the PLC–PKC pathway may be involved. However, depletion of PKC only partially inhibits activation of MAP kinase, raising the possibility that a PKC-independent pathway may participate as well. Studies of Ettehadieh *et al.* suggest that the CD4/p56^{lck} complex may be involved, since they found that cross-linking of CD3 molecules activated MAP kinase in a CD4+ T cell line but not in a matched CD4-non-expressing line (119). MAP kinase also serves as a substrate for p56^{lck} *in vitro*; however, it has not been demonstrated that p56^{lck} phosphorylates MAP kinase directly *in vivo*. In addition, the tyrosine phosphatase CD45 may play a role in turning off MAP kinase after cell activation (117, 120). Thus, tyrosine phosphorylation and dephosphorylation may mediate both the positive and negative regulation of MAP kinase activity.

CYCLOSPORIN A AND FK 506

The immunosuppressants cyclosporin A (CSA), FK 506, and rapamycin have provided substantial insight into later signal transduction events following TCR stimulation (121, 122). Many studies have shown that these agents selectively inhibit calcium-dependent pathways of T cell activation that lead to lymphokine gene transcription (123). These agents are relatively selective for T cells, and their effects are specific for the mode of T cell activation, in that they are ineffective at preventing T cell activation by calcium-independent pathways (124). CSA and FK 506 inhibit essentially identical aspects of T cell activation, while rapamycin has distinct effects. Both CSA and FK 506 efficiently inhibit TCR-induced lymphokine gene transcription, T cell proliferation, and TCR-induced apoptosis (125, 126). In contrast, rapamycin interferes with lymphokine signal transduction, a process not inhibited by CSA or FK 506. Indeed, Sigal and co-workers made the intriguing observation that rapamycin is able to reverse the effects of FK 506 by competitive binding to the same intracellular receptor (127).

Both CSA and FK 506 bind to distinct families of intracellular immunophilin receptors: the cyclophilins and FK binding proteins (FKBP), respectively (128, 129). Cyclophilin and FKBPs are peptidyl-prolyl *cis–trans* isomerases (rotamases) that are expressed at abundant levels in many tissues, and are thought to be involved in the assembly of newly translated proteins (130). CSA inhibits the rotamase activity of cyclophilin, although it has never been clear as to how this would confer the relatively specific effects of CSA on lymphokine gene transcription. Several lines of evidence indicate that CSA and FK 506 do not function simply by inhibiting the function of their respective intracellular immunophilin receptors. For example, analogs of CSA exist that bind to and inhibit rotamase activity of cyclophilin, and yet are not immunosuppressive (131). Thus, rotamase inhibition cannot explain the immunosuppressive effects of these agents.

A current model to explain the immunosuppressive effects of CSA on T cell activation is shown in Figure 5.2. Calcineurin is a calcium- and calmodulin-dependent serine/threonine phosphatase that is expressed in the brain and in T lymphocytes. Recently, it was found that both cyclophilin and FKBPs can bind to calcineurin, forming a ternary complex of immunosuppressant, immunophilin, and calmodulin (132, 133). Thus, the effector complex potentially consists of at least six components, as calcineurin consists of a 61 kDa A subunit, containing the catalytic phosphatase site and a binding site for calmodulin, and a regulatory 19 kDa B subunit, containing a calcium binding site (Figure 5.2). The model to explain the effects of FK 506 is essentially the same, except that FK 506 would encounter calcineurin via an FKBP. This model is likely to become even more complex. For example,

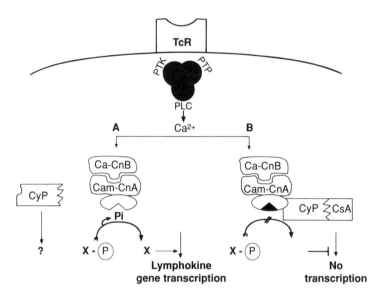

Figure 5.2. Model of cyclosporin A-mediated immunosuppression. The interaction of the TCR with antigenic ligand on APC results in protein tyrosine kinase (PTK), protein tyrosine phosphatase (PTP) and phospholipase C (PLC) activity, generating increased $[Ca^{2+}]i$. (A) In the absence of cyclosporin A (CsA), calcium interacts with calcineurin B (CnB) and forms a complex with calmodulin and calcineurin A (Cam–CnA). Calcineurin phosphatase activity results in dephosphorylation of protein X, which is required for the induction of cytokine gene transcription. The physiological function of the rotamase cyclophilin (CyP) is unknown. (B) In the presence of CsA, CsA binds to CyP, and the resulting complex binds to the calcineurin (Ca^{2+}–CnB–Cam–CnA) complex, inhibiting phosphatase activity. Protein X remains phosphorylated, and cytokine gene transcription is prevented

both cyclophilin and FK 506 belong to distinct families of proteins, of which new members are continually being appreciated (133, 134).

Both CSA and FK 506 inhibit calcineurin phosphatase activity (135). The inhibition of cellular calcineurin phosphatase activity occurs at similar or identical concentration of CSA or FK 506 to those required to inhibit cellular IL-2 production (135). Thus, calcineurin appears to be the relevant intracellular target of CSA and FK 506. Furthermore, these findings indicate that the calcineurin phosphatase is likely to play a crucial role in signal transduction in T cell activation (136). Finally, the physiological functions of immunophilins in the absence of immunosuppressants remains unknown.

CO-STIMULATORY RECEPTORS

Normal T cells or T cell clones do not proliferate in response to TCR ligation by antigen unless other signals are provided by antigen-presenting cells

(APC) (13). In most cases, the co-stimulatory signal provided by the APC requires cell contact, while in some instances soluble factors have been shown to provide an efficient co-stimulatory signal. For example, in the mouse, interleukin 1 (IL-1) produced by APC appears to provide a co-stimulatory signal to T_H2 clones that produce IL-4 (137). However, soluble factors do not appear to provide the co-stimulatory signals in the case of mouse T_H1 clones that produce IL-2. Most normal human and mouse CD4+ T cells appear to require the interaction of adhesion receptors between the T cell and the APC in order to deliver the co-stimulatory signal, as purified CD4+ T cells or T cell clones do not produce IL-2 when cultured on planar lipid membranes that contain antigen-bearing MHC class II ligands unless APC are also present (13).

Results from several laboratories indicate that the signal provided by the CD28 adhesion receptor is capable of providing a co-stimulatory signal. CD28 is a 44 kDa glycoprotein expressed as a homodimer on the surface of most peripheral blood T cells and thymocytes (138). CD28 is a member of a receptor family that also includes CTLA-4, a molecule that is expressed in activated T cells (139). In both mouse and man, anti-CD28 mAbs have stimulatory effects that greatly enhance IL-2 production and proliferation of T cells stimulated with anti-CD3 mAb or mitogenic lectins (138, 140).

The B7 or BB-1 receptor is a 45 kDa antigen that is expressed on activated B cells and monocytes (141, 142). B7 is the counter-receptor for both the CD28 and CTLA-4 receptors that are expressed on T cells (143, 144). The cross-linking of MHC class II molecules on APC induces B7 expression (145). Transfection of non-lymphoid cells with B7 cDNA confers co-stimulatory properties to the cells in conjunction with anti-CD3 mAb or lectins (146). Alloantigen-induced T cell proliferation can be prevented if the interaction between CD28 and B7 is blocked (145). Further evidence for the role of CD28 and B7 interaction in providing a second signal during T cell activation is derived from observations that the efficiency of APC function correlates with B7 expression: the ability of B cell lymphoma lines to stimulate T cell proliferation in a mixed lymphocyte culture is correlated with the density of B7 expression (147). Furthermore, small B cells that have little or no B7 expression stimulate T cells poorly, and in some instances may even elicit T cell tolerance (148). In contrast, activated B cells display efficient APC function.

The biochemical pathway used by the CD28 receptor remains poorly understood. In resting T cells, ligation of CD28 by mAb does not induce calcium mobilization, in contrast to TCR or CD2 cross-linking (149). Inhibition of protein tyrosine kinase activity by herbimycin A prevents CD28-induced IL-2 production, and ligation of the CD28 receptor by anti-CD28 mAb induces tyrosine phosphorylation in T cells (150). Chinese hamster ovary (CHO) cells transfected with B7 cDNA induce tyrosine phosphorylation in T cells. CD28-induced tyrosine phosphorylation differs from TCR-induced tyrosine phosphorylation in several aspects. The pattern of substrate tyrosine phosphorylation differs after CD28 and TCR ligation. TCR ligation induces tyrosine phosphorylation of the TCR ζ chain, while CD28 ligation does not. Resting T cells do not respond to CD28 ligation, while resting T cells respond to TCR ligation. In contrast, after activation by anti-TCR or PMA, T cells have a strong response to CD28 ligation.

A central question concerning the role of accessory molecules in T cell activation is whether or not the accessory signal is enhancing the signals provided by the T cell receptor, or whether the signal is distinct from the T cell receptor. Several studies indicate that CD28 functions independently from the T cell receptor during the course of T cell activation. CD28 appears to initiate a signal transduction pathway distinct from the T cell receptor, in part because CD28 stimulation was shown to enhance lymphokine production even in the presence of maximal phorbol ester and calcium ionophore stimulation, signals that mimic those provided by the TCR (151). In addition, increased mRNA levels and secretion of IL-2, interferon-γ, GM-CSF, and TNF-α can all be induced by a combination of PMA and anti-CD28 stimulation (152). This means of producing IL-2 is completely resistant to suppression by cyclosporin A in normal T cells. In contrast, the major transcriptional stimulation of IL-2 mediated by the T cell receptor or phorbol ester plus calcium ionophore can be completely abolished by cyclosporin A.

The primary mechanism by which anti-CD28 augments lymphokine production in mature T cells is by inhibiting the degradation of lymphokine mRNAs (153). As a result of the stabilization of mRNA, the steady state levels of lymphokines increase, leading to enhanced translation and protein secretion. In addition to a primary effect on mRNA stability, co-stimulation of quiescent T cells with anti-CD3 and anti-CD28 does appear to have a number of secondary effects on T cell responses. Late after stimulation, IL-2 mRNA levels appear to be enhanced by a CD28-dependent increase in transcription as well as mRNA stability. This appears to be the major mechanism whereby CD28 stimulation increases lymphokine production in the Jurkat leukemia line (154). Weiss and colleagues have identified a DNA binding protein that binds to a site in the IL-2 promotor that is distinct from the previously described sites and is required for CD28-mediated responses (154). Thus, it appears that CD28 may increase lymphokine production by several mechanisms. The binding site mediating CD28 effects is functional in primary T cells (155) as well as in Jurkat cells; however, the biochemical signal provided by CD28 appears to differ in that the transcriptional increases in IL-2 production are cyclosporin A sensitive in Jurkat cells while in primary T cells they are cyclosporin A resistant (156). It remains to be determined whether this reflects heterogeneity of signal transduction among primary T cells, or whether this is a phenomenon limited to transformed cell lines.

CD28 appears to have other effects beyond its role in lymphokine secretion. The binding of CD28 mAb to T cells induces increased adhesion of several integrin receptors (157), and it is possible that these receptors might induce some of the effects attributed to CD28 stimulation. CD28 stimulation by mAb or by B7-expressing cells induces cytotoxic activity in resting CD8+ T cells (158). It is not yet clear if this is a direct effect of CD28-mediated signal transduction, or if lymphokines produced consequent to CD28 activation might play a role in the cytotoxicity.

OTHER SIGNALING MOLECULES INVOLVED IN T CELL ACTIVATION

There is a growing number of surface molecules other than growth factor receptors that are involved in T cell activation (Table 5.2). The molecules listed in the table are candidate receptors that are currently known or suspected to be involved in T cell activation. Some of the molecules are expressed on activated and resting T cells, while others are found on activated T cells only, so it is likely that some of the molecules have distinct functions that may be limited to certain phases of the cell cycle. For most of the receptors, a ligand has been discovered that is present on accessory cells or

Table 5.2 Cell surface accessory receptors involved in signal transduction and T cell activation

T cell accessory receptor	Counter-receptor[a]	Ref.[b]
CD2	LFA-3 (CD58)	159–168
CD4	MHC class II	46–48, 55, 169, 170
CD8	MHC class I	171–172
CD5 (Ly-1)	CD72 (Lyb-2)	173–175
CD6	?	176, 177
LFA-1 (CD11a/CD18)	ICAM (CD54)	183–186, 192
CD28	B7	140–158
CTLA-4[c]	B7	139
Thy-1[d]	?	187–189
Ly-6[d]	?	190
Heat-stable antigen[d]	?	191
CD69[c]	?	197–200
MHC class II[c]	?CD4	178
CD26	Collagen	180–182
VLA-4[c]	Fibronectin	192, 194, 195
VLA-5[c]	Fibronectin	193, 194
VLA-6[c]	Laminin	192, 195, 196

[a]In some cases the existence of a ligand (counter-receptor) is not known (?).
[b]References selected indicate potential *in vitro* or *in vivo* role of T cell surface molecules in T cell activation.
[c]Surface expression in activated T cells and not on resting T cells.
[d]Antigens expressed on mouse T cells.

in the extracellular matrix, while in other cases a ligand (soluble or cell bound) is not known to exist, and the function of the molecule on T cells is inferred from the *in vitro* effects of monoclonal antibodies that are presumed to mimic physiological ligands upon binding. In almost all cases it is not yet known if the receptors are involved in physiological T cell activation that occurs *in vivo*. These receptors should also be considered as potential candidates that might be involved in certain forms of pathological T cell activation.

In many cases it is difficult to distinguish whether the molecules function by increasing intracellular adhesion, thereby augmenting or sustaining signals delivered through the TCR, or, alternatively, by transmitting a signal independent of the TCR. Shaw and colleagues have addressed this question by immobilizing ligands for accessory receptors on beads, and asking whether the ligand can deliver a co-stimulatory signal to T cells when immobilized on a different bead, or only when immobilized on the same bead that is coated with anti-CD3 mAb (159). Co-stimulation occurring only when the two ligands are immobilized on the same bead is termed "local co-stimulation" while co-stimulation occurring with the ligands on different beads is termed "remote co-stimulation", and indicates that the accessory signal cannot function simply by increasing adhesion and thereby promoting TCR signaling.

CD2 is an adhesion receptor that is expressed on T cells and NK cells. The physiological role of CD2 remains unknown, and it has been argued that the early expression of CD2 in T cell ontogeny may signify a role in T cell differentiation (160). Treatment of mice with anti-CD2 mAbs *in vivo* is able to induce T cell unresponsiveness (168). There appear to be several counter-receptors for CD2, one of which is CD58 (LFA-3). CD2 is able to activate phospholipase C in T cells and NK cells (160, 164), and it appears that CD2 can increase phospholipase A2 activity (165). It remains controversial as to whether CD2 can function independent of the TCR in T cells; however, most studies indicate that it cannot (162). Antigen-specific T cell responses were found to be augmented in T cells that were transfected with CD2 cDNA that lacked the cytoplasmic tail, suggesting that adhesion rather than signaling is a primary function of CD2 (163). On the other hand, Shaw and co-workers found that CD2 could deliver "remote co-stimulation" (159), implying that a component of the signal delivered by CD2 is independent of adhesion.

CD4 and CD8 function in MHC-restricted antigen presentation by binding to invariant regions of the MHC molecules on APC, and these interactions promote antigen recognition and signaling by the TCR. As discussed above, CD4 transmits signals important for T cell activation via the associated protein tyrosine kinase p56^{lck} (169, 170). CD4 cross-linking increases activity of the *lck* kinase but it does not activate phospholipase C. CD8 is expressed as a homodimer or a heterodimer, and transmits signals after interaction with the counter-receptor MHC class I molecule that is expressed on APC. The binding of CD8 to MHC class I proteins is increased upon signal transduction through the TCR (172). There is evidence that the signal delivered by CD8-αβ heterodimers differs from that of cells that express CD8-αα homodimers (171).

CD5 is expressed on T cells, and at low levels on some B cells. The counter-receptor for CD5 is CD72, which is found on B cells (173). Cross-linking of CD5 with mAbs co-stimulates with CD3, and activates PI metabolism and tyrosine phosphorylation (174, 175). In some cases CD5 stimulation by particular CD5 mAbs is able to activate protein kinase C in the absence of detectable PI breakdown or calcium mobilization (175). Signal transduction by CD5 appears to require surface expression of the TCR on T cells. It is not yet known if the binding of the natural ligand to CD5 also activates T cells. In the mouse, the homologous molecule Ly-1 appears to have similar functional effects.

The binding of mAb to LFA-1, or the addition of its purified ligand ICAM-1 to T cells, causes "remote" co-stimulation (159). TCR-mediated signal transduction increases adhesion of T cells, in part, by an increase in the avidity of LFA-1 for ICAM-1 (183). LFA-1 cross-linking on T cells results in increased $[Ca^{2+}]_i$ when CD11a (LFA-1 α) but not when anti-CD18 (LFA-1 β) chain mAbs are used (186). Furthermore, LFA-1 mAbs prolong CD3-induced calcium signals over that observed when CD3 alone is used (185). The administration of mAbs to LFA-1 and ICAM-1 prevents cardiac allograft rejection, and appears to result in the induction of specific tolerance (184). Thus, while the mechanism for this very interesting effect remains to be determined, it is likely that the signal delivered by the interaction between LFA-1 and ICAM-1 provides an important co-stimulatory signal in the context of alloantigen presentation, and may be important in regulating T cell proliferation and tolerance induction.

In the mouse, monoclonal antibodies to Thy-1 or Ly-6 cause potent co-stimulatory effects on T cells, and activate phospholipase C (188–190). Unlike other co-stimulatory molecules, these molecules have a glycosyl PI linkage, and are associated with tyrosine kinases of the *src* family (187). Studies to date indicate that Thy-1 and Ly-6 require the presence of the TCR in order to provide a complete signal, although, as discussed below, these molecules appear to be able to activate programmed cell death in the absence of TCR expression.

Antibodies to CD69 augment CD3-induced proliferation of T cells (197, 198). CD69 is associated with a GTP binding protein (199). While the signal transduction pathway used by CD69 remains unknown, the binding of anti-CD69 increases transcription factor AP-1 activity (200). Heat-stable antigen is a mouse antigen that provides a co-stimulatory effect for CD4+ T cells during antigen-induced activation (191). Ligands for CD69 and heat-stable antigen have not yet been discovered.

MHC class I and class II molecules are expressed on APC and are thought to play an important role in antigen-mediated T cell activation via their associated counter-receptors on T cells, CD8 and CD4. MHC class I products are expressed on all T cells, while activated human T cells express MHC class II, and evidence is accumulating that these molecules themselves might function as signal transduction molecules on T cells. For example, the cross-linking of MHC class I and II molecules on T cells causes increased calcium and increased cellular tyrosine phosphorylation (178, 179). Surprisingly, the cytoplasmic domain of the MHC class I molecule is not required for signal transduction (179). The physiological relevance of this form of activation is unknown, although it is possible that super-antigens, as ligands for MHC class II molecules, may be able to directly activate T cells that express MHC class II molecules. Further studies will be required to explore whether signal transduction by these molecules on T cells might contribute to certain forms of immunopathology.

The integrins VLA-4, VLA-5 and VLA-6 (very late antigen) are able to provide co-stimulatory effects to T cells (193–195). The ligands for these molecules are components of the extracellular matrix. The mechanism of the co-stimulatory effects are not yet clear but these interactions may be important in various aspects of tissue inflammation.

LYMPHOKINE-MEDIATED SIGNALING

While TCR stimulation prepares T cells for proliferation by promoting the movement of cells into the G1 phase of the cell cycle (201–203), completion of the cell cycle requires stimulation by growth-promoting lymphokines. Both IL-2 and IL-4 can induce proliferation in receptor-bearing cells. The receptor for IL-4 and the β chain of the IL-2 receptor belong to the cytokine receptor super-family (204–206). This family is quite large and includes the receptors for GM-CSF, IL-3, IL-5 and IL-6. These receptors share certain motifs in their extracellular domain, including the short stretch Trp-Ser-X-Trp-Ser (where X can be any amino acid) seen in all members of this family (207). None of these receptors encode enzymatic activity in their cytosolic tails, so it is believed that they couple indirectly to signal transduction pathways. Many members of this receptor family, including both the IL-2 and IL-4 receptor, activate tyrosine phosphorylation (208–210). While little is known about the early events following stimulation of cells with IL-4, a great deal of information is available regarding the molecular events underlying IL-2 effects.

Many of the same signal-transducing elements found to be activated by tyrosine kinase–growth factor receptors have been implicated in the action of IL-2. In particular, it has been shown that $p21^{ras}$ is activated, as measured by an increase in the ratio of the active GTP- to the inactive GDP-bound forms

(98, 211). In contrast, IL-4 stimulation does not activate *ras*, suggesting clear differences in the actions of these receptors in spite of their structural homologies (211). Phosphatidyl inositol 3-kinase (PI-3K) is activated rapidly in response to IL-2 stimulation (212). In fact, this enzyme also becomes associated with the IL-2 receptor in a ligand-dependent manner. PI-3K has been shown to associate with tyrosine kinase–growth factor receptors by a specific association between its SH2 domain and a tyrosine phosphate residue in the tyrosine kinase (81). However, the region of the IL-2 receptor responsible for PI-3K binding has not yet been defined. The serine/threonine kinase *raf-1* has also been shown to be activated in response to IL-2 (213).

A novel signal transduction pathway involving the generation of inositol phosphoglycan has also been implicated in the proliferative response to IL-2. This pathway was initially described as a component of the cellular response to insulin (214–216) and nerve growth factor (217). In responsive cells, the substrate is a distinctive glycosylphosphatidyl inositol (GPI) situated in the plasma membrane. On ligand binding, GPI is hydrolyzed by a specific PLC, generating the hydrophobic myristylated diacylglycerol (myr-DAG) and the soluble product inositol phosphoglycan (IP-glycan). In T and B lymphocyte lines expressing high-affinity IL-2 receptors, it has been found that IL-2 induces the hydrolysis of GPI in a dose-dependent manner, as measured by the generation of both products (218, 219). The induction is rapid, with peak effects seen at 2 minutes in the B lymphocyte line BCL_1 and at 30 seconds in the T lymphocyte line CTLL. The biological importance of GPI hydrolysis is suggested by two observations. First, GPI hydrolysis parallels proliferation in the BCL_1 line (218). In these cells, IL-4 antagonizes both the proliferative effects of IL-2 and the ability of IL-2 to induce GPI hydrolysis. Second, purified IP-glycan synergizes with IL-2 in CTLL cells, as demonstrated by a shift in the EC_{50} for IL-2 from 20 to 7 pM (219). This last study suggests that GPI hydrolysis is a rate-limiting component of the response to IL-2 but is not by itself sufficient for proliferation. The mechanism by which IL-2 induces GPI hydrolysis and the relationship (if any) with tyrosine phosphorylation is currently unknown.

Several lines of evidence suggest that tyrosine kinase activation is important in the action of IL-2. IL-2 induces rapid phosphorylation of a number of substrates in responsive cells (208, 210, 213), including the β chain of the IL-2 receptor itself (Table 5.1) (210, 220). A potential mechanism of coupling of the receptor to tyrosine phosphorylation is suggested by the finding that the β chain is physically associated with a tyrosine kinase activity. One component of this activity appears to be the cytosolic tyrosine kinase p56[lck], as shown by its co-precipitation with the receptor (221). In fact, p56[lck] is activated in response to IL-2 stimulation (222). The region of the β chain responsible for p56[lck] association is a serine-rich region in the cytosolic tail. Currently the significance of the association is unclear since deletion mutants have shown that it is an acidic domain and not this serine-rich region that is required for signal transduction through the IL-2 receptor (223). Fung *et al.* have also explored the association of protein kinases with the high-affinity IL-2 receptor (224). They found both a tyrosine kinase and a serine/threonine kinase activity co-precipitating with the receptor. Interestingly, association with the tyrosine kinase required the presence of the same acidic region previously shown to be required for IL-2 signaling. In contrast, the serine/threonine kinase associated with a different region situated in the C-terminus which was also required for growth. The identity of these protein kinases has not yet been determined. These data indicate that the cytosolic tail of the β chain of the IL-2 receptor is composed of multiple domains which independently associate with a variety of protein kinases. The observation that domains involved in binding the protein kinases are also essential for growth suggests that these kinases are critical components of IL-2 signaling.

POTENTIAL ORPHAN PATHWAYS OF SIGNAL TRANSDUCTION IN T CELL ACTIVATION

Historically, the first well-characterized signal transduction pathway involved the cyclic nucleotide-dependent kinase family. However, today the functional role of cyclic nucleotides in lymphocyte activation and metabolism remains unknown. Cross-linking of the TCR with mAbs causes increases in cAMP concentration, and mitogenic lectins increase T cell cAMP levels (149, 225, 226). Lectins also increase the activity of cyclic nucleotide-dependent phosphodiesterases in T cells (227). The mechanisms and significance of these effects remain poorly understood.

A diverse group of phospholipases, in addition to PLC, have been shown to be activated in lymphocytes. Phospholipase D is activated in T cells after TCR stimulation (228). A magnesium-dependent PLC is activated in a subset of mouse B cells after antigen receptor cross-linking (229).

Various metabolic products of sphingomyelin may function in signal transduction. Ceramide is produced by sphingomyelinase and is an inhibitor of PKC. Ceramide analogs stimulate threonine phosphorylation of the EGF-R in A431 carcinoma cells (230). Ceramide treatment results in the differentiation of the HL-60 leukemic cell line (231). TNF-α stimulates a rapid increase in ceramide concentration in cell-free lysates of HL-60 cells, and an increase in ceramide-activated protein kinase activity (232, 233). Thus this pathway may be important for TNF signal transduction, and might play a role in T cell activation.

Diverse biochemical pathways are involved in lymphocyte activation. The emphasis of this chapter has been on the regulation of the signal transduction cascades that are thought to be most relevant to subsequent function of

T cells. It is likely that still other pathways of major significance are yet to be appreciated.

SIGNAL TRANSDUCTION AND APOPTOSIS

Apoptosis or programmed cell death is a multi-step biochemical process that eventuates in cell suicide (234). This process is distinct from necrosis—the death of cells from non-specific injury. Apoptosis is important in immune function, and is thought to be critical in T cell development as a means of selecting the T cell repertoire by removing self-reactive T cells. The bcl-2 proto-oncogene is expressed in the inner mitochondrial membrane, and the transforming mechanism of the bcl-2 oncogene appears to involve inhibiting cell death rather than by stimulating cell proliferation. Over-expression of the bcl-2 gene can protect thymocytes from many forms of cell death, such as corticosteroid, radiation and anti-CD3-induced apoptosis. However, bcl-2 cannot protect thymocytes from antigen-induced cell death, leading to the conclusion that there are multiple pathways in T cells leading to apoptosis (235).

The signal transduction pathways involved in the activation of programmed T cell death are only beginning to be understood. Antigen or anti-CD3 stimulation induces programmed cell death in thymocytes and transformed T cell lines (236–238). Thus, a basic paradox has emerged concerning how the signals delivered by the TCR result in either cellular proliferation or cell death. It is not yet resolved whether the differentiation state of the T cell determines the outcome, or whether there are differences in the signals delivered. Newell and co-workers found that mouse splenic T cells could be induced to proliferate or undergo cell death, depending on whether CD4 and the TCR were cross-linked independently or together, arguing that signals, in addition to the state of cellular differentiation, control the functional outcome (239). The signals delivered by cytokines also appear to select whether TCR stimulation by antigen leads to cell death or cell proliferation (240).

The induction of cell death in T cell hybridomas appears to be biphasic. The first phase is the establishment of cell cycle arrest at the G1/S interface, and occurs within an hour of anti-CD3 stimulation. This phase does not require extracellular calcium and is cyclosporin A insensitive. The second phase eventuates in cell lysis, and can be prevented by EGTA (ethyline bis[oxyethylenenitrilo]tetraacetic acid) and cyclosporin A, indicating that signal transduction involving calcium is required (241).

As was mentioned above, there appear to be distinct biochemical pathways leading to programmed T cell death. Both anti-CD3 and corticosteroids are able to induce cell death in thymocytes, yet these pathways are mutually antagonistic, as anti-CD3-induced cell death is prevented in the presence of corticosteroids (242). Furthermore, cyclosporin A blocked anti-CD3-induced cell death but enhanced corticosteroid-induced cell death (242, 243). Agents that increase cAMP concentration cause apoptosis in thymocytes, while agents that activate PKC are able to inhibit programmed cell death (244, 245). The signals provided by IL-1 and anti-CD28 are also able to inhibit programmed cell death in some instances (246, 247). Thus, many receptor-mediated signal transduction events are able to inhibit TCR-induced cell death. Further studies will be required to determine whether these signals are involved in the decision to select T cell proliferation or cell death after antigen encounter. It is also possible that the inadvertent delivery of some of these signals could operate pathologically to prevent cell death, and thereby permit the emergence of autoreactive T cell clones and subsequent autoimmune disease.

Heat shock or ionizing radiation are able to induce apoptosis in lymphoma cell lines. Baxter and Lavin found that the induction of apoptosis in these lines was associated with dephosphorylation of a specific set of proteins (248). Okadaic acid, an inhibitor of protein serine/threonine phosphatases, was able to prevent apoptosis and the dephosphorylation of the proteins, suggesting that activation of phosphatases or loss of kinase activity are important in some forms of apoptosis.

The mouse accessory activation receptors Thy-1 and Ly-6 are able to trigger T cell proliferation and IL-2 production, as was mentioned above. This proliferative signal is dependent on the surface expression of the TCR. Nickas and co-workers found that Thy-1 and Ly-6 are also able to trigger programmed cell death. In contrast to T cell activation, the cell death induced by Thy-1 and Ly-6 occurs in the absence of the TCR, further indicating that the signals regulating cellular activation and apoptosis are distinct (249).

The Fas antigen is a 52 kDa transmembrane protein that has structural homology to tumor necrosis factor receptor and to the low-affinity nerve growth factor receptor. A ligand for this receptor has not yet been discovered. The antigen is expressed in various tissues, including thymocytes and a number of mature T cell lines. Cross-linking of the Fas antigen can lead to apoptosis in thymocytes and activated T cells (250). Recently, *lpr* mice were shown to have mutations in the Fas gene (251). As this strain of mice develops a lymphoproliferative disorder of T cells and is prone to autoimmune disease, the results indicate that the Fas antigen may have an important role in the form of programmed cell death that occurs in the thymus to remove autoreactive T cells. There is as yet no information concerning the signal transduction pathway controlled by the Fas receptor.

There is increasing evidence to indicate that HIV-1 infection may kill T cells by inducing apoptosis (252). CD4+T cells isolated from HIV-1-infected patients early in the course of the illness undergo apoptosis when stimulated with antigen (247). Interestingly, the signal delivered by anti-CD28 was able to prevent cell death in these cells. Thus, the immunodeficiency associated with this infection may result, in part, from a signal delivered by HIV-1 to the T cell that programs the cells for suicide upon subsequent antigen activation. Together with the results of Newell and co-workers, who found that CD4 cross-linking with mAb could prime mature T cells to undergo cell death after anti-TCR stimulation (239), these findings suggest that one function of the CD4 receptor might be to modulate the TCR signal to result in cellular proliferation or cell death.

SIGNALS INVOLVED IN INDUCTION OF T CELL TOLERANCE

Tolerance is an example of a situation where engagement of the TCR, typically by self antigen, leads to inactivation of the receptor-bearing cells. In some cases self tolerance is maintained by the functional inactivation (anergy) of T cells expressing TCR specific for certain self antigens, while in other cases there is deletion of the reactive clones. Bretcher and Cohn first proposed a two-signal model of lymphocyte activation to explain how antigen-specific T cell activation could either result in T cell proliferation or anergy (253). Schwartz and colleagues have developed an *in vitro* cell culture model of anergy that displays many of the features predicted by the Bretcher and Cohn hypothesis. In this model, signal 1 is delivered by TCR occupancy, and signal 2 is delivered by the interaction of a co-stimulatory receptor on APC with a counter-receptor on T cells. If signal 1 is delivered in the absence of signal 2, a long-lasting state of unresponsiveness in mouse T_H1 clones and in some human CD4+ T cell clones is produced (13). The cells remain viable and will proliferate if exogenous IL-2 is added; however, the cells do not produce IL-2 or proliferate when subsequently exposed to APC pulsed with antigen. Conversely, T cell proliferation results when both signal 1 and signal 2 are delivered.

During the induction of anergy, signals are transduced by the TCR, including production of the second messengers calcium and Ins(1,4,5)P3, leading to the conclusion that signal 1 is normal during the induction of this form of anergy. Further, the TCR does not appear to be desensitized in anergic T cells, as antigen-unresponsive T cells transduce normal signals after reexposure to antigen or after anti-CD3 mAb cross-linking. Efforts to date have not identified a specific co-stimulatory signal, although co-stimulatory signals do not appear to involve PLC (13). The transcription factors that are thought to regulate IL-2 gene expression may provide a biochemical signature to indicate the induction of unresponsiveness or T cell proliferation. When T cell clones are cultured in conditions that induce anergy, NFAT is not induced, and only one of two subunits of NK-κB are induced (254). These changes appear to be specific, as other transcription factors such as

AP-1 appear to be normally induced in the same cell cultures. The signal transduction cascades responsible for the induction of these transcription factors remain to be elucidated.

Several candidate receptors on APC have been proposed to function as the co-stimulatory receptor involved in T cell activation. In the mouse T_H1 model of anergy, the CD28 receptor appears to deliver a co-stimulatory signal, as anti-CD28 mAb is able to prevent the induction of non-responsiveness (140). Furthermore, a soluble fusion protein consisting of CTLA-4 and the IgG FcR can prevent or delay cardiac allograft rejection in the rat (255). Presumably, the mechanism responsible for this effect is that soluble CTLA-4 is able to prevent the interaction of B7 and endogenous cell surface CD28, as CTLA-4 is a higher-affinity ligand for B7 than is CD28. The *in vivo* administration of mouse anti-CD2 mAb can result in the induction of unresponsiveness to antigens (168). In a rat allograft model of heart transplantation, the administration of anti-LFA-3 and anti-ICAM-1 mAbs is able to induce antigen-specific tolerance (184). Thus it is likely that multiple mechanisms may be employed to induce T cell anergy, and that several phenotypic states of unresponsiveness exist. To date, there is no evidence to indicate which mechanisms are operating *in vivo* in the various states of tolerance described above.

CONCLUSIONS

Substantial progress has been made in defining signal transduction pathways activated in response to stimulation through T lymphocyte cell surface receptors. Yet, in several important ways, gaps remain in our understanding of how T cells respond on the molecular level. Currently, many components have been identified in signal transduction through the various receptors. Further work will be required to order these components into coherent pathways and to determine in each case whether signaling proceeds in a linear manner from one component to the next or if multiple independent pathways operate in parallel. In addition, more experiments will be required to specify which of the signaling components are essential and which are dispensable. The goal of signal transduction studies is to derive a complete picture of how receptor engagement at the plasma membrane ultimately leads to the important nuclear events which underlie new gene expression. At the present, the mechanism by which the different signal transduction components interact has not been defined. However, the biochemical basis for interactions between different components is becoming better understood. Clearly, kinases—which regulate a multitude of substrates—and subdomains of proteins which participate in protein–protein interactions—like the SH2 domains—represent examples of how connections are made between different signaling molecules in responses mediated by many different receptors.

The picture which emerges from our current understanding of signal transduction appears quite complex. What is the utility to the immune system of having so many different elements involved in signaling? One likely explanation is that these signaling pathways originally evolved as part of the response to quite different stimuli. During evolution, receptors specific for T lymphocytes became coupled to several of these pre-existing signal transduction pathways and acquired their specificity based at least in part on the particular combination of pathways activated. Such a combinatorial mechanism of receptor specificity is likely since distinct receptors can activate some of the same signaling pathways yet retain their distinct effector function. The activation of p21^{ras} by stimulation of both the TCR and the IL-2 receptor provides just one example. Another result of the complexity is to provide multiple levels at which signaling pathways can interact with each other. Such interactions may cause synergistic or inhibitory effects when two different receptors are activated simultaneously. Further studies of this form of receptor crosstalk may help to explain the complex interactions between the many different T lymphocyte receptors and accessory molecules. Such studies will undoubtedly help to extend our molecular understanding of the complex phenomena of T cell biology.

ACKNOWLEDGEMENTS

This report was supported by NMRDC #M0095.007-1003. The views expressed in this chapter are those of the authors and do not reflect the official policy or position of the Department of the Navy, Department of Defense, or the United States Government.

REFERENCES

1. Ullrich, A. and Schlessinger, J. (1990) Signal transduction by receptors with tyrosine kinase activity. *Cell*, **61**, 203–212.
2. Taga, T., Hibi, M., Hirata, Y., Yamasaki, K., Yasukawa, K., Matsuda, T., Hirano, T. and Kishimoto, T. (1989) Interleukin-6 triggers the association of its receptor with a possible signal transducer, gp130. *Cell*, **58**, 573–581.
3. Crabtree, G.R. (1989) Contingent genetic regulatory events in T lymphocyte activation. *Science*, **243**, 355–361.
4. Ullman, K.S., Northrop, J.P., Verweij, C.L. and Crabtree, G.R. (1990) Transmission of signals from the T lymphocyte antigen receptor to the genes responsible for cell proliferation and immune function: The missing link. *Annu. Rev. Immunol.*, **8**, 421–452.
5. Finkel, T.H., Marrack, P., Kappler, J.W., Kubo, R.T. and Cambier, J.C. (1989) Alpha beta T cell receptor and CD3 transduce different signals in immature T cells: Implications for selection and tolerance. *J. Immunol.*, **142**, 3006–3012.
6. Lewis, D.B., Larsen, A. and Wilson, C.B. (1986) Reduced interferon-gamma mRNA levels in human neonates: Evidence for an intrinsic T cell deficiency

independent of other genes involved in T cell activation. *J. Exp. Med.*, **163**, 1018–1023.

7. Gajewski, T.F., Schell, S.R. and Fitch, F.W. (1990) Evidence implicating utilization of different T cell receptor-associated signaling pathways by TH1 and TH2 clones. *J. Immunol.*, **144**, 4110–4120.

8. Betz, M. and Fox, B.S. (1991) Prostaglandin E2 inhibits production of Th1 lymphokines but not of Th2 lymphokines. *J. Immunol.*, **146**, 108–113.

9. Makgoba, M.W., Sanders, M.E. and Shaw, S. (1989) The CD2–LFA-3 and LFA-1-ICAM pathways: Relevance to T-cell recognition. *Immunol. Today*, **10**, 417–422.

10. Horgan, K.J., Van Seventer, G.A., Shimizu, Y. and Shaw, S. (1990) Hyporesponsiveness of "naive" (CD45RA+) human T cells to multiple receptor-mediated stimuli but augmentation of responses by co-stimuli. *Eur. J. Immunol.*, **20**, 1111–1118.

11. Sanders, M.E., Makgoba, M.W., June, C.H., Young, H.A. and Shaw, S. (1989) Enhanced responsiveness of human memory T cells to CD2 and CD3 receptor-mediated activation. *Eur. J. Immunol.*, **19**, 803–808.

12. Blackman, M.A., Finkel, T.H., Kappler, J., Cambier, J. and Marrack, P. (1991) Altered antigen receptor signaling in anergic T cells from self-tolerant T-cell receptor beta-chain transgenic mice. *Proc. Nat. Acad. Sci. USA*, **88**, 6682–6686.

13. Schwartz, R.H. (1990) A cell culture model for T lymphocyte clonal anergy. *Science*, **248**, 1349–1356.

14. Ashwell, J.D. and Klausner, R.D. (1990) Genetic and mutational analysis of the T-cell antigen receptor. *Annu. Rev. Immunol.*, **8**, 139–167.

15. Klausner, R.D., Lippincott-Schwartz, J. and Bonifacino, J.S. (1990) The T cell antigen receptor: Insights into organelle biology. *Annu. Rev. Cell. Biol.*, **6**, 403–431.

16. Samelson, L.E., Patel, M.D., Weissman, A.M., Harford, J.B. and Klausner, R.D. (1986) Antigen activation of murine T cells induce tyrosine phosphorylation of a polypeptide associated with the T cell antigen receptor. *Cell*, **46**, 1083–1090.

17. Baniyash, M., Garcia-Morales, P., Bonifacino, J.S., Samelson, L.E. and Klausner, R.D. (1988) Disulfide linkage of the zeta and eta chains of the T cell receptor: Possible identification of two structural classes of receptors. *J. Biol. Chem.*, **263**, 9874–9878.

18. Orloff, D.G., Ra, C.S., Frank, S.J., Klausner, R.D. and Kinet, J.P. (1990) Family of disulphide-linked dimers containing the zeta and eta chains of the T-cell receptor and the gamma chain of Fc receptors. *Nature*, **347**, 189–191.

19. Saito, H., Koyama, T., Georgopoulos, K., Clevers, H., Haser, W.G., LeBien, T., Tonegawa, S. and Terhorst, C. (1987) Close linkage of the mouse and human CD3 gamma- and delta-chain genes suggests that their transcription is controlled by common regulatory elements. *Proc. Nat. Acad. Sci. USA*, **84**, 9131–9134.

20. Gold, D.P., Clevers, H., Alarcon, B., Dunlap, S., Novotny, J., Williams, A.F. and Terhorst, C. (1987) Evolutionary relationship between the T3 chains of the T-cell receptor complex and the immunoglobulin supergene family. *Proc. Nat. Acad. Sci. USA*, **84**, 7649–7653.

21. Weissman, A.M., Baniyash, M., Hou, D., Samelson, L.E., Burgess, W.H. and Klausner, R.D. (1988). Molecular cloning of the zeta chain of the T cell antigen receptor. *Science*, **239**, 1018–1021.

22. Weissman, A.M., Hou, D., Orloff, D.G., Modi, W.S., Seuanez, H., O'Brien, S.J. and Klausner, R.D. (1988) Molecular cloning and chromosomal localization of

the human T-cell receptor zeta chain: Distinction from the molecular CD3 complex. *Proc. Nat. Acad. Sci. USA*, **85**, 9709–9713.

23. Kuster, H., Thompson, H. and Kinet, J.P. (1990) Characterization and expression of the gene for the human Fc receptor gamma subunit: Definition of a new gene family. *J. Biol. Chem.*, **265**, 6448–6452.

24. Clayton, L.K., D'Adamio, L., Howard, F.D., Sieh, M., Hussey, R.E., Koyasu, S. and Reinherz, E.L. (1991) CD3 eta and CD3 zeta are alternatively spliced products of a common genetic locus and are transcriptionally and/or post-transcriptionally regulated during T-cell development. *Proc. Nat. Acad. Sci. USA*, **88**, 5202–5206.

25. Raulet, D.H. (1989) The structure, function, and molecular genetics of the gamma/delta T cell receptor. *Annu. Rev. Immunol.*, **7**, 175–207.

26. Allison, J.P. and Raulet, D.H. (1990) The immunobiology of gamma delta+ T cells. *Semin. Immunol.*, **2**, 59–65.

27. Blumberg, R.S., Ley, S., Sancho, J., Lonberg, N., Lacy, E., McDermott, F., Schad, V., Greenstein, J.L. and Terhorst, C. (1990) Structure of the T-cell antigen receptor: Evidence for two CD3 epsilon subunits in the T-cell receptor–CD3 complex. *Proc. Nat. Acad. Sci. USA*, **87**, 7220–7224.

28. Coulie, P.G., Uyttenhove, C., Wauters, P., Manolios, N., Klausner, R.D., Samelson, L.E. and Van Snick, J. (1991) Identification of a murine monoclonal antibody specific for an allotypic determinant on mouse CD3. *Eur. J. Immunol.*, **21**, 1703–1709.

29. Alarcon, B., Ley, S.C., Sanchez-Madrid, F., Blumberg, R.S., Ju, S.T., Fresno, M. and Terhorst, C. (1991) The CD3-gamma and CD3-delta subunits of the T cell antigen receptor can be expressed within distinct functional TCR/CD3 complexes. *EMBO J.*, **10**, 903–912.

30. Bauer, A., McConkey, D.J., Howard, F.D., Clayton, L.K., Novick, D., Koyasu, S. and Reinherz, E.L. (1991) Differential signal transduction via T-cell receptor CD3 zeta 2, CD3 zeta–eta, and CD3 eta 2 isoforms. *Proc. Nat. Acad. Sci. USA*, **88**, 3842–3846.

31. Irving, B.A. and Weiss, A. (1991) The cytoplasmic domain of the T cell receptor zeta chain is sufficient to couple receptor-associated signal transduction pathways. *Cell*, **64**, 891–901.

32. Romeo, C. and Seed, B. (1991) Cellular immunity to HIV activated by CD4 fused to T cell or Fc receptor polypeptides. *Cell*, **64**, 1037–1046.

33. Letourneur, F. and Klausner, R.D. (1992) Activation of T cells by a tyrosine kinase activation domain in the cytoplasmic tail of CD3 epsilon. *Science*, **255**, 79–82.

34. Wegener, A.M., Letourneur, F., Hoeveler, A., Brocker, T., Luton, F. and Malissen, B. (1992) The T cell receptor/CD3 complex is composed of at least two autonomous transduction modules. *Cell*, **68**, 83–95.

35. Romeo, C., Amiot, M. and Seed, B. (1992) Sequence requirements for induction of cytolysis by the T cell antigen/Fc receptor zeta chain. *Cell*, **68**, 889–897.

36. Keegan, A.D. and Paul, W.E. (1992) Multichain immune recognition receptors: Similarities in structure and signaling pathways. *Immunol. Today*, **13**, 63–68.

37. Patel, M.D., Samelson, L.E. and Klausner, R.D. (1987) Multiple kinases and signal transduction: Phosphorylation of the T cell antigen receptor complex. *J. Biol. Chem.*, **262**, 5831–5838.

38. Klausner, R.D. and Samelson, L.E. (1991) T cell antigen receptor activation pathways: The tyrosine kinase connection. *Cell*, **64**, 875–878.

39. Siegel, J.N., Egerton, M., Phillips, A.F. and Samelson, L.E. (1991) Multiple signal transduction pathways activated through the T cell receptor for antigen. *Semin. Immunol.*, **3**, 325–334.

40. Weiss, A., Irving, B.A., Tan, L.K. and Koretzky, G.A. (1991) Signal transduction by the T cell antigen receptor. *Semin. Immunol.*, **3**, 313–324.

41. Weiss, A., Imboden, J., Hardy, K., Manger, B., Terhorst, C. and Stobo, J. (1986) The role of the T3/antigen receptor complex in T-cell activation. *Annu. Rev. Immunol.*, **4**, 593–619.

42. June, C.H., Fletcher, M.C., Ledbetter, J.A. and Samelson, L.E. (1990) Increases in tyrosine phosphorylation are detectable before phospholipase C activation after T cell receptor stimulation. *J. Immunol.*, **144**, 1591–1599.

43. June, C.H., Fletcher, M.C., Ledbetter, J.A., Schieven, G.L., Siegel, J.N., Phillips, A.F. and Samelson, L.E. (1990) Inhibition of tyrosine phosphorylation prevents T-cell receptor-mediated signal transduction. *Proc. Nat. Acad. Sci. USA*, **87**, 7722–7726.

43a. Mustelin, T., Coggeshall, K.M., Isakov, N. and Altman, A. (1990) T cell antigen receptor-mediated activation of phospholipase C requires tyrosine phosphorylation. *Science*, **247**, 1584–1587.

44. Hunter, T. (1990) Protein-tyrosine phosphatases: The other side of the coin. *Cell*, **58**, 1013–1016.

45. Eiseman, E. and Bolen, J.B. (1990) src-related tyrosine protein kinases as signaling components in hematopoietic cells. *Cancer Cells*, **20**, 303–310.

46. Rudd, C.E., Trevillyan, J.M., Dasgupta, J.D., Wong, L.L. and Schlossman, S.F. (1988) The CD4 receptor is complexed in detergent lysates to a protein-tyrosine kinase (pp58) from human T lymphocytes. *Proc. Nat. Acad. Sci. USA*, **85**, 5190–5194.

47. Veillette, A., Bookman, M.A., Horak, E.M. and Bolen, J.B. (1988) The CD4 and CD8 T cell surface antigens are associated with the internal membrane tyrosine-protein kinase p56lck. *Cell*, **55**, 301–308.

48. Turner, J.M., Brodsky, M.H., Irving, B.A., Levin, S.D., Perlmutter, R.M. and Littman, D.R. (1990) Interaction of the unique N-terminal region of tyrosine kinase p56lck with cytoplasmic domains of CD4 and CD8 is mediated by cysteine motifs. *Cell*, **60**, 755–765.

49. Shaw, A.S., Chalupny, J., Whitney, J.A., Hammond, C., Amrein, K.E., Kavathas, P., Sefton, B.M. and Rose, J.K. (1990) Short related sequences in the cytoplasmic domains of CD4 and CD8 mediate binding to the amino-terminal domain of the p56lck tyrosine protein kinase. *Mol. Cell. Biol.*, **10**, 1853–1862.

50. Frankel, A.D., Bredt, D.S. and Pabo, C.O. (1988) Tat protein from human immunodeficiency virus forms a metal-linked dimer. *Science*, **240**, 70–73.

50a. Glaichenhaus, N., Shastri, N., Littman, D.R. and Turner, J.M. (1991) Requirement for association of p56lck with CD4 in antigen-specific signal transduction in T cells. *Cell*, **64**, 511–520.

51. Saizawa, K., Rojo, J. and Janeway, C.A., Jr (1987) Evidence for a physical association of CD4 and the CD3:alpha:beta T-cell receptor. *Nature*, **328**, 260–263.

52. Kupfer, A., Singer, S.J., Janeway, C.A., Jr and Swain, S.L. (1987) Coclustering of CD4 (L3T4) molecule with the T-cell receptor is induced by specific direct interaction of helper T cells and antigen-presenting cells. *Proc. Nat. Acad. Sci. USA*, **84**, 5888–5892.

53. Anderson, P., Blue, M.L. and Schlossman, S.F. (1988) Comodulation of CD3 and CD4: Evidence for a specific association between CD4 and approximately

5% of the CD3:T cell receptor complexes on helper T lymphocytes. *J. Immunol.,* **140**, 1732–1737.

54. Mittler, R.S., Goldman, S.J., Spitalny, G.L. and Burakoff, S.J. (1989) T-cell receptor–CD4 physical association in a murine T-cell hybridoma: Induction by antigen receptor ligation. *Proc. Nat. Acad. Sci. USA,* **86**, 8531–8535.

54a. Telfer, J.C. and Rudd, C.E. (1991) A 32-kD GTP-binding protein associated with the CD4–p56lck and CD8–p56lck T cell receptor complexes. *Science,* **254**, 439–441.

55. Abraham, N., Miceli, M.C., Parnes, J.R. and Veillette, A. (1991) Enhancement of T-cell responsiveness by the lymphocyte-specific tyrosine protein kinase p56lck. *Nature,* **350**, 62–66.

56. Molina, T.J., Kishihara, K., Siderovski, D.P., van Ewijk, W., Narendran, A., Timms, E., Wakeham, A., Paige, C.J., Hartmann, K.U., Veillette, A. *et al.* (1992) Profound block in thymocyte development in mice lacking p56lck. *Nature,* **357**, 161–164.

57. Samelson, L.E., Phillips, A.F., Luong, E.T. and Klausner, R.D. (1990) Association of the fyn protein–tyrosine kinase with the T-cell antigen receptor. *Proc. Nat. Acad. Sci. USA,* **87**, 4358–4362.

58. Cooke, M.P. and Perlmutter, R.M. (1989) Expression of a novel form of the fyn proto-oncogene in hematopoietic cells. *New Biol.,* **1**, 66–74.

59. Cooke, M.P., Abraham, K.M., Forbush, K.A. and Perlmutter, R.M. (1991) Regulation of T cell receptor signaling by a src family protein–tyrosine kinase (p59fyn). *Cell,* **65**, 281–291.

60. Chan, A.C., Irving, B.A., Fraser, J.D. and Weiss, A. (1991) The zeta chain is associated with a tyrosine kinase and upon T-cell antigen receptor stimulation associates with ZAP-70, a 70-kDa tyrosine phosphoprotein. *Proc. Nat. Acad. Sci. USA,* **88**, 9166–9170.

61. Charbonneau, H., Tonks, N.K., Walsh, K.A. and Fischer, E.H. (1988) The leukocyte common antigen (CD45): A putative receptor-linked protein tyrosine phosphatase. *Proc. Nat. Acad. Sci. USA,* **85**, 7182–7186.

62. Trowbridge, I.S. (1991) CD45: A prototype for transmembrane protein tyrosine phosphatases. *J. Biol. Chem.,* **266**, 23517–23520.

63. Pingel, J.T. and Thomas, M.L. (1989) Evidence that the leukocyte-common antigen is required for antigen-induced T lymphocyte proliferation. *Cell,* **58**, 1055–1065.

64. Koretzky, G.A., Picus, J., Thomas, M.L. and Weiss, A. (1990) Tyrosine phosphatase CD45 is essential for coupling T-cell antigen receptor to the phosphatidyl inositol pathway. *Nature,* **346**, 66–86.

65. Koretzky, G.A., Picus, J., Schultz, T. and Weiss, A. (1991) Tyrosine phosphatase CD45 is required for T-cell antigen receptor and CD2-mediated activation of a protein tyrosine kinase and interleukin 2 production. *Proc. Nat. Acad. Sci. USA,* **88**, 2037–2041.

66. Garcia-Morales, P., Minami, Y., Luong, E., Klausner, R.D. and Samelson, L.E. (1990) Tyrosine phosphorylation in T cells is regulated by phosphatase activity: Studies with phenylarsine oxide. *Proc. Nat. Acad. Sci. USA,* **87**, 9255–9259.

67. Ledbetter, J.A., Schieven, G.L., Uckun, F.M. and Imboden, J.B. (1991) CD45 cross-linking regulates phospholipase C activation and tyrosine phosphorylation of specific substrates in CD3/Ti-stimulated T cells. *J. Immunol.,* **146**, 1577–1583.

68. Ostergaard, H.L., Shackelford, D.A., Hurley, T.R., Johnson, P., Hyman, R., Sefton, B.M. and Trowbridge, I.S. (1989) Expression of CD45 alters

phosphorylation of the lck-encoded tyrosine protein kinase in murine lymphoma T-cell lines. *Proc. Nat. Acad. Sci. USA*, **86**, 8959–8963.

69. Ostergaard, H.L. and Trowbridge, I.S. (1990) Coclustering CD45 with CD4 or CD8 alters the phosphorylation and kinase activity of p56lck. *J. Exp. Med.*, **172**, 347–350.
70. Weiss, A., Koretzky, G., Schatzman, R.C. and Kadlecek, T. (1991) Functional activation of the T-cell antigen receptor induces tyrosine phosphorylation of phospholipase C-gamma 1. *Proc. Nat. Acad. Sci. USA*, **88**, 5484–5488.
71. Park, D.J., Min, H.K. and Rhee, S.G. (1992) Inhibition of CD3-linked phospholipase C by phorbol ester and by cAMP is associated with decreased phosphotyrosine and increased phosphoserine contents of PLC-gamma 1. *J. Biol. Chem.*, **267**, 1496–1501.
72. Secrist, J.P., Karnitz, L. and Abraham, R.T. (1991) T-cell antigen receptor ligation induces tyrosine phosphorylation of phospholipase C-gamma 1. *J. Biol. Chem.*, **266**, 12135–12139.
73. Nishibe, S., Wahl, M.I., Hernandez-Sotomayor, S.M., Tonks, N.K., Rhee, S.G. and Carpenter, G. (1990) Increase of the catalytic activity of phospholipase C-gamma 1 by tyrosine phosphorylation. *Science*, **250**, 1253–1256.
74. Goldschmidt-Clermont, P.J., Kim, J.W., Machesky, L.M., Rhee, S.G. and Pollard, T.D. (1991) Regulation of phospholipase C-gamma 1 by profilin and tyrosine phosphorylation. *Science*, **251**, 1231–1233.
75. Kim, H.K., Kim, J.W., Zilberstein, A., Margolis, B., Kim, J.G., Schlessinger, J. and Rhee, S.G. (1991) PDGF stimulation of inositol phospholipid hydrolysis requires PLC-gamma 1 phosphorylation on tyrosine residues 783 and 1254. *Cell*, **65**, 435–441.
76. Bustelo, X.R., Ledbetter, J.A. and Barbacid, M. (1992) Product of vav proto-oncogene defines a new class of tyrosine protein kinase substrates. *Nature*, **356**, 68–71.
77. Margolis, B., Hu, P., Katzav, S., Li, W., Oliver, J.M., Ullrich, A., Weiss, A. and Schlessinger, J. (1992) Tyrosine phosphorylation of vav proto-oncogene product containing SH2 domain and transcription factor motifs. *Nature*, **356**, 71–74.
78. Koch, C.A., Anderson, D., Moran, M.F., Ellis, C. and Pawson, T. (1991) SH2 and SH3 domains: Elements that control interactions of cytoplasmic signaling proteins. *Science*, **252**, 668–674.
79. Stover, D.R., Charbonneau, H., Tonks, N.K. and Walsh, K.A. (1991) Protein-tyrosine-phosphatase CD45 is phosphorylated transiently on tyrosine upon activation of Jurkat T cells. *Proc. Nat. Acad. Sci. USA*, **88**, 7704–7707.
80. Cantley, L.C., Auger, K.R., Carpenter, C., Duckworth, B., Graziani, A., Kapeller, R. and Soltoff, S. (1991) Oncogenes and signal transduction. *Cell*, **64**, 281–302.
81. Shen, S.H., Bastien, L., Posner, B.I. and Chretien, P. (1991) A protein–tyrosine phosphatase with sequence similarity to the SH2 domain of the protein–tyrosine kinases [published erratum appears in *Nature* (1991), **353**, 868]. *Nature*, **352**, 736–739.
82. Furuichi, T., Yoshikawa, S., Miyawaki, A., Wada, K., Maeda, N. and Mikoshiba, K. (1989) Primary structure and functional expression of the inositol 1,4,5-trisphosphate-binding protein P400. *Nature*, **342**, 32–38.
83. Nishizuka, Y. (1988) The molecular heterogeneity of protein kinase C and its implications for cellular regulation. *Nature*, **334**, 661–665.
84. Masmoudi, A., Labourdette, G., Mersel, M., Huang, F.L., Huang, K.P., Vincendon, G. and Malviya, A.N. (1989) Protein kinase C located in rat liver nuclei:

Partial purification and biochemical and immunochemical characterization. *J. Biol. Chem.*, **264**, 1172–1179.

85. Davies, A.A., Cantrell, D.A., Hexham, J.M., Parker, P.J., Rothbard, J. and Crumpton, M.J. (1987) The human T3 gamma chain is phosphorylated at serine 126 in response to T lymphocyte activation. *J. Biol. Chem.*, **262**, 10918–10921.

86. Jain, J., McCaffrey, P.G., Valge-Archer, V.E. and Rao, A. (1992) Nuclear factor of activated T cells contains Fos and Jun. *Nature*, **356**, 801–804.

87. Desai, D.M., Newton, M.E., Kadlecek, T. and Weiss, A. (1990) Stimulation of the phosphatidylinositol pathway can induce T-cell activation. *Nature*, **348**, 66–69.

88. Sussman, J.J., Mercep, M., Saito, T., Germain, R.N., Bonvini, E. and Ashwell, J.D. (1988) Dissociation of phosphoinositide hydrolysis and Ca^{2+} fluxes from the biological responses of a T-cell hybridoma. *Nature*, **334**, 625–628.

89. O'Shea, J.J., Ashwell, J.D., Bailey, T.L., Cross, S.L., Samelson, L.E. and Klausner, R.D. (1991) Expression of v-src in a murine T-cell hybridoma results in constitutive T-cell receptor phosphorylation and interleukin 2 production. *Prod. Nat. Acad. Sci. USA*, **88**, 1741–1745.

90. Barbacid, M. (1987) ras genes. *Annu. Rev. Biochem.*, **56**, 779–827.

91. Downward, J., Graves, J.D., Warne, P.H., Rayter, S. and Cantrell, D.A. (1990) Stimulation of p21ras upon T-cell activation. *Nature*, **346**, 719–723.

92. Martegani, E., Vanoni, M., Zippel, R., Coccetti, P., Brambilla, R., Ferrari, C., Sturani, E. and Alberghina, L. (1992) Cloning by functional complementation of a mouse cDNA encoding a homologue of CDC25, a *Saccharomyces cerevisiae* RAS activator. *EMBO J.*, **11**, 2151–2158.

93. Hall, A. (1990) ras and GAP—who's controlling whom? *Cell*, **61**, 921–923.

94. Wigler, M.H. (1990) Oncoproteins: GAPs in understanding Ras. *Nature*, **346**, 696–697.

95. Ballester, R., Marchuk, D., Boguski, M., Saulino, A., Letcher, R., Wigler, M. and Collins, F. (1990) The NF1 locus encodes a protein functionally related to mammalian GAP and yeast IRA proteins. *Cell*, **63**, 851–859.

96. Martin, G.A., Viskochil, D., Bollag, G., McCabe, P.C., Crosier, W.J., Haubruck, H., Conroy, L., Clark, R., O'Connell, P., Cawthon, R.M. *et al.* (1990) The GAP-related domain of the neurofibromatosis type 1 gene product interacts with ras p21. *Cell*, **63**, 843–849.

97. Viskochil, D., Buchberg, A.M., Xu, G., Cawthon, R.M., Stevens, J., Wolff, R.K., Culver, M., Carey, J.C., Copeland, N.G., Jenkins, N.A. *et al.* (1990) Deletions and a translocation interrupt a cloned gene at the neurofibromatosis type 1 locus. *Cell*, **62**, 187–192.

98. Downward, J., Graves, J. and Cantrell, D. (1992) The regulation and function of p21^{ras} in T cells. *Immunol. Today*, **13**, 89–92.

99. Baldari, C.T., Macchia, G. and Telford, J.L. (1992) Interleukin-2 promoter activation in T-cells expressing activated Ha-ras. *J. Biol. Chem.*, **267**, 4289–4291.

100. Siegel, J.N., Klausner, R.D., Rapp, U.R. and Samelson, L.E. (1990) T cell antigen receptor engagement stimulates c-raf phosphorylation and induces c-raf-associated kinase activity via a protein kinase C-dependent pathway. *J. Biol. Chem.*, **265**, 18472–18480.

101. Li, P., Wood, K., Mamon, H., Haser, W. and Roberts, T. (1991) Raf-1: A kinase currently without a cause but not lacking in effects. *Cell*, **64**, 479–482.

102. Rapp, U.R. (1991) Role of Raf-1 serine/threonine protein kinase in growth factor signal transduction. *Oncogene*, **6**, 495–500.

103. Morrison, D.K. (1990) The Raf-1 kinase as a transducer of mitogenic signals. *Cancer Cells*, **2**, 377–382.

104. Bruder, J.T., Heidecker, G. and Rapp, U.R. (1992) Serum-, TPA-, and Ras-induced expression from Ap-1/Ets-driven promoters requires Raf-1 kinase. *Genes Dev.*, **6**, 545–556.

105. Kolch, W., Heidecker, G., Lloyd, P. and Rapp, U.R. (1991) Raf-1 protein kinase is required for growth of induced NIH/3T3 cells. *Nature*, **349**, 426–428.

106. Jamal, S. and Ziff, E. (1990) Transactivation of c-fos and beta-actin genes by raf as a step in early response to transmembrane signals. *Nature*, **344**, 463–466.

107. Wasylyk, C., Wasylyk, B., Heidecker, G., Huleihel, M. and Rapp, U.R. (1989) Expression of raf oncogenes activates the PEA1 transcription factor motif. *Mol. Cell. Biol.*, **9**, 2247–2250.

108. Morrison, D.K., Kaplan, D.R., Rapp, U. and Roberts, T.M. (1988) Signal transduction from membrane to cytoplasm: Growth factors and membrane-bound oncogene products increase Raf-1 phosphorylation and associated protein kinase activity. *Proc. Nat. Acad. Sci. USA*, **85**, 8855–8859.

109. Mihaly, A., Olah, Z., Krug, M., Kuhnt, U., Matthies, H., Rapp, U.R. and Joo, F. (1990) Transient increase of raf protein kinase-like immunoreactivity in the rat dentate gyrus during the long-term potentiation. *Neurosci. Lett.*, **116**, 45–50.

110. Olah, Z., Komoly, S., Nagashima, N., Joo, F., Rapp, U.R. and Anderson, W.B. (1991) Cerebral ischemia induces transient intracellular redistribution and intranuclear translocation of the raf proto-oncogene product in hippocampal pyramidal cells. *Exp. Brain Res.*, **84**, 403–410.

111. Calvo, V., Bierer, B.E. and Vik, T.A. (1992) T cell receptor activation of a ribosomal S6 kinase activity. *Eur. J. Immunol.*, **22**, 457–462.

112. Thomas, G. (1992) MAP kinase by any other name smells just as sweet. *Cell*, **68**, 3–6.

113. Anderson, N.G., Maller, J.L., Tonks, N.K. and Sturgill, T.W. (1990) Requirement for integration of signals from two distinct phosphorylation pathways for activation of MAP kinase. *Nature*, **343**, 651–653.

114. Boulton, T.G., Nye, S.H., Robbins, D.J., Ip, N.Y., Radziejewska, E., Morgenbesser, S.D., DePinho, R.A., Panayotatos, N., Cobb, M.H. and Yancopoulos, G.D. (1991) ERKs: A family of protein–serine/threonine kinases that are activated and tyrosine phosphorylated in response to insulin and NGF. *Cell*, **65**, 663–675.

115. Nakielny, S., Cohen, P., Wu, J. and Sturgill, T. (1992) MAP kinase activator from insulin-stimulated skeletal muscle is protein threonine/tyrosine kinase. *EMBO J.*, **11**, 2123–2130.

116. Rossomando, A., Wu, J., Weber, M.J. and Sturgill, T.W. (1992) The phorbol ester-dependent activator of the mitogen-activated protein kinase p42^{mapk} is a kinase with specificity for the threonine and tyrosine regulatory sites. *Proc. Nat. Acad. Sci. USA*, **89**, 5221–5225.

117. Nel, A.E., Ledbetter, J.A., Williams, K., Ho, P., Akerley, B., Franklin, K. and Katz, R. (1991) Activation of MAP-2 kinase activity by the CD2 receptor in Jurkat T cells can be reversed by CD45 phosphatase. *Immunology*, **73**, 129–133.

118. Nel, A.E., Hanekom, C., Rheeder, A., Williams, K., Pollack, S., Katz, R. and Landreth, G.E. (1990) Stimulation of MAP-2 kinase activity in T lymphocytes by anti-CD3 or anti-Ti monoclonal antibody is partially dependent on protein kinase C. *J. Immunol.*, **144**, 2683–2689.

119. Ettehadieh, E., Sanghera, J.S., Pelech, S.L., Hess-Bienz, D., Watts, J., Shastri, N. and Aebersold, R. (1992) Tyrosyl phosphorylation and activation of MAP kinases by p56lck. *Science*, **255**, 853–855.

120. Pollack, S., Ledbetter, J.A., Katz, R., Williams, K., Akerley, B., Franklin, K., Schieven, G. and Nel, A.E. (1991) Evidence for involvement of glycoprotein-CD45 phosphatase in reversing glycoprotein-CD3-induced microtubule-associated protein-2 kinase activity in Jurkat T-cells. *Biochem. J.*, **276**, 481–485.

121. Bierer, B.E., Jin, Y.J., Fruman, D.A., Calvo, V. and Burakoff, S.J. (1991) FK 506 and rapamycin: Molecular probes of T-lymphocyte activation. *Transplant. Proc.*, **23**, 2850–2855.

122. Sigal, N.H., Siekierka, J.J. and Dumónt, F.J. (1990) Observations on the mechanism of action of FK-506: A pharmacologic probe of lymphocyte signal transduction. *Biochem. Pharmacol.*, **40**, 2201–2208.

123. Baldari, C.T., Macchia, G., Heguy, A., Melli, M. and Telford, J.L. (1991) Cyclosporin A blocks calcium-dependent pathways of gene activation. *J. Biol. Chem.*, **266**, 19103–19108.

124. June, C.H., Ledbetter, J.A., Gillespie, M.M., Lindsten, T. and Thompson, C.B. (1987) T cell proliferation involving the CD28 pathway is associated with cyclosporine-resistant interleukin-2 gene expression. *Mol. Cell. Biol.*, **7**, 4472–4481.

125. Bierer, B.E., Mattila, P.S., Standaert, R.F., Herzenberg, L.A., Burakoff, S.J., Crabtree, G. and Schreiber, S.L. (1990) Two distinct signal transmission pathways in T lymphocytes are inhibited by complexes formed between an immunophilin and either FK506 or rapamycin. *Proc. Nat. Acad. Sci. USA*, **87**, 9231–9235.

126. Dumont, F.J., Staruch, M.J., Koprak, S.L., Melino, M.R. and Sigal, N.H. (1990) Distinct mechanisms of suppression of murine T cell activation by the related macrolides FK-506 and rapamycin. *J. Immunol.*, **144**, 251–258.

127. Dumont, F.J., Melino, M.R., Staruch, M.J., Koprak, S.L., Fischer, P.A. and Sigal, N.H. (1990) The immunosuppressive macrolides FK-506 and rapamycin act as reciprocal antagonists in murine T cells. *J. Immunol.*, **144**, 1418–1424.

128. Handschumacher, R.E., Harding, M.W., Rice, J., Drugge, R.J. and Speicher, D.W. (1984) Cyclophilin: A specific cystolic binding protein for cyclosporin A. *Science*, **226**, 544–547.

129. Harding, M.W., Galat, A., Uehling, D.E. and Schreiber, S.L. (1989) A receptor for the immunosuppressed FK506 is a *cis–trans* peptidyl-prolyl isomerase. *Nature*, **341**, 758–760.

130. Schreiber, S.L. (1991) Chemistry and biology of the immunophilins and their immunosuppressive ligands. *Science*, **251**, 283–287.

131. Sigal, N.H., Dumont, F., Durette, P., Siekierka, J.J., Peterson, L., Rich, D.H., Dunlap, B.E., Staruch, M.J., Melino, M.R., Koprak, S.L. *et al.* (1991) Is cyclophilin involved in the immunosuppressive and nephrotoxic mechanism of action of cyclosporin A? *J. Exp. Med.*, **173**, 619–628.

132. Liu, J., Farmer, J.D., Jr, Lane, W.S., Friedman, J., Weissman, I. and Schreiber, S.L. (1991) Calcineurin is a common target of cyclophilin–cyclosporin A and FKBP–FK506 complexes. *Cell*, **66**, 807–815.

133. Friedman, J. and Weissman, I. (1991) Two cytoplasmic candidates for immunophilin action are revealed by affinity for a new cyclophilin: One in the presence and one in the absence of CsA. *Cell*, **66**, 799–806.

134. Jin, Y.J., Albers, M.W., Lane, W.S., Bierer, B.E., Schreiber, S.L. and Burakoff, S.J. (1991) Molecular cloning of a membrane-associated human FK506- and rapamycin-binding protein, FKBP-13. *Proc. Nat. Acad. Sci. USA*, **88**, 6677–6812.

135. Fruman, D.A., Klee, C.B., Bierer, B.E. and Burakoff, S.J. (1992) Calcineurin phosphatase activity in T lymphocytes is inhibited by FK 506 and cyclosporin A. *Proc. Nat. Acad. Sci. USA,* **89**, 3686–3690.

136. McKeon, F. (1990) When worlds collide: Immunosuppressants meet protein phosphatases. *Cell,* **66**, 823–826.

137. Weaver, C.T. and Unanue, E.R. (1990) The costimulatory function of antigen-presenting cells. *Immunol. Today,* **11**, 49–55.

138. June, C.H., Ledbetter, J.A., Linsley, P.S. and Thompson, C.B. (1990) Role of the CD28 receptor in T-cell activation. *Immunol. Today,* **11**, 211–216.

139. Harper, K., Balzano, C., Rouvier, E., Mattei, M.G., Luciani, M.F. and Golstein, P. (1991) CTLA-4 and CD28 activated lymphocyte molecules are closely related in both mouse and human as to sequence, message expression, gene structure, and chromosomal location. *J. Immunol.,* **147**, 1037–1044.

140. Harding, F.A., McArthur, J.G., Gross, J.A., Raulet, D.H. and Allison, J.P. (1992) CD28-mediated signalling co-stimulates murine T cells and prevents induction of anergy in T-cell clones. *Nature,* **356**, 607–609.

141. Freeman, G.J., Freedman, A.S., Segil, J.M., Lee, G., Whitman, J.F. and Nadler, L.M. (1989) B7, a new member of the Ig superfamily with unique expression on activated and neoplastic B cells. *J. Immunol.,* **143**, 2714–2722.

142. Freedman, A.S., Freeman, G.J., Rhynhart, K. and Nadler, L.M. (1991) Selective induction of B7/BB-1 on interferon-gamma stimulated monocytes: A potential mechanism for amplification of T cell activation through the CD28 pathway. *Cell Immunol.,* **137**, 429–437.

143. Linsley, P.S., Clark, E.A. and Ledbetter, J.A. (1990) T-cell antigen CD28 mediates adhesion with B cells by interacting with activation antigen B7/BB-1. *Proc. Nat. Acad. Sci. USA,* **87**, 5031–5035.

144. Linsley, P.S., Brady, W., Urnes, M., Grosmaire, L.S., Damle, N.K. and Ledbetter, J.A. (1991) CTLA-4 is a second receptor for the B cell activation antigen B7. *J. Exp. Med.,* **174**, 561–569.

145. Koulova, L., Clark, E.A., Shu, G. and Dupont, B. (1991) The CD28 ligand B7/BB1 provides costimulatory signal for alloactivation of CD4+ T cells. *J. Exp. Med.,* **173**, 759–762.

146. Gimmi, C.D., Freeman, G.J., Gribben, J.G., Sugita, K., Freedman, A.S., Morimoto, C. and Nadler, L.M. (1991) B-cell surface antigen B7 provides a costimulatory signal that induces T cells to proliferate and secrete interleukin 2. *Proc. Nat. Acad. Sci. USA,* **88**, 6575–6579.

147. Jenkins, M.K., Taylor, P.S., Norton, S.D. and Urdahl, K.B. (1991) CD28 delivers a costimulatory signal involved in antigen-specific IL-2 production by human T cells. *J. Immunol.,* **147**, 2461–2466.

148. Eynon, E.E. and Parker, D.C. (1992) Small B cells as antigen-presenting cells in the induction of tolerance to soluble protein antigens. *J. Exp. Med.,* **175**, 131–138.

149. Ledbetter, J.A., Parsons, M., Martin, P.J., Hansen, J.A., Rabinovitch, P.S. and June, C.H. (1986) Antibody binding to CD5 (Tp67) and Tp44 molecules: Effects in cyclic nucleotides, cytoplasmic free calcium, and cAMP-mediated suppression. *J. Immunol.,* **137**, 3299–3305.

150. Vandenberghe, P., Freeman, G.J., Nadler, L.M., Fletcher, M.C., Kamoun, M., Turka, L., Ledbetter, J.A., Thompson, C.B. and June, C.H. (1992) Antibody and B7/BB1-mediated ligation of the CD28 receptor induces tyrosine phosphorylation in human T cells. *J. Exp. Med.,* **175**, 951–960.

151. June, C.H., Ledbetter, J.A., Lindsten, T. and Thompson, C.B. (1989) Evidence for the involvement of three distinct signals in the induction of IL-2 gene expression in human T lympocytes. *J. Immunol.*, **143**, 153–161.

152. Thompson, C.B., Lindsten, T., Ledbetter, J.A., Kunkel, S.L., Young, H.A., Emerson, S.G., Leiden, J.M. and June, C.H. (1989) CD28 activation pathway regulates the production of multiple T-cell-derived lymphokines/cytokines. *Proc. Nat. Acad. Sci. USA*, **86**, 1333–1337.

153. Lindsten, T., June, C.H., Ledbetter, J.A., Stella, G. and Thompson, C.B. (1989) Regulations of lymphokine messenger RNA stability by a surface-mediated T cell activation pathway. *Science*, **244**, 339–343.

154. Fraser, J.D., Irving, B.A., Crabtree, G.R. and Weiss, A. (1991) Regulation of interleukin-2 gene enhancer activity by the T cell accessory molecule CD28. *Science*, **251**, 313–316.

155. Fraser, J.D., Newton, M.E. and Weiss, A. (1992) CD28 and T cell antigen receptor signal transduction coordinately regulate interleukin 2 gene expression in response to superantigen stimulation. *J. Exp. Med.*, **175**, 1131–1134.

156. Williams, T.M., Moolten, D.M., Makni, H., Kim, H.W., Kant, J.A. and Kamoun, M. (1992) CD28-stimulated IL-2 gene expression in Jurkat T cells occurs in part transcriptionally and is cyclosporine-A sensitive. *J. Immunol.*, **148**, 2609–2616.

157. Shimizu, Y., van Seventer, G.A., Ennis, E., Newman, W., Horgan, K.J. and Shaw, S. (1992) Crosslinking of the T cell-specific accessory molecules CD7 and CD28 modulates T cell adhesion. *J. Exp. Med.*, **175**, 577–582.

158. Azuma, M., Cayabyab, M., Buck, D., Phillips, J.H. and Lanier, L.L. (1992) CD28 interaction with B7 costimulates primary allogeneic proliferative responses and cytotoxicity mediated by small, resting T lymphocytes. *J. Exp. Med.*, **175**, 353–360.

159. Van Seventer, G.A., Shimizu, Y., Horgan, K.J., Luce, G.E., Webb, D. and Shaw, S. (1991) Remote T cell co-stimulation via LFA-1/ICAM-1 and CD2/LFA-3: Demonstration with immobilized ligand/mAb and implication in monocyte-mediated co-stimulation. *Eur. J. Immunol.*, **21**, 1711–1718.

160. Haynes, B.F., Denning, S.M., Singer, K.H. and Kurtzberg, J. (1989) Ontogeny of T-cell precursors: A model for the initial stages of human T-cell development. *Immunol. Today*, **10**, 87–91.

161. June, C.H., Ledbetter, J.A., Rabinovitch, P.S., Martin, P.J., Beatty, P.G. and Hansen, J.A. (1986) Distinct patterns of transmembrane Ca^{2+} flux and intracellular Ca^{2+} mobilization after differentiation antigen 2 (E rosette receptor) or 3 (T3) stimulation of human lymphocytes. *J. Clin. Invest.*, **77**, 1224–1232.

162. Desai, D.M., Goldsmith, M.A. and Weiss, A. (1990) A transfected human muscarinic receptor fails to substitute for the T cell antigen receptor complex in CD2-initiated signal transduction. *Int. Immunol.*, **2**, 615–620.

163. Moingeon, P., Chang, H.C., Wallner, B.P., Stebbins, C., Frey, A.Z. and Reinherz, E.L. (1989) CD2-mediated adhesion facilitates T lymphocyte antigen recognition function. *Nature*, **339**, 312–314.

164. Kanner, S.B., Damle, N.K., Blake, J., Aruffo, A. and Ledbetter, J.A. (1992) CD2/LFA-3 ligation induces phospholipase-C gamma 1 tyrosine phosphorylation and regulates CD3 signaling. *J. Immunol.*, **148**, 2023–2029.

165. Le Gouvello, S., Colard, O., Theodorou, I., Bismuth, G., Tarantino, N. and Debre, P. (1990) CD2 triggering stimulates a phospholipase A2 activity besides the phospholipase C pathway in human T lymphocytes. *J. Immunol.*, **144**, 2359–2364.

166. Samelson, L.E., Fletcher, M.C., Ledbetter, J.A. and June, C.H. (1990) Activation of tyrosine phosphorylation in human T cells via the CD2 pathway: Regulation by the CD45 tyrosine phosphatase. *J. Immunol.,* **145**, 2448–2454.

167. Spruyt, L.L., Glennie, M.J., Beyers, A.D. and William, A.F. (1991) Signal transduction by the CD2 antigen in T cells and natural killer cells: Requirement for expression of a functional T cell receptor or binding of antibody Fc to the Fc receptor, Fc gamma RIIIA (CD16). *J. Exp. Med.,* **174**, 1407–1415.

168. Guckel, B., Berek, C., Lutz, M., Altevogt, P., Schirrmacher, V. and Kyewski, B.A. (1991) Anti-CD2 antibodies induce T cell unresponsiveness *in vivo. J. Exp. Med.,* **174**, 957–967.

169. Veillette, A., Bookman, M.A., Horak, E.M., Samelson, L.E. and Bolen, J.B. (1989) Signal transduction through the CD4 receptor involves the activation of the internal membrane tyrosine-protein kinase p56lck. *Nature,* **338**, 257–259.

170. Barber, E.K., Dasgupta, J.D., Schlossman, S.F., Trevillyan, J.M. and Rudd, C.E. (1989) The CD4 and CD8 antigens are coupled to a protein-tyrosine kinase (p56lck) that phosphorylates the CD3 complex. *Proc. Nat. Acad. Sci. USA,* **86**, 3277–3281.

171. Wheeler, C.J., von Hoegen, P. and Parnes, J.F. (1992) An immunological role for the CD8 β-chain. *Nature,* **357**, 247–249.

172. O'Rourke, A.M., Rogers, J. and Mescher, M.F. (1990) Activated CD8 binding to class I protein mediated by the T-cell receptor results in signalling. *Nature,* **346**, 187–189.

173. Van de Velde, H., von Hoegen, I., Luo, W., Parnes, J.R. and Thielemans, K. (1991) The B-cell surface protein CD72/Lyb-2 is the ligand for CD5. *Nature ,* **351**, 662–665.

174. June, C.H., Rabinovitch, P.S. and Ledbetter, J.A. (1987) Anti-CD5 antibodies increase cytoplasmic calcium concentration and augment CD3-stimulated calcium mobilization in T cells. *J. Immunol.,* **138**, 2782–2792.

175. Alberola-Ila, J., Places, L., Cantrell, D.A., Vives, J. and Lozano, F. (1992) Intracellular events involved in CD5-induced human T cell activation and proliferation. *J. Immunol.,* **148**, 1287–1293.

176. Swack, J.A., Gangemi, R.M., Rudd, C.E., Morimoto, C., Schlossman, S.F. and Romain, P.L. (1989) Structural characterization of CD6: Properties of two distinct epitopes involved in T cell activation. *Mol. Immunol.,* **26**, 1037–1049.

177. Aruffo, A., Melnick, M.B., Linsley, P.S. and Seed, B. (1991) The lymphocyte glycoprotein CD6 contains a repeated domain structure characteristic of a new family of cell surface and secreted proteins. *J. Exp. Med.,* **174**, 949–952.

178. Odum, N., Martin, P.J., Schieven, G.L., Masewicz, S., Hansen, J.A. and Ledbetter, J.A. (1991) HLA-DR molecules enhance signal transduction through the CD3/Ti complex in activated T cells. *Tissue Antigens,* **38**, 72–77.

179. Gur, H., el-Zaatari, F., Geppert, T.D., Wacholtz, M.C., Taurog, J.D. and Lipsky, P.E. (1990) Analysis of T cell signaling by class I MHC molecules: The cytoplasmic domain is not required for signal transduction. *J. Exp. Med.,* **172**, 1267–1270.

180. Torimoto, Y., Dang, N.H., Vivier, E., Tanaka, T., Schlossman, S.F. and Morimoto, C. (1991) Coassociation of CD26 (dipeptidyl peptidase IV) with CD45 on the surface of human T lymphocytes. *J. Immunol.,* **147**, 2514–2517.

181. Dang, N.H., Torimoto, T., Sugita, K., Daley, J.F., Schow, P., Prado, C., Schlossman, S.F. and Morimoto, C. (1990) Cell surface modulation of CD26 by anti-IF7 monoclonal antibody: Analysis of surface expression and human T cell activation. *J. Immunol.,* **145**, 3963–3971.

182. Dang, N.H., Torimoto, Y., Shimamura, K., Tanaka, T., Daley, J.F., Schlossman, S.F. and Morimoto, C. (1991) 1F7 (CD26): A marker of thymic maturation involved in the differential regulation of the CD3 and CD2 pathways of human thymocyte activation. *J. Immunol.*, **147**, 2825–2832.

183. Dustin, M.L. and Springer, T.A. (1989) T-cell receptor cross-linking transiently stimulates adhesiveness through LFA-1. *Nature,* **341**, 619–624.

184. Isobe, M., Yagita, H., Okumura, K. and Ihara, A. (1992) Specific acceptance of cardiac allograft after treatment with antibodies to ICAM-1 and LFA-1. *Science,* **255**, 1125–1127.

185. Wacholtz, M.C., Patel, S.S. and Lipsky, P.E. (1989) Leukocyte function-associated antigen 1 is an activation molecule for human T cells. *J. Exp. Med.,* **170**, 431–448.

186. Pardi, R., Bender, J.R., Dettori, C., Giannazza, E. and Engleman, E.G. (1989) Heterogeneous distribution and transmembrane signaling properties of lymphocyte function-associated antigen (LFA-1) in human lymphocyte subsets. *J. Immunol.,* **143**, 3157–3166.

187. Stefanova, I., Horejsi, V., Ansotegui, I.J., Knapp, W. and Stockinger, H. (1991) GPI-anchored cell-surface molecules complexed to protein tyrosine kinases. *Science,* **254**, 1016–1019.

188. Gunter, K.C., Germain, R.N., Kroczek, R.A., Saito, T., Yokoyama, W.M., Chan, C., Weiss, A. and Shevach, E.M. (1987) Thy-1-mediated T-cell activation requires co-expression of CD3/Ti complex. *Nature,* **326**, 505–507.

189. Kroczek, R.A., Gunter, K.C., Germain, R.N. and Shevach, E.M. (1986) Thy-1 functions as a signal transduction molecule in T lymphocytes and transfected B lymphocytes. *Nature,* **322**, 181–184.

190. Rock, K.L., Reiser, H., Bamezai, A., McGrew, J. and Benacerraf, B. (1989) The LY-6 locus: A multigene family encoding phosphatidylinositol-anchored membrane proteins concerned with T-cell activation. *Immunol. Rev.,* **111**, 195–224.

191. Liu, Y., Jones, B., Aruffo, A., Sullivan, K.M., Linsley, P.S. and Janeway, C.A., Jr (1992) Heat-stable antigen is a costimulatory molecule for CD4 T cell growth. *J. Exp. Med.,* **175**, 437–445.

192. Shimizu, Y., van Seventer, G.A., Horgan, K.J. and Shaw, S. (1990) Roles of adhesion molecules in T-cell recognition: Fundamental similarities between four integrins on resting human T cells (LFA-1, VLA-4, VLA-5, VLA-6) in expression, binding, and costimulation. *Immunol. Rev.,* **114**, 109–143.

193. Matsuyama, T., Yamada, A., Kay, J., Yamada, K.M., Akiyama, S.K., Schlossman, S.F. and Morimoto, C. (1989) Activation of CD4 cells by fibronectin and anti-CD3 antibody: A synergistic effect mediated by the VLA-5 fibronectin receptor complex. *J. Exp. Med.,* **170**, 1133–1148.

194. Davis, L.S., Oppenheimer-Marks, N., Bednarczyk, J.L., McIntyre, B.W. and Lipsky, P.E. (1990) Fibronectin promotes proliferation of naive and memory T cells by signaling through both the VLA-4 and VLA-5 integrin molecules. *J. Immunol.,* **145**, 785–793.

195. Shimizu, Y., van Seventer, G.A., Horgan, K.J. and Shaw, S. (1990) Costimulation of proliferative responses of resting CD4+ T cells by the interaction of VLA-4 and VLA-5 with fibronectin or VLA-6 with laminin. *J. Immunol.,* **145**, 59–67.

196. Shimizu, Y., van Seventer, G.A., Horgan, K.J. and Shaw, S. (1990) Regulated expression and binding of three VLA (beta 1) integrin receptors on T cells. *Nature,* **345**, 250–253.

197. Nakamura, S., Sung, S.S., Bjorndahl, J.M. and Fu, S.M. (1989) Human T cell activation. IV. T cell activation and proliferation via the early activation antigen EA 1. *J. Exp. Med.*, **169**, 677–689.

198. Testi, R., Phillips, J.H. and Lanier, L.L. (1989) T cell activation via Leu-23 (CD69). *J. Immunol.*, **143**, 1123–1128.

199. Risso, A., Smilovich, D., Capra, M.C., Baldissarro, I., Yan, G., Bargellesi, A. and Cosulich, M.E. (1991) CD69 in resting and activated T lymphocytes: Its association with a GTP binding protein and biochemical requirements for its expression. *J. Immunol.*, **146**, 4105–4114.

200. Tugores, A., Alonso, M.A., Sanchez-Madrid, F. and de Landazuri, M.O. (1992) Human T cell activation through the activation-inducer molecule/CD69 enhances the activity of transcription factor AP-1. *J. Immunol.*, **148**, 2300–2306.

201. Stern, J.B. and Smith, K.A. (1986) Interleukin-2 induction of T-cell G1 progression and c-myb expression. *Science*, **233**, 203–206.

202. Meuer, S.C., Hussey, R.E., Cantrell, D.A., Hodgdon, J.C., Schlossman, S.F., Smith, K.A. and Reinherz, E.L. (1984) Triggering of the T3–Ti antigen–receptor complex results in clonal T-cell proliferation through an interleukin 2-dependent autocrine pathway. *Proc. Nat. Acad. Sci. USA*, **81**, 1509–1513.

203. Gromo, G., Geller, R.L., Inverardi, L. and Bach, F.H. (1987) Signal requirements in the step-wise functional maturation of cytotoxic T lymphocytes. *Nature*, **327**, 424–426.

204. Galizzi, J.P., Zuber, C.E., Harada, N., Gorman, D.M., Djossou, O., Kastelein, R., Banchereau, J., Howard, M. and Miyajima, A. (1990) Molecular cloning of a cDNA encoding the human interleukin 4 receptor. *Int. Immunol.*, **2**, 669–675.

205. Harada, N., Castle, B.E., Gorman, D.M., Itoh, N., Schreurs, J., Barrett, R.L., Howard, M. and Miyajima, A. (1990) Expression cloning of a cDNA encoding the murine interleukin 4 receptor based on ligand binding. *Proc. Nat. Acad. Sci. USA*, **87**, 857–861.

206. Bazan, J.F. (1990) Haemopoietic receptors and helical cytokines. *Immunol. Today*, **11**, 350–354.

207. Bazan, J.F. (1990) Structural design and molecular evolution of a cytokine receptor superfamily. *Proc. Nat. Acad. Sci. USA*, **87**, 6934–6938.

208. Saltzman, E.M., Thom, R.R. and Casnellie, J.E. (1988) Activation of a tyrosine protein kinase is an early event in the stimulation of T lymphocytes by interleukin-2. *J. Biol. Chem.*, **263**, 6956–6959.

209. Morla, A.O., Schreurs, J., Miyajima, A. and Wang, J.Y. (1988) Hematopoietic growth factors activate the tyrosine phosphorylation of distinct sets of proteins in interleukin-3-dependent murine cell lines. *Mol. Cell. Biol.*, **8**, 2214–2218.

210. Mills, G.B., May, C., McGill, M., Fung, M., Baker, M., Sutherland, R. and Greene, W.C. (1990) Interleukin 2-induced tyrosine phosphorylation: Interleukin 2 receptor beta is tyrosine phosphorylated. *J. Biol. Chem.*, **265**, 3561–3567.

211. Satoh, T., Nakafuku, M., Miyajima, A. and Kaziro, Y. (1991) Involvement of ras p21 protein in signal-transduction pathways from interleukin 2, interleukin 3, and granulocyte/macrophage colony-stimulating factor, but not from interleukin 4. *Proc. Nat. Acad. Sci. USA*, **88**, 3314–3318.

212. Remillard, B., Petrillo, R., Maslinski, W., Tsudo, M., Strom, T.B., Cantley, L. and Varticovski, L. (1991) Interleukin-2 receptor regulates activation of phosphatidylinositol 3-kinase. *J. Biol. Chem.*, **266**, 14167–14170.

213. Turner, B., Rapp, U., App, H., Greene, M., Dobashi, K. and Reed, J. (1991) Interleukin 2 induces tyrosine phosphorylation and activation of p72–74 Raf-1 kinase in a T-cell line. *Proc. Nat. Acad. Sci. USA*, **88**, 1227–1231.

214. Saltiel, A.R., Fox, J.A., Sherline, P. and Cuatrecasas, P. (1986) Insulin-stimulated hydrolysis of a novel glycolipid generates modulators of cAMP phosphodiesterase. *Science,* **233**, 967–972.

215. Saltiel, A.R., Sherline, P. and Fox, J.A. (1987) Insulin-stimulated diacylglycerol production results from the hydrolysis of a novel phosphatidylinositol glycan. *J. Biol. Chem.,* **262**, 1116–1121.

216. Gaulton, G.N., Kelly, K.L., Pawlowski, J., Mato, J.M. and Jarett, L. (1988) Regulation and function of an insulin-sensitive glycosyl-phosphatidylinositol during T lymphocyte activation. *Cell,* **53**, 963–970.

217. Chan, B.L., Chao, M.V. and Saltiel, A.R. (1989) Nerve growth factor stimulates the hydrolysis of glycosylphosphatidylinositol in PC-12 cells: A mechanism of protein kinase C regulation. *Proc. Nat. Acad. Sci. USA,* **86**, 1756–1760.

218. Eardley, D.D. and Koshland, M.E. (1991) Glycosylphosphatidylinositol: A candidate system for interleukin-2 signal transduction. *Science,* **251**, 78–81.

219. Merida, I., Pratt, J.C. and Gaulton, G.N. (1990) Regulation of interleukin 2-dependent growth responses by glycosylphosphatidylinositol molecules. *Proc. Nat. Acad. Sci. USA,* **87**, 9421–9425.

220. Sharon, M., Gnarra, J.R. and Leonard, W.J. (1989) The beta-chain of the IL-2 receptor (p70) is tyrosine-phosphorylated on YT and HUT-102B2 cells. *J. Immunol.,* **143**, 2530–2533.

221. Hatakeyama, M., Kono, T., Kobayashi, N., Kawahara, A., Levin, S.D. and Perlmutter, R.M. (1991) Taniguchi T Interaction of the IL-2 receptor with the src-family kinase p56lck: Identification of novel intermolecular association. *Science,* **252**, 1523–1528.

222. Horak, I.D., Gress, R.E., Lucas, P.J., Horak, E.M., Waldmann, T.A. and Bolen, J.B. (1991) T-lymphocyte interleukin 2-dependent tyrosine protein kinase signal transduction involves the activation of p56lck. *Proc. Nat. Acad. Sci. USA,* **88**, 1996–2000.

223. Hatakeyama, M., Mori, H., Doi, T. and Taniguchi, T. (1989) A restricted cytoplasmic region of IL-2 receptor beta chain is essential for growth signal transduction but not for ligand binding and internalization. *Cell,* **59**, 837–845.

224. Fung, M.R., Scearce, R.M., Hoffman, J.A., Peffer, N.J., Hammes, S.R., Hosking, J.B., Schmandt, R., Kuziel, W.A., Haynes, B.F., Mills, G.B. *et al.* (1991) A tyrosine kinase physically associates with the beta-subunit of the human IL-2 receptor. *J. Immunol.,* **147**, 1253–1260.

225. Wang, T., Sheppard, J.R. and Foker, J.E. (1978) Rise and fall of cyclic AMP required for onset of lymphocyte DNA synthesis. *Science,* **201**, 155–157.

226. Wacholtz, M.C., Minakuchi, R. and Lipsky, P.E. (1991) Characterization of the 3',5'-cyclic adenosine monophosphate-mediated regulation of IL2 production by T cells and Jurkat cells. *Cell Immunol.,* **135**, 285–298.

227. Meskini, N., Hosni, M., Nemoz, G., Lagarde, M. and Prigent, A.F. (1992) Early increase in lymphocyte cyclic nucleotide phosphodiesterase activity upon mitogenic activation of human peripheral blood mononuclear cells. *J. Cell Physiol.,* **150**, 140–148.

228. Stewart, S.J., Cunningham, G.R., Strupp, J.A., House, F.S., Kelley, L.L., Henderson, G.S., Exton, J.H. and Bocckino, S.B. (1991) Activation of phospholipase D: A signaling system set in motion by perturbation of the T lymphocyte antigen receptor/CD3 complex. *Cell Regul.,* **2**, 841–850.

229. Chien, M.M. and Cambier, J.C. (1990) Divalent cation regulation of phosphoinositide metabolism: Naturally occurring B lymphoblasts contain a

Mg^{2+}-regulated phosphatidylinositol-specific phospholipase C. *J. Biol. Chem.*, **265**, 9201–9207.

230. Goldkorn, T., Dressler, K.A., Muindi, J., Radin, N.S., Mendelsohn, J., Menaldino, D., Liotta, D. and Kolesnick, R.N. (1991) Ceramide stimulates epidermal growth factor receptor phosphorylation in A431 human epidermoid carcinoma cells: Evidence that ceramide may mediate sphingosine action. *J. Biol. Chem.*, **266**, 16092–16097.

231. Okazaki, T., Bielawska, A., Bell, R.M. and Hannun, Y.A. (1990) Role of ceramide as a lipid mediator of 1 alpha,25-dihydroxyvitamin D3-induced HL-60 cell differentiation. *J. Biol. Chem.*, **265**, 15823–15831.

232. Dressler, K.A., Mathias, S. and Kolesnick, R.N. (1992) Tumor necrosis factor-alpha activates the sphingomyelin signal transduction pathway in a cell-free system. *Science*, **255**, 1715–1718.

233. Candela, M., Barker, S.C. and Ballon, L.B. (1991) Sphingosine synergistically stimulates tumor necrosis factor alpha-induced prostaglandin E2 production in human fibroblasts. *J. Exp. Med.*, **174**, 1363–1369.

234. Williams, G.T. (1991) Programmed cell death: Apoptosis and oncogenesis. *Cell*, **65**, 1097–1098.

235. Sentman, C.L., Shutter, J.R., Hockenbery, D., Kanagawa, O. and Korsmeyer, S.J. (1991) bcl-2 inhibits multiple forms of apoptosis but not negative selection in thymocytes. *Cell*, **67**, 879–888.

236. Smith, C.A., Williams, G.T., Kingston, R., Jenkinson, E.J. and Owen, J.J. (1989) Antibodies to CD3/T-cell receptor complex induce death by apoptosis in immature T cells in thymic cultures. *Nature*, **337**, 181–184.

237. Murphy, K.M., Heimberger, A.B. and Loh, D.Y. (1990) Induction by antigen of intrathymic apoptosis of CD4+CD8+TCRlo thymocytes *in vivo*. *Science*, **250**, 1720–1723.

238. Sambhara, S.R. and Miller, R.G. (1991) Programmed cell death of T cells signaled by the T cell receptor and the alpha 3 domain of class I MHC. *Science*, **252**, 1424–1427.

239. Newell, M.K., Hghn, L.J., Maroun, C.R. and Julius, M.H. (1990) Death of mature T cells by separate ligation of CD4 and the T-cell receptor for antigen. *Nature*, **347**, 286–289.

240. Lenardo, M.J. (1991) Interleukin-2 programs mouse alpha beta T lymphocytes for apoptosis. *Nature*, **353**, 858–861.

241. Mercep, M., Noguchi, P.D. and Ashwell, J.D. (1989) The cell cycle block and lysis of an activated T cell hybridoma are distinct processes with different Ca^{2+} requirements and sensitivity to cyclosporine A. *J. Immunol.*, **142**, 4085–4092.

242. Zacharchuk, C.M., Mercep, M., Chakraborti, P.K., Simons, S.S., Jr and Ashwell, J.D. (1990) Programmed T lymphocyte death: Cell activation and steroid-induced pathways are mutually antagonistic. *J. Immunol.*, **145**, 4037–4045.

243. Shi, Y.F., Sahai, B.M. and Green, D.R. (1989) Cyclosporin A inhibits activation-induced cell death in T-cell hybridomas and thymocytes. *Nature*, **339**, 625–626.

244. McConkey, D.J., Orrenius, S. and Jondal, M. (1990) Agents that elevate cAMP stimulate DNA fragmentation in thymocytes. *J. Immunol.*, **145**, 1227–1230.

245. McConkey, D.J., Hartzell, P., Chow, S.C., Orrenius, S. and Jondal, M. (1990) Interleukin 1 inhibits T cell receptor-mediated apoptosis in immature thymocytes. *J. Biol. Chem.*, **265**, 3009–3011.

246. McConkey, D.J., Hartzell, P., Jondal, M. and Orrenius, S. (1989) Inhibition of DNA fragmentation in thymocytes and isolated thymocyte nuclei by agents that stimulate protein kinase C. *J. Biol. Chem.*, **264**, 13399–13402.

247. Groux, H., Torpier, G., Monte, D., Mouton, Y., Capron, A. and Ameisen, J.C. (1992) Activation-induced death by apoptosis in CD4+ T cells from human immunodeficiency virus-infected asymptomatic individuals. *J. Exp. Med.,* **175,** 331–340.

248. Baxter, G.D. and Lavin, M.F. (1992) Specific protein dephosphorylation in apoptosis induced by ionizing radiation and heat shock in human lymphoid tumor lines. *J. Immunol.,* **148,** 1949–1954.

249. Nickas, G., Meyers, J., Hebshi, L.D., Ashwell, J.D., Gold, D.P., Sydora, B. and Ucker, D.S. (1992) Susceptibility to cell death is a dominant phenotype: Triggering of activation-driven T-cell death independent of the T-cell antigen receptor complex. *Mol. Cell. Biol.,* **12,** 379–385.

250. Itoh, N., Yonehara, S., Ishii, A., Yonehara, M., Mizushima, S., Sameshima, M., Hase, A., Seto, Y. and Nagata, S. (1991) The polypeptide encoded by the cDNA for human cell surface antigen Fas can mediate apoptosis. *Cell,* **66,** 233–243.

251. Watanabe-Fukunaga, R., Brannan, C.I., Copeland, N.G., Jenkins, N.A. and Nagata, S. (1992) Lymphoproliferation disorder in mice explained by defects in Fas antigen that mediates apoptosis. *Nature,* **356,** 314–317.

252. Ameisen, J.C. and Capron, A. (1991) Cell dysfunction and depletion in AIDS: The programmed cell death hypothesis. *Immunol. Today,* **12,** 102–105.

253. Bretscher, P. and Cohn, M. (1970) A theory of self–nonself discrimination. *Science,* **169,** 1042–1049.

254. Go, C. and Miller, J. (1992) Differential induction of transcription factors that regulate the interleukin 2 gene during anergy induction and restimulation. *J. Exp. Med.,* **175,** 1327–1336.

255. Turka, L.A., Linsey, P.S., Lin, H., Brady, W., Leiden, H.M., Wei, R.-Q., Gibson, M.L., Zheng, X.-G., Myrdal, S., Gordon, D., Bailey, T., Bolling, S.F. and Thompson, C.B. (1992) T cell activation by the CD28-ligand B7 is required for cardiac allograft rejection *in vivo. Proc. Natl. Acad. Sci. (USA),* **89,** 11102–11105.

Chapter 6

Adhesion Molecules which Guide Neutrophil–Endothelial Cell Interactions at Sites of Inflammation

TAKASHI KEI KISHIMOTO and ROBERT ROTHLEIN

Boehringer-Ingelheim Pharmaceuticals Inc., Immunology Department, Ridgefield, Connecticut, USA

Neutrophils are the primary front-line defense against most microbial pathogens. The circulatory system provides the network by which the neutrophil can gain access to virtually any tissue in the body. Thus neutrophil interactions with vascular endothelial cells are of central importance in guiding the acute inflammatory response. Three families of adhesion molecules have emerged as key players in neutrophil–endothelial cell interactions: (a) the leukocyte or CD18 integrins—LFA-1 (CD11a/CD18), Mac-1 (CD11b/CD18), and p150,95 (CD11C/CD18); (b) the intercellular adhesion molecules (ICAMs)—ICAM-1, ICAM-2, and ICAM-3; and (c) the selectins—L-selectin, E-selectin, and P-selectin. It has become increasingly clear that the process of neutrophil localization is a dynamic one, involving multiple steps. The orchestration of these steps must be precisely regulated to ensure a rapid response to isolate and destroy the invading pathogen yet with minimal damage to healthy tissues. This review will briefly introduce the key adhesion molecules involved in this process and then focus on a dynamic model of neutrophil–endothelial cell interactions at sites of inflammation.

New Concepts in Immunodeficiency Diseases. Edited by S. Gupta and C. Griscelli
© 1993 John Wiley & Sons Ltd

THE CD18 INTEGRINS

CD18 Structure and Function

LFA-1, Mac-1 and p150,95 are structurally related $\alpha\beta$ heterodimers which share a common subunit (1–3). The CD18 integrins are in turn related to a larger family of integrin adhesion molecules, which include primarily extracellular matrix receptors, such as the fibronectin receptor, vitronectin receptor, and platelet glycoprotein IIbIIIa. The α subunits of the CD18 integrins, like other integrins, contain multiple divalent cation-binding domains which are similar to the Ca^{2+}-binding domains of calmodulin and troponin C (4–7). Not surprisingly, CD18 adhesion functions are Mg^{2+} and Ca^{2+} dependent. In contrast to members of other integrin families, except for VLA-2 (very late antigen), the leukocyte integrin α subunits contain a unique domain, designated "I" or "inserted" domain, which is homologous to similar domains found in von Willebrand factor, complement proteins C2 and B, and cartilage matrix protein. The leukocyte integrin subunit, like other integrin subunits, is a cysteine-rich transmembrane protein, with a fourfold repeat of an unusual cysteine motif (8, 9).

CD18 integrin expression is restricted to white blood cells. LFA-1 is expressed by lymphocytes, monocytes, and granulocytes; while Mac-1 and p150,95 are primarily restricted to myeloid cells, although they are also expressed by some lymphocytes and natural killer (NK) cells. The CD18 integrins have a broad role in many leukocyte adhesion-related functions. LFA-1 has been implicated in cell-mediated cytolysis, antigen presentation, lymphocyte homotypic aggregation, and leukocyte adhesion to a variety of cytokine-activated cells, including endothelial cells (1–3). Mac-1 has been implicated in neutrophil homotypic aggregation, adhesion to substrates, binding and phagocytosis of iC3b-coated particles, adhesion-dependent respiratory burst, neutrophil locomotion, and leukocyte adhesion to cytokine-activated cells.

Both LFA-1 and Mac-1 mediate adhesion through multiple ligands. LFA-1 binds to the intercellular adhesion molecules ICAM-1 (10), ICAM-2 (11), and ICAM-3 (see below). Mac-1 also binds to ICAM-1 (12, 13), although at a site distinct from that of LFA-1 (14). In addition, Mac-1 recognizes a wide spectrum of unrelated molecules, including the iC3b fragment of complement, fibrinogen, factor X, and several microbial antigens. The molecular basis for the promiscuous nature of ligand recognition is not well defined.

CD18 Regulation

The broad range of functions that the CD18 integrins mediate suggests that the functional activity of these receptors must be closely regulated to prevent inappropriate adhesion. Mac-1 can be regulated both quantitatively and qualitatively. Mac-1 is stored in intracellular granules of neutrophils and monocytes (15). Upon stimulation with low levels of chemotactic agents, these pools are rapidly recruited to the cell surface, resulting in a three- to tenfold increase in surface Mac-1 expression. In addition, Mac-1 functional activity is qualitatively regulated by chemoattractant-induced neutrophil activation (16, 17). On resting neutrophils, the CD18 integrins are in an inactive state. Upon cellular activation, the CD18 integrins are induced into an active conformation, perhaps through cytoskeletal interactions. This active state can be mimicked by mAbs which recognize an activation epitope and can hold the CD18 integrins in an active conformation in the absence of cellular activation (18). The active state conformation is transient, resulting in rapid de-adhesion. This transient adhesiveness enables leukocytes to migrate and to engage multiple target cells in cell-mediated cytolysis. Finally, the integrins have been implicated in signaling directly or co-signaling through other receptors. For example, signaling through the T cell receptor is markedly enhanced by co-ligation of LFA-1 (19, 20).

Leukocyte Adhesion Deficiency

The most dramatic demonstration of the importance of CD18 integrins in neutrophil localization to inflamed sites was the discovery and characterization of a group of patients who are genetically deficient in CD18 integrin expression (21, 22). Defects in the β subunit common to LFA-1, Mac-1, and p150,95 prevent surface expression of all three leukocyte integrins (23–26). The hallmarks of this disease, termed leukocyte adhesion deficiency, is the recurrent, life-threatening bacterial infections, and a lack of neutrophils in the infected lesions despite chronically high levels of circulating neutrophils. These observations suggest that the CD18 integrins are crucial for neutrophil extravasation.

CD18 *In Vivo* Studies

Insight from the study of leukocyte adhesion deficiency also led investigators to hypothesize that anti-CD18 antagonists may be potent therapeutics in disease states which are compounded by inappropriate tissue damage by activated neutrophils. Neutrophil-mediated tissue damage is prominent in ischemia-reperfusion type injury, as seen in cardiac infarction, hemorrhagic shock, organ transplantation, burn, and frostbite. Numerous animal models of these disease states clearly demonstrate the efficacy of anti-CD18 antibodies in minimizing healthy tissue damage. Anti-CD11b mAb significantly reduced cardiac reperfusion injury in dogs (27), and anti-CD18 mAb was protective in a model of hemorrhagic shock (28). Furthermore, Vedder *et al.* reported that anti-CD18 mAb protected rabbits in a model of limb reattachment, where a rabbit ear is severed except for the central artery and vein

(29). The central artery is then clamped for 10 hours and reperfusion is allowed to occur. Anti-CD18 antibody given either just prior to clamping or just prior to reperfusion was effective in reducing swelling of the ear and in allowing the tissue to survive.

Anti-CD18 mAb has been tested in a model of antigen-reduced arthritis in rabbits (30). Rabbits sensitized to ovalbumin and then given intra-articular ovalbumin develop an acute form of joint inflammation reminiscent of rheumatoid arthritis, which is marked by a severe granulocyte infiltration. Anti-CD18 mAbs inhibit this infiltration 2 and 4 weeks post-challenge. Interestingly, rabbits treated with anti-CD18 mAb and control animals had the same degree of anti-ovalbumin antibodies, suggesting that the anti-CD18 antibody affected the initial damage mediated by the leukocyte infiltrate, which in turn had prolonged effects in mitigating joint damage.

INTERCELLULAR ADHESION MOLECULES

All three members of the intercellular adhesion molecule (ICAM) family were originally functionally defined as LFA-1 ligands. ICAM-1 and ICAM-2 are known to be structurally related members of the immunoglobulin (Ig) super-gene family. They are most closely related to other Ig-like adhesion molecules such as vascular cell adhesion molecule-1 (VCAM-1) and NCAM. ICAM-1 has five Ig-like domains, with a short hinge region separating the third and fourth Ig-like domains (31, 32). ICAM-1 is a ligand for Mac-1 as well as LFA-1. Interestingly, the binding sites for LFA-1 and Mac-1 are distinct. LFA-1 binds to domains 1 and 2 (33), while Mac-1 binds to domain 3 (14). ICAM-1 also serves as receptor for rhinovirus (34) and malaria-infected red blood cells. ICAM-2, in contrast, has only two Ig-like domains which are most closely related to domains 1 and 2 of ICAM-1 (11). ICAM-3 is defined only functionally by mAb (35): its primary structure is still unresolved.

The distribution and regulation of the ICAM molecules are quite distinct. ICAM-1 is expressed basally only at low levels on some vascular endothelial cells and on lymphocytes (10, 36). However, ICAM-1 expression can be induced to high levels on a variety of cells by stimulation with inflammatory cytokines, such as interleukin 1 (IL-1), tumor necrosis factor (TNF), and interferon-γ (IFNγ) (36). Induced or greatly increased expression of ICAM-1 has been reported on vascular endothelial cells, keratinocytes, epithelial cells, hepatocytes, and myocytes. In addition, ICAM-1 expression is increased on activated lymphocytes. Induction of ICAM-1 requires *de novo* synthesis. As a counter-receptor for LFA-1, ICAM-1 has been implicated in guiding leukocyte migration, cell-mediated cytolysis, antigen presentation, and lymphocyte homotypic aggregation. Additionally, ICAM-1 as a receptor for Mac-1 is involved in neutrophil–endothelial cell interactions, transendothelial migration, and adhesion-dependent respiratory burst.

ICAM-2 expression, in contrast to that of ICAM-1, is constitutive and restricted to endothelial cells and mononuclear leukocytes (37, 38). Functionally it is not clear what role ICAM-2 plays in the inflammatory response. ICAM-3 is even more restricted in expression. It is expressed only on monocytes, lymphocytes, and granulocytes (35). Interestingly, ICAM-3 is the only ICAM molecule expressed by neutrophils.

ICAM-1 *In Vivo* Studies

ICAM-1, as a major ligand for both Mac-1 and LFA-1, is a good target for therapeutic intervention. In contrast to anti-CD18 mAbs, which react with all leukocytes, resting or activated, anti-ICAM-1 mAbs would preferentially target cells at the site of inflammation. One mAb, R6.5, is unique in that it blocks ICAM-1 binding to both LFA-1 and Mac-1 (14). The R6.5 mAb has been tested in a variety of animal models. Like anti-CD18 mAb, anti-ICAM-1 is effective in mitigating cardiac reperfusion injury in rabbits (39). Recently anti-ICAM-1 has been found to enable the prolongation of ischemic time to rabbit spinal cords without causing paralysis over the next 24 hours (40). Anti-ICAM-1 has been found to inhibit Shwartzman reactions in rabbits, where rabbits are injected intradermally with lipopolysaccharide (LPS) and 18 hours later challenged systemically with zymosan. In the absence of antibody there is hemorrhaging at the site of LPS injection following the systemic challenge, as monitored by influx of radiolabeled red blood cells. This hemorrhaging is greatly reduced in the presence of or anti-ICAM-1 mAb (41). Anti-ICAM-1 also inhibits eosinophil influx and airway hyperresponsiveness in a primate model of antigen-induced airway hyperresponsiveness in non-human primates (42). Finally it was recently reported that anti-ICAM-1, when given to non-human primates daily for 12 days, more than doubled the survival time of kidney allografts in a primate model of kidney transplantation (43). Furthermore, anti-ICAM-1 mAb reversed acute kidney allograft rejection episodes in monkeys given suboptimal doses of cyclosporin A. Comparable data were established in heterotopic heart transplants (44).

THE SELECTINS

Selectin Structure and Function

All three members of the selectin family share common structural features (45–51), most prominently an N-terminal C-type lectin domain. As discussed below, the lectin domain is central to the carbohydrate-binding properties of all three selectins. The lectin domain motif belongs to the C-type lectin family described by Drickamer *et al.* (52). This Ca^{2+}-dependent lectin domain accounts for, at least in part, the requirement of Ca^{2+} in adhesion mediated by all three selectins. The lectin domain is followed by a domain homologous to epidermal growth factor (EGF), a variable number of short consensus repeats (SCRs), which is a motif found in many complement regulatory proteins, a conventional transmembrane domain, and a C-terminal cytoplasmic domain. Much of the size difference between the selectins is accounted for by the number of SCRs: L-selectin, the smallest member, has two SCRs, E-selectin has six SCRs, and P-selectin has alternatively spliced forms of eight and nine SCRs. This is a highly conserved gene family, with over 60% amino acid identity lectin and EGF domains.

L-selectin was first described as a lymphocyte homing molecule involved in tissue-specific migration to peripheral lymph nodes (53, 54). More recently, L-selectin has been demonstrated on myeloid cells and is involved in neutrophil–endothelial cell and monocyte–endothelial cell interactions at sites of inflammation. Monoclonal antibodies against L-selectin reduce neutrophil adhesion to cytokine-stimulated endothelial cell cultures. Interestingly, L-selectin-mediated adhesion appears to be most readily measured when neutrophils are subjected to shear stress (55–57) (see below). A role for carbohydrate binding by L-selectin was demonstrated by Rosen and colleagues (54) many years before the lectin domain structure was elucidated by gene cloning.

E-selectin was first defined as a cytokine-inducible adhesion molecule on endothelial cells (58). Monoclonal antibodies against E-selectin specifically block neutrophil and myeloid cell lines (HL-60) adhesion to IL-1 and TNF-stimulated endothelial cells (58, 59). E-selectin expression is prominent in acute inflammatory lesions *in vivo* and correlates with the large influx of neutrophils (60–64). Although E-selectin appears to be primarily associated with acute inflammatory lesions, where it can be induced almost anywhere, recent studies have shown E-selectin expression in some chronic inflammatory lesions, notably the inflamed skin (63, 65) and the synovium from patients with arthritis (66). Furthermore, a small subset of memory T lymphocytes, defined by the HECA-452 mAb, bind specifically to E-selectin (65). These studies indicate that in some circumstances E-selectin can mediate lymphocyte traffic to chronic inflammatory sites.

P-selectin was first defined as a marker for activated platelets (67, 68). P-selectin was localized to the α granules of platelets (69, 70) and later to the Weibel–Palade bodies of endothelial cells (71–73). In both cell types, cell activation results in a rapid recruitment of these granules to the cell surface (69, 70, 73). P-selectin is involved in mediating neutrophil–platelet interactions (74–76) and in neutrophil–endothelial cell interactions *in vitro* (77–79). These results indicate that P-selectin may play a central role in bridging hemostasis and acute inflammation very early in the response to vascular injury or insult.

Selectin Ligands

Since L-selectin was first described as a lymphocyte homing receptor the most intense search for an L-selectin ligand has been on high endothelial venules (HEVs) of lymph nodes. In a series of elegant studies, Rosen and colleagues demonstrated a clear role for carbohydrates in L-selectin-mediated adhesion (54). Lymphocyte adhesion to HEVs is sensitive to neuraminidase treatment of the HEVs (80, 81). Charged sugars, such as mannose 6-phosphate, and polymers of charged sugars such as polyphospho mannan ester (PPME) (mannose 6-phosphate rich) and fucoidin (fucose sulfate rich) bind specifically to L-selectin and block lymphocyte adhesion to HEVs (82–84). Rosen, Lasky and colleagues have recently utilized soluble L-selectin, in the form of a bivalent L-selectin–IgG chimeric molecule, to immunopurify a 50 kDa protein from lymph node tissue. This protein is heavily glycosylated and contains sulfated sugars (85). In a parallel line of research, Butcher and colleagues have developed an mAb, MECA-79, which specifically stains peripheral lymph node HEVs, but not mucosal HEVs, and blocks lymphocyte adhesion to peripheral node HEVs (86). The MECA-79 mAb is an IgM and appears to recognize a carbohydrate determinant. Western blot analysis and immunoaffinity purification of reactive antigen shows several distinct bands: a major band of 105 kDa, with minor bands of 65, 90, 150, and 200 kDa. The purified MECA-79 antigen supports tissue-specific lymphocyte binding, which is blocked by both MECA-79 and by anti-L-selectin mAb. Interestingly, the major 50 kDa product isolated with the L-selectin–IgG chimeric molecule by Rosen *et al.* also immunoreacts with the MECA-79 mAb.

A ligand for L-selectin on stimulated human umbilical veins endothelial cells (HUVEC) has not been defined. The MECA-79 mAb, which cross-reacts with human lymph node HEVs, does not appear to stain stimulated HUVEC. Yet L-selectin-dependent adhesion of neutrophils to stimulated HUVEC has been demonstrated by several independent groups. There is general consensus that L-selectin-dependent neutrophil adhesion to HUVEC occurs only with cytokine stimulation of the endothelium (55–57). The adhesion occurs readily at low temperature, and appears to be enhanced by mild, rotational shear force (55, 57). Spertini *et al.* (57) have shown that neuraminidase treatment of the stimulated endothelial cells inhibits L-selectin-mediated adhesion. Curiously, *in vivo* intravital microscopy studies in normal animals demonstrate L-selectin-dependent adhesion in the absence of any applied cytokine stimulation (87, 88). These results suggest that at least one L-selectin ligand is constitutively expressed or is rapidly inducible (within minutes) simply by the anesthesia or surgical manipulation necessary to prepare the animal for intravital microscopy.

The identification of a lectin domain in the E-selectin structure led to an intense, focused search for a carbohydrate ligand expressed by myeloid cells.

Numerous independent groups reported that sialyl Lewis X (SLEX), or related sialylated, fucosylated sugars, serve as specific ligands for E-selectin. SLEX is appropriately expressed by neutrophils and monocytes. Several complementary lines of evidence support these claims. Phillips *et al.* demonstrated that liposomes composed of glycolipids containing the SLEX structure are capable of inhibiting E-selectin-mediated adhesion (89). Furthermore, the LEC11 cell line, a variant CHO cell, expresses SLEX and binds to HUVEC in an E-selectin-dependent manner. Monoclonal antibodies against the SLEX determinant inhibit E-selectin-mediated adhesion (89, 90). Transfection of a 1,3-fucosyltransferase into COS or CHO cells confers upon these cells the ability to synthesize SLEX and to bind E-selectin (91, 92). However, the identity of the endogenous myeloid fucosyltransferase is still controversial (92, 93). Brandley *et al.* purified glycolipids from myeloid cells and identified fractions which support E-selectin adhesion (94). More recently, sialyl Lewis A, an SLEX-related carbohydrate, has been implicated as a ligand for E-selectin (95, 96). Computer modeling suggests that the sialic acid and fucose residues are oriented in the same manner in both SLEX and sialyl Lewis A. Both SLEX and sialyl Lewis A are recognized by the HECA-452 mAb which defines a subpopulation of lymphocytes capable of binding to E-selectin (95).

A similar search for carbohydrate ligands of P-selectin followed the recognition that P-selectin possessed an N-terminal lectin domain. Initially it was reported that Lewis X antigen (CD15) was a major ligand for P-selectin (76). However, several groups have shown that P-selectin-dependent adhesion is sensitive to neuraminidase treatment of the target cell, suggesting a requirement for sialic acid (97–99). Indeed, P-selectin shows significantly higher affinity for sialyl Lewis X than for Lewis X (96). Although both E-selectin and P-selectin bind to SLEX, the binding characteristics are distinct (96). Thus E-selectin and P-selectin are not identical in ligand specificity. More recently, Aruffo *et al.* (100) have reported that soluble P-selectin–IgG chimeric molecules bind specifically to sulfatides (3-sulfated galactosyl ceramides) derived from myeloid cells and some tumor cell lines. Treatment of HL-60 cells with selenate, an inhibitor of sulfation, reduces binding to P-selectin but not to E-selectin. These studies suggest that sulfatides may be the major ligand for P-selectin.

While it is clear that SLEX, either on proteins or lipids, can support E-selectin-mediated adhesion *in vitro*, it is unclear whether all SLEX on the neutrophil cell surface can bind with equal efficiency and affinity to E-selectin. One possibility is that SLEX may be added to a variety of proteins and lipids, but only a subset is presented in a favorable conformation, thus creating a hierarchy where E-selectin preferentially binds to a subset of the total available SLEX. This hierarchy might reflect the accessibility of the SLEX or the protein sequences adjacent to the SLEX. Alternatively, some proteins may be presented on microvilli and pseudopods which are more likely to mediate cell–cell contact. Based primarily on mAb blocking data, we have found evidence that L-selectin and E-selectin appear to operate in the same CD18-independent adhesion pathway (101). Anti-L-selectin and anti-E-selectin mAb have non-additive blocking effects, while both are additive in combination with anti-CD18 and anti-ICAM-1 mAb. Picker *et al.* (102) extended these studies and showed that L-selectin isolate from neutrophils but not from lymphocytes bears the SLEX carbohydrate and can support E-selectin-dependent adhesion. Moreover, neutrophils treated with chymotrypsin, which cleaves L-selectin from the cell surface but does not significantly affect overall SLEX levels, bind poorly to E-selectin. Similarly activated neutrophils, which have significant SLEX on their surface, bind significantly less than unstimulated neutrophils to E-selectin. Moore *et al.* (98) have found that protease treatment of neutrophils completely eliminates binding of fluid-phase P-selectin, even though significant SLEX remains on glycolipids. Siegelmann *et al.* have hypothesized that the lectin domain of the selectins provides the carbohydrate specifity while the EGF domain may bind to protein determinants (103). Thus it may be possible to observe adhesion to carbohydrate alone *in vitro*, but optimal adhesion activity may require both protein and carbohydrate determinants. What specific protein determinants are necessary still remains to be resolved.

Selectin Regulation

L-selectin is constitutively expressed on resting neutrophils in a seemingly functional form. Freshly isolated neutrophils can bind to stimulated endothelium at a reduced temperature (4–7°C) *in vitro* (55, 57). However, within minutes of neutrophil exposure to low levels of chemotactic factors, L-selectin is rapidly down-regulated from the cell surface (104). Near-complete down-regulation of L-selectin can be detected within minutes *in vitro*. A large fragment of L-selectin can be recovered from the supernatant of activated cells, suggesting that L-selectin is proteolytically clipped close to the transmembrane domain (104). A broad range of activating agents including C5a, N-formylmethionyl-leucyl-phenylalanine (fMLP), TNF, GM-CSF and IL-8, are effective at inducing this response (56, 104–106). Interestingly, the rapid shedding of L-selectin follows the kinetics of Mac-1 up-regulation from intracellular stores. Analysis of neutrophils which are recovered from the inflamed peritoneum *in vivo* (105), and immunohistological analysis of neutrophils in inflamed skin sites (104), suggest that this inverse regulation of adhesion molecules occurs *in vivo* as well. These observations led to the proposal of a two-step adhesion model (see below).

A second major means by which L-selectin function is regulated is an increased affinity for ligand. Tedder and colleagues have reported that, just prior to L-selectin shedding, there is a transient increased affinity for carbohydrate ligands, such as PPME (107), and adhesion to HEVs. This increased affinity is presumably transmitted through a conformational change in the L-selectin extracellular domain. This "inside-out" signaling is reminiscent of that seen with the leukocyte integrins (108).

E-selectin is normally absent from endothelial cells. However, upon stimulation with inflammatory cytokines, endothelial cells express E-selectin within several hours. E-selectin is synthesized *de novo*, and is blocked by protein synthesis inhibitors (58). This up-regulation of E-selectin is similar to that seen with other endothelial adhesion molecules, such as ICAM-1 and VCAM-1. However, in contrast to these other adhesion molecules which remain highly expressed for over 24 hours, E-selectin expression peaks at 3–4 hours and then is down-modulated by 8–24 hours *in vitro* (58, 109). The mechanism of E-selectin down-modulation is not well characterized. The time course of E-selectin expression is similar to that of neutrophil infiltration into acute inflammatory sites *in vivo*. These results suggest that E-selectin is involved primarily in the acute inflammatory response. E-selectin expression is also rapidly inducible *in vivo* and coincides with the influx of neutrophils (60–64, 110). However, in some chronic inflammatory lesions, notably some inflamed skin and synovial sites, E-selectin expression is quite prominent (60, 65, 66, 110).

P-selectin, like E-selectin, are expressed by activated endothelium. However, the activation signals and the kinetics of expression are completely different for these two events. P-selectin is stored in intracellular Weibel–Palade bodies (71–73). Stimulation of endothelial cells with histamine or thrombin induces a rapid recruitment of Weibel–Palade bodies to the cell surface, resulting in surface expression of P-selectin within minutes after stimulation. Similarly, P-selectin is also stored in the α granules of platelets, which are recruited to the cell surface within seconds of platelet activation (69, 70). This near-instantaneous up-regulation of P-selectin suggests a critical role in the earliest events of inflammation and hemostasis. Surface expression of P-selectin on endothelium is also extremely transient. Within 30 minutes P-selectin is down-modulated, apparently by receptor endocytosis rather than surface proteolysis. Low levels of hydrogen peroxide induces prolonged expression of P-selectin; however, this may be at least in part associated with endothelial cell damage (78). However, Stoolman and colleagues find that chronic levels of P-selectin may be important in some disease states, such as arthritis(110a).

Selectin *In Vivo* Studies

Lewinsohn *et al.* (111) showed that *in vivo* administration of anti-L-selectin mAb inhibits neutrophil localization to cutaneous sites of inflammation. Jutila *et al.* further demonstrated that neutrophil migration to the inflamed

peritoneum is inhibited to the same extent by *in vivo* administration of antibodies against Mac-1 or L-selectin (105). Watson *et al.* found that an L-selectin–
IgG chimeric molecule, containing two L-selectin extracellular domains genetically engineered onto the Fc portion of immunoglobulin, directly blocks neutrophil response to acute inflammation (112). Although neutrophils do not
normally migrate to peripheral lymph nodes, they do bind specifically to
HEVs in the Stamper–Woodruff assay (105, 111). These results suggest that *in
vivo* a second signal, perhaps a chemotactic factor, is required for neutrophil
migration across the endothelium. This factor would be present in an acute
inflammatory lesion, but not in normal lymphoid tissues.

Recent studies have demonstrated that *in vivo* administration of mAb
against E-selectin inhibits neutrophil accumulation in the lung in a primate
model of late-phase response (113) and in a rat model of immune complex-
mediated lung injury (114). Currently there are no *in vivo* studies with anti-
P-selectin mAbs demonstrating inhibition of inflammation or hemostasis.

A MODEL FOR NEUTROPHIL–ENDOTHELIAL CELL INTERACTIONS

In 1989, a two-step adhesion model for neutrophil interaction with endothelium was proposed, based primarily on the observation that Mac-1 and
L-selectin are inversely regulated by exposure to chemotactic factors (105,
115, 116) (Figure 6.1). The rapid down-regulation of L-selectin with a concomitant up-regulation of Mac-1 suggested that these adhesion molecules
mediate distinct but complementary adhesion events. We had proposed that
L-selectin mediates the initial interaction of the resting, circulating neutrophil with the activated endothelium, thus guiding the unstimulated neutrophil to the appropriate site of inflammation. This initial binding or rolling
event would slow the neutrophil down and expose it to low levels of chemotactic factors released at the site of inflammation. The chemoattractants
would provide the signal for the neutrophil to enter the inflamed tissue and
trigger the transition from L-selectin-mediated adhesion to CD18-mediated
adhesion. The CD18 integrins, LFA-1 and Mac-1, are largely responsible for
subsequent adhesion strengthening, neutrophil aggregation, and transendothelial migration. The appeal of this model is that it provides a mechanism
to closely regulate neutrophil localization and neutrophil activation, thus
ensuring minimal damage to surrounding healthy tissue. Data from a number of independent investigators support and extend this model.

Induction of Vascular Adhesion Molecules

The laboratories of Gimbrone and Pober showed that inflammatory
cytokines, such as IL-1, IFN-γ, and TNF, induced profound changes in
cultured endothelial cells, including induction of class II MHC antigens (in

142

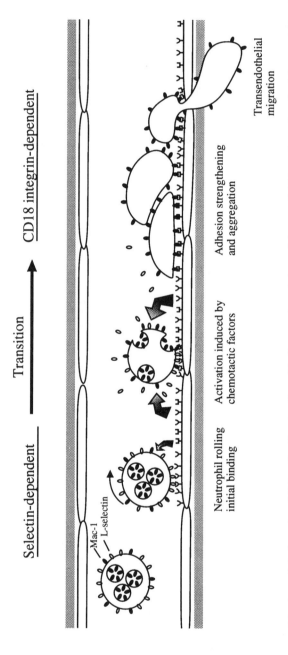

Figure 6.1. A model of neutrophil localization to sites of inflammation. Adapted from ref. 116, and reprinted with permission from *The Journal of NIH Research*, Washington, DC

response to IFNγ), procoagulatant activity, and, perhaps most strikingly, a dramatic increase in the ability of endothelial cells to support neutrophil adhesion (117–120). These studies indicated that activation of endothelial cells by cytokines induces expression of cell adhesion molecules, which enables leukocytes in circulation to differentiate between normal vascular endothelium and vascular endothelium adjacent to a site of infection. Cytokines such as IL-1 and TNF induce *de novo* synthesis of ICAM-1, VCAM-1, and E-selectin, resulting in their surface expression 3–4 hours after the initial stimulus. In contrast, histamine or thrombin can induce rapid mobilization of the P-selectin stored in Weibel–Palade bodies, resulting in surface expression of P-selectin within seconds after activation.

Initial Binding Event

Neutrophils in circulation must resist tremendous shear forces in order to stop along the vascular endothelium. The phenomenon of neutrophil rolling has been known for over a century in classic intravital microscopy studies (121). Neutrophils can be seen to roll and stop along the exteriorized venule but not in any arterioles. The slow movement of rolling neutrophils is accentuated by the blur of erythrocytes in the mainstream of the venules. The molecular basis of this rolling behavior has been unknown until recently; however, several lines of evidence now suggest a direct role for the selectin adhesion molecules in mediating neutrophil rolling.

Arfors *et al.* (122) used intravital microscopy to demonstrate that anti-CD18 mAb inhibits leukocyte extravasation into sites of inflammation but had no effect on neutrophil rolling behavior. In an independent line of investigation, Smith and colleagues developed an *in vitro* flow model to simulate shear stress on neutrophils interacting with cultured endothelial cells (123). Interestingly, neutrophils exhibited rolling and sticking behavior, but only on cytokine-stimulated endothelium, not on unstimulated endothelium. While neutrophil adhesion to endothelial cells in the absence of shear stress is partially CD18 dependent, adhesion under a shear stress of 2 dynes/cm^2 is CD18 independent. Neutrophils from leukocyte adhesion deficiency (LAD) patients deficient in CD18 expression roll and adhere under flow as well as normal neutrophils. These observations, together with our own observations that L-selectin and Mac-1 are inversely regulated on stimulated neutrophils, led to the hypothesis that L-selectin is involved in these early adhesion events under flow conditions (104, 105). To test this model, we developed mAb against human L-selectin (124) and examined their ability to inhibit neutrophil adhesion to stimulated endothelium under shear stress *in vitro*. Anti-L-selectin mAb dramatically reduced, but did not totally inhibit, neutrophil rolling and adhesion under flow conditions which are CD18 independent (1.85 dynes/cm^2) (56). Neutrophil activation with fMLP, which results in rapid shedding of L-selectin, substantially reduced neutrophil rolling and adhesion under flow. Anti-L-selectin mAb did not further reduce adhesion of activated neutrophils.

In a parallel line of investigation, two groups have used intravital microscopy to show a role for L-selectin in mediating neutrophil rolling *in vivo*. Ley *et al.* (88) showed that a polyclonal sera against L-selectin significantly reduces neutrophil rolling in the rat mesentery. Furthermore a soluble, bivalent L-selectin–IgG chimera also blocks neutrophil rolling, while a CD4–IgG control had no effect. These studies utilized a technique to inject the antagonists into venules directly upstream. Thus the inhibition is reversible if the antagonist is no longer administered. Similarly von Adnrian *et al.* found that the DREG-200 mAb, which cross-reacts with rabbit L-selectin, inhibits the number of neutrophils rolling as well as their velocity of rolling (87).

Since L-selectin is involved in neutrophil rolling and adhesion under flow, it seems reasonable to propose that the other selectins, P-selectin and E-selectin, may also mediate neutrophil rolling. Lawrence *et al.* showed that purified P-selectin, incorporated into lipid planar membranes, supports neutrophil rolling in a flow chamber *in vitro* (125). Similarly we have shown that mouse L cell fibroblasts, transfected with the E-selectin gene, supports neutrophil rolling and adhesion under flow to levels comparable to that seen with IL-1-stimulated endothelial cells (Abbassi *et al.*, submitted). The interaction of neutrophils with the E-selectin transfectants was completely blocked with anti-E-selectin mAb. Significantly, ICAM-1-transfected L cells did not support neutrophil rolling or adhesion under flow. Further intravital microscopy studies will be required to demonstrate E-selectin and P-selectin involvement in neutrophil rolling *in vivo*.

The Trigger

The transition from selectin-mediated adhesion to CD18-mediated adhesion occurs rapidly *in vitro*. A variety of chemotactic factors can cause quantitative down-regulation of L-selectin at the same time that Mac-1 is upregulated. This transition is reflected in neutrophil adhesion to endothelial cells *in vitro*. Under static conditions, where no shear stress is applied, resting neutrophil adhesion is partially selectin dependent and partially CD18/ICAM-1 dependent (56, 57, 59, 101). Upon activation of the neutrophil, the adhesion becomes almost entirely CD18/ICAM-1 dependent (126, 127). Similarly, activated neutrophils bind poorly under conditions of flow (127). The physiologically relevant trigger of this transition *in vivo* is unknown. It is likely that there are multiple mediators, perhaps utilized in different types of inflammatory events. It would be most efficient if the stimulated endothelial cells, themselves, could produce the appropriate chemoattractant. This would ensure appropriate localization of the neutrophil to the inflammatory site. Endothelial cells are capable of producing several neutrophil chemoat-tractants, including IL-8, GM-CSF, and platelet-activating factor (PAF).

Smith and co-workers demonstrated that co-culture of freshly isolated neutrophils with IL-1-stimulated endothelial cells for 30 minutes induced a dramatic down-regulation of L-selectin, up-regulation of Mac-1, and an accompanying neutrophil shape change response (56). Furthermore, the conditioned media from IL-1-stimulated endothelial cells can directly induce this transition in neutrophils (56). Huber *et al.* (128) recently reported that an anti-IL-8 serum significantly blocked neutrophil transmigration across stimulated endothelial cells. Immunolocalization of IL-8 demonstrates association with both the endothelial cells and the underlying collagen gel matrix. These results suggest that in 3–4 hour stimulated endothelial cultures IL-8 is the major chemotactic factor involved. Another interesting possibility is that neutrophil adhesion to E-selectin is sufficient to trigger activation of the CD18 integrins.

Zimmerman, McIntyre and colleagues have studied the role of PAF in neutrophil adhesion and activation (129, 130). Both PAF and P-selectin are induced within minutes on thrombin- or histamine-activated endothelium, correlating with increased neutrophil adhesiveness (131, 132). These results suggest that in the earliest events in vascular insult, PAF and P-selectin may function cooperatively to mediate neutrophil localization. These investigators propose that P-selectin acts as a tether to stop the circulating neutrophil, allowing PAF to induce the transition to CD18-dependent transmigration (79).

Neutrophil Adhesion Strengthening and Aggregation

As neutrophils are exposed to chemotactic factors, the inverse regulation of L-selectin and Mac-1 begins. During this transition, L-selectin and Mac-1 must work cooperatively to ensure that the primed neutrophil is not released by shear forces. Both L-selectin and the CD18 integrins undergo a conformational change resulting in a transient increase in affinity for ligand. This increased adhesiveness strengthens the interaction of neutrophils with the endothelium. At the same time, these activated neutrophils show increased adhesiveness for each other, resulting in neutrophil aggregation. Some vessels at sites of inflammation are so filled with neutrophils that the vessels become occluded. This aggregation of the neutrophils presumably helps to slow blood flow and allow for further neutrophil accumulation. Neutrophil aggregation is a Mac-1-dependent event (1–3). Recent data suggest that L-selectin may serve as a counter-receptor for Mac-1 in neutrophil aggregation (133). Interestingly, the rate of L-selectin down-regulation coincides with the kinetics of neutrophil disaggregation. The transient nature of neutrophil aggregation is important, since the ultimate goal of the neutrophil is to migrate into the inflammatory site.

Neutrophil Transendothelial Migration

Neutrophils enter the inflamed tissue by first migrating between endothelial junctions and then through the basement membrane. Both neutrophil aggregation (2, 3) and transendothelial migration (59, 127, 134, 135) are CD18 integrin-dependent events. Neutrophils treated with anti-CD18 mAb and neutrophils isolated from CD18-deficient patients fail to aggregate and to transmigrate *in vitro*. Thus these later stages of neutrophil localization to inflammatory sites require CD18 function. These events require distinct CD18 ligands, since mAbs against ICAM-1 block neutrophil transendothelial migration but do not affect neutrophil aggregation.

Whether CD18–ICAM-1 interactions are sufficient for neutrophil transmigration is controversial. It is widely agreed that anti-CD18 mAb both reduces the number of adherent neutrophils and inhibits all transmigration of the remaining adherent cells (56, 57, 101, 134–136). Furthermore both anti-L-selectin and anti-E-selectin mAb reduce the number of neutrophils which can bind to stimulated endothelial cells. However, Smith and colleagues find that those neutrophils that are adherent in the presence of anti-selectin mAb are not affected in their ability to migrate across the endothelial monolayer (56, 101). Furie *et al.* find similar results in neutrophil migration across the endothelium in response to an applied chemotactic gradient. In contrast, Luscinskas and colleagues find profound inhibition of transmigration with anti-E-selectin (136) and, to a lesser extent, with anti-L-selectin mAb (57). The reason for this discrepancy is not clear, but may reflect differences in the culture and assay systems used.

SUMMARY

Neutrophil interactions with endothelium have become a topic of intense study. Over the years specific molecules involved in this process have been elucidated. A dynamic model has been proposed based upon the wealth of data in the literature. This division of labor between selectins and integrins provides an efficient means to regulate the site of neutrophil localization and activation. The addition of triggering factors, such as chemoattractants, provides an additional degree of specificity. This basic model can be expanded to monocyte–endothelial cell and lymphocyte–endothelial cell interactions. Cell-specific chemoattractants may dictate whether a response is dominated by neutrophils or mononuclear leukocytes. Not surprisingly, numerous biotechnology and pharmaceutical companies are intensely focused on adhesion molecules and chemoattractants. The use of existing mAbs in a variety of animal models has already shown the efficacy of targeting adhesion molecules to prevent the inflammatory response. Novel biological anti-inflammatory drugs might include small molecule antagonists which are non-immunogenic and highly specific.

REFERENCES

1. Kishimoto, T.K., Larson, R.S., Corbi, A.L., Dustin, M.L., Staunton, D.E. and Springer, T.A. (1989) The leukocyte integrins. *Adv. Immunol.*, **46**, 149–182.
2. Kishimoto, T.K. and Anderson, D.C. (1992) The role of integrins in inflammation. In Gallin, J.I., Goldstein, I.M. and Snyderman, R. (eds) *Inflammation: Basic Principals and Clinical Correlates*, 2nd edn. Raven Press, New York, pp. 353–406.
3. Arnaout, M.A. (1990) Structure and function of the leukocyte adhesion molecules CD11/CD18. *Blood*, **75**, 1037–1050.
4. Corbi, A.L., Miller, L.J., O'Connor, K., Larson, R.S. and Springer, T.A. (1987) cDNA cloning and complete primary structure of the alpha subunit of a leukocyte adhesion glycoprotein, p150,95. *EMBO J.*, **6**, 4023–4028.
5. Corbi, A.L., Kishimoto, T.K., Miller, L.J. and Springer, T.A. (1988) The human leukocyte adhesion glycoprotein Mac-1 (complement receptor type 3, CD11b) alpha subunit: Cloning, primary structure, and relation to the integrins, von Willebrand factor and factor B. *J. Biol. Chem.*, **263**, 12403–12411.
6. Arnaout, M.A., Gupta, S.K., Pierce, M.W. and Tenen, D.G. (1988) Amino acid sequence of the alpha subunit of human leukocyte adhesion receptor Mo1 (complement receptor type 3). *J. Cell Biol.*, **106**, 2153–2158.
7. Larson, R.S., Corbi, A.L., Berman, L. and Springer, T.A. (1989) Primary structure of the LFA-1 alpha subunit: An integrin with an embedded domain defining a protein superfamily. *J. Cell Biol.*, **108**, 703–712.
8. Kishimoto, T.K., O'Connor, K., Lee, A., Roberts, T.M. and Springer, T.A. (1987) Cloning of the beta subunit of the leukocyte adhesion proteins: Homology to an extracellular matrix receptor defines a novel supergene family. *Cell*, **48**, 681–690.
9. Law, S.K.A., Gagnon, J., Hildreth, J.E.K., Wells, C.E., Willis, A.C. and Wong, A.J. (1987) The primary structure of the beta subunit of the cell surface adhesion glycoproteins LFA-1, CR3 and p150,95 and its relationship to the fibronectin receptor. *EMBO J.*, **6**, 915–919.
10. Rothlein, R., Dustin, M.L., Marlin, S.D. and Springer, T.A. (1986) A human intercellular adhesion molecule (ICAM-1) distinct from LFA-1. *J. Immunol.*, **137**, 1270–1274.
11. Staunton, D.E., Dustin, M.L. and Springer, T.A. (1989) Functional cloning of ICAM-2, a cell adhesion ligand for LFA-1 homologous to ICAM-1. *Nature*, **339**, 61–64.
12. Diamond, M.S., Staunton, D.E., De Fougerolles, A.R., Stacker, S.A., Garcia-Aguilar, J., Hibbs, M.L. and Springer, T.A. (1990) ICAM-1 (CD54): A counter-receptor for Mac-1 (CD11b/CD18). *J. Cell Biol.*, **111**, 3129–3139.
13. Smith, C.W., Marlin, S.D., Rothlein, R., Toman, C. and Anderson, D.C. (1989) Cooperative interactions of LFA-1 and Mac-1 with intercellular adhesion molecule-1 in facilitating adherence and transendothelial migration of human neutrophils *in vitro*. *J. Clin. Invest.*, **83**, 2008–2017.
14. Diamond, M.S., Staunton, D.E., Marlin, S.D. and Springer, T.A. (1991) Binding of the integrin Mac-1 (CD11b/CD18) to the third immunoglobulin-like domain of ICAM-1 (CD54) and its regulation by glycosylation. *Cell*, **65**, 961–971.
15. Todd, R.F., III, Arnaout, M.A., Rosin, R.E., Crowley, C.A., Peters, W.A. and Babior, B.M. (1984) Subcellular localization of the large subunit of Mo1 (Mo1 alpha; formerly gp 110), a surface glycoprotein associated with neutrophil adhesion. *J. Clin. Invest.*, **74**, 1280–1290.
16. Buyon, J.P., Abramson, S.B., Philips, M.R., Slade, S.G., Ross, G.D., Weissman, G. and Winchester, R.J. (1988) Dissociation between increased surface expression

of Gp165/95 and homotypic neutrophil aggregation. *J. Immunol.,* **140,** 3156–3160.

17. Vedder, N.B. and Harlan, J.M. (1988) Increased surface expression of CD11b/CD18 (Mac-1) is not required for stimulated neutrophil adherence to cultured endothelium. *J. Clin. Invest.,* **81,** 676–682.

18. Keizer, G.D., Visser, W., Vliem, M. and Figdor, C.G. (1988) A monoclonal antibody (NKI-L16) directed against a unique epitope on the alpha-chain of human leukocyte function-associated antigen 1 induces homotypic cell–cell interactions. *J. Immunol.,* **140,** 1393–1400.

19. Wacholtz, M.C., Patel, S.S. and Lipsky, P.E. (1989) Leukocyte function-associated antigen 1 is an activation molecule for human T cells. *J. Exp. Med.,* **170,** 431–448.

20. Van Seventer, G.A., Shimizu, Y., Horgan, K.J. and Shaw, S. (1990) The LFA-1 ligand ICAM-1 provides an important costimulatory signal for T cell receptor-mediated activation of resting T cells. *J. Immunol.,* **144,** 4579–4586.

21. Anderson, D.C. and Springer, T.A. (1987) Leukocyte adhesion deficiency: An inherited defect in the Mac-1, LFA-1, and p150,95 glycoproteins. *Annu. Rev. Med.,* **38,** 175–194.

22. Fischer, A., Lisowska-Grospierre, B., Anderson, D.C. and Sprinter, T.A. (1988) The leukocyte adhesion deficiency: Molecular basis and functional consequences. *Immunodef. Rev.,* **1,** 39–54.

23. Kishimoto, T.K., O'Connor, K. and Springer, T.A. (1989) Leukocyte adhesion deficiency: Aberrant splicing of a conserved integrin sequence causes a moderate deficiency phenotype. *J. Biol. Chem.,* **264,** 3588–3595.

24. Kishimoto, T.K., Hollander, N., Roberts, T.M., Anderson, D.C. and Springer, T.A. (1987) Heterogenous mutations in the beta subunit common to the LFA-1, Mac-1, and p150,95 glycoproteins cause leukocyte adhesion deficiency. *Cell,* **50,** 193–202.

25. Arnaout, M.A., Dana, N., Gupta, S.K., Tenen, D.G. and Fathallah, D.M. (1990) Point mutations impairing cell surface expression of the common β subunit (CD18) in a patient with leukocyte adhesion molecule (Leu-CAM) deficiency. *J. Clin. Invest.,* **85,** 977–981.

26. Dimanche, M.T., Le Deist, F., Fischer, A., Arnaout, M.A., Griscelli, C. and Lisowska-Grospierre, B. (1987) LFA-1 beta-chain synthesis and degradation in patients with leukocyte adhesive protein deficiency. *Eur. J. Immunol.,* **17,** 417–419.

27. Simpson, P.J., Todd, R.F., III, Fantone, J.C., Mickelson, J.K., Griffin, J.D., Lucchesi, B.R., Adams, M.D., Hoff, P., Lee, K. and Rogers, C.E. (1988) Reduction of experimental canine myocardial reperfusion injury by a monoclonal antibody (anti-Mo1, anti-CD11b) that inhibits leukocyte adhesion. *J. Clin. Invest.,* **81,** 624–629.

28. Mileski, W.J., Winn, R.J., Vedder, N.B., Pohlman, T.H., Harlan, J.M. and Rice, C.L. (1990) Inhibition of CD18-dependent neutrophil adherence reduces organ injury after hemorrhagic shock in primates. *Surgery,* **108,** 206–212.

29. Vedder, N.B., Winn, R.K., Rice, C.L., Chi, E.Y., Artors, K.-E. and Harlan, J.M. (1988) A monoclonal antibody to the adherence-promoting leukocyte glycoprotein, CD18, reduces organ injury and improves survival from hemorrhagic shock and resuscitation in rabbits. *J. Clin. Invest.,* **81,** 939–944.

30. Jasin, H.E., Lightfoot, E., Kavanaugh, A., Rothlein, R., Faanes, R.B. and Lipsky, P.E. (1990) Successful treatment of chronic antigen-induced arthritis in rabbits

with monoclonal antibodies to leukocyte adhesion molecules. *Arthritis Rheum.,* **33**, suppl. s34 (Abstract).

31. Staunton, D.E., Marlin, S.D., Stratowa, C., Dustin, M.L. and Springer, T.A. (1988) Primary structure of intercellular adhesion molecule 1 (ICAM-1) demonstrates interaction between members of the immunoglobulin and integrin supergene families. *Cell,* **52**, 925–933.
32. Simmons, D., Makgoba, M.W. and Seed, B. (1988) ICAM, an adhesion ligand of LFA-1, is homologous to the neural cell adhesion molecule NCAM. *Nature,* **331**, 624–627.
33. Staunton, D.E., Dustin, M.L., Erickson, H.P. and Springer, T.A. (1990) The arrangement of the immunoglobulin-like domains of ICAM-1 and the binding sites for LFA-1 and rhinovirus. *Cell,* **61**, 243–254.
34. Staunton, D.E., Merluzzi, V.J., Rothlein, R., Barton, R., Marlin, S.D. and Springer, T.A. (1989) A cell adhesion molecule, ICAM-1, is the major surface receptor for rhinoviruses. *Cell,* **56**, 849–853.
35. De Fougerolles, A.R. and Springer, T.A. (1992) Intercellular adhesion molecule 3, a third adhesion counter-receptor for lymphocyte function-associated molecule 1 on resting lymphocytes. *J. Exp. Med.,* **175**, 185–190.
36. Dustin, M.L., Rothlein, R., Bhan, A.K., Dinarello, C.A. and Springer, T.A. (1986) Induction by IL-1 and interferon, tissue distribution, biochemistry, and function of a natural adherence molecule (ICAM-1). *J. Immunol.,* **137**, 245–254.
37. De Fougerolles, A.R., Stacker, S.A., Schwarting, R. and Springer, T.A. (1991) Characterization of ICAM-2 and evidence for a third counter-receptor for LFA-1. *J. Exp. Med.,* **174**, 253–267.
38. Nortamo, P., Salcedo, R., Timonen, T., Patarroyo, M. and Gahmberg, C.G. (1991) A monoclonal antibody to the human leukocyte adhesion molecule intercellular adhesion molecule-2: Cellular distribution and molecular characterization of the antigen. *J. Immunol.,* **146**, 2530–2535.
39. Seewaldt-Becker, E., Rothlein, R. and Dammgen, J. (1990) CDw18 dependent adhesion of leukocytes to endothelium and its relevance for cardiac reperfusion. In Springer, T.A., Anderson, D.C., Rosenthal, A.S. and Rothlein, R. (eds) *Leukocyte Adhesion Molecules: Structure, Function, and Regulation.* Springer-Verlag, New York, pp. 138–148.
40. Clark, W.M., Madden, K.P., Rothlein, R. and Zivin, J.A. (1991) Reduction of central nervous system ischemic injury by monoclonal antibody to intracellular adhesion molecule. *J. Neurosurg.,* **75**, 623–627.
41. Argenbright, L.W. and Barton, R.W. (1991) The Shwartzman response: A model of ICAM-1 dependent vasculitis. *Agents Actions,* **34**, 208–210.
42. Wegner, C.D., Gundel, R.H., Reilly, P., Haynes, N., Letts, L.G. and Rothlein, R. (1990) Intercellular adhesion molecule-1 (ICAM-1) in the pathogenesis of asthma. *Science,* **247**, 456–459.
43. Cosimi, A.B., Conti, D., Delmonico, F.L., Preffer, F.I., Wee, S.-L., Rothlein, R., Faanes, R. and Colvin, R.B. (1990) *In vivo* effects of monoclonal antibody to ICAM-1 (CD54) in nonhuman primates with renal allografts. *J. Immunol.,* **144**, 4604–4612.
44. Flavin, T., Rothlein, R., Faanes, R., Ivens, K. and Starnes, V. (1990) Monoclonal antibody against intercellular adhesion molecule (ICAM)-1 prolongs cardiac allograft survival in cynomologus monkeys. *Transplant. Proc.,* **23**, 533–534.
45. Johnston, G.I., Cook, R.G. and McEver, R.P. (1989) Cloning of GMP-140, a granule membrane protein of platelets and endothelium: Sequence similarity to proteins involved in cell adhesion and inflammation. *Cell,* **56**, 1033–1044.

46. Lasky, L.A., Singer, M.S., Yednock, T.A., Dowbenko, D., Fennie, C., Rodriguez, H., Nguyen, T., Stachel, S. and Rosen, S.D. (1989) Cloning of a lymphocyte homing receptor reveals a lectin domain. *Cell,* **56,** 1045–1055.
47. Siegelman, M.H., Van de Rijn, M. and Weissman, I.L. (1989) Mouse lymph node homing receptor cDNA clone encodes a glycoprotein revealing tandem interaction domains. *Science,* **243,** 1165–1172.
48. Bevilacqua, M.P., Stengelin, S., Gimbrone, M.A. and Seed, B. (1989) Endothelial leukocyte adhesion molecule 1: An inducible receptor for neutrophils related to complement regulatory proteins and lectins. *Science,* **243,** 1160–1165.
49. Siegelman, M.H. and Weissman, I.L. (1989) Human homologue of mouse lymph node homing receptor: Evolutionary conservation at tandem cell interaction domains. *Proc. Nat. Acad. Sci. USA,* **86,** 5562–5566.
50. Tedder, T.F., Isaacs, C.M., Ernst, T.J., Demetri, G.D., Adler, D.A. and Disteche, C.M. (1989) Isolation and chromosomal localization of cDNAs encoding a novel human lymphocyte cell surface molecule, LAM-1: Homology with the mouse lymphocyte homing receptor and other human adhesion proteins. *J. Exp. Med.,* **170,** 123–133.
51. Bowen, B.R., Nguyen, T. and Lasky, L.A. (1989) Characterization of a human homologue of the murine peripheral lymph node homing receptor. *J. Cell Biol.,* **109,** 421–427.
52. Drickamer, K. (1988) Two distinct classes of carbohydrate-recognition domains in animal lectins. *J. Biol. Chem.,* **263,** 9557–9560.
53. Butcher, E.C. (1986) The regulation of lymphocyte traffic. *Curr. Topics Microbiol. Immunol.,* **128,** 85–122.
54. Yednock, T.A. and Rosen, S.D. (1989) Lymphocyte homing. *Adv. Immunol.,* **44,** 313–378.
55. Hallmann, R., Jutila, M.A., Smith, C.W., Anderson, D.C., Kishimoto, T.K. and Butcher, E.C. (1991) The peripheral lymph node homing receptor, LECAM-1, is involved in CD18-independent adhesion of neutrophils to endothelium. *Biochem. Biophys. Res. Commun.,* **174,** 236–243.
56. Smith, C.W., Kishimoto, T.K., Abbassi, O., Hughes, B.J., Rothlein, R., McIntire, L.V., Butcher, E.C. and Anderson, D.C. (1991) Chemotactic factors regulate lectin adhesion molecule-1 (LECAM-1)-dependent neutrophil adhesion to cytokine-stimulated endothelial cells *in vitro. J. Clin. Invest.,* **87,** 609–618.
57. Spertini, O., Luscinskas, F.W., Kansas, G.S., Munro, J.M., Griffin, J.D., Gimbrone, M.A., Jr and Tedder, T.F. (1991) Leukocyte adhesion molecule-1 (LAM-1, L-selectin) interacts with an inducible endothelial cell ligand to support leukocyte adhesion. *J. Immunol.,* **147,** 2565–2573.
58. Bevilacqua, M.P., Pober, J.S., Mendrick, D.L., Cotran, R.S. and Gimbrone, M.A. (1987) Identification of an inducible endothelial–leukocyte adhesion molecule, E-LAM 1. *Proc. Nat. Acad. Sci. USA,* **84,** 9238–9242.
59. Luscinskas, F.W., Brock, A.F., Arnaout, M.A. and Gimbrone, M.A. (1989) Endothelial–leukocyte adhesion molecule-1-dependent and leukocyte (CD11/CD18)-dependent mechanisms contribute to polymorphonuclear leukocyte adhesion to cytokine-activated human vascular endothelium. *J. Immunol.,* **142,** 2257–2263.
60. Cotran, R.S., Gimbrone, M.A., Bevilacqua, M.P., Mendrick, D.L. and Pober, J.S. (1986) Induction and detection of a human endothelial activation antigen *in vivo. J. Exp. Med.,* **164,** 661–666.

61. Munro, J.M., Pober, J.S. and Cotran, R.S. (1991) Recruitment of neutrophils in the local endotoxin response: Association with *de novo* endothelial expression of endothelial leukocyte adhesion molecule-1. *Lab Invest.,* **64**, 295–298.
62. Redl, H., Dinges, H.P., Buurman, W.A., Van der Linden, C.J., Pober, J.S., Cotran, R.S. and Schlag, G. (1991) Expression of endothelial leukocyte adhesion molecule-1 in septic but not traumatic/hypovolemic shock in the baboon. *Am. J. Pathol.,* **139**, 461–466.
63. Munro, J.M., Pober, J.S. and Cotran, R.S. (1989) Tumor necrosis factor and interferon-gamma induce distinct patterns of endothelial activation and leukocyte accumulation in skin of *Papio anubis. Am. J. Pathol.,* **135**, 121–133.
64. Leung, D.Y.M., Pober, J.S. and Cotran, R.S. (1991) Expression of endothelial–leukocyte adhesion molecule-1 in elicited late phase allergic reactions. *J. Clin. Invest.,* **87**, 1805–1809.
65. Koch, A.E., Burrows, J.C., Haines, G.K., Carlos, T.M., Harlan, J.M. and Leibovich, S.J. (1991) Immunolocalization of endothelial and leukocyte adhesion molecules in human rheumatoid and osteoarthritic synovial tissues. *Lab. Invest.,* **64**, 313–320.
66. Picker, L.J., Kishimoto, T.K., Smith, C.W., Warnock, R.A. and Butcher, E.C. (1991) ELAM-1 is an adhesion molecule for skin-homing T cells. *Nature,* **349**, 796–799.
67. McEver, R.P. and Martin, M.N. (1984) A monoclonal antibody to a membrane glycoprotein binds only to activated platelets. *J. Biol. Chem.,* **259**, 9799–9804.
68. Hsu-Lin, S.-C., Berman, C.L., Furie, B.C., August, D. and Furie, B. (1984) A platelet membrane protein expressed during platelet activation and secretion. Studies using a monoclonal antibody specific for thrombin-activated platelets. *J. Biol. Chem.,* **259**, 9121–9126.
69. Stenberg, P.E., McEver, R.P., Shuman, M.A., Jacques, Y.V. and Bainton, D.F. (1985) A platelet alpha granule membrane protein (GMP-140) is expressed on the plasma membrane after activation. *J. Cell Biol.,* **101**, 880–886.
70. Berman, C.L., Yeo, E.L., Wencel-Drake, J.D., Furie, B.C., Ginsberg, M.H. and Furie, B. (1986) A platelet alpha granule membrane protein that is associated with the plasma membrane after activation. *J. Clin. Invest.,* **78**, 130–137.
71. McEver, R.P., Beckstead, J.H., Moore, K.L., Marshall, C.L. and Bainton, D.F. (1989) GMP-140, a platelet alpha-granule membrane protein, is also synthesized by vascular endothelial cells and is localized in Weibel–Palade bodies. *J. Clin. Invest.,* **84**, 92–99.
72. Bonfanti, R., Furie, B.C., Furie, B. and Wagner, D.D. (1989) PADGEM (GMP140) is a component of Weibel–Palade bodies of human endothelial cells. *Blood,* **73**, 1109–1112.
73. Hattori, R., Hamilton, K.K., Fugate, R.D., McEver, R.P. and Sims, P.J. (1989) Stimulated secretion of endothelial von Willebrand factor is accompanied by rapid redistribution to the cell surface of the intracellular granule membrane protein (GMP-140). *J. Biol. Chem.,* **264**, 7768–7771.
74. Hamburger, S.A. and McEver, R.P. (1990) GMP-140 mediates adhesion of stimulated platelets to neutrophils. *Blood,* **75**, 550–554.
75. Larsen, E., Celi, A., Gilbert, G.E., Furie, B.C., Erban, J.K., Bonfanti, R., Wagner, D.D. and Furie, B. (1989) PADGEM protein: A receptor that mediates the interaction of activated platelets with neutrophils and monocytes. *Cell,* **59**, 305–312.
76. Larsen, E., Palabrica, T., Sajer, S., Gilbert, G.E., Wagner, D.D., Furie, B.C. and Furie, B. (1990) PADGEM-dependent adhesion of platelets to monocytes and

neutrophils is mediated by a lineage-specific carbohydrate, LNF III (CD15). *Cell*, **63**, 467–474.

77. Geng, J.-G., Bevilacqua, M.P., Moore, K.L., McIntyre, T.M., Prescott, S.M., Kim, J.M., Bliss, G.A., Zimmerman, G.A. and McEver, R.P. (1990) Rapid neutrophil adhesion to activated endothelium mediated by GMP-140. *Nature*, **343**, 757–760.

78. Patel, K.D., Zimmerman, G.A., Prescott, S.M., McEver, R.P. and McIntyre, T.M. (1991) Oxygen radicals induce human endothelial cells to express GMP-140 and bind neutrophils. *J. Cell Biol.*, **112**, 749–759.

79. Lorant, D.E., Patel, K.D., McIntyre, T.M., McEver, R.P., Prescott, S.M. and Zimmerman, G.A. (1991) Coexpression of GMP-140 and PAF by endothelium stimulated by histamine or thrombin: A juxtacrine system for adhesion and activation of neutrophils. *J. Cell Biol.*, **115**, 223–234.

80. Rosen, S.D., Singer, M., Yednock, T.A. and Stoolman, L.M. (1985) Involvement of sialic acid on endothelial cells in organ-specific lymphocyte recirculation. *Science*, **228**, 1005–1007.

81. True, D.D., Singer, M.S., Lasky, L.A. and Rosen, S.D. (1990) Requirement for sialic acid on the endothelial ligand of a lymphocyte homing receptor. *J. Cell Biol.*, **111**, 2757–2764.

82. Yednock, T.A., Stoolman, L.M. and Rosen, S.D. (1987) Phosphomannosyl-derivatized beads detect a receptor involved in lymphocyte homing. *J. Cell Biol.*, **104**, 713–723.

83. Stoolman, L.M., Tenforde, T. and Rosen, S.D. (1984) Phosphomannosyl receptors may participate in the adhesive interaction between lymphocytes and high endothelial venules. *J. Cell Biol.*, **99**, 1535–1549.

84. Yednock, T.A., Butcher, E.C., Stoolman, L.M. and Rosen, S.D. (1987) Receptors involved in lymphocyte homing: Relationship between a carbohydrate-binding receptor and the MEL-14 antigen. *J. Cell Biol.*, **104**, 725–731.

85. Imai, Y., Singer, M.S., Fennie, C., Lasky, L.A. and Rosen, S.D. (1991) Identification of a carbohydrate-based endothelial ligand for a lymphocyte homing receptor. *J. Cell Biol.*, **113**, 1213–1221.

86. Streeter, P.R., Rouse, B.T. and Butcher, E.C. (1988) Immunohistologic and functional characterization of a vascular addressin involved in lymphocyte homing into peripheral lymph nodes. *J. Cell Biol.*, **107**, 1853–1862.

87. Von Andrian, U.H., Chambers, J.D., McEvoy, L.M., Bargatze, R.F., Arfors, K.-E. and Butcher, E.C. (1991) Two-step model of leukocyte–endothelial cell interaction in inflammation: Distinct roles for LECAM-1 and the leukocyte β_2 integrins *in vivo*. *Proc. Nat. Acad. Sci. USA*, **88**, 7538–7542.

88. Ley, K., Gaehtgens, P., Fennie, C., Singer, M.S., Lasky, L.A. and Rosen, S.D. (1991) Lectin-like cell adhesion molecule 1 mediates leukocyte rolling in mesenteric venules *in vivo*. *Blood*, **77**, 2553–2555.

89. Phillips, M.L., Nudelman, E., Gaeta, F.C.A., Perez, M., Singhal, A.K., Hakomori, S. and Paulson, J.C. (1990) ELAM-1 mediates cell adhesion by recognition of a carbohydrate ligand, sialyl-Le^x. *Science*, **250**, 1130–1132.

90. Walz, G., Aruffo, A., Kolanus, W., Bevilacqua, M.P. and Seed, B. (1990) Recognition by ELAM-1 of the sialyl-Lex determinant on myeloid and tumor cells. *Science*, **250**, 1132–1134.

91. Lowe, J.B., Stoolman, L.M., Nair, R.P., Larsen, R.D., Berhend, T.L. and Marks, R.M. (1990) ELAM-1-dependent cell adhesion to vascular endothelium determined by a transfected human fucosyltransferase cDNA. *Cell*, **63**, 475–484.

92. Goelz, S.E., Hession, C., Goff, D., Griffiths, B., Tizard, R., Newman, B., Chi-Rosso, G. and Lobb, R. (1990) ELFT: A gene that directs the expression of an ELAM-1 ligand. *Cell*, **63**, 1349–1356.

93. Lowe, J.B., Stoolman, L.M., Nair, R.P., Larsen, R.D., Behrend, T.L. and Marks, R.M. (1991) A transfected human fucosyltransferase cDNA determines biosynthesis of oligosaccharide ligand(s) for endothelial-leukocyte adhesion molecule I. *Biochem. Soc. Trans.*, **19**, 649–654.

94. Tiemeyer, M., Swiedler, S.J., Ishihara, M., Moreland, M., Schweingruber, H., Hirtzer, P. and Brandley, B.K. (1991) Carbohydrate ligands for endothelial–leukocyte adhesion molecule-1. *Proc. Nat. Acad. Sci. USA*, **88**, 1138–1142.

95. Berg, E.L., Robinson, M.K., Mansson, O., Butcher, E.C. and Magnani, J.L. (1991) A carbohydrate domain common to both sialyl Le^a and sialyl Le^x is recognized by the endothelial cell leukocyte adhesion molecule ELAM-1. *J. Biol. Chem.*, **266**, 14869–14872.

96. Tyrrell, D., James, P., Rao, N., Foxall, C., Abbas, S., Dasgupta, F., Nashed, M., Hasegawa, A., Kiso, M., Asa, D., Kidd, J. and Brandley, B.K. (1991) Structural requirements for the carbohydrate ligand of E-selectin. *Proc. Nat. Acad. Sci. USA*, **88**, 10372–10376.

97. Polley, M.J., Phillips, M.L., Wayner, E., Nudelman, E., Singhal, A.K., Hakomori, S. and Paulson, J.C. (1991) CD62 and endothelial cell–leukocyte adhesion molecule 1 (ELAM-1) recognize the same carbohydrate ligand, sialyl-Lewis x. *Proc. Nat. Acad. Sci. USA*, **88**, 6224–6228.

98. Moore, K.L., Varki, A. and McEver, R.P. (1991) GMP-140 binds to a glycoprotein receptor on human neutrophils: Evidence for a lectin-like interaction. *J. Cell Biol.*, **112**, 491–499.

99. Corral, L., Singer, M.S., Macher, B.A. and Rosen, S.D. (1990) Requirement for sialic acid on neutrophils in a GMP-140 (PADGEM) mediated adhesive interaction with activated platelets. *Biochem. Biophys. Res. Commun.*, **172**, 1349–1356.

100. Aruffo, A., Kolanus, W., Walz, G., Fredman, P. and Seed, B. (1991) CD62/P-selectin recognition of myeloid and tumor cell sulfatides. *Cell*, **67**, 35–44.

101. Kishimoto, T.K., Warnock, R.A., Jutila, M.A., Butcher, E.C., Lane, C., Anderson, D.C. and Smith, C.W. (1991) Antibodies against human neutrophil LECAM-1 (LAM-1/Leu-8/DREG- 56 antigen) and endothelial cell ELAM-1 inhibit a common CD18-independent adhesion pathway *in vitro*. *Blood*, **78**, 805–811.

102. Picker, L.J., Warnock, R.A., Burns, A.R., Doerschuk, C.M., Berg, E.L. and Butcher, E.C. (1991) The neutrophil selectin LECAM-1 presents carbohydrate ligands to the vascular selectins ELAM-1 and GMP-140. *Cell*, **66**, 921–933.

103. Siegelman, M.H., Cheng, I.C., Weissman, I.L. and Wakeland, E.K. (1990) The mouse lymph node homing receptor is identical with the lymphocyte cell surface marker Ly-22: Role of the EGF domain in endothelial binding. *Cell*, **61**, 611–622.

104. Kishimoto, T.K., Jutila, M.A., Berg, E.L. and Butcher, E.C. (1989) Neutrophil Mac-1 and MEL-14 adhesion proteins inversely regulated by chemotactic factors. *Science*, **245**, 1238–1241.

105. Jutila, M.A., Rott, L., Berg, E.L. and Butcher, E.C. (1989) Function and regulation of the neutrophil MEL-14 antigen *in vivo*: Comparison with LFA-1 and Mac-1. *J. Immunol.*, **143**, 3318–3324.

106. Griffin, J.D., Spertini, O., Ernst, T.J., Belvin, M.P., Levine, H.B., Kanakura, Y. and Tedder, T.F. (1990) Granulocyte–macrophage colony-stimulating factor and other cytokines regulate surface expression of the leukocyte adhesion

molecule-1 on human neutrophils, monocytes, and their precursors. *J. Immunol.*, **145**, 576–584.

107. Spertini, O., Kansas, G.S., Munro, J.M., Griffin, J.D. and Tedder, T.F. (1991) Regulation of leukocyte migration by activation of the leukocyte adhesion molecule-1 (LAM-1) selectin. *Nature*, **349**, 691–694.

108. Dustin, M.L. and Springer, T.A. (1989) T cell receptor cross-linking transiently stimulates adhesiveness through LFA-1. *Nature*, **341**, 619–624.

109. Pober, J.S., Gimbrone, M.A., Jr, Lapierre, L.A., Mendrick, D.L., Fiers, W., Rothlein, R. and Springer, T.A. (1986) Overlapping patterns of activation of human endothelial cells by interleukin 1, tumor necrosis factor and immune interferon. *J. Immunol.*, **137**, 1893–1896.

110. Norris, P., Poston, R.N., Thomas, D.S., Thornhill, M., Hawk, J. and Haskard, D.O. (1991) The expression of endothelial leukocyte adhesion molecule-1 (ELAM-1), intercellular adhesion molecule-1 (ICAM-1), and vascular cell adhesion molecule-1 (VCAM-1) in experimental cutaneous inflammation: A comparison of ultraviolet B erythema and delayed hypersensitivity. *J. Invest. Dermatol.*, **96**, 763–770.

110a. Stoolman, L.M., Grober, J., Bowen, B., Reddy, P., Shih, J., Thompson, C., Fox, D.A. and Ebling, H. (1992) Selectin-dependent monocyte adhesion in frozen sections of rheumatoid synovitis. In Lipsky, P.E., Rothlein, R., Kishimoto, T.K., Faanes, R.B. and Smith, C.W. (Eds.), Structure, Function and Regulation of Molecules involved in Leukocyte Adhesion. Springer-Verlag, New York.

111. Lewinsohn, D.M., Bargatze, R.F. and Butcher, E.C. (1987) Leukocyte–endothelial cell recognition: Evidence of a common molecular mechanism shared by neutrophils, lymphocytes, and other leukocytes. *J. Immunol.*, **138**, 4313–4321.

112. Watson, S.R., Fennie, C. and Lasky, L.A. (1991) Neutrophil influx into an inflammatory site inhibited by a soluble homing receptor–IgG chimaera. *Nature*, **349**, 164–167.

113. Gundel, R.H., Wegner, C.D., Torcellini, C.A., Clarke, C.C., Haynes, N., Rothlein, R., Smith, C.W. and Letts, L.G. (1991) Endothelial leukocyte adhesion molecule-1 mediates antigen-induced acute airway inflammation and late-phase airway obstruction in monkeys. *J. Clin. Invest.*, **88**, 1407–1411.

114. Mulligan, M.S., Varani, J., Dame, M.K., Lane, C.L., Smith, C.W., Anderson, D.C. and Ward, P.A. (1991) Role of endothelial-leukocyte adhesion molecule 1 (ELAM-1) in neutrophil-mediated lung injury in rats. *J. Clin. Invest.*, **88**, 1396–1406.

115. Kishimoto, T.K., Jutila, M.A., Berg, E.L. and Butcher, E.C. (1989) Neutrophil Mac-1 and MEL-14 adhesion proteins inversely regulated by chemotactic factors. *Science*, **245**, 1238–1241.

116. Kishimoto, T.K. (1991) A dynamic model for neutrophil localization to inflammatory sites. *J. NIH Res.*, **3**, 75–77.

117. Bevilacqua, M.P., Pober, J.S., Wheeler, M.E., Cotran, R.S. and Gimbrone, M.A., Jr (1985) Interleukin 1 acts on cultured human vascular endothelium to increase the adhesion of polymorphonuclear leukocytes, monocytes, and related leukocyte cell lines. *J. Clin. Invest.*, **76**, 2003–2011.

118. Bevilacqua, M.P., Pober, J.S., Majeau, G.R., Cotran, R.S. and Gimbrone, M.A., Jr (1984) Interleukin 1 (IL-1) induces biosynthesis and cell surface expression of procoagulant activity in human vascular endothelial cells. *J. Exp. Med.*, **160**, 618–623.

119. Pober, J.S. and Gimbrone, M.A., Jr (1982) Expression of Ia-like antigens by human vascular endothelial cells is inducible *in vitro*: demonstration by monoclonal antibody binding and immunoprecipitation. *Proc. Nat. Acad. Sci. USA*, **79**, 6641–6645.

120. Pober, J.S., Bevilacqua, M.P., Mendrick, D.L., Lapierre, L.A., Fiers, W. and Gimbrone, M.A., Jr (1986) Two distinct monokines, interleukin 1 and tumor necrosis factor, each independently induce biosynthesis and transient expression of the same antigen on the surface of cultured human vascular endothelial cells. *J. Immunol.*, **136**, 1680–1687.

121. Cohnheim, J. (1889) *Lectures on General Pathology: A Handbook for Practitioners and Students*. The New Sydenham Society, London.

122. Arfors, K.-E., Lundberg, C., Lindbom, L., Lundberg, K., Beatty, P.G. and Harlan, J.M. (1987) A monoclonal antibody to the membrane glycoprotein complex CD18 inhibits polymorphonuclear accumulation and plasma leakage *in vivo*. *Blood*, **69**, 338–340.

123. Lawrence, M.B., Smith, C.W., Eskin, S.G. and McIntire, L.V. (1988) Effect of venous shear stress on CD18-mediated neutrophil adhesion to culture endothelium. Manuscript.

124. Kishimoto, T.K., Jutila, M.A. and Butcher, E.C. (1990) Identification of a human peripheral lymph node homing receptor: A rapidly down-regulated adhesion molecule. *Proc. Nat. Acad. Sci. USA*, **87**, 2244–2248.

125. Lawrence, M.B. and Springer, T.A. (1991) Leukocytes roll on a selectin at physiologic flow rates: Distinction from and prerequisite for adhesion through integrins. *Cell*, **65**, 1–20.

126. Dobrina, A., Carlos, T.M., Schwartz, B.R., Beatty, P.G., Ochs, H.D. and Harlan, J.M. (1990) Phorbol ester causes down-regulation of CD11/CD18-independent neutrophil adherence to endothelium. *Immunology*, **69**, 429–434.

127. Smith, C.W., Marlin, S.D., Rothlein, R., Lawrence, M.B., McIntire, L.V. and Anderson, D.C. (1989) Role of ICAM-1 in the adherence of human neutrophils to human endothelial cells *in vitro*. In Springer, T.A., Anderson, D.C., Rosenthal, A.S. and Rothlein, R. (eds) *Leukocyte Adhesion Molecules*, Springer-Verlag, New York, pp. 170–189.

128. Huber, A.R., Kunkel, S.L., Todd, R.F. and Weiss, S.J. (1991) Regulation of transendothelial neutrophil migration by endogenous Il-8. *Science*, **254**, 99–102.

129. Prescott, S.M., Zimmerman, G.A. and McIntyre, T.M. (1984) Human endothelial cells in culture produce platelet-activating factor when stimulated with thrombin. *Proc. Nat. Acad. Sci. USA*, **81**, 3534–3538.

130. Zimmerman, G.A., McIntyre, T.M., Mehra, M. and Prescott, S.M. (1990) Endothelial cell-associated platelet-activating factor: a novel mechanism for signalling intercellular adhesion. *J. Cell. Biol.*, **110**, 529–540.

131. Zimmerman, G.A. and McIntyre, T.M. (1988) Neutrophil adherence to human endothelium *in vitro* occurs by CDw18 (Mo1, Mac-1/LFA-1/gp150,95) glycoprotein-dependent and independent mechanisms. *J. Clin. Invest.*, **81**, 531–537.

132. Zimmerman, G.A., McIntyre, T.M. and Prescott, S.M. (1985) Thrombin stimulates the adherence of neutrophils to human endothelial cells *in vitro*. *J. Clin. Invest.*, **76**, 2235–2246.

133. Simon, S.I., Rochen, Y.R., Anderson, D.C., Smith, C.W. and Sklar, L.A. (1992) Are beta-2 integrin and L-selectin counter-receptors in neutrophil aggregation? *Fed. Am. Soc. Exp. Biol. J.*, **6**, A1689 (Abstract).

134. Smith, C.W., Rothlein, R., Hughes, B.J., Mariscalco, M.M., Schmalstieg, F.C. and Anderson, D.C. (1988) Recognition of an endothelial determinant for CD18-dependent neutrophil adherence and transendothelial migration. *J. Clin. Invest.*, **82**, 1746–1756.
135. Smith, C.W., Marlin, S.D., Rothlein, R., Toman, C. and Anderson, D.C. (1989) Cooperative interactions of LFA-1 and Mac-1 with intercellular adhesion molecule-1 in facilitating adherence and transendothelial migration of human neutrophils *in vitro*. *J. Clin. Invest.*, **83**, 2008–2017.
136. Luscinskas, F.W., Cybulsky, M.I., Kiely, J.-M., Peckins, C.S., Davis, V.M. and Gimbrone, M.A., Jr (1991) Cytokine-activated human endothelial monolayers support enhanced neutrophil transmigration via a mechanism involving both endothelial-leukocyte adhesion molecule-1 and intercellular adhesion molecule-1. *J. Immunol.*, **146**, 1617–1625.

Part B

IMMUNODEFICIENCY DISEASES

Chapter 7

X-linked Severe Combined Immunodeficiency

MARY ELLEN CONLEY

Department of Pediatrics, University of Tennessee, Memphis; and Department of Immunology, St Jude Children's Research Hospital, Memphis, Tennessee, USA

Severe combined immunodeficiency (SCID) is a term that came into common usage in the early 1970s to refer to a group of disorders in which the affected infants had profound defects of both cellular and humoral immunity (1). Although no specific diagnostic criteria have been developed that permit a uniform definition of SCID, this diagnosis is usually limited to children with genetic disorders who present to medical attention with an opportunistic infection, or an unusually severe or persistent infection, at less than 1 year of age. Laboratory evaluation usually demonstrates lymphopenia, hypogammaglobulinemia and markedly reduced proliferative responses to mitogens (1–6). A somewhat more liberal definition would include children who fail to make antibodies to antigens they have encountered and whose T cells do not proliferate in response to antigens (2).

As increasingly sophisticated diagnostic studies and therapeutic options have become available, it has become both possible and necessary to dissect out the various genetic disorders that result in SCID. It has been clear since the earliest use of the term SCID that there were both autosomal recessive and X-linked forms of the disorder (1). Adenosine deaminase deficiency, which can be demonstrated in 10–20% of patients with SCID (3, 7), was the first specific gene defect associated with SCID (8). Studies of patients with this autosomal recessive disorder continue to provide models for the analysis of normal lymphocyte development (9, 10), as well as diagnosis and treatment of specific genetic defects (11–15). It is likely that some of the lessons learned in attempts to provide the missing or defective gene product (13, 14), or a normal copy of the gene itself (15), can be generalized to other immunodeficiencies.

New Concepts in Immunodeficiency Diseases. Edited by S. Gupta and C. Griscelli
© 1993 John Wiley & Sons Ltd

Other single gene defects that affect both cellular and humoral immunity have been described. These include defects in another enzyme in the purine salvage pathway, purine nucleoside phosphorylase (PNP) (16), and defects in either the γ or the ε chain of the T cell antigen receptor-associated complex (17–19). However, in these disorders, the patients tend to have a milder course and many immunologists would not give them the diagnosis of SCID. Affected children usually do not have overwhelming problems in the first year of life and many survive without heroic measures (16–19).

There remain very few other specific genetic defects that are known to cause SCID. Small numbers of patients with SCID have what is referred to as the bare lymphocyte syndrome; cells from these patients fail to express class II HLA antigens (20–22). Analysis of the enhancer region of class II genes in cell lines from these patients indicates that some patients lack a DNA binding protein, RFX, that is required for transcription of the class II genes (20). However, complementation studies and DNA footprinting analysis suggest that there are several different genetic defects that result in failure to express class II genes, and in none of them has the primary lesion been identified (21, 22). A distinct subset of patients with SCID lack both T cells and B cells. Schwarz *et al.* have recently suggested that these patients have defective assembly of antigen receptor genes (23), as is seen in the murine model of SCID (24). However, the defective gene in the murine model of SCID has not yet been identified and it is not clear that all of the patients who lack T cells and B cells have the same gene defect. Patients who have defective production of T cell-derived lymphokines (25, 26), abnormal signal transduction (27, 28), or failure to express CD7 (29) have also been described; but in these patients as well the primary genetic lesion remains unknown.

In all large series of patients with SCID, affected males outnumber females. In Europe, the ratio of males to females is approximately 2 : 1 (6), whereas in North America the ratio is closer to 4 : 1 (3, 4). These figures suggest that about 30% of patients with SCID in Europe and 60% of patients with SCID in North America have X-linked forms of the disease. However, as is true with all X-linked disorders that are lethal without medical intervention, only about half of the affected males have a positive family history of immunodeficiency (30). The remaining patients represent the first manifestation in their family of a new mutation. Based on comparisons with other immunodeficiencies (7, 31, 32), it can be estimated that the frequency of XSCID is approximately 1–5 per million male births.

CLINICAL AND LABORATORY CHARACTERISTICS OF X-LINKED SEVERE COMBINED IMMUNODEFICIENCY

Most infants with XSCID are born at term after an uncomplicated pregnancy. The perinatal period is usually uneventful, but sometime between 1 and

6 months of age the patient comes to medical attention, sometimes because of fulminant sepsis, but more often because of persistent candidiasis, diarrhea, tachypnea and/or pyoderma (2, 3, 33, 34). More than one organ system is usually involved, and by 4–6 months of age the patient is almost invariably below the expected weight for age (2, 3). The onset of symptoms is often insidious and, early in the clinical course, patients with documented viral infections, such as respiratory syncytial virus, parainfluenza or rotavirus, may have minimal secondary symptoms such as fever and irritability, underlining the importance of the normal immune response in eliciting these symptoms. In infants with a positive family history of immunodeficiency, the mean age at diagnosis of XSCID is 3.3 months, whereas in patients who represent the first manifestation of a new mutation the mean age at diagnosis of SCID in the United States is 6.3 months (34).

Laboratory findings in XSCID depend, in part, on the patient's age and clinical status. Most patients have mild lymphopenia, with lymphocyte counts of 1500–3000/mm^3 (33). In the absence of overwhelming infection or severe failure to thrive, the hemoglobin, neutrophil count and platelet count are usually normal. Beyond the newborn period the serum IgG and IgA are markedly decreased, whereas in approximately 50% of patients the IgM is in the normal range (33). Paraproteins involving any isotype may be seen and are not necessarily indicative of a bad prognosis.

Analysis of lymphocyte cell surface markers in patients with XSCID demonstrate markedly reduced or absent T cells, as identified with monoclonal antibodies to CD2, CD3, CD4 or CD8 (33–36). T cells that are detected are usually of maternal origin (33). O'Reilly *et al.* have shown that as many as 50% of patients with SCID have engraftment of maternal cells that enter the infant's circulation before or during the birth process (5). These maternally acquired cells usually do not cause graft-versus-host disease, although they may be responsible for rejections of a T cell-depleted transplant from a third-party donor (5). Lymphocytes from patients with XSCID, even those with maternally acquired lymphocytes, generally do not proliferate in response to T cell mitogens or allogeneic stimulation (33).

B cells are present in the blood of patients with XSCID in normal or elevated numbers. These cells express the surface markers characteristic of B cells, including surface IgM and IgD, CD19, CD20, CD21, CD22 and CD24 (33, 35, 36). In addition, peripheral blood B cells from these patients express p120, a marker detected with the monoclonal antibody AL1 (36). This marker is usually expressed on pre-B cells, along with common acute lymphatic leukemia antigen (CALLA), and it is not seen on cells in the peripheral circulation. However, XSCID B cells do not bear CALLA, nor do they express two activation antigens, 4F2 and the transferrin receptor, which are characteristically seen on B cells from age-matched controls (36). B cells from patients with XSCID will proliferate and secrete IgM in response to combinations of cytokines, mitogens and anti-IgM (35, 36), but the amount of proliferation or immunoglobulin production tends to be decreased compared to age-matched controls. The unusual phenotype and diminished B cell activation and differentiation could be attributed to either the absence of T cell or to expression of the gene defect in B cells as well as T cells.

Although there are some discrepancies in the literature, the most recent studies indicate that natural killer (NK) cells are not seen in the peripheral circulation of patients with XSCID (36). Again, this could be attributed to either an absolute requirement for T cells, or T cell-derived cytokines in NK cell production, or to expression of the gene defect in the NK lineage. There is no evidence of defects in monocyte or neutrophil number or function in XSCID.

In the absence of a family history of immunodeficiency, it may be difficult to make the diagnosis of XSCID. Several groups have described females with a disorder that is identical to XSCID in both clinical and laboratory findings; a review of several large series suggests that females constitute about 10% of patients with SCID who have B cells but no T cells (4, 35, 37). This suggests that there is an autosomal recessive disorder that cannot easily be distinguished from XSCID. A male infant who has B cells but no T cells and who has no family history of immunodeficiency may have the autosomal recessive form of SCID that is phenotypically identical to XSCID; or the child may be the first manifestation of a new mutation of the XSCID gene. At the present time, it is important to distinguish between these two possibilities in order to provide the most informative genetic counselling. In the future, it is likely that therapy will be influenced by the patient's specific genetic defect.

THERAPY

At the present time, bone marrow transplantation is the only therapy for XSCID that results in long-term survival (2–6, 38, 39). However, many of the signs and symptoms of XSCID are amenable to symptomatic treatment. The poor weight gain that is typical of XSCID may be due to increased energy expenditures necessitated by chronic pulmonary infections or to occult infections of the gastrointestinal tract (38). Patients with SCID have been documented to have as many as five different gastrointestinal viral infections (40). Intravenous hyperalimentation is often required to provide these patients with sufficient calories and nutrients to maintain or gain weight. Pneumocystis pneumonia, which is frequently the presenting complaint in patients with XSCID, usually responds promptly to appropriate doses of trimethoprim and sulfamethoxazole. Fungal and viral infections may improve when the patient is treated with appropriate agents; but until the patient has successfully engrafted T cells, these infections usually return when the antimicrobial is discontinued.

In 1968 the first successful HLA-matched bone marrow transplant for XSCID was reported (41). This patient subsequently experienced pancytopenia as a result of graft-versus-host disease involving the bone marrow. A second bone marrow transplant from the same donor resulted in complete engraftment of all hematopoietic cell lineages (42). This bone marrow recipient remains well more than 20 years after the second transplant.

Since 1968, at least 300 patients with SCID have been treated with bone marrow transplants. However, in published studies describing outcome, it is usually not possible to distinguish the patients with XSCID from those with other forms of the disease. In addition to survival, the outcomes that should be considered include: (a) time until T cell engraftment; (b) the breadth and depth of T cell engraftment; (c) the adequacy of B cell function; (d) incidence of complications of transplant such as graft-versus-host disease, Epstein–Barr virus (EBV)-induced lymphoproliferation, and autoimmune disease; and (e) cost of transplant. These outcomes are influenced by the age and clinical status of the patient at the time of transplant and by the type of transplant used to treat the patient.

Approximately 30% of patients with SCID treated with bone marrow transplant have received HLA-matched transplants from a sibling or another closely related family member (6). In these patients T cell engraftment may be seen as early as 1–2 weeks after transplant (4, 38, 41, 43). However, graft-versus-host disease, as described in the patient who was transplanted in 1968, remains a significant risk (38, 41). Most patients do not have an HLA-matched related donor. In 1981 Reisner *et al.* showed that these patients could be treated with a T cell-depleted transplant from a parent who shared a single HLA haplotype with the patient (44).

Since that time a variety of protocols have been used to prepare the patient for transplant, to deplete the marrow of donor T cells and to protect the patient from graft-versus-host disease and EBV-induced lymphoproliferative disease (4–6, 38, 39). T cells are usually removed either by treatment with anti-T cell antibodies and complement (6, 39) or by selective agglutination with soybean agglutinin and/or sheep red blood cells (4–6). There is no strong evidence to indicate that one mechanism of depleting T cells is preferable to others. Engraftment may be somewhat delayed when the donor marrow is depleted of T cells by agglutination with soybean lectin and sheep erythrocytes; however, this may be balanced by a decreased incidence or severity of graft-versus-host disease and possibly by a lower incidence of EBV-induced lymphoproliferative disease. Recent studies suggest that over 60% of patients with SCID who receive a T cell-depleted transplant and 80–90% of those who receive an HLA-matched transplant achieve long-term survival (6). The younger the patient is at the time of transplant, the greater the chances are of success (6, 38).

Patients with XSCID usually engraft donor T cells readily (4–6, 34).

However, unless the patient receives cytoreductive therapy, donor B cells do not engraft (4–6, 34). Residual abnormalities of the immune system are common in both patients who are treated with HLA-matched and T cell-depleted transplants (34). In a review of 10 patients with XSCID, none of whom were treated with cytoreductive therapy, we found that only 3 had normal concentrations of serum immunoglobulins and 5 had normal percentages of CD3+, CD4+, CD8+ T cells, B cells and NK cells, more than 2 years after transplant. Data from the European centers suggest that cytoreductive therapy may result in improved outcome, particularly in patients who are without significant infection at the time of transplant (6).

CARRIER DETECTION

Obligate carriers of XSCID, the mothers of affected boys, are normal by all immunological criteria (33, 45). They have normal numbers of lymphocytes, normal proliferation in response to mitogens and they do not have a history of unusual infections. The failure of these women to show signs of their gene defect can be explained by selective use of the normal, non-mutant X as the active X in the cell lineages primarily affected by the gene defect (33, 34, 46–50).

Early in embryogenesis of the female, there is random inactivation of one of the two X chromosomes in each somatic cell (51). The mechanisms by which this inactivation occur are not well understood, but once it occurs it is maintained, at least in part, by differences in methylation between the active and inactive X (52). As a result of X inactivation, the normal female is a mosaic. Approximately half the cells in any lineage have the maternally derived X as the active X and half have the paternally derived X as the active X. However, if one of the two X chromosomes carries a defect that is detrimental to the proliferation or survival of cells of a particular lineage, then, by default, the cells of that lineage will be derived from the precursors that have the other X—the normal X—as the active X. Several laboratories have demonstrated that certain cell lineages from obligate carriers of XSCID demonstrate non-random X chromosome inactivation (46–50). This observation can be used both to provide carrier detection and to examine the nature of the gene defect itself.

To evaluate patterns of X chromosome inactivation, one must be able to distinguish the maternal versus paternal X, and the active versus the inactive X. There are several techniques that accomplish these tasks. We have used a technique in which the cells of interest, for example T cells, are fused to cells from a Chinese hamster cell line that is deficient in the X-linked enzyme hypoxanthine phosphoribosyl transferase (HPRT). The cell line that we use, RJK88, is an efficient fusion partner but the hybrids tend to throw off human chromosomes. If the hybrids are grown in selective media, they must retain the active human X to provide the HPRT (33, 47, 53, 54). When a series of 10–30 somatic cell hybrids is produced, DNA from each hybrid can be analyzed with any X-linked restriction fragment length polymorphism for which the woman in question is heterozygous. If there is random X chromosome inactivation, some hybrids will contain the maternally derived X and others will contain the paternally derived X. In T cell hybrids from carriers of XSCID there is non-random X inactivation; all, or almost all, of the hybrids have the normal, non-mutant X as the active X (46, 47).

Other techniques to analyze X chromosome inactivation patterns depend on the differences in methylation between the active and inactive X. In the upstream of 5' region of many "housekeeping" genes on the X chromosome are sites that differ in methylation between the active and inactive X (52, 55). If these variably methylated sites are close to polymorphic DNA sequences, it may be possible to use a methylation-sensitive enzyme to distinguish the active and inactive X and a second technique to demonstrate the polymorphism. HPRT at Xq26, phosphoglycerate kinase (PGK) at Xq13 and DXS255 at Xp11.2 are all polymorphic loci that differ in methylation between the active and inactive X chromosome (52, 55, 56). It is possible to digest DNA with a restriction enzyme to reveal the polymorphism, and then digest an aliquot of that DNA with a methylation-sensitive enzyme. Both aliquots are then examined in a Southern blot. If the DNA was taken from cells demonstrating a random pattern of X inactivation, then both alleles will be seen in the sample digested with the methylation-sensitive enzyme; in contrast, in non-random X inactivation, one allele completely disappears because it has been digested with the methylation-sensitive enzyme.

Recently, a variation on the methylation technique has been described using polymerase chain reaction (PCR). The methylation site and the polymorphic restriction site at the PGK locus are within 500 base pairs of each other. This makes it possible to use oligonucleotide primers that flank both sites to amplify the DNA in this region. An aliquot of DNA is first digested with the methylation-sensitive enzyme, then both the digested and undigested DNA are amplified by PCR and separated by size using gel electrophoresis (57). If the subject is heterozygous for PGK and her cells demonstrate random X inactivation, both alleles will be seen in the sample digested with the methylation-sensitive enzyme; however, if she has non-random X chromosome inactivation, one allele will be lost because no intact DNA is available for the primers to amplify. Unfortunately, only 33% of women are heterozygous for PGK (57), making this approach uninformative in most women.

Another locus that is particularly useful for PCR X inactivation analysis is the androgen receptor gene, where a site that is always methylated in the inactive X but never methylated in the active X is 20 nucleotides away from a trinucleotide repeat that is highly polymorphic (58, 59). Seventeen alleles have been detected at this site, with 90% of women being heterozygous (59). Both the PGK and androgen receptor loci have the added advantage that they are linked to the gene for XSCID (see below); the PGK locus shows no recombination with XSCID and the androgen receptor locus is approximately 10 cM proximal to XSCID.

In evaluating patterns of X chromosome inactivation, it is important to keep in mind that random X chromosome inactivation can result in a pattern that differs from the expected mean of 50% of cells with the maternally derived X as the active X and 50% with the paternally derived X as the active X. In as many as 10% of normal women, random X inactivation results in one X being active in 80% of cells, with the remaining cells having the other X as the active X (60, 61). In most women the pattern of X chromosome inactivation in all cell lineages tends to be similar (60). Thus, if one finds preferential but not exclusive use of one X chromosome as the active X in a particular cell lineage, it is helpful to examine cell lineages that are not affected by the gene defect. If all cell lineages demonstrate the same degree of skewing, it is likely that the woman is at the far end of the normal spectrum of random X inactivation. In contrast, skewing in one lineage but not others suggests selection against the X not used as the active X in the cell lineage demonstrating skewing.

THE NATURE OF THE GENE DEFECT

X chromosome inactivation analysis has also been used to examine the nature of the gene defect in XSCID. Exclusive use of the normal X as the active X in T cells from carriers of XSCID indicates that the gene product is intrinsic to the T cell lineage (46–50). Only T cell precursors that have the normal X as the active X are able to survive or proliferate. It is unlikely that the gene product is secreted. If the gene product were transportable between cells, one would expect the normal gene product to interact with cells having the abnormal X as the active X and thus permit these cells to survive or proliferate.

To determine whether the hypogammaglobulinemia in patients with XSCID was secondary to the T cell deficiency or due to expression of the gene defect in B cells as well as T cells, we evaluated X inactivation patterns in polyclonal EBV-transformed cell lines from obligate carriers of XSCID (47). B cell hybrids from all of the women showed preferential use of a single X as the active X; this X was always the same X that was used as the active X in the T cell hybrids. These results indicate that the XSCID gene defect is intrinsic to B cells as well as T cells. There were a small number of B cell hybrids from some of the women that had the mutant X as the active X. One possible explanation for this finding is that the XSCID defect might result in a relative but not absolute block in B cell proliferation or differentiation. If this were true, one would expect that the B cells having the mutant X as the active X would be the least mature B cells—those that had undergone the least proliferation or differentiation. To examine this possibility, peripheral blood B cells were separated into immature B cells, expressing a high intensity of surface IgM, and surface IgM-negative B cells. Both subpopulations were transformed with EBV and grown in multiple aliquots.

B cell hybrids that were derived from the sIgM– cells, the cells committed to IgG and IgA, demonstrated exclusive use of the normal X as the active X, whereas B cell hybrids derived from the immature, sIgM+ cells showed frequent use of the mutant X as the active X (47). The finding of random X inactivation in the sIgM+ hybrids rules out the possibility that the XSCID gene defect is expressed only in a precursor common to both T and B cells. If the gene were expressed only in a precursor, then all the cells past this early stage in differentiation would show the same degree of skewing. Nor is the defect likely to be involved in isotype switching. The B cell hybrids derived from the unselected EBV transformed cells, which were predominantly IgM+, did show significant skewing. We have interpreted our findings as indicating that the XSCID gene defect results in a disadvantage in B cell proliferation or differentiation at multiple stages of B cell development. At each successive stage in B cell differentiation, it is less and less likely that a B cell with the mutant X as the active X will be found.

In contrast, monocytes from obligate carriers of XSCID demonstrate random X inactivation (47), indicating that a defective XSCID gene product is not detrimental to proliferation or survival of these cells. Because the XSCID gene product is expressed in T and B cells but not monocytes, we have been particularly interested in its expression in NK cells. Preliminary results, using the PCR technique described above, suggest that NK cells from obligate carriers of XSCID, like T and B cells, exhibit non-random X inactivation. Expression of the XSCID gene defect in NK cells would indicate that the gene product does not involve production of a rearranged antigen receptor gene.

X inactivation patterns in T cells, B cells, granulocytes and fibroblasts from carriers of XSCID have also been examined by Goodship *et al.*, who found exclusive use of the normal X as the active X in T cells, preferential use of the normal X as the active X in EBV-transformed B cell lines from all carriers and preferential use of the normal X as the active X in granulocytes and fibroblasts from some but not all carriers (49). These investigators have interpreted their findings as indicating that the XSCID gene product is expressed in all of these cell lineages and they have proposed that the defect involves an enzyme in a metabolic pathway that is more critical to T cells than other cell lineages.

An alternative interpretation of the preferential use of the normal X as the active X in granulocytes and fibroblasts from some carriers of XSCID is that these women may be at the far end of the spectrum of normal random X inactivation, with the majority of cells in all tissues having the normal X as the active X. Although a defect in a metabolic enzyme might explain the pattern of X inactivation in T cells, B cells and NK cells, other possibilities fit the data as well. For example, the gene product could be a transcription factor, a receptor for a growth factor, or a second messenger. The fact that there is an autosomal recessive disorder that is phenotypically identical to XSCID suggests that the products of the XSCID gene and the autosomal recessive gene may be functionally related. One can postulate that the products might form a dimer, a receptor–ligand complex, or two components of a protein cascade in which the product of one gene precedes that of the other.

LINKAGE ANALYSIS

By studying a large number of multi-generation families, it has been possible to map the gene for XSCID to the proximal part of the long arm of the X at Xq13 (62–64). The gene for XSCID has shown no recombination with PGK or three other closely linked polymorphic loci—DXS441, DXS347 and DXS325 (64)—although no deletions or altered fragment size have been detected when probes at these loci have been used to analyze DNA from affected males. The proximal and distal flanking markers, DXS159 and DXS72 respectively, are both approximately 3–5 cM from the gene (1 cM is equal to 1% probability of recombination). The availability of these closely linked markers makes carrier detection and prenatal diagnosis relatively straightforward in families with a clear diagnosis of XSCID. However, certain caveats should be kept in mind. (a) If the underlying diagnosis is in error, then the results of linkage analysis will be misleading. Both X-linked hyper-IgM syndrome and X-linked agammaglobulinemia can result in a family history of several baby boys who died of infection. As noted above, there is probably an autosomal recessive disorder that is phenotypically identical to XSCID. (b) Linkage analysis will not be helpful in individuals who have inherited a cross-over between flanking markers. (c) The mutation may have come from an unexpected source. Several families have been described in which a healthy male has transmitted an X-linked immunodeficiency to more than one of his daughters (65, 66 and personal observation). It can be assumed that these males were gonadal chimeras.

In the past, linkage studies were usually performed using probes that detected two allele polymorphisms on Southern blot analysis. More recently, there has been a trend towards using PCR probes that reveal multi-allele polymorphisms. Throughout the human genome there are short tandem repeats (STR) of sequences two to four nucleotides long (59, 67, 68). These STRs occur with a frequency of about 1 per 60–300 kb, and in approximately half the STRs the number of times the repeat occurs is polymorphic

(68). Oligonucleotide primers that flank the polymorphic site can be used to amplify the alleles.

There is no evidence at this time that there is more than one gene that results in XSCID. In all of the families that demonstrate a clear X-linked pattern of inheritance and in whom the proband has the clinical and laboratory features of XSCID, the defect maps to the same locus at Xq13 and the obligate carriers demonstrate non-random X inactivation in T cells and B cells. Several families have been described that may have milder allelic variants of XSCID (69–72). In these families the affected males usually have reduced numbers of T cells and reduced T cell function (71, 72). In one such family, linkage analysis and X chromosome inactivation studies were identical to those seen in families with typical XSCID (72).

GENETIC COUNSELLING

Families may request genetic counselling under a variety of circumstances. If a woman wants to learn whether she is a carrier of XSCID because she had a brother, cousin or uncle with SCID, linkage analysis is the fastest and least costly means of providing carrier detection if the following requirements can be met. (a) There must be a clear pattern of X-linked inheritance with males of more than one generation affected. (b) Laboratory studies on a proband should demonstrate markedly decreased or absent T cells with minimal proliferation in response to mitogen stimulation and increased proportions of B cells with hypogammaglobulinemia. If the proband was born more than 15 years ago, the laboratory studies are less reliable. However, autopsy evidence of severe thymic dysplasia in a boy with hypogammaglobulinemia provides strong support for the diagnosis of XSCID in a child with a family history of additional early male deaths. (c) To identify the X chromosome haplotype bearing the XSCID mutation, DNA from an obligate carrier and an affected or unaffected son of an obligate carrier in the subject's family must be available.

If the mother of a boy with sporadic SCID or a member of her family is interested in carrier detection, then one must analyze X inactivation patterns in lymphocytes from the mother of the affected boy (33). If her T cells demonstrate non-random X chromosome inactivation with random X inactivation of non-lymphoid lineages, she is a carrier of XSCID and her daughters are at 50% risk of being carriers. Informative flanking markers at the XSCID locus can be determined by examining DNA from the carrier and from the affected son, an unaffected son, or a T cell hybrid that contains the non-mutant maternal X. Once the flanking markers have been identified, prenatal diagnosis is possible for the mother's future pregnancies (73, 74).

If the maternal aunts or cousins of a boy with sporadic SCID desire carrier detection, and the boy's mother has been shown to be a carrier by X inactivation analysis, one should evaluate the maternal grandparents. If T cells from the maternal grandmother demonstrate non-random X inactivation, then linkage analysis can be used to provide carrier detection for her descendants. However, if T cells from the maternal grandmother show random X inactivation, the maternal aunts and cousins may still be at risk. As noted above, gonadal chimerism, in which an individual who does not have the signs or symptoms of a genetic defect has passed that defect on to several offspring, has been described in families with X-linked agammaglobulinemia, Wiskott–Aldrich syndrome and XSCID (65, 66 and J.M. Puck, personal communication). Therefore, in this situation, carrier detection for maternal aunts should include X inactivation analysis.

Genetic counselling is more difficult for the mother of a boy who has what appears to be XSCID but whose T cells exhibit random X chromosome inactivation. This woman may be a carrier of the autosomal recessive form of SCID that is similar to XSCID. It may be that her son has XSCID on the basis of a new mutation that occurred in the ovum that gave rise to this child. Alternatively, she may be a gonadal chimera, in which case she could pass the gene defect on to future children. At this time it is not possible to distinguish these possibilities. Prenatal diagnosis in this situation can be provided by analysis of a fetal blood sample.

FUTURE TRENDS

The rapid advancements in molecular genetics suggest that the gene for XSCID will be identified, isolated and characterized in the next 5–10 years, perhaps sooner. The most immediate benefit of this accomplishment will be improved genetic counselling. PCR techniques that permit amplication of specific exons and detection of single base pair changes should make it possible to detect most mutant alleles (75, 76). This is critically important in identifying new mutations. In most families with well-established disease, linkage analysis using PCR probes that are very close to the gene defect will continue to be the mainstay of genetic counselling.

Characterization of the XSCID gene, that is, comparison of the sequence of this gene to other known genes, localization of the gene product to a particular site within the cell, and analysis of mutations that result in altered gene function, will increase our understanding not only of this specific gene defect but also of normal lymphocyte development. In recent years several ''knock out'' experiments, in which genes that are considered central to the immune system have been crippled, have had less impressive effects than expected (77, 78). In contrast, the XSCID gene appears to be essential for normal lymphoid development and function.

A better understanding of the structure and function of the XSCID gene will eventually result in improved therapy for affected patients. It is possible that ways will be discovered to compensate for an abnormal or missing gene product or to increase production of a labile or partially functioning gene product. It is more likely that targeted gene therapy will depend on the ability to replace the defective gene with a normal copy. Although it has been possible to treat patients with adenosine deaminase deficiency with a normal gene or gene product in a vehicle external to the affected cells (79), X chromosome inactivation studies suggest that the normal XSCID gene or gene product must be found within the affected cells. Because the XSCID gene product is expressed in T cells, B cells and NK cells, it will be necessary to replace the defective gene in a stem cell that gives rise to all lymphoid subpopulations. Replacing the defective gene with a normal copy will place the gene in the appropriate regulatory context. In patients who are diagnosed as having XSCID early in gestation, it will probably be possible to replace the defective gene several months prior to birth so that at the time of birth the patient will have been cured of his disease.

Although these possibilities may seem overly optimistic, remarkable progress has been made in the last 5 years in each of the areas required to provide targeted gene therapy. The next 5 years are likely to be equally exciting.

REFERENCES

1. Fudenberg, H., Good, R.A., Goodman, H.C., Hitzig, W., Kunkel, H.G., Roitt, I.M., Rosen, F.S., Rowe, D.S., Seligmann, M. and Soothill, J.R. (1971) Primary immunodeficiencies: Report of a World Health Organization Committee. *Pediatrics*, **47**, 927–946.
2. Ammann, A.J. and Hong, R. (1989) Disorders of the T-cell system. In Stiehm, E.R. (ed.) *Immunologic Disorders in Infants and Children*. Saunders, Philadelphia, pp. 257–315.
3. Gelfand, E.W. and Dosch, H.-M. (1983) Diagnosis and classification of severe combined immunodeficiency disease. *Birth Defects*, **19**, 65–72.
4. Buckley, R.H., Schiff, S.E., Sampson, H.A., Schiff, R.I., Markert, M.L., Knutsen, A.P., Hershfield, M.S., Huang, A.T., Mickey, G.H. and Ward, F.E. (1986) Development of immunity in human severe primary T cell deficiency following haploidentical bone marrow stem cell transplantation. *J. Immunol.*, **136**, 2398–2407.
5. O'Reilly, R.J., Keever, C.A., Small, T.N. and Brochstein, J. (1989) The use of HLA-non-identical T-cell-depleted marrow transplants for correction of severe combined immunodeficiency disease. *Immunodef. Rev.*, **1**, 273–309.
6. Fischer, A., Landais, P., Friedrich, W., Morgan, G., Gerritsen, B., Fasth, A., Porta, F., Griscelli, C., Goldman, S.F., Levinsky, R. and Vossen, J. (1990) European experience of bone-marrow transplantation for severe combined immunodeficiency. *Lancet*, **ii**, 850–854.
7. Hirschhorn, R. (1990) Adenosine deaminase deficiency. *Immunodef. Rev.*, **2**, 175–198.
8. Giblett, E.R., Anderson, J.E., Cohen, F., Pollara, B. and Meuwissen, H.J. (1972) Adenosine-deaminase deficiency in two patients with severely impaired cellular immunity. *Lancet*, **ii**, 1067–1069.

9. Carson, D.A., Wasson, D.B., Lakow, E. and Kamatani, N. (1982) Possible metabolic basis for the different immunodeficient states associated with genetic deficiencies of adenosine deaminase and purine nucleoside phosphorylase. *Proc. Nat. Acad. Sci. USA*, **79**, 3848–3852.

10. Cohen, A., Barankiewicz, J., Lederman, H.M. and Gelfand, E.W. (1983) Purine and pyrimidine metabolism in human T lymphocytes. *J. Biol. Chem.*, **258**, 12334–12340.

11. Akeson, A.L., Wiginton, D.A. and Hutton, J.J. (1989) Normal and mutant human adenosine deaminase genes. *J. Cell. Biochem.*, **39**, 217–228.

12. Hirschhorn, R., Chakravarti, V., Puck, J.M. and Douglas, S.D. (1991) Homozygosity for a newly identified missense mutation in a patient with very severe combined immunodeficiency due to adenosine deaminase deficiency (ADA–SCID). *Am. J. Hum. Genet.*, **49**, 878–885.

13. Polmar, S.H., Stern, R.C., Schwartz, A.L., Wetzler, E.M., Chase, P.A. and Hirschhorn, R. (1976) Enzyme replacement therapy for adenosine deaminase deficiency and severe combined immunodeficiency. *N. Engl. J. Med.*, **295**, 1337–1343.

14. Hershfield, M.S., Buckley, R.H., Greenberg, M.L., Melton, A.L., Schiff, R., Hatem, C., Kurtzberg, J., Markert, M.L., Kobayashi, R.H., Kobayashi, A.L. and Abuchowski, A. (1987) Treatment of adenosine deaminase deficiency with polyethylene glycol-modified adenosine deaminase. *N. Engl. J. Med.*, **316**, 589–596.

15. Culver, K.W., Osborne, W.R.A., Miller, A.D., Fleisher, T.A., Berger, M., Anderson, W.F. and Blaese, R.M. (1991) Correction of ADA deficiency in human T lymphocytes using retroviral-mediated gene transfer. *Transplant. Proc.*, **23**, 170–171.

16. Giblett, E.R., Ammann, A.J., Wara, D.W., Sandman, R. and Diamond, L.K. (1975) Nucleoside-phosphorylase deficiency in a child with severely defective T-cell immunity and normal B-cell immunity. *Lancet*, **i**, 1010–1013.

17. Alarcon, B., Regueiro, J.R., Arnaiz-Villena, A. and Terhorst, C. (1988) Familial defect in the surface expression of the T-cell receptor–CD3 complex. *N. Engl. J. Med.*, **319**, 1203–1208.

18. Pérez-Aciego, P., Alarcón, B., Arnaiz-Villena, A., Terhorst, C., Timón, M., Seguardo, O.G. and Regueiro, J.R. (1991) Expression and function of a variant T cell receptor complex lacking CD3-gamma. *J. Exp. Med.*, **174**, 319–326.

19. Le Deist, F., Thoenes, G., Corado, J., Lisowska-Grospierre, B. and Fischer, A. (1991) Immunodeficiency with low expression of the T cell receptor/CD3 complex: Effect on T lymphocyte activation. *Eur. J. Immunol.*, **21**, 1641–1647.

20. Reith, W., Satola, S., Herrero Sanchez, C., Amaldi, I., Lisowska-Grospierre, B., Griscelli, C., Hadam, M.R. and Mach, B. (1988) Congenital immunodeficiency with a regulatory defect in MHC class II gene expression lacks a specific HLA-DR promoter binding protein, RF-X. *Cell*, **53**, 897–906.

21. Kara, C.J. and Glimcher, L.H. (1991) *In vivo* footprinting of MHC class II genes: Bare promoters in the bare lymphocyte syndrome. *Science*, **252**, 709–712.

22. Seidl, C., Saraiya, C., Osterweil, Z., Fu, Y.P. and Lee, J.S. (1992) Genetic complexity of regulatory mutants defective for HLA class II gene expression. *J. Immunol.*, **148**, 1576–1584.

23. Schwarz, K., Hansen-Hagge, T.E., Knobloch, C., Friedrich, W., Kleihauer, E. and Bartram, C.R. (1991) Severe combined immunodeficiency (SCID) in man: B cell-negative (B−) SCID patients exhibit an irregular recombination pattern at the J_H locus. *J. Exp. Med.*, **174**, 1039–1048.

24. Schuler, W., Weiler, I.J., Schuler, A., Phillips, R.A., Rosenberg, N., Mak, T.W., Kearney, J.F., Perry, R.P. and Bosma, M.J. (1986) Rearrangement of antigen receptor genes is defective in mice with severe combined immune deficiency. *Cell,* **46**, 963–972.

25. Chatila, T., Castigli, E., Pahwa, R., Pahwa, S., Chirmule, N., Oyaizu, N., Good, R.A. and Geha, R.S. (1990) Primary combined immunodeficiency resulting from defective transcription of multiple T-cell lymphokine genes. *Proc. Nat. Acad. Sci. USA,* **87**, 10033–10037.

26. Weinberg, K. and Parkman, R. (1990) Severe combined immunodeficiency due to a specific defect in the production of interleukin-2. *N. Engl. J. Med.,* **322**, 1718–1723.

27. Chatila, T., Wong, R., Young, M., Miller, R., Terhorst, C. and Geha, R.S. (1989) An immunodeficiency characterized by defective signal transduction in T lymphocytes. *N. Engl. J. Med.,* **320**, 696–702.

28. Rijker, G.T., Scharenberg, J.G.M., Van Dongen, J.J.M., Neijens, H.J. and Zegers, B.J.M. (1991) Abnormal signal transduction in a patient with severe combined immunodeficiency disease. *Pediatr. Res.,* **29**, 306–309.

29. Jung, L.K.L., Fu, S.M., Hara, T., Kapoor, N. and Good, R.A. (1986) Defective expression of T cell-associated glycoprotein in severe combined immunodeficiency. *J. Clin. Invest.,* **77**, 940–946.

30. Haldane, J.B.S. (1935) The rate of spontaneous mutation of a human gene. *J. Genet.,* **31**, 317–326.

31. Perry, G.S., Spector, B.D., Schuman, L.M., Mandel, J.S., Anderson, V.E., McHugh, R.B., Hanson, M.R., Fahlstrom, S.M., Krivit, W. and Kersey, J.H. (1980) The Wiskott–Aldrich syndrome in the United States and Canada (1892–1979). *J. Pediatr.,* **97**, 72–78.

32. Fasth, A. (1979) Primary immunodeficiency disorders in Sweden: Cases among children, 1974–1979. *J. Clin. Immunol.,* **2**, 86–92.

33. Conley, M.E., Buckley, R.H., Hong, R., Guerra-Hanson, C., Roifman, C.M., Brochstein, J.A., Pahwa, S. and Puck, J.M. (1990) X-linked severe combined immunodeficiency: Diagnosis in males with sporadic severe combined immunodeficiency and clarification of clinical findings. *J. Clin. Invest.,* **85**, 1548–1554.

34. Conley, M.E. (1991) X-linked severe combined immunodeficiency. *Clin. Immunol. Immunopathol.,* **61**, S94–S99.

35. Small, T.N., Keever, C., Collins, N., Dupont, B., O'Reilly, R.J. and Flomenberg, N. (1989) Characterization of B cells in severe combined immunodeficiency disease. *Human Immunol.,* **25**, 181–193.

36. Gougeon, M.-L., Drean, G., Le Deist, F., Dousseau, M., Fevrier, M., Diu, A., Theze, J., Griscelli, C. and Fischer, A. (1990) Human severe combined immunodeficiency disease: Phenotypic and functional characteristics of peripheral B lymphocytes. *J. Immunol.,* **145**, 2873–2879.

37. Griscelli, C., Durandy, A., Virelizier, J.L., Ballet, J.J. and Daguillard, F. (1978) Selective defect of precursor T cells associated with apparently normal B lymphocytes in severe combined immunodeficiency disease. *J. Pediatr.,* **93**, 404–411.

38. Bortin, M.M. and Rimm, A.A. (1977) Severe combined immunodeficiency disease. *JAMA,* **238**, 591–600.

39. Moen, R.C., Horowitz, S.D., Sondel, P.M., Borcherding, W.R., Trigg, M.E., Billing, R. and Hong, R. (1987) Immunologic reconstitution after haploidentical bone marrow transplantation for immune deficiency disorders: Treatment of bone

marrow cells with monoclonal antibody CT-2 and complement. *Blood*, **70**, 664–669.

40. Chrystie, I.L., Booth, I.W., Kidd, A.H., Marshall, W.C. and Banatvala, J.E. (1982) Multiple faecal virus excretion in immunodeficiency. *Lancet*, **i**, 282.

41. Gatti, R.A., Meuwissen, H.J., Allen, H.D., Hong, R. and Good, R.A. (1968) Immunological reconstitution of sex-linked lymphopenic immunological deficiency. *Lancet*, **ii**, 1366–1369.

42. Meuwissen, H.J., Gatti, R.A., Terasaki, P.I., Hong, R. and Good, R.A. (1969) Treatment of lymphopenic hypogammaglobulinemia and bone-marrow aplasia by transplantation of allogeneic marrow. *N. Engl. J. Med.*, **281**, 691–697.

43. DeVoe, P.W., Buckley, R.H., Shirley, L.R., Darby, C.P., Ward, F.E., Mickey, G.H., Raab-Traub, N. and Vandenbark, G.R. (1985) Successful immune reconstitution in severe combined immunodeficiency despite Epstein–Barr virus and cytomegalovirus infections. *Clin. Immunol. Immunopathol.*, **34**, 48–59.

44. Reisner, Y., Kapoor, N., Kirkpatrick, D., Pollack, M.S., Dupont, B., Good, R.A. and O'Reilly, R.J. (1981) Transplantation for acute leukaemia with HLA-A and B nonidentical parental marrow cells fractionated with soybean agglutinin and sheep red blood cells. *Lancet*, **ii**, 327–331.

45. Goldblum, R.M., Lord, R.A., Dupree, E., Weinberg, A.G. and Goldman, A.S. (1973) Transfer factor induced delayed hypersensitivity in X-linked combined immunodeficiency. *Cell. Immunol.*, **9**, 297–305.

46. Puck, J.M., Nussbaum, R.L. and Conley, M.E. (1987) Carrier detection in X-linked severe combined immunodeficiency based on patterns of X chromosome inactivation. *J. Clin. Invest.*, **79**, 1395–1400.

47. Conley, M.E., Lavoie, A., Briggs, C., Brown, P., Guerra, C. and Puck, J.M. (1988) Nonrandom X chromosome inactivation in B cells from carriers of X chromosome-linked severe combined immunodeficiency. *Proc. Nat. Acad. Sci. USA*, **85**, 3090–3094.

48. Goodship, J., Lau, Y.L., Malcolm, S., Pembrey, M.E. and Levinsky, R.J. (1988) Use of X chromosome inactivation analysis to establish carrier status for X-linked severe combined immunodeficiency. *Lancet*, **i**, 729–732.

49. Goodship, J., Malcolm, S. and Levinsky, R.J. (1991) Evidence that X-linked severe combined immunodeficiency is not a differentiation defect of T lymphocytes. *Clin. Exp. Immunol.*, **83**, 4–9.

50. de Saint Basile, G. and Fischer, A. (1991) X-linked immunodeficiencies: Clues to genes involved in T- and B-cell differentiation. *Immunol. Today*, **12**, 456–461.

51. Lyon, M.F. (1974) Mechanisms and evolutionary origins of variable X-chromosome activity in mammals. *Proc. R. Soc. Lond.*, **187**, 243–268.

52. Wolf, S.F., Jolly, D.J., Lunnen, K.D., Friedmann, T. and Migeon, B.R. (1984) Methylation of the hypoxanthine phosphoribosyltransferase locus on the human X chromosome: Implications for X-chromosome inactivation. *Proc. Nat. Acad. Sci. USA*, **81**, 2806–2810.

53. Conley, M.E. and Puck, J.M. (1988) Definition of the gene loci in X-linked immunodeficiencies. *Immunol. Invest.*, **17**, 425–463.

54. Conley, M.E. (1992) Molecular approaches to analysis of X-linked immunodeficiencies. *Annu. Rev. Immunol.*, **10**, 215–238.

55. Vogelstein, B., Fearon, E.R., Hamilton, S.R., Presinger, A.C., Willard, H.F., Michelson, A.M., Riggs, A.D. and Orkin, S.H. (1987) Clonal analysis using recombinant DNA probes from the X-chromosome. *Cancer Res.*, **47**, 4806–4813.

56. Boyd, Y. and Fraser, N.J. (1990) Methylation patterns at the hypervariable X-chromosome locus DXS255 (M27β): Correlation with X-inactivation status. *Genomics*, **7**, 182–187.

57. Gilliland, D.G., Blanchard, K.L., Levy, J., Perrin, S. and Bunn, H.F. (1991) Clonality in myeloproliferative disorders: Analysis by means of the polymerase chain reaction. *Proc. Nat. Acad. Sci. USA*, **88**, 6848–6852.

58. Allen, R.C., Edwards, A.O., Caskey, C.T. and Belmont, J.W. (1991) Methylation status of an X-linked *HpaII* site 20 base pairs from a polymorphic trimeric repeat correlates with X-inactivation. *Am. J. Hum. Genet.*, **49**, 181S (Abstract).

59. Edwards, A., Civitello, A., Hammond, H.A. and Caskey, C.T. (1991) DNA typing and genetic mapping with trimeric and tetrameric tandem repeats. *Am. J. Hum. Genet.*, **49**, 746–756.

60. Fialkow, P.J. (1973) Primordial cell pool size and lineage relationships of five human cell types. *Ann. Hum. Genet. Lond.*, **37**, 39–48.

61. Puck, J.M. and Stewart, C.C. (1992) Maximum likelihood analysis of T-cell X chromosome inactivation: Normal women vs. carriers of X-linked severe combined immunodeficiency. *Am. J. Hum. Genet.*, **50**, 742–748.

62. de Saint Basile, G., Arveiler, B., Oberlé, I., Malcolm, S., Levinsky, R.J., Lau, Y.L., Hofker, M., Debre, M., Fischer, A., Griscelli C. and Mandel, J.L. (1987) Close linkage of the locus for X chromosome-linked severe combined immunodeficiency to polymorphic DNA markers in Xq11–q13. *Proc. Nat. Acad. Sci. USA*, **84**, 7576–7579.

63. Puck, J.M., Nussbaum, R.L., Smead, D.L. and Conley, M.E. (1989) X-linked severe combined immunodeficiency: Localization within the region Xq13.1–q21.1 by linkage and deletion analysis. *Am. J. Hum. Genet.*, **44**, 724–730.

64. Puck, J.M., Bailey, L.C. and Conley, M.E. (1991) Update on linkage of X-linked severe combined immunodeficiency (SCIDX1) to loci in Xq13. *Cytogenet. Cell Genet.*, **58**, 2082–2083.

65. Hendriks, R.W., Mensink, E.J.B.M., Kraakman, M.E.M., Thompson, A. and Schuurman, R.K.B. (1989) Evidence for male X chromosomal mosaicism in X-linked agammaglobulinemia. *Hum. Genet.*, **83**, 267–270.

66. Arveiler, B., de Saint Basile, G., Fischer, A., Griscelli, C. and Mandel, J.L. (1990) Germ-line mosaicism simulates genetic heterogeneity in Wiskott–Aldrich syndrome. *Am. J. Hum. Genet.*, **46**, 906–911.

67. Weber, J.L. and May, P.E. (1989) Abundant class of human DNA polymorphisms which can be typed using the polymerase chain reaction. *Am. J. Hum. Genet.*, **44**, 388–396.

68. Luty, J.A., Guo, Z., Willard, H.F., Ledbetter, D.H., Ledbetter, S. and Litt, M. (1990) Five polymorphic microsatellite VNTRs on the human X chromosome. *Am. J. Hum. Genet.*, **46**, 776–783.

69. Powell, B.R., Buist, N.R.M. and Stenzel, P. (1982) An X-linked syndrome of diarrhea, polyendocrinopathy, and fatal infection in infancy. *J. Pediatr.*, **100**, 731–737.

70. Shigeoka, A.O., Araneo, B.A., Carey, J.C. and Rallison, M.L. (1991) An X-linked T cell activation syndrome: Immunologic evaluation and response to cyclosporin A therapy in one affected infant. *Pediatr. Res.*, **29**, 163A (Abstract).

71. Brooks, E.G., Schmalstieg, F.C., Wirt, D.P., Rosenblatt, H.M., Adkins, L.T., Lookingbill, D.P., Rudloff, H.E., Rakusan, T.A. and Goldman, A.S. (1990) A novel X-linked combined immunodeficiency disease. *J. Clin. Invest.*, **86**, 1623–1631.

72. de Saint Basile, G., Le Deist, F., Caniglia, M., Lebranchu, Y., Griscelli, C. and Fischer, A. (1992) Genetic study of a new X-linked recessive immunodeficiency syndrome. *J. Clin. Invest.*, **89**, 861–866.

73. Puck, J.M., Krauss, C.M., Puck, S.M., Buckley, R.H. and Conley, M.E. (1990) Prenatal test for X-linked severe combined immunodeficiency by analysis of maternal X-chromosome inactivation and linkage analysis. *N. Engl. J. Med.*, **322**, 1063–1066.
74. Goodship, J., Levinsky, R. and Malcolm, S. (1989) Linkage of PGK1 to X-linked severe combined immunodeficiency (IMD4) allows predictive testing in families with no surviving male. *Hum. Genet.*, **84**, 11–14.
75. Erlich, H.A., Gelfand, D. and Sninsky, J.J. (1991) Recent advances in the polymerase chain reaction. *Science*, **252**, 1643–1650.
76. Rossiter, B.J.F. and Caskey, C.T. (1991) Molecular studies of human genetic disease. *FASEB J.*, **5**, 21–27.
77. Koller, B.H., Marrack, P., Kappler, J.W. and Smithies, O. (1990) Normal development of mice deficient in β_2M MHC class I proteins, and CD8+ T cells. *Science*, **248**, 1227–1230.
78. Schorle, H., Holtschke, T., Hünig, T., Schimpl, A. and Horak, I. (1991) Development and function of T cells in mice rendered interleukin-2 deficient by gene targeting. *Nature*, **352**, 621–624.
79. Blaese, R.M. (1991) Progress toward gene therapy. *Clin. Immunol. Immunopathol.*, **61**, S47–S55.

Chapter 8

Combined Immunodeficiency with Defective Expression in MHC Class II Genes

CLAUDE GRISCELLI and BARBARA LISOWSKA-GROSPIERRE
Paediatric Immunology and Haematology unit and INSERM U 132, Department of
Paediatrics, Hôpital des Enfants Malades, 149, rue de Sèvres, Paris, France

BERNARD MACH
Department of Microbiology, University of Geneva, Switzerland

Primary immunodeficiencies in humans are a heterogeneous group of diseases mostly characterized by abnormal differentiation of T and/or B lymphocytes. In the 1980s, several patients with inherited immunodeficiencies, with normal number of T and B lymphocytes, were described. Among them we described a combined immunodeficiency syndrome characterized by an abnormal expression of HLA class II antigens and abnormal cellular and humoral responses to foreign antigens (1–3). The knowledge of the role exerted by the major histocompatibility complex (MHC) in all specific immune responses (4, 5) allowed us to predict the relationship between the absence of MHC class II molecules at the cell membrane of leucocytes and the susceptibility to infections. Indeed, the proper recognition of foreign antigens depends on their presentation, together with MHC class II molecules, on the cell membrane of antigen-presenting cells (APC) (6). MHC class II-deficient combined immunodeficiency (CID) confirmed the important role of MHC gene products in immune defence mechanisms since all patients lacking these molecules have abnormal cellular and humoral responses to specific antigen and suffer from repeated and severe infections that are frequently the cause of death. A certain confusion

New Concepts in Immunodeficiency Diseases. Edited by S. Gupta and C. Griscelli
© 1993 John Wiley & Sons Ltd

persists in the terms used to designate immunodeficiencies associated to an abnormal membrane expression of MHC molceules. The "bare lymphocyte syndrome" which was first reported by Touraine *et al.* (7) is characterized by abnormal MHC class I antigen expression, while MHC class II expression was normally expressed on patient cell lines. The same membrane abnormalities were described in non-immunodeficient or normal individuals (8, 9). Studies performed at the protein and RNA levels showed that the defect involves MHC class I gene expression (10).

The syndrome we described differs from the bare lymphocyte syndrome by (a) an inconsistent reduced expression of MHC class I antigens at the cell membrane level, always corrected by interferon (α, β or γ); (b) a consistent and profound defect of all MHC class II molecule expression; and (c) a combined immunodeficiency.

This disease was named MHC class II deficiency by the WHO committee for classification of inherited immunodeficiencies. In our opinion, the patients described by Schuurman *et al.* (11) had the same disease, not recognized at the time when well-defined anti-MHC class II reagents had not yet been developed.

Recently, an experimental model of transgenic MHC class II-deficient mice was obtained by two groups (12, 13) and allows comparison with the observations made in humans. This review is based on a study of 39 observations of MHC class II deficiency (from 29 families) including 31 patients followed in our unit at the Necker-Enfants Malades Hospital (1, 3, 14–24) and 8 patients reported from The Netherlands (including the Schuurman patient) (14, 22–31), Germany (32–34) and the USA (35–38).

CLINICAL MANIFESTATIONS

All 39 patients suffered with severe infections that occurred within the first year of life (Table 8.1). Bacterial infections in various locations were dominant: intestinal infections, pneumonitis, bronchitis and septicaemias. In the majority of patients intestinal tract bacterial infections together with candidiasis and/or cryptosporidiosis were responsible for protracted diarrhoea, malabsorption with osteoporosis and severe failure to thrive. These intestinal manifestations were associated with sclerosing cholangitis in patients suffering from long-term chronic diarrhoea, especially when cryptosporidosis was present. Histological examination of intestinal mucosa frequently showed partial or profound atrophy with a normal infiltration of lymphocytes and macrophages and some plasma cells. Intestinal involvement was not modified by gliadin exclusion or by antibiotics used in an attempt to decontaminate the intestinal tract. The marked intestinal involvement needed chronic parenteral nutrition in several patients.

Table 8.1   HLA class II deficiency: clinical manifestations[a]

Repeated severe infections	39
Protracted diarrhoea	36
Lower respiratory tract infections	29
Failure to thrive	25
Severe viral infections	19
Mucocutaneous candidiasis	10
Cryptosporidiosis	10
Autoimmune cytopenia	9
Sclerosing cholangitis	5

[a]31 patients examined in Necker-Enfants Malades hospital group and 8 reported patients.

The majority of patients suffered from severe viral infections. Adenovirus, herpes simplex virus, respiratory syncytial virus and cytomegalovirus (CMV) were the most frequent causes of respiratory manifestations and, for hepatitis, CMV was the most frequent cause. Coxsackie virus, adenovirus and poliovirus were also frequently responsible for meningoencephalitis. Two patients developed poliomyelitis, despite previous vaccination with inactivated virus. In addition, one patient developed a fatal postvaccinal poliomyelitis with encephalitis after a vaccination with live attenuated virus vaccine. Fungal infections due to *Candida albicans* were frequent. *Pneumocystis carinii* was isolated from bronchial lavage of 7 patients. Interestingly enough, none of the 9 patients who received BCG at birth developed disseminated BCG infection, indicating residual immune functions to mycobacteria. Nine patients developed an autoimmune cytopenia (anaemia, neutropenia and/or thrombocytopenia) of severe nature, sensitive only to high doses of steroids and justifying splenectomy in one case. Finally, it is to be pointed out that none of the 11 patients who had received transfusion(s) of fresh blood cells before diagnosis developed graft-versus-host disease.

The disease is very severe since, at the time of publication, 23 out of the 39 patients have died. The oldest of the deceased patients was 17 years old, but most of them died between 6 months and 5 years of age. Eleven of our patients are still alive. Because of the severity of the disease a bone marrow transplantation (BMT) was performed in 14 patients (2 cases already reported in ref. 20). Seven patients were transplanted with an HLA-identical donor but only two had a complete reconstitution and are well. In these fully grafted patients, the epithelial cells of intestinal mucosa and the endothelium of vessels remain MHC class II deficient. Yet they have no clinical symptoms involving the intestinal functions or vessels, an observation which raises the question of the role of MHC class II molecules on the surface of these cells. Seven patients received T lymphocyte-depleted BMT from HLA-mismatched (haplo-identical) family donors, after myelodepletion and immunosuppression (20). Three of them are partially (2 patients) or fully (1 patient) reconstituted and are alive. Four remaining patients who did not receive BMT are in a poor condition despite considerable medical care.

ABNORMAL MEMBRANE EXPRESSION OF MHC ANTIGENS

MHC class I (A, B, C) and β_2-microglobulin (β_2) were detected on the membrane of leucocytes and platelets of all patients but were found to be reduced in several patients. Percentages of immunofluorescent cells (1, 2, 27, 32) as well as mean fluorescence intensity of the anti-MHC class I molecules (30, 33) were often decreased. In addition, variations in MHC class I expression were observed on PBL and PHA-induced blasts from patient to patient and from time to time, in a given patient (1). In all patients studied, correction in MHC class I expression was obtained by *in vitro* treatment of blood by interferon (IFN)α, -β or -γ (15, 28, 31). All Epstein–Barr virus (EBV)-induced B cell lines or phytohaemagglutinin (PHA)-induced interleukin 2 (IL-2)-dependent T cell lines, as well as dermal fibroblasts, expressed MHC class I antigens. However, a lower mean fluorescence intensity with anti-MHC class I staining was frequently observed on the patients' EBV lymphoblasts as compared to controls. These data were confirmed by immunoprecipitation of membrane-labelled patients' cells (21).

Membrane expression of MHC class II antigens was defective. Although a few (less than 1%) cells were able to react with anti-MHC class II antibody occasionally, a MHC class II expression was abnormal on all cells that expressed them; B lymphocytes, monocytes and PHA-activated T blast cells were DR, DQ and DP negative (29). MHC class II molecules were also absent at the membrane of EBV-derived B cell or IL-2-dependent T cell lines. All cells of macrophage lineage, i.e. skin Langerhans cells, Kupffer cells and monocytic cells from spleen and intestinal mucosa had an abnormal expression of MHC class II molecules. In some tissue sections, few (estimated to be 1% of normal) MHC class II-positive Langerhans cells were observed. This abnormal expression of MHC class II molecules was also shown on endothelial and epithelial cells of the intestinal mucosa.

Because it is well known that the thymic environment plays an important role in the differentiation of T cells and in self-recognition, it was interesting to assess the HLA expression on the various thymic cells. The expression of MHC molecules was abnormal in the thymus of four patients (26, 29, and in two of our patients). Very few cells were found to be MHC class II positive. Schuurman *et al.* (28) observed the presence of only few positive stromal cells. Both dendritic and stromal cells were positive in very few numbers in the thymus of two of our patients. These last anomalies were also observed in our unit in fetal thymuses obtained after therapeutic abortion of fetuses at risk following prenatal diagnosis of the disease. Besides these results, it is interesting to note that the thymic architecture was normal, including the presence of Hassal's corpuscles (29, 32).

MEMBRANE EXPRESSION OF NON-MHC MOLECULES

Numbers of blood lymphocytes were normal in all patients at the time of diagnosis, with few exceptions of patients presenting with severe viral infections. CD3+ cells are occasionally decreased. CD8+ cells are generally increased (27–65% versus 15–25% in controls). All but two patients investigated (29 in the our series and 3 reported patients) had low CD4+ cells counts (5–35% versus 45–65% in controls) (19). This feature appears to be an important characteristic of the disease since it is independent of the clinical status. Similar reduction (14) or near-complete absence (12) of the CD4+ cells was observed in the periphery of transgenic class II-deficient mice. This is in accordance with the results of Kruisbeek *et al.* (39), who demonstrated that *in vivo* treatment of mice with antibody to MHC class II molecules prevents the differentiation of thymocytes into CD4+ lymphocytes. Expression of T cell receptors (TCR) for antigen was easily detected in 14 patients investigated.

The number of B cells detected by surface immunoglobulin expression (sIg) was normal in 31 patients and decreased, at time of diagnosis in 3 others. Rijkers *et al.* (30) and Hadam *et al.* (32) reported that patients' cells, as neonatal B lymphocytes, expressed a higher density of sIgM than sIgD. In a single patient, Clement *et al.* (36) observed the normal number of CD20 and CD5 B cells, whereas CD38+ immature B cells were increased. In this patient, B cells poorly expressed CD21 that corresponds to the receptors for EBV/C3d. This latter observation may explain the difficulty in establishing EBV-derived cell lines from several of these patients.

IMMUNOLOGICAL CONSEQUENCES OF THE ABNORMAL EXPRESSION OF MHC MOLECULES

The constant feature is a combined cellular and humoral deficiency of specific immune responses. The absence of delayed type hypersensitivity, observed in all patients investigated, correlated with an *in vitro* absence of T cell responses to antigens with which the patients were immunized (tetanus and diphtheria toxoid or purified protein derivative (PPD)) or sensitized after infections such as *Candida albicans* (19, 29, 35). In contrast, most patients have a normal allogeneic response as measured by proliferative response and the generation of cytotoxic T cell (CTC) response in mixed leucocyte reaction (19). Study of patients' leucocytes to stimulate allogeneic cells gave surprisingly variable results. Although in most patients this capacity was absent or reduced (15–25% of controls), it was inconsistent at times for a given patient and was found almost normal (60–80% of controls) in some occasions. These results do not correlate with the degree of MHC class II antigen expression and are difficult to understand: either residual MHC class II molecules are sufficient in number to allow alloreactivity or MHC class I molecules are involved instead of class II molecules under such circumstances. The mitogen as well as anti-CD3 and anti-CD2-induced proliferations were generally normal. In severely infected patients, a transitory reduced proliferative response can be observed.

As judged from the level of serum immunoglobulins, there was a variable expression of humoral immunity from patient to patient. While most of them were hypogammaglobulinaemic (or almost agammaglobulinaemic) (2, 25, 32), we have observed normal concentrations of immunoglobulins in 8 patients and even elevated IgM levels in 2 (19). In 4 patients IgG2, IgG4 and IgA levels were low (23). Antibody responses to immunization antigens (tetanus and diphtheria toxoids and polioviruses) were never observed even in patients with normal immunoglobulin levels. Isohaemagglutinins (anti-A and anti-B blood group substances) were normal in 50% of our patients, as were anti-*Candida albicans* antibodies of IgM isotype in most patients. This suggests that antibody response to T-independent antigens is preserved in MHC class II-deficient patients, in agreement with similar findings in transgenic class II-deficient mice model (12, 13). Antibody responses following infection were dissociated. Some chronically infected patients had antibodies to viruses (CMV or adenovirus). The interpretation of such an observation is not clear. It is possible that residual membrane expression of MHC class II molecules may allow antibody response in the course of certain chronic stimulation. Several *in vitro* studies were performed in order to analyse the mechanisms of the abnormal antibody production. Antibody synthesis in response to antigen-specific stimuli was studied in two distinct systems using mannan of *Candida albicans* or influenza virus haemagglutinin (19, 24). Only IgM antibody to mannan could be detected in 6 out of 14 patients studied, while cells from 4 patients did not produce IgG anti-influenza virus antibodies. *In vitro* cell-to-cell interactions involved in antibody production were studied in various systems. Zegers *et al.* (26), using a primary antigen (ovalbumin or sheep red blood cells (SRBC)) system, reported that antigen presentation by monocytes and interactions between antigen-pulsed normal monocytes and T or B cells were impaired in their patients.

INHERITANCE

The MHC class II deficiency is an autosomal recessive disorder. Consanguinity is frequently documented in families, suggesting that the mutation is rare. This high rate of consanguinity is explained by the predominance of families of North African origin: 18 families were from North Africa or the Mediterranean. Because MHC class I typing is possible in patients with this disorder, analysis of frequencies of MHC class I phenotypes were performed. There was no indication of a predominant haplotype in the 18 families studied. Twelve families were also informative for the segregation study of inheritance of the genetic abnormality and of HLA phenotype: 2 affected siblings had different MHC class I phenotypes in 3 families and an affected individual had a MHC class I identical healthy sibling or father in 9 other families. These results were confirmed in 5 of them by studying their genotypes (18). As judged by cytotoxicity and confirmed in several instances by cytofluorometry, MHC class II expression was normal in all obligatory heterozygous parents investigated.

MOLECULAR DEFECT UNDERLYING THE HLA CLASS II DEFICIENCY

The characteristic feature of MHC class II deficiency is an absence of cell surface MHC class II molecules of all specificities (1–4). In order to understand the mechanism of the defect, studies of synthesis of MHC class II molecules were performed. Lymphocytes from patients do not synthesize any MHC class II α and β chains (3, 15, 16). This was demonstrated by an analysis of MHC class II molecules in lymphoytes from controls and patients that were biosynthetically labelled with [^{35}S]methionine. Studies were thus performed in order to analyse messenger RNA (mRNA) in patients' cells. An absence of all different MHC class II mRNAs was observed in all patients investigated. (15, 16). Even PHA-activated lymphocytes were totally negative. Furthermore, the expression of MHC class II mRNA could not be induced by stimulation with IFNγ (16). Patients' cells contained mRNA for the HLA-associated invariant chain (Inv), which is normally co-regulated with class II genes. The level of mRNA for MHC class I was either normal or slightly reduced in certain patients (16, 17). Further studies of the defect in MHC class II gene expression in MHC class II deficiency was greatly facilitated by the establishment of EBV-transformed permanent B cell lines. Several such lines derived from different patients in different laboratories in France, Germany and Holland conserve an MHC class II-negative phenotype at the membrane level. In some cell lines, however, a low level of DR α mRNA can be detected (21, 40, 41).

The global nature of the class II defect, affecting all of the α and β chain genes, strongly suggest a general MHC class II regulatory defect. As mentioned above, this was formally established in family studies where the inheritance of MHC class I alleles was followed and shown to segregate independently of the disease. This simple observation allowed the conclusion that the genetic defect of MHC class II deficiency must be located outside the MHC and probably outside chromosome 6 (19). Accordingly, it was also shown that no major deletion in MHC class II region has occurred in these patients (18). The absence of mRNA does not establish the nature of the block in gene expression, which could result from abnormalities in the processing and splicing of RNA transcripts or in the stability of RNA. Direct transcription assays performed with control and cell lines from patients have shown that the disease is characterized by an absence of MHC class II gene transcription (22).

It is now well demonstrated that expression of MHC class II genes is under the control of several nuclear proteins that bind to conserved nucleic acid sequence located on promotor regions (42–44). It was shown in various regulatory systems that such interactions between nuclear proteins or regulatory factors to promotor regions may result in the generation of specific DNase I hypersensitive sites. Thus, the chromatin structure of MHC class II genes for DNase I was studied in normal and patients' B cells. A lack of two specific DNase sites in HLA-DR A promoter was observed in patients' cells. This strongly suggests an abnormality in the chromatin structure, possibly due to an abnormal binding of a given nuclear protein to MHC class II promoter (22).

A study of specific binding of nuclear proteins from patient cell lines to the MHC class II promoter was performed in several patients. Several groups have identified specific factors that bind to MHC class II promoters (43, 44). Binding of individual proteins known to bind to either the Y box to the TRE/CRE element or to the X box itself was studied in detail. With nuclear extracts from patient cell lines, no difference was noted in the binding to the Y box or to the TRE/CRE element, but a remarkable difference was noted for the X box: the DNA/protein complex formed with the X box was specifically absent in these patients (22). Direct analysis of the contact points of MHC class II X box binding protein (RF-X) to the promoter sequence by footprinting and methylation interference experiments confirmed that the protein affected binds to the X box (22). From these experiments, it was possible to conclude that a specific RF-X, which normally binds to a regulatory sequence common to class II promoters, is affected in the hereditary defect in MHC class II regulation. MHC class II deficiency therefore represents the first genetic disease involving a regulatory DNA-binding protein. The recent cloning of an RF-X gene has revealed a novel type of DNA-binding factor, with a novel DNA-binding domain (40, 45). There exists a family of RF-X factors, all having an almost identical DNA-binding domain and all binding to the X box of MHC class II promoters with the same characteristics (46).

Two of the cloned RF-X genes map to the short arm of chromosome (19, 47). The gene affected in patients is thus a member of this new RF-X family but has not yet been identified. An extensive characterization of the entire family of RFX genes is an urgent task, in order to identify the particular X box-binding protein responsible for the complex which is specifically missing in patients with MHC class II deficiency.

Comparison of a large number of B cell lines derived from individual patients (8 from Paris and 4 from Germany) has shown that one can detect traces of MHC class II mRNA in certain lines. Interestingly, this "leakiness" in the class II expression genetic defect is also reflected at the level of the binding of RFX on the class II promoter. It can therefore be concluded that there is a correlation between various levels of class II mRNA production and residual binding of RFX. This correlation reinforces the functional significance of the molecular defect observed at the level of gene regulation. These data also suggest that the genetic defect in this disease is not always the same. This heterogeneity could reflect, for instance, different types of amino acid substitution in the DNA-binding domain of RFX.

DISTINCT MOLECULAR DEFECTS IN DIFFERENT FORMS OF MHC CLASS II REGULATORY MUTATIONS

Regulatory defect in the control of class II gene expression has also been proposed in the case of certain *in vitro* generated human and mouse B cells mutants (48–51). In these cases, fusion of the MHC class II-deficient mutant with normal class II-positive cells could restore the expression of class II antigens of the mutant specificity. The *in vitro* generated mutant human cell lines exhibit an identical phenotype, with no expression of class II mRNA, but with the presence of mRNA for the invariant chain. An analysis of one such *in vitro* mutant (50, 58) at the level of DNase I sites and of promoter-binding proteins has demonstrated that it is not affected with the same genetic defect as MHC class II-deficient patients (Satola *et al.*, in preparation). In particular, the binding of RFX is observed normally and the DNase I sites of the class II promoter are normally present. This indicates that the molecular defect responsible for the lack of class II gene expression is different in the inherited disease and in the *in vitro* generated mutant. This conclusion concerning distinct molecular defects is in agreement with recent results of fusion experiments between the B cell lines of an MHC class II-deficient patient and the *in vitro* mutant which has shown reciprocal complementation and re-expression of HLA-DR molecules (52). More recent fusion experiments show that genes governing the expression of class II antigens fall into at least four complementation groups (53).

It is expected that rapid progress will make it possible to identify and characterize gene(s) affected in MHC class II deficiency. This will allow better knowledge of the mechanisms controlling the expression of MHC class II genes and trials of gene therapy in order to correct the abnormal expression of MHC class II in this severe disease.

CONCLUSIONS

In summary, MHC class II deficiency is an inherited immunodeficiency disease characterized by the presence of normal numbers of T and B lymphocytes and profound anomaly of cellular and humoral responses to foreign antigens. Almost all bone marrow-derived cells (including B lymphocytes, monocytes and activated T lymphocytes), and epithelial and endothelial cells lack expression of all HLA class II molecules (DR, DQ and DP) on their membrane. It is known that the proper recognition of foreign antigens depends on their presentation, together with HLA class II molecules, on the membrane of antigen-presenting cells. The MHC class II-deficient combined immunodeficiency confirms the important role of MHC gene products in immune defence mechanisms. The patients suffer from repeated and severe infections that are frequently the cause of death.

The defect in HLA class II expression is the consequence of a lack of synthesis of HLA class II α and β chains. There is no major abnormality of MHC class II genes and mRNA of all HLA molecules that were not detected in patients' cells. These results, together with segregation studies performed in several families, suggested that the defect in HLA class II gene expression involves a transacting regulatory factor. An analysis of the binding of nuclear proteins from patient cell lines to HLA class II promoters showed that RFX, a factor that normally binds to the X box motive shared by all HLA class II promoters, is specifically affected in MHC class II combined immunodeficiency. This disease therefore represents the first example of a genetic defect involving a DNA-binding regulatory protein.

REFERENCES

1. Griscelli, C., Durandy, A. and Virelizier, J. (1980) Impaired cell to cell interaction in partial immunodeficiency with variable expression of HLA antigens. In Seligmann, M. and Hitzig, W.H. (eds) *Primary Immunodeficiencies*. Elsevier/North-Holland, Amsterdam, pp. 499–503.

2. Griscelli, C., Fischer, A., Grospierre, B., Durandy, A., Bremard, C., Charron, D., Vilmer, E. and Virelizier, J.L. (1984) Clinical and immunological aspects of combined immunodeficiency with defective expression of HLA antigens. In Griscelli, C. and Vossen, J. (eds) *Progress in Immunodeficiency Research and Therapy I*. Excerpta Medica, Amsterdam, pp. 19–26.

3. Lisowska-Grospierre, B., Durandy, A., Virelizier, J.L., Fischer, A. and Griscelli, C. (1983) Combined immunodeficiency with defective expression of HLA: Modulation of an abnormal HLA and functional studies. *Birth Defects*, **19**, 87–92.

4. Benacerraff, B. (1981) Cellular interactions. In Dorf, M.E. (ed.) *The Role of the Major Histocompatibility Complex in Immunobiology*. Garland, New York, p. 255.

5. Schwartz, R.H. (1984) The role of gene products of the MHC in T cell activation and cellular interactions. In Paul, W.E. (ed.) *Fundamental Immunology*. Raven Press, New York, pp. 379–439.

6. Kappler, J.W. and Marrack, P. (1976) Helper T cells recognize antigen and macrophage surface components simultaneously. *Nature*, **262**, 797–799.

7. Touraine, J.L., Betuel, H. and Souillet, G. (1978) Combined immunodeficiency disease associated with absence of cell-surface HLA A and B antigens. *J. Physiol.*, **93**, 47–51.

8. Payne, R., Brodsky, F.M., Peterlin, B.M. and Young, L.M. (1963) "Bare lymphocytes" without immunodeficiency. *Hum. Immunol.*, **6**, 219–227.

9. Maeva, H., Hirata, R., Chen, R.F., Suzaki, H., Kudoh, S. and Tohyama, H. (1985) Defective expression of HLA class I antigens: A case of the Bare lymphocyte without immunodeficiency. *Immunogenetics*, **21**, 549–558.

10. Sullivan, K.E., Stobo, J.D. and Peterlin, B.M. (1976) Molecular analysis of the Bare lymphocyte syndrome. *J. Clin. Invest.*, **76**, 75–79.

11. Schuurman, R.K.B., Van Rood, J.J., Vossen, J.M., Schellekens, P.T.A., Feltkamp-Vroom, T.M., Doyer, E., Gmelig-Meyling, F. and Visser, H.K.A. (1979) Failure of lymphocyte-membrane HLA A and B expression in two siblings with combined immunodeficiency. *Clin. Immunol. Immunopathol.*, **14**, 418–434.

12. Cosgrove, D., Gray, D., Dieriech, A., Kaufman, J., Lemeur, M., Benoist, C. and Mathis, D. (1991) Mice lacking MHC class II molecules. *Cell*, **66**, 1052–1066.

13. Grusby, M.J., Johnson, R.S., Papaionnou, V.E. and Glimcher, L.H. (1991) Depletion of CD4 (+) T cells in major histocompatibility complex class II-deficient mice. *Nature*, **253**, 1417–1420.

14. Durandy, A., Virelizier, J. and Griscelli, C. (1983) Enhancement by interferon of membrane HLA antigens in patients with combined immunodeficiency with defective HLA expression. *Clin. Exp. Immunol.*, **52**, 173–178.

15. Lisowska-Grospierre, B., Charron, D.J., de Préval, C., Durandy, A., Griscelli, C. and Mach, B. (1985) A defect in the regulation of major histocompatibility complex class II gene expression in human HLA DR negative lymphocytes from patients with combined immunodeficiency syndrome. *J. Clin. Invest.*, **26**, 381–385.

16. Lisowska-Grospierre, B., Charron, D.J., de Préval, C., Durandy, A., Griscelli, C. and Mach, B. (1985) A defect in the regulation of major histocompatibility complex class II gene expression in human HLA DR negative lymphocytes from patients with combined immunodeficiency syndrome. *J. Clin. Invest.*, **26**, 381–385.

17. de Préval, C., Lisowska-Grospierre, B., Loche, M., Griscelli, C. and Mach, B. (1985) A transacting class II regulatory gene unlinked to the MHC controls expression of HLA class II genes. *Nature*, **318**, 291–295.

18. Marcadet, A., Cohen, D., Dausset, J., Fischer, A., Durandy, A. and Griscelli, C. (1985) Genotyping with DNA probes in combined immunodeficiency syndrome with defective expression of HLA. *N. Engl. J. Med.*, **312**, 1287–1292.

19. Griscelli, C., Fischer, A., Lisowska-Grospierre, B., Durandy, A., Bremard, C., Cerf-Bensussan, N., Le Deist, F., Marcadet, A. and de Préval, C. (1985) Defective synthesis of HLA class I and II molecules associated with a combined immunodeficiency. In Aiuti, F., Rosen, E. and Cooper, M.D. (eds) *Recent Advances in Primary and Acquired Immunodeficiencies*, Vol. 28. Serano Symposia from Raven Press, New York, pp. 176–183.

20. Fischer, A., Griscelli, C., Blanche, S., Le Deist, F., Veber, F., Lopez, M., De Laage, M., Olive, D., Mawas, C. and Janossy, G. (1986) Prevention of graft failure by an anti-LFA-1 monoclonal antibody in HLA-mismatched bone marrow transplantation. *Lancet*, **ii**, 1058–1062.

21. Lisowska-Grospierre, B., Guyot, A., Dimanche, M.T., Mach, B. and Griscelli, C. (1988) Low level re-expression of the silent MHC class II genes in the lymphoblasts from patients with the HLA-class II deficient SCID. In Mani, J.C. and

Dornand, J. (eds) *Lymphocyte Activation and Differentiation*. de Gruyter, Berlin, pp. 449–452.

22. Reith, W., Satola, S., Sanchez, C.H., Amaldi, I., Lisowska-Grospierre, B., Hadams, M.R., Griscelli, C. and Mach, B. (1988) Congenital immunodeficiency with a regulatory defect in MHC class II gene expression lacks a specific HLA-DR promoter binding proteins, RF-X. *Cell*, **53**, 897–907.

23. Smith, C.I.E., Bremard-Oury, C., Le Desit, F., Griscelli, C., Aucouturier, P., Moller, G., Hammarstrom, L., Preud'Homme, J.L. and Weening, R.S. (1988) The antibody spectrum in individuals with defect expression of HLA class II and the LFA-1 glycoprotein family genes. *Clin. Exp. Immunol.*, **74**, 449–453.

24. Durandy, A., Mangeney, M., Griscelli, C., Forveille, M., Le Deist, F. and Fischer, A. (1989) Activation of genetically MHC class II deficient B lymphocytes. *J. Clin. Immunol.*, **9**, 125–131.

25. Kuis, W., Roord, J., Zegers, B.J.M., Schuurman, R.K.B., Heijnen, C.J., Baldwin, W.M., Goulmy, E., Claas, F., Van de Griend, R.J., Rijkers, G.T., Van Rood, J.J., Vossen, J.M., Ballieux, R.E. and Stoop, J.W. (1981) Clinical and immunological studies in a patient with the "Bare lymphocyte" syndrome. In Touraine, J.L., Gluckman, E. and Griscelli, C. (eds) *Bone Marrow Transplantation in Europe*. Excerpta Medica, Amsterdam, pp. 210–208.

26. Zegers, B.J.M., Heijnen, C.J., Roord, J.J., Kuis, W., Schuurman, R.K.B., Stoop, J.W. and Ballieux, R.E. (1983) Defective expression of mononuclear cell membrane HLA antigens associated with combined immunodeficiency: Impaired cellular interactions. *Birth Defects*, **19**, 93–96.

27. Zegers, B.J.M., Heijnen, C.J., Roord, J.J., Kuis, W., Stoop, J.W. and Ballieux, R.E. (1984) Combined immunodeficiency with defective expression of HLA-antigens: Analysis of the nature of defective monocyte–T cell interaction. In Griscelli, I.C. and Vossen, J. (eds) *Progress in Immunodeficiency Research and Therapy*. Excerpta Medica, Amsterdam, pp. 35–42.

28. Schuurman, H.J., Van de Wijngaert, F.P., Huber, J., Schuurman, R.K.B., Zegers, B.J.M., Roord, J.J. and Kater, L. (1985) The thymus in "Bare lymphocyte" syndrome: Significance of expression of major histocompatibility complex antigens on thymic epithelial cells in intrathymic T-cell maturation. *Hum. Immunol.*, **13**, 69–82.

29. Zegers, B.J.M., Rijkers, G.T., Roord, J.J., Koning, F., Schuurman, H.J., Heijnen, C.H., Kuis, W., Van de Berg, H. and Stoop, J.W. (1986) Defective expression of MHC antigens on mononuclear cells in two siblings with combined immunodeficiency: Delineation of the class II antigen defect. In Vossen, J. and Griscelli, C. (eds) *Progress in Immunodeficiency Research and Therapy II*. Elsevier, Amsterdam, p. 97.

30. Rijkers, G.T., Roord, J.J., Koning, F., Kuis, W. and Zegers, B.J.M. (1987) Phenotypal and functional analysis of B lymphocytes of two siblings with combined immunodeficiency and defective expression of major histocompatibility complex (MHC) class II antigens on mononuclear cells. *J. Clin. Immunol.*, **7**, 98–106.

31. Schuurman, H.J., Van de Wijngaert, F.P., Huber, J., Zegers, B.J.M., Schuurman, R.K.B., Roord, J.J. and Kater, L. (1985) The thymus in "Bare lymphocyte" syndrome. In Klaus, G.G.B. (ed.) *Microenvironments in the Lymphoid System*. Plenum Publishing Corporation, New York, pp. 921–928.

32. Hadam, M.R., Dopfer, R., Peter, H.H. and Niethammer, D. (1984) Congenital agammaglobulinemia associated with lack of expression of HLA D– region antigens. In Griscelli, C. and Vossen, J. (eds) *Progress in Immunodeficiency Research and Therapy*. Excerpta Medica, Amsterdam, pp. 19–24.

33. Hadam, M.R., Dofer, R., Dammer, G., Peter, H.H., Schlesier, M., Müller, C. and Niethammer, D. (1984) Defective expression of HLA-D– region determinants in children with congenital agammaglobulinemia and malabsorption: A new syndrome. In Albert, E.D. *et al.* (eds) *Histocompatibility Testing.* Springer-Verlag, Berlin, pp. 645–650.

34. Niethammer, D., Dopfer, R., Dammer, G., Peter, H., de Préval, C., Mach, B. and Hadam, M.R. (1985) Congenital agammaglobulinemia associated with malabsorption: No expression of MHC class II antigens due to a regulatory gene defect. In Aiuti, F., Rosen, F. and Cooper, M.D. (eds) *Recent Advances in Primary and Acquired Immunodeficiencies*, Vol. 28. Serano Symposia from Raven Press, New York, pp. 185–193.

35. Haas, A. and Stiehm, E.R. (1987) Failure to thrive, thrush and hypogammaglobulinemia in a 6 months-old infant. *Ann. Allergy.*, **59**, 141–144.

36. Clement, L.T., Plaeger-Marshall, S., Haas, A., Saxon, A. and Martin, A.M. (1988) Lymphocyte syndrome: Consequences of absent class II major histocompatibility antigen expression for B lymphocyte differentiation and function. *J. Clin. Invest.*, **81**, 669–675.

37. Plager-Marshal, S., Haas, A., Clement, L.T., Glogi, J.V., Chen, I.S.Y., Quan, S.G., Garti, R.A. and Stiehm, E.R. (1988) Interferon-induced expression of class II major histocompatibility antigens in the MHC class II deficiency syndrome. *J. Clin. Immunol.*, **8**, 285–295.

38. Hume, C.R., Shookster, L.A., Collins, N., O'Reilly, R. and Lee, J.S. (1989) Bare lymphocyte syndrome altered class II expression in two B cell lines. *Hum. Immunol.*, **25**, 1–11.

39. Kruisbeek, A. M., Mond, J.J., Fowlkes, B.J., Carmen, Y.A., Bridges, S. and Longo, D.L. (1985) Absence of Lyt-2– L3T4+ lineage of T-cells in mice treated neonatally with anti-I-A correlates with absence of intrathymic I-A-bearing antigen presenting cells. *J. Exp. Med.*, 1029–1047.

40. Reith, W., Barras, E., Satola, S., Kobr, M., Reinharz, D., Herrero Sanchez, C. and Mach, B. (1989) Cloning of the MHC class II promoter binding protein affected in a hereditary defect in class II gene regulation. *Proc. Nat. Acad. Sci. USA*, **86**, 4200–4204.

41. de Préval, C., Hadam, M.R. and Mach, B. (1988) Regulation of genes for HLA class II antigens in cell lines from patients with severe combined immunodeficiency. *N. Engl. J. Med.*, **318**, 1295–1300.

42. Dorn, A., Durand, B., Marfing, C., Le Meur, M., Benoist, C. and Mathis, D. (1987) The conserved MHC class II boxes X and Y are transcriptional control elements and specifically bind nuclear proteins. *Proc. Nat. Acad. Sci. USA*, **84**, 6249–6253.

43. Benoist, C. and Mathis, D. (1990) Regulation of major histocompatibility complex class II genes: X, Y and other letters of the alphabet. *Annu. Rev. Immunol.*, **8**, 681–715.

44. Glimcher, L.H. and Kara, C.J. (1992) Sequences and factors: a guide to MHC class II transcription. *Annu. Rev. Immunol.* 10113–49.

45. Reith, W., Herrero Sanchez, C., Kobr, M., Silacci, P., Berte, C., Barras, E., Fey, S. and Mach, B. (1990) MHC class II regulatory factor RFX has a novel DNA binding-domain and a functionally independent dimerization domain. *Genes Dev.*, **4**, 1528–1540.

46. Mach, B. *et al.* In Sasazuki, T., *et al.* (eds) *Hal 1991*, Vol. 2. Oxford University Press, Oxford (in press).

47. Pugliatti, L., Derré, J., Berger, R., Ucla, C., Reigh, W. and Mach, B. (1992) The genes for MHC class II regulatory factors RFX1 and RFX2 are located on the short arm of chromosome 19. *Genomics*, **13**, 1307–1310.
48. Gladstone, P. and Plous, D. (1978) Stable variants affecting B cell alloantigens in human lymphoid cells. *Nature*, **271**, 459–461.
49. Levins, F. and Pious, D. (1984) Revertans from the HLA class II regulatory mutant 6.1.6: Implications for the regulation of Ia gene expression. *J. Immunol.*, **132**, 959–963.
50. Accola, R.S. (1983) Human B cell variants immunoselected against a single Ia antigen subset have lost expression of several Ia antigen subsets. *J. Exp. Med.*, **157**, 1053–1058.
51. Carra, G. and Guardiola, J. (1985) Reactivation by a transacting factor of human major histocompatibility complex Ia gene expression in interspecies hybrids between an Ia-negative human B-cell variant and an Ia-positive mouse B-cell lymphoma. *Proc. Nat. Acad. Sci. USA*, **82**, 5145–5149.
52. Yang, Zhi, Accola, R.S., Pious, D., Zegers, B.J.M. and Strominger, J.L. (1988) Two distinct genetic loci regulating class II gene expression are defective in human mutant and patient cell lines. *EMBO J.*, **7**, 1965–1972.
53. Hume, C.R. and Lee, J.S. (1989) Congenital immunodeficiencies associated with absence of HLA class II antigens on lymphocytes result from distinct mutations in transacting factors. *Hum. Immunol.*, **26**, 288–309.

Chapter 9

Genetic Abnormalities in Leukocyte Adhesion Molecule Deficiency

M. AMIN ARNAOUT* and MASAHIRO MICHISHITA

Leukocyte Biology and Inflammation Program, Renal Unit and Department of Medicine, Harvard Medical School, and Massachusetts General Hospital, East 149 13th Street, Charlestown, Massachusetts, USA

It has long been appreciated that immune cells (polymorphonuclear cells, monocytes and lymphocytes) play a pivotal role in defending host tissues against a myriad of "foreign" bodies that are a threat to host survival. In an age where the concept of "foreignness" is being challenged by rapid introduction of "life-preserving" material into the host biological environment (artificial organs, hemodialysis, allografts) or through rapid resuscitation of damaged (now "foreign") tissues, the "slowly" adapting immune system often constitutes an impediment rather than a preserver of host survival. In such a "new" environment, immune cells are activated to maintain the "old self" status, thus rejecting the new means of life to the host through release of toxic chemicals, phagocytosis and target killing. Diverse as these immune functions are, a common thread ties them together, namely the need for immune cells to adhere to each other and to extracellular matrix.

The first indication of the impact of the process of cell adhesion on function of immune cells came from the discovery of a rare disease in humans—Leu-CAM deficiency—where diverse functional impairments in leukocyte migration to inflammatory sites, phagocytosis, release of proteolytic enzymes and oxidants were all related to an inability of leukocytes to adhere

---

*Author to whom correspondence should be addressed.

New Concepts in Immunodeficiency Diseases. Edited by S. Gupta and C. Griscelli
© 1993 John Wiley & Sons Ltd

firmly to each other, to endothelial cells, to components of extracellular matrix and to their targets. This commonality raised hopes that manipulation of this cellular process could be useful in helping immune cells "adapt" to the introduction of life-saving measures in their midst.

In this chapter, the major features of Leu-CAM deficiency and the insights it provided in understanding the role of cell adhesion in immune reactions will be briefly reviewed, with emphasis on recent progress into the genetic defects leading to this disease.

Leu-CAM (CD11/CD18) DEFICIENCY

Leu-CAM deficiency is a disease of leukocyte adhesion whereby affected cells lose the ability to emigrate to inflamed organs and to eliminate invading microorganisms through phagocytosis and target cell killing (1). The disease has an autosomal recessive mode of inheritance, with few cases probably representing *de novo* mutations. Leu-CAM deficiency affects all races and both sexes. Clinically, patients present in the pediatric age group with recurrent episodes of infections involving any organ and often culminating in fatal septicemias. The humeral response is preserved and manifested by intense vasodilation, redness and swelling of inflamed tissues. However, examination of all infected tissues (with the exception of lung) (2), characteristically shows a paucity of neutrophils in the interstitium despite the abundant presence of bacteria. Neutrophils instead are seen entrapped within the microvasculature unable to cross the endothelial cell barrier. The increased susceptibility of these patients to pneumonias despite the ability of neutrophils to emigrate to this tissue is reflective of the importance of Leu-CAM not only in extravasation but also in phagocytosis and target cell killing. Leu-CAM deficiency has little or no impact on lymphocyte functions *in vivo*, as reflected by normal skin testing to antigens and mitogens, intact delayed hypersensitivity reactions and normal levels of immunoglobulins (3), and by the lack of increased susceptibility to viral infections. These findings suggested the presence of alternative pathways that can compensate for Leu-CAM deficiency in lymphocytes *in vivo* (4), an interpretation borne out by recent data (5). Leu-CAM deficiency is not restricted to humans, but has also been described in dogs (6) and in Holstein cattle (7), where the disease is much more prevalent (due to inbreeding), with a carrier rate of 15%, making it the most common mutation known in animal agriculture.

Leu-CAM deficiency is caused by the partial (type 1) or complete (type II) absence of three leukocyte adhesion molecules (Leu-CAM, CD11/CD18) now known to be members of the integrin superfamily (β2 integrins). The three members—CD11a/CD18, CD11b/CD18 and CD11c/CD18—are heterodimers each with a distinct α subunit (CD11a, b or c) non-covalently associated with an identical β subunit (CD18) (8). CD11a/CD18 is expressed on all leukocytes. CD11b and CD11c expression is normally restricted to myelomonocytic cells and natural killer (NK) cells. Association between the CD11 and CD18 subunits occurs in the endoplasmic reticulum (ER) and is a requirement for transfer of these glycoproteins to the Golgi compartment for additional processing to their mature membrane-bound form. Leu-CAM deficiency is caused by structural defects in the CD18 subunit, leading to little or no heterodimer formation and resulting in entrapment and degradation of the subunits in the ER.

The primary structure of CD11/CD18 has been derived from molecular cloning of the individual subunits (8) and the gene structure of several subunits has been elucidated (9, 10). The CD11 subunits are homologous glycoproteins each with one membrane-spanning region and a short cytoplasmic C-terminal tail. The N-terminal halves of the large extracellular segments of each CD11 subunit contain seven short repeats, three of which (repeats five to seven) each contain a consensus divalent cation binding site with a lock-washer configuration (8). In addition, a single A-type motif first identified in the adhesive protein vWF is present between the second and third repeats of each CD11 subunit. The shorter and structurally distinct CD18 subunit has a short cytoplasmic tail, spans the plasma membrane once and has a characteristic protease-resistant cysteine-rich segment in the extracellular region in common with all integrin β subunits (11).

ROLE OF CD11/CD18 IN LEUKOCYTE FUNCTIONS

Recruitment of inflammatory cells to tissues to fight or contain "foreign" antigens is a complex process with at least three components: homing or *targeting* of circulating cells to sites of inflammation; *adhesion* and *migration* across endothelial cells to tight junctions; and *invasion* of the underlying diseased or damaged tissue. These stages are also seen during formation and remodeling of tissues, metastasis of tumors and recirculation/seeding of lymphocytes in lymphoid organs.

Recent evidence suggests that in neutrophils—the major cells affected in Leu-CAM deficiency—*targeting* is mediated by a distinct class of adhesion molecules, the selectins (12). These C-type lectins are expressed on leukocytes (L-selectin) or vascular endothelium (E- and P-selectins). Inflammatory mediators released at damaged sites increase expression of vascular selectins on adjacent endothelia within minutes to hours. Expression of vascular selectins causes circulating neutrophils at the respective site to "roll", net effect of selectin binding to their cognate ligands on neutrophils and the shear stress of blood flow. Rolling brings the circulating neutrophils close to the endothelial surface but is not sufficient to mediate the second and third phases of neutrophil extravasation, namely *migration* along the endothelial lining and *invasion* (penetration) at tight junctions into the subendothelial space. These phases as well as the subsequent phagocytosis of target cells are mediated in neutrophils by CD11/CD18, the major integrins expressed on these cells. In other cell types (e.g. lymphocytes), additional members of the integrin super-family as well as other adhesion molecule families (5) are also expressed which tend to compensate for deficiency of CD11/CD18 on these cells. The differential cell distribution of adhesion molecules and the critical role of CD11/CD18 in phagocytosis explain why Leu-CAM deficiency presents clinically as a phagocytic cell defect but not a lymphocytic cell defect.

CD11/CD18 integrins bind to several ligands. These include serum-derived proteins as complement iC3b, fibrinogen and factor X, plasma membrane-bound receptors (e.g. CD54 and ICAM-2) and other protein or lipid moieties expressed by bacteria, fungi and certain parasites (e.g. lipid A, polysaccharides, *Leishmania* gp 63) (8). CD11b/CD18 is the major receptor expressed on activated neutrophils and is responsible for the majority of CD11/CD18 functions in these cells.

REGULATION OF CD11/CD18

To serve its vital role in chemotaxis, transendothelial migration and phagocytosis, CD11/CD18 ($\beta2$ integrins) receptors must rapidly and rever-sibly modulate their avidity state to various ligands in response to agonists, redistribute on the surface membrane locomoting cells and tether to the force-generating cytoskeleton. In addition to these functional adaptations of existing surface-membrane receptors, phagocytic cells can also rapidly re-cruit to the cell surface additional receptors from secondary and tertiary intracellular granules (4, 13). Given the spectrum of pro-inflammatory func-tions mediated by CD11/CD18, rigorous control of their activation state is mandatory to maintain the non-adhesive phenotype of circulating immune cells and avoid the pathological consequences of hyperadherence (self-aggregation, pulmonary embolization, tissue damage, vasculopathy).

The mechanisms by which CD11/CD18 receptors are maintained in a non-adhesive state are poorly understood, as are the mechanisms which rapidly and reversibly change these receptors into an active form. Recent data suggest that the adhesive phenotype is an intrinsic property of the receptors. Upon truncation of the cytoplasmic and transmembrane regions, constitutively active forms of CD11/CD18 are generated, suggesting that the deleted segments have a net negative effect on receptor avidity. More selec-tive truncations or point mutations in the cytoplasmic tail of CD18 also modify receptor avidity to extracellular ligands (14). Agonist-induced tran-sient phosphorylation of the cytoplasmic tail of CD18 has also been demon-strated, occurring with kinetics that mirror the transition of these receptors from low to high avidity states. Phosphorylation occurs on several serines, threonines and a single tyrosine residue (15), is thus mediated by more than one kinase and reflects a more complex and perhaps hierarchic role of receptor phosphorylation in regulating the avidity state of CD11/CD18.

As in other integrins (16), increased CD11/CD18 avidity also results from direct conformational changes in the extracellular domain induced in the purified receptors by certain divalent cations, mAbs and lipid extracts. Mn^{2+} millimolar concentrations and certain lipid moieties increase avidity of purified CD11b/CD18 to iC3b (17, 18) and the avidity of CD11a/CD18 to CD54 (19). Agonists also induce expression of a Ca^{2+}-dependent epitope for the NKI-L16 mAb on CD11a/CD18 in a temperature- and energy-independent manner (20). Induction of these conformational states in intact cells, however, often requires metabolic energy (19, 21), arguing that post-translational modifications play important roles in receptor function under physiological conditions.

The CD11b/CD18 receptor has been shown to undergo recycling through coated pits (22), an event which may be important in the role of this receptor in cell migration and phagocytosis. This physical recycling is mediated by structural motifs present in the cytoplasmic tail of CD18 since deletions within this segment abolish coated-pit internalization of the recombinant receptor (14). The role of CD18 and CD11 phosphorylation in receptor endocytosis has not yet been evaluated.

HETEROGENEITY OF Leu-CAM DEFICIENCY AND ITS STRUCTURAL BASIS

In the majority of cases of Leu-CAM deficiency, normal amounts of normal-sized CD18 precursors are made which fail to associate with the CD11 subunits, suggesting that point mutations, small deletions or insertions in the coding region of the protein are the most common genetic abnormalities (23). Less common mutations include absence of CD18 mRNA and deletions/insertions large enough to be detected by northern blot analysis of CD18 mRNA. Although it is quite possible that patients with structural mutations in the CD11 subunits may exist, as observed in Glanzmann's thrombasthenia (24), no such cases have been reported to date. In addition, no patients were described in which deficiency is due to normal surface expression of dysfunctional heterodimers, probably owing to the difficulty of establishing the diagnosis in such cases.

The underlying structural mutations in CD18 reported to date are summarized in Figure 9.1. Several of the patients studied were found to be compound heterozygous for mutations that impair to various degrees the surface expression of CD18 (25–28). In other cases, where more than one family member is affected, a single mutation is commonly found. This appears to be the case in Holstein cattle, where inbreeding for high milk

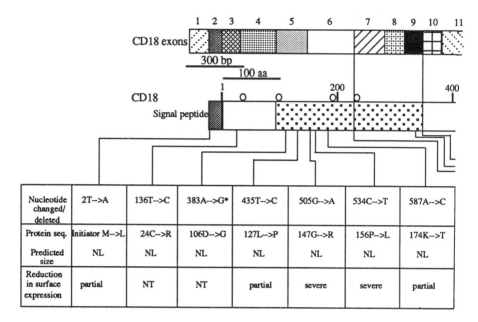

Figure 9.1. Mutations in the CD18 gene identified to date in patients with Leu-CAM deficiency. The CD18 gene contains 16 exons and spans a region of approximately 40 kb (10). In numbering nucleotides and amino acids, the adenine of the initiation codon and the N-terminus of the mature protein were used as first residues respectively. For mutations that result in frame shifts, the predicted number of out-of-frame amino acids is indicated in parentheses. The boundaries of exon 13 were delineated since the cause for deletion of this exon have not been

production in dairy farms led inadvertently to the high prevalence of the [106]D/G mutant allele (29). The majority of mutations found in patients with Leu-CAM deficiency involve two regions of the CD18 gene, one spanning exons five to nine (eight mutations) and a second spanning exon 13 (four mutations). Three other mutations have been discovered that are outside these two regions (Figure 9.1). The region encoded by exons 5 to 9 consists of 251 amino acids (amino acids 88 to 339) and is highly conserved among β integrins, suggesting that this region subserves common structural and/or functional requirements. Single amino acid substitutions with this segment impair either partially ([127]L/P, [174]K/T) (25, 30) or completely ([106]D/G, [147]G/R, [156]P/L, [329]N/S) (26, 27, 29, 30), the non-covalent association of CD11 subunits with CD18 suggesting a vital role for this region (H, heterodimer domain) in heterodimer complex formation. Of interest is the fact that mutations in the H domain which abolish surface expression involve amino acid residues that are conserved in all other β subunits, while others producing a partial phenotype involve non-conserved amino acids ([127]L/P, [174]K/T).

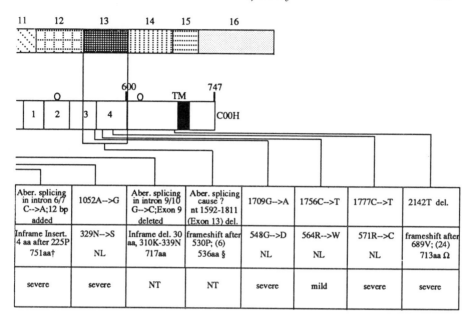

Aber. splicing in intron 6/7 C-->A;12 bp added	1052A-->G	Aber. splicing in intron 9/10 G-->C;Exon 9 deleted	Aber. splicing cause? nt 1592-1811 (Exon 13) del.	1709G-->A	1756C-->T	1777C-->T	2142T del.
Inframe Insert. 4 aa after 225P 751aa†	329N-->S NL	Inframe del. 30 aa, 310K-339N 717aa	frameshift after 530P; (6) 536aa §	548G-->D NL	564R-->W NL	571R-->C NL	frameshift after 689V; (24) 713aa Ω
severe	severe	NT	NT	severe	mild	severe	severe

determined. NL indicates a predicted normal size of the mature protein. *This mutation has only been shown in cattle. †In-frame amino acids are SSPE. §Out-of-frame amino acids are APAPSA. ΩOut-of-frame amino acids are ERAESVW-QAPTSPPSSGAPWQASC. Single-letter code is used to indicate individual amino acids. Reduction in surface expression is based on data derived from transfection studies in COS cells or leukocytes in which cDNA encoding for each mutation was used

A role for the H domain in heterodimer formation is also supported by electron microscopy studies of several integrins (31, 32), which revealed that association of the subunits occurs in their N-terminal regions. In other integrins, the H domain is also important for ligand binding. In the β3 integrin IIb/IIIa (CD41/CD61), the H domain contains an RGD binding site (amino acids 83–145 of the mature β3 protein) (33), a fibrinogen binding site localized to (amino acids 185–196 of mature β3) (34) and a putative divalent cation binding site involving [119]D (35). A mutation changing this residue to a Y in a patient with Glanzmann's thrombasthenia interfered with RGD (Arg-Gly-Asp) binding of IIb/IIIa and altered its divalent cation-dependent conformation (35).

In addition to the point mutations described above, two splicing mutations have been identified within the H domain, resulting in one case in an in-frame addition of four amino acids (26) and in the other in an in-frame deletion of 30 amino acids (exon 9) (36). The in-frame insertion was directly shown to abolish surface expression in COS cells transfected with the mutant cDNA (26). Both the insertion as well as the deletion alleles are capable of generating small amounts of normally spliced products contributing to the type I phenotype in the respective patients' leukocytes.

The second major cluster of mutations in the CD18 gene involve exon 13 (Figure 9.1). Three amino acid substitutions ([548]G/D, [564]R/W and [571]R/C) (25, 26, 37) and one out-of-frame deletion of the whole exon (27) have been identified in four unrelated patients. Of the three point mutations, two involve conserved amino acids in all β integrins ([548]G/D and [571]R/C), while the third ([564]R/W) involves a non-conserved amino acid. While the effect of the [548]G/D alteration on receptor expression has not yet been evaluated, that of [571]R/C was found to abolish surface membrane receptor expression (25). The [564]R/W substitution had small effects on receptor expression. These data again suggest that replacement of certain conserved amino acids in this region is deleterious to formation of heterodimers. The mechanisms by which mutations within this region affect heterodimer formation despite its location outside the contact area in the αβ complex is unclear. Since this segment is a component of the rigid cysteine-rich repeats in the β subunits, mutations here may impair heterodimer formation by inducing conformational changes that preclude proper or stable associations of the H domain with the respective CD11 subunits.

Three additional mutations have been described in other parts of the CD18 gene. In one case, an M to L substitution of the initiator codon results in reduced copies of the gene product, probably owing to low levels of initiation of translation at the second codon (28). A second allele in the same patient as well as in an unrelated patient ([2142]T deleted) resulted in a frameshift mutation and truncation of the transmembrane and cytoplasmic regions of CD18. The gene product in this case was not detected on the cell surface of leukocytes, suggesting that the 24 out-of-frame amino acids added to the C-terminus (which include a cysteine residue) may alter, through formation of aberrant cysteine bridges, the N-terminal conformation required for heterodimer formation.

The heterogeneity of the mutations described above offer an explanation for the wide ranges of receptor expression (<2% to 20% of normal levels) in this disease. These and other mutations generate a spectrum of affinities of the altered CD18 subunit to the CD11 subunits which in turn determine the extent of complex formation and subsequent surface expression of the particular heterodimer. In addition, variability is created by the modifications of epitopes for certain mAbs. In both the [127]L/P and [329]N/S, for example, the mAb TS1/18 does not bind to the expressed mutant protein (26, 30). Binding of the anti-CD18 mAbs CLB54, MHM23, GRF1 and M232 to [127]L/P mutant is also reduced or absent (30). In another patient with an as yet uncharacterized defect, the TS1/18 mAb also failed to immunoprecipitate a CD18 precursor (38) present in normal amounts (39). These findings stress the need for comprehensive functional as well as immunochemical phenotyping in evaluating therapeutic alternatives in Leu-CAM deficiency.

PROGNOSIS AND TREATMENT

In its complete form, Leu-CAM deficiency is invariably fatal. Several patients diagnosed with the partial form of the disease (10–20% surface expression and diminished but not absent neutrophil functions) are now young adults. These patients have been managed similar to other patients with neutropenia. They are aggressively treated with antibiotics when they develop an infection and several are kept on long-term suppressive doses of antibiotics. In these individuals, infections become less frequent as they grow, perhaps due to development of specific immunoglobulins to common pathogens which are then eliminated through Fc receptor-mediated phagocytosis and killing.

Bone marrow transplantation is curative in this disease (40). In Holstein cattle, screening for carriers of the [106]D/G allele will soon lead to eradication of this disease through selection. In humans, given the large and expanding list of heterogeneous mutations discovered, genetic counselling can only be offered to parents with affected children. Correction of the gene defect in cells from afflicted patients has been achieved *in vitro* using retroviral vectors (41). Gene therapy using homologous recombination will be the ultimate treatment in this and many other genetic diseases.

CD11/CD18 AS TARGETS OF ANTI-INFLAMMATORY DRUGS

Since the CD11/CD18 adhesion molecules mediate final common pathways in exudation of immune cells at inflammatory sites, it was logical to assume that induction of an acquired form of Leu-CAM deficiency using reagents which block CD11/CD18 functions may be beneficial when inflammation becomes a foe rather than a friend to the host, as in ischemia–reperfusion injury and rejection of transplanted organs. In several models of ischemia–reperfusion injury (e.g. myocardial infarction, thermal injury, hemorrhagic shock, prolonged preservation time of harvested donor kidneys) use of anti-CD11/CD18 mAbs have markedly reduced the degree of tissue damage (2). More recently, preclinical trials examining renal survival in allograft recipients with high risk for delayed graft function (cadaveric kidneys with prolonged preservation time) have also shown significant improvement in graft survival when patients were pretreated with anti-CD54 (a ligand for CD11a/CD18 and CD11b/CD18) mAbs. These encouraging results suggest that comprehensive understanding of the structure and function of CD11/CD18 may allow development of synthetic drugs that can tame harmful inflammatory reactions and redefine the boundaries of self and non-self.

ACKNOWLEDGEMENTS

The authors wish to thank Ms Robin Parsons for expert secretarial assistance. This work was supported by grant AI-21964 from the National Institutes of Health, a grant from the March of Dimes and a fellowship award to M.M. from the American Heart Association.

REFERENCES

1. Arnaout, M.A. (1990) Leukocyte adhesion molecules deficiency: Its structural basis, pathophysiology and implications for modulating the inflammatory response. *Immunol. Rev.*, **114**, 145–180.
2. Carlos, T.M. and Harlan, J.M. (1990) Membrane proteins involved in phagocyte adherence to endothelium. *Immunol. Rev.*, **114**, 5–28.
3. Arnaout, M.A., Pitt, J., Cohen, H.J., Melamed, J., Rosen, F.S. and Colten, H.R. (1982) Deficiency of a granulocyte-membrane glycoprotein (gp 150) in a boy with recurrent bacterial infections. *N. Engl. J. Med.*, **306**, 693–699.
4. Arnaout, M.A., Spits, H., Terhorst, C., Pitt, J. and Todd, R.F., III (1984) Deficiency of a leukocyte surface glycoprotein (LFA-1) in two patients with Mo1 deficiency: Effects of cell activation on Mo1/LFA-1 surface expression in normal and deficient leukocytes. *J. Clin. Invest.*, **74**, 1291–1300.
5. Stoolman, L.M. (1989) Adhesion molecules controlling lymphocyte migration. *Cell*, **56**, 907–910.
6. Giger, U., Boxer, L.A., Simpson, P.J., Lucchesi, B.R. and Todd, R.F., III (1987) Deficiency of leukocyte surface glycoproteins Mo1, LFA-1, and Leu-M5 in a dog with recurrent bacterial infections: An animal model. *Blood*, **69**, 1622–1630.
7. Kehrli, M.E., Shuster, D.E. and Ackermann, M.R. (1992) Leukocyte adhesion deficiency among Holstein cattle. *Cornell Vet.*, **82**, 103–109.
8. Arnaout, M.A. (1990) Structure and function of the leukocyte adhesion molecules CD11/CD18. *Blood*, **75**, 1037–1050.
9. Corbi, A.L., Garcia-Aguilar, J. and Springer, T.A. (1990) Genomic structure of an integrin α subunit, the leukocyte p150,95 molecule. *J. Biol. Chem.*, **265**, 2782–2788.
10. Weitzman, J.B., Wells, C.E., Wright, A.H., Clark, P.A. and Law, A.S.K. (1992) The gene organization of the human β2 integrin subunit (CD18). *FEBS Lett.*, **294**, 97–103.
11. Hynes, R.O. (1987) Integrins: A family of cell surface receptors. *Cell*, **48**, 549–554.
12. Hynes, R.O. and Lander, A.D. (1992) Contact and adhesive specificities in the association, migrations, and targeting of cells and axons. *Cell*, **68**, 303–322.
13. Todd, R.F., III, Arnaout, M.A., Rosin, R.E., Crowley, C.A., Peters, W.A., Curnutte, J.T. and Babior, B.M. (1984) Subcellular localization of the subunit of Mo1 (Mo1 alpha; formerly gp110), a surface glycoprotein associated with neutrophil adhesion. *J. Clin. Invest.*, **74**, 1280–1290.
14. Rabb, H., Michishita, M., Sharma, C.P., Brown, D. and Arnaout, M.A. (1992) The cytoplasmic tails of human complement receptor type 3 (CR 3, CD 11b/CD 18) regulate ligand avidity and the internalization of occupied receptors (submitted).
15. Chatila, T., Geha, R.S. and Arnaout, M.A. (1989) Constitutive and stimulus-induced phosphorylation of CD11/CD18 leukocyte adhesion molecules. *J. Cell Biol.*, **109**, 3435–3444.
16. Sims, P.J., Ginsberg, M.H., Plow, E.F. and Shattil, S.J. (1991) Effect of platelet activation on the conformation of the plasma membrane glycoprotein IIb–IIIa complex. *J. Biol. Chem.*, **266**, 7345–7352.

17. Altieri, D.C. (1991) Occupancy of CD11b/CD18 (Mac-1) divalent ion binding site(s) induces leukocyte adhesion. *J. Immunol.*, **147**, 1891–1896.

18. Hermanowski-Vosatka, A., Van Strip, J.A.G., Swiggard, W.J. and Wright, S.D. (1992) Integrin modulation factor-1: A lipid that alters the function of leukocyte integrins. *Cell*, **68**, 341–352.

19. Dransfield, I., Cabanas, C., Craig, A. and Hogg, N. (1992) Divalent cation regulation of the function of the leukocyte integrin LFA-1. *J. Cell Biol.*, **116**, 219–226.

20. van Kooyk, Y., Weder, P., Hogervorst, F., Verhoeven, A.J., van Seventer, G., te Velde, A.A., Borst, J., Keizer, G.D. and Figdor, C.G. (1991) Activation of LFA-1 through a Ca^{2+}-dependent epitope stimulates lymphocyte adhesion. *J. Cell Biol.*, **112**, 345–354.

21. Altieri, D.C., Bader, R., Mannucci, P.M. and Edgington, T.S. (1988) Oligospecificity of the cellular adhesion receptor MAC-1 encompasses an inducible recognition specificity for fibrinogen. *J. Cell Biol.*, **107**, 1893–1900.

22. Bretscher, M.S. (1992) Circulating integrins: $\alpha5\beta1$, $\alpha6\beta4$ and Mac-1, but not $\alpha3\beta1$, $\alpha4\beta1$ or LFA-1. *EMBO J.*, **11**, 405–410.

23. Arnaout, M.A. (1992) Molecular basis for leukocyte adhesion deficiency. In Horton, M. (ed.) *Biochemistry of Macrophages and Related Cell Types*, Plenum Press, New York (in press).

24. Newman, P.J., Seligsohn, U., Lyman, S. and Coller, B.S. (1991) The molecular genetic basis of Glanzmann thrombasthenia in the Iraqi–Jewish and Arab populations in Israel. *Proc. Nat. Acad. Sci. USA*, **88**, 3160–3164.

25. Arnaout, M.A., Dana, N., Gupta, S.K., Tenen, D.G. and Fathallah, D.F. (1990) Point mutations impairing cell surface expression of the common β subunit (CD18) in a patient with Leu-CAM deficiency. *J. Clin. Invest.*, **85**, 977–981.

26. Nelson, C., Rabb, H. and Arnaout, M.A. (1992) Genetic cause of leukocyte adhesion molecule deficiency: Abnormal splicing and a missense mutation in a conserved region of CD18 impair cell surface expression of $\beta2$ integrins. *J. Biol. Chem.*, **267**, 3351–3357.

27. Back, A.L., Kwok, W.W. and Hickstein, D.D. (1992) Identification of two molecular defects in a child with leukocyte adherence deficiency. *J. Biol. Chem.*, **267**, 5482–5487.

28. Sligh, J.E., Hurwitz, M.Y., Zhu, C., Anderson, D.C. and Beaudet, A.L. (1992) An initiation codon mutation in CD18 in association with the moderate phenotype of leukocyte adhesion deficiency. *J. Biol. Chem.*, **267**, 714–718.

29. Shuster, D.E., Kehrli, M.E., Ackermann, M.R. and Gilbert, R.O. (1992) Identification and prevalence of a genetic defect that causes leukocyte adhesion deficiency in Holstein cattle. *Proc. Natl. Acad. Sci. (USA)*, **89**, 9225–9229.

30. Wardlaw, A.J., Hibbs, M.L., Stacker, S.A. and Springer, T.A. (1990) Distinct mutations in two patients with leukocyte adhesion deficiency and their functional correlates. *J. Exp. Med.*, **172**, 335–345.

31. Kelly, T., Molony, L. and Burridge, K. (1987) Purification of two smooth muscle glycoproteins related to integrin. *J. Biol. Chem.*, **262**, 17189–17199.

32. Nermut, M.V., Green, N.M., Eason, P., Yamada, S.S. and Yamada, K.M. (1988) Electron microscopy and structural model of human fibronectin receptor. *EMBO J.*, **7**, 4093–4099.

33. D'Souza, S.E., Ginsberg, M.H., Burke, T.A., Lam, S.C.-T. and Plow, E.F. (1988) Localization of an Arg-Gly-Asp recognition site within an integrin adhesion receptor. *Science*, **242**, 91–93.

34. Kieffer, N. and Phillips, D.R. (1990) Platelet membrane glycoproteins: Functions in cellular interactions. *Annu. Rev. Cell Biol.*, **6**, 329–357.

35. Loftus, J.C., O'Toole, T.E., Plow, E.F., Glass, A., Frelinger, A.L., III and Ginsberg, M.H. (1990) A β3 integrin mutation abolishes ligand binding and alters divalent cation-dependent conformation. *Science*, **249**, 915–918.
36. Kishimoto, T.K., Hollander, N., Roberts, T.M., Anderson, D.C. and Springer, T.A. (1989) Leukocyte adhesion deficiency: Aberrant splicing of a conserved integrin sequence causes a moderate deficiency phenotype. *J. Biol. Chem.*, **264**, 3588–3595.
37. Law, S.K.A. (1992) Complement receptors. In Horton, M. (ed.) *Biochemistry of Macrophages and Related Cell Types*. Plenum Press, New York (in press).
38. Springer, T.A., Thompson, W.S., Miller, L.J., Schmalstieg, F.C. and Anderson, D.C. (1984) Inherited deficiency of the Mac-1, LFA-1, p150,95 glycoprotein family and its molecular basis. *J. Exp. Med.*, **160**, 1901–1918.
39. Dana, N., Tenen, D., Clayton, L., Pierce, M., Lachmann, P. and Arnaout, M.A. (1987) Leukocytes from four patients with complete or partial Leu-CAM deficiency contain the common beta subunit precursor and beta subunit messenger RNA. *J. Clin. Invest.*, **79**, 1010–1015.
40. Fisher, A., Trung, P.H., Descamps-Latscha, B., Lisowska-Grospierre, B., Gerota, I., Perez, N., Scheinmetzler, C., Durandy, A., Virelizier, J.L. and Griscelli, C. (1983) Bone marrow transplantation for inborn error of phagocytic cells associated with defective adherence, chemotaxis and oxidative response during opsonized particle phagocytosis. *Lancet*, **ii**, 473–476.
41. Wilson, J.M., Ping, A.J., Krauss, J.C., Mayo-Bond, L., Rogers, C.E., Anderson, D.C. and Todd, R.F. (1990) Correction of CD18-deficient lymphocytes by retrovirus-mediated gene transfer. *Science*, **248**, 1413–1416.

Chapter 10

Ataxia–Telangiectasia: Genetic Studies

RICHARD A. GATTI

UCLA School of Medicine, Department of Pathology, Los Angeles, California, USA

The syndrome of ataxia–telangiectasia (A–T) is complex and, despite the fact that it results from a single autosomal recessive gene defect, includes such apparently unrelated findings as: (a) a progressive cerebellar ataxia with onset around 1–2 years of age, involving Purkinje cells and granule cells (1, 2); (b) subsequent onset of dilated peripheral blood vessels (telangiectasia), usually over the eyes and ears; (c) maldevelopment of the thymus, with immunodeficiency; (d) cancer susceptibility, involving 38% of patients (3); and (e) hypersensitivity to ionizing radiation. The syndrome was described rather comprehensively in some of the first reports by Boder and Sedgwick (4, 5), who selected the name "ataxia–telangiectasia" (A–T). The ensuing years have added further complexity to the syndrome but have made little contribution to a unifying hypothesis for its pathogenesis (6–11). A brief historical review follows.

In 1961, Thieffry et al. (12) described IgA deficiency in A–T patients. Soon after, Hecht and co-workers (13) noted a chromosomal translocation, involving chromosome 14. A propensity to develop cancer, mainly lymphoid, was noted early by Boder and Sedgwick (4) and then further documented by Gatti and Good (14). In 1972, an elevated alfafetoprotein (AFP) was described that involved almost all patients (15).

Gotoff et al. (16) launched yet another level of complexity for A–T research when they reported an "untoward reaction to ionizing radiation" in a patient who developed fatal complications while being treated for lymphoma. This led to reports of in vitro radiosensitivity of A–T fibroblasts (17, 18) and lymphoblasts (19). An intermediate level of radiosensitivity exists in A–T heterozygotes.

New Concepts in Immunodeficiency Diseases. Edited by S. Gupta and C. Griscelli
© 1993 John Wiley & Sons Ltd

Murnane and Painter (20), and Jaspers *et al.* (21) discovered that if the fibroblasts of two unrelated patients were fused, by Sendai virus or polyethylene glycol treatment, the resulting heterodikaryons were often of normal radiosensitivity. After a large international effort involving 40 A–T families, four clinically indistinguishable complementation groups were defined: A (55%), C (28%), D (14%), and E (3%) (22). A similar radiosensitivity (i.e. radioresistant DNA synthesis) was defined in a few patients without ataxia or telangiectasia who had Nijmegen breakage syndrome (NBS) (23–25); "breakage", in this case, referred to the translocations of chromosomes 7 and 14 that were observed, which were indistinguishable from those seen in A–T patients. Despite this similarity, the fibroblasts of typical A–T patients always corrected NBS fibroblasts, as would the fibroblasts of normal controls. Thus, A–T and NBS patients appeared to have different genetic defects, until a set of Mexican twins was described who had both A–T *and* NBS (26), i.e. their fibroblasts did not correct the radiosensitivity of NBS patients, thereby suggesting that at least one form of A–T shared a gene with NBS. This complementation group is called "variant 1" or "V1", and the combined syndrome is called A–T$_{Fresno}$.

By the early 1980s, numerous types of immunodeficiency had been described in A–T patients, ranging from: (a) IgA deficiency in 60% (12), (b) IgG2 deficiency in 80% (27–29); (c) IgE deficiency in 50% (30); and (d) occasionally elevated B cell levels (31); to (e) skin anergy (32); (f) occasionally decreased T cell levels (29, 31, 33–36); (g) decreased or absent responses to antigens, such as tetanus, and mitogens (29, 36); (h) very poor mixed leukocyte culture responses (35); (i) poor cytotoxic responses to influenza-infected target cells (37); (j) abnormal T cell killing (29, 36); (k) rapid "capping" of concanavalin A receptors by peripheral lymphocytes (29); and (l) extremely elevated intracellular levels of cAMP *and* cGMP in isolated T cells (29). Neutrophil chemotaxis was decreased in some studies and within normal range in others, as were NK cell activity and NK cell levels (29, 35, 38). Later, a suggestion was made that T$\gamma\delta$ cell proportions were elevated in some patients, but this was apparently an artifact of poorly defined normal ranges.

Thus, before genetic studies got underway, the challenge was to decipher the pathogenesis of a very complex syndrome that, although monogenic (in any one family), involved organ systems and physiological phenomena with no apparent relationship to one another. No disease-specific protein had been identified to allow a biochemical approach. Immunological findings explained little. Chromosomal analyses of many, many patients failed to reveal a single constitutional translocation or deletion that might aid in pinpointing the location of the A–T gene(s). Later even using high-resolution analysis of chromosome 11q, we have not seen a constitutional chromosomal defect in over 40 patients (unpublished data).

LINKAGE ANALYSES

Historically there were two very weak genetic leads to locating the A–T gene(s) in the human genome. First, AFP levels are elevated in almost all A–T patients (although not in NBS), implicating the AFP gene region in the pathogenesis of A–T; and second, the chromosomal translocations and inversions almost exclusively involved breakpoints at 7q35, 14q12 and 14q32 (39, 40), all sites of gene rearrangements, implicating perhaps a common recombinase.

The AFP gene is on chromosome 4. It was hypothesized that the A–T gene(s) might be nearby. Linkage studies later excluded this region (unpublished data).

The data indicating the region of translocation breakpoints were even less compelling since the chromosomal translocations and inversions seen in A–T are all somatic changes, not inherited ones. Further, only one of these sites could contain the A–T gene, and even 10 years ago it seemed clear that a single common mechanism was influencing all of the reciprocal translocations. Thus, it seemed unlikely that the defective A–T protein would be coded by a gene near any of these translocation sites. In this regard, the TCRβ (T cell receptor β chain) region at 7q35 was soon excluded by linkage analysis (unpublished data), using a set of Vβ gene polymorphisms that had just been developed by Concannon *et al.* (41). Linkage to the IHG (immunoglobulin heavy chain) region at 14q32 was also excluded (42).

On clinical grounds, most of the X chromosome could be excluded since both males and females were affected. HLA technology allowed the major histocompatibility complex region on chromosome 6p to be excluded as well (43).

However, an important caveat weakened the validity of most of the early linkage analyses. Combining the segregation data from different A–T families, without knowing their complementation groups, ignored the fact that complementation studies suggest genetic heterogeneity, i.e. that more than one A–T gene exists, and it was unlikely that the different complementation genes would be clustered into a single chromosomal region (although this may in fact prove to be the case!).

To circumvent the potential heterogeneity problem, a single large family was selected for screening the genome with a battery of genetic markers. This family was of Amish–Mennonite background, with carefully documented genealogy dating back 200 years and including 11 generations (44, 45). Subsequent complementation studies assigned the family to group A, the most common A–T group.

Before a linked marker could be found, approximately 35% of the genome was screened and excluded, using 171 markers (45). The marker that was finally found to co-segregate with the disease in the Amish–Mennonite family was THY1/MspI (46); it was located on chromosome 11q22–23. THY1 itself was actually an interesting candidate gene for A–T, since it is involved in neurological and immunological development, but recombinants between THY1/MspI and the A–T gene were subsequently identified in group A families, thereby excluding it as the ATA gene. A second genetic marker in this region also linked to ATA; this probe has had several names (45): MCT128, pYNB3.12, and finally D11S144 (Figure 10.1). (The D11 prefix indicates the chromosome 11 location of a marker; because all subsequent discussion involves only chromosome 11, the D11 prefix has been omitted elsewhere in this chapter.)

(The statistical evaluation of co-segregation (linkage) is expressed as LOD scores, i.e., the logarithm of the odds of the difference between observed pedigree data and free recombination within the same genetic model. The parameters of A–T model were: (a) autosomal recessive inheritance; (b) no interference; (c) complete penetrance; (d) known population frequencies for

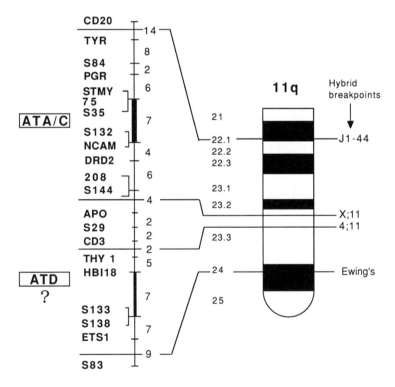

Figure 10.1. Linkage map (left) and cytogenic map (right) of the distal long arm of chromosome 11, including the regions of the A–T genes (bold lines). Numbers in linkage map depict distances (in centimorgans) between genetic markers. Characterized breakpoints of mouse–human hybrid cells anchor the two maps

the disease and for each allele of the tested marker and the ATA gene. Typically, six distances or recombination fractions (θ) are evaluated for each marker: ≈ 0, 0.05, 0.10, 0.20, 0.30 and 0.40. A LOD score greater than 3.0 (considered equivalent to a *p* value of 0.001) is the international minimum standard to establish linkage or co-segregation between any two genetic markers. If the original observation of linkage is correct, and additional "comparable" families are studied, the LOD score will increase.)

Using only the original eight group A families (45) gave LOD scores of 3.63 and 2.47 for THY1 and S144, respectively. Unexpectedly, when data from all families were combined (including not only group A families, but also two group C families, one V1 family, and 20 other unassigned A–T families from Turkey and the USA), the LOD scores were actually higher: 4.34 at θ = 0.10 for THY1, and 5.58 at θ = 0.08 for S144. This suggested three alternatives: (a) most of the unassigned families were also group A; (b) other complementation group genes were clustered near ATA; and/or (c) the complementation studies might not in fact be identifying different A–T genes.

FURTHER LOCALIZATION OF THE A–T GENE(S) AT 11q22–23

The next priority was to develop a better, i.e. higher-resolution, map of the 11q22–23 region, so that the ATA gene could be localized between two flanking markers that were close enough to allow serious cloning studies to begin. For this, the A–T families were set aside and, with the assistance of Charmley *et al.* (47) and Julier *et al.* (48), a set of 40 large, three-generation families were typed with all markers suspected of localizing to the distal long arm of chromosome 11. The 40 families were provided by the Centre d'Etude du Polymorphisme Humain (CEPH), a Paris-based international consortium of 20 charter laboratories (49), of which ours was one, aimed at creating a linkage map of the entire human genome. Within a year, the consortium had established a mathematically derived linkage map 11q22–23 with interval-specific sex-averaged distances established between about ten markers. Other laboratories also made significant contributions to the map of 11q (50, 51).

Using this map, we could return to analyzing the A–T families. Three-point location scores localized the A–T gene(s) proximal to both THY1 and S144, in a 21 cM region flanked by STMY (the gene for stromelysin) and S144 (52). This work was confirmed and extended by McConville *et al.* (53, 54), using a group of 41 British A–T families. Shortly thereafter, Ziv *et al.* (55) showed that the 11q22–23 markers also linked to the inheritance of A–T in a large group C family from Israel, thus placing the ATC gene and the ATA gene close to one another (if, indeed, they are separate genes).

In preparing the Sanal *et al.* (52) report, we became aware of the statistical weakness of location scores generated by conventional linkage analysis algorithms and on a data set of only 31 A–T families. Before serious cloning attempts could be initiated, we needed to localize the gene(s) to within 1 cM or less. This goal seemed very far off! To close this gap, Lange and Sobel developed a Monte Carlo simulation method that increased location scores by 5–6 log units (56). Monte Carlo simulations handled missing data (e.g. on unstudied family members) much more efficiently than standard deterministic calculations of LOD scores.

We also established collaborations with other A–T investigators in England, Italy, Israel, and Istanbul that added 60 more families to the database. We added more American families as well. By 1991, Foroud *et al.* (57) were able to report the localization of the A–T gene(s) to within a 2.8 cM male-specific interval flanked by STMY and S132 (Figure 10.1). This localization was 100 000 000 times more likely than the ''next best interval'' and was based on Monte Carlo simulations involving 91 A–T families (Figure 10.2A).

GENETIC HETEROGENEITY

The statistical power of Monte Carlo analysis, and the addition of new families, now allowed us to address the question of genetic heterogeneity. Was there one A–T gene at 11q22–23, or several; and if so, did they all localize to a single region? We had noticed a second peak in the location scores depicted in Figure 1 of Foroud *et al.* (57) (reproduced here as Figure 10.2A). When we recalculated the location scores using only sixteen families known to be group A or C, the second peak was no longer observed, i.e. the location scores in this region were now zero, while the first peak remained between the markers STMY and S132 (Figure 10.2B). (The first peak was now lower because the data set was based on only 16 rather than 94 families.) Since the only remaining complementation group of significant proportions in the previous Jaspers analysis (22) would be group D (i.e. 14% of tested families were group D, while only 3% were group E), we presumed that this second peak indicated the location of the ATD gene (58). Conversely, when the 16 group A and group C families were excluded from the 94 families, the second peak was now increased by several log units, suggesting that the removal of group A and group C families enriched the proportion of group D families in the remaining families and increased the location scores contributing to that peak (data not shown). However, caution remains in making this interpretation of a presumptive group D peak since conventional tests for heterogeneity in our database are not yet statistically significant!

If a second A–T region exists, it maps approximately 30 cM distal to the ATA/ATC region, is still within the 11q22–23 region. This putative evidence for heterogeneity of the A–T genes has several important implications. First, it necessitates a reanalysis of the fine mapping of the ATA/ATC gene(s), now excluding group D families. However, without actually being able to assign families by complementation studies, a tedious task that by present methods could take several years, we are attempting to create a probabilistic group assignment based on how strongly each family's location scores contribute to each peak. Needless to say, this is a somewhat circular approach and may not prove valid. Nonetheless, we are presently calculating these tentative group D assignments with the hope that by excluding a "probable group D" subset, and adding additional genetic markers, we will be better able to sublocalize the ATA/ATC genes.

A second implication of finding heterogeneity would be that the syntenic homology between markers on human chromosome 11q22–24 (H11) and mouse chromosome 9 (M9) clearly includes the putative group D region between genes THY1 and ETS1 but does not necessarily include the more centromeric ATA/ATC region, since the syntenic homology between H11 and M9 appears to end just proximal to the human gene NCAM (neural adhesion molecule) (Figure 10.1) (59). Exactly how far proximal is not known. Thus, M9 may or may not contain the homologous ATA/ATC gene(s). This important comparative mapping question is being addressed (a) by fluorescent *in situ* hybridization (FISH) with genes conserved in mouse and human, and (b) by linkage mapping of homologous genes in genetically divergent mouse strains.

HAS THE ATD GENE BEEN CLONED?

A candidate group D gene, ATDC, has been isolated by Kapp *et al.*, by "shotgun" transfection and complementation (60, 61), which would simplify the above analyses of genetic heterogeneity—if it indeed is the ATD gene! The ATDC gene localizes to the same region as the second peak of location scores shown in Figure 10.2. It was localized independently by polymerase chain reaction (PCR) experiments using DNA from radiation hybrid cells as templates, and primers from the partially-sequenced ATDC gene. Unfortunately, as of this writing, no significant mutations of the ATDC gene have been identified in three known group D patients (L. Kapp, personal communication).

Clearly, if the ATD gene has yet to be cloned, a full-scale linkage project to further localize the gene (similar to what has been done for ATA/ATC) will be necessary before definitive cloning studies can be initiated. Unfortunately, it will be very difficult to identify group D families for such a study. Complementational cloning, despite its extremely slow pace, may be the best approach to cloning the ATD gene, if it is indeed a different gene from ATA/ATC (see below).

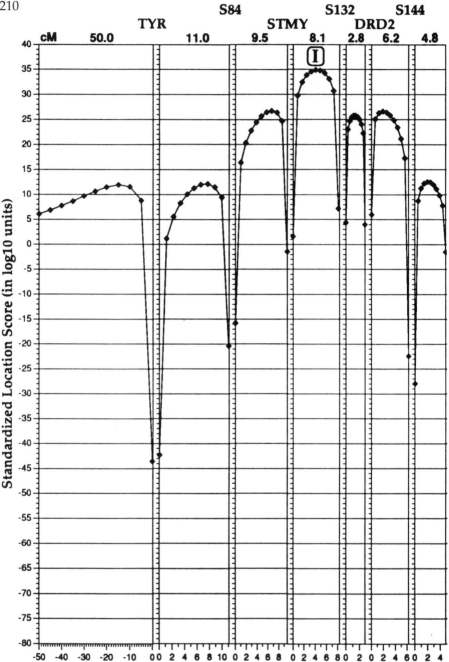

A   Position of AT Gene Relative to Marker Loci (in cM)

Figure 10.2A. Standardized location score estimates, derived by Monte Carlo likely interval'' (labelled I) for an A–T gene. Note second peak (II) between S147 and

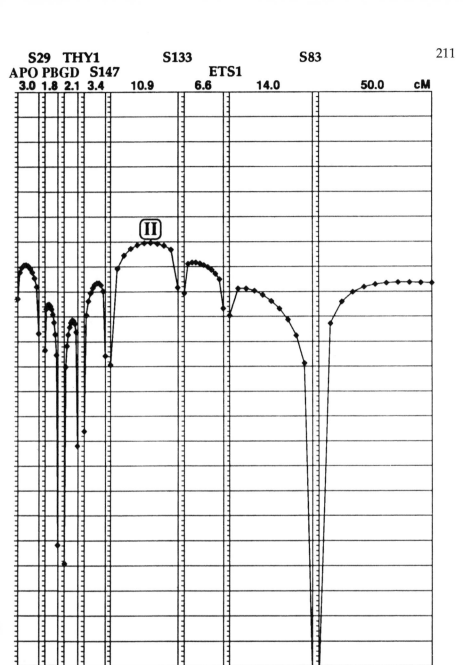

simulations and using 91 families, identify the STMY–S132 segment as the ''most
S133

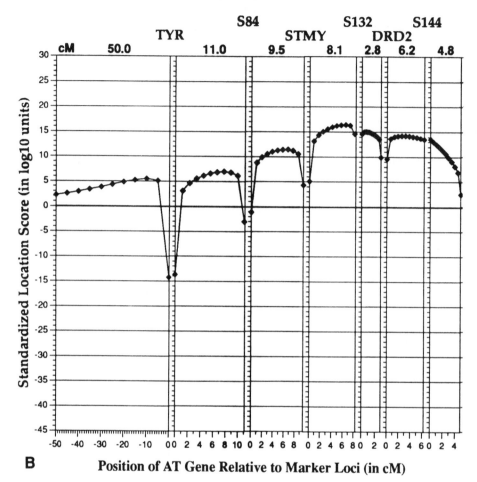

B   **Position of AT Gene Relative to Marker Loci (in cM)**

(B) (above and opposite) Standardized location score estimates, using only 14 A–T families known to be either complementation group A or group C. Note complete disappearance of second peak. Reprinted from Sobel and Lange (56), by permission of University of Chicago Press

ISOLATING THE AT GENE(S)

Returning to the ATA/ATC region, a region that should contain the gene(s) for approximately 83% of A–T families worldwide (22), present efforts are aimed at: (a) improving the fine map of the region flanked by STMY and DRD2 by developing new polymorphic markers within that region; (b) producing libraries of small segments of 11q22–23, such as from YAC clones localized to the region by pertinent probes, and mRNA (and thereby cDNA) enriched for the ATA/ATC gene(s) by various strategies;

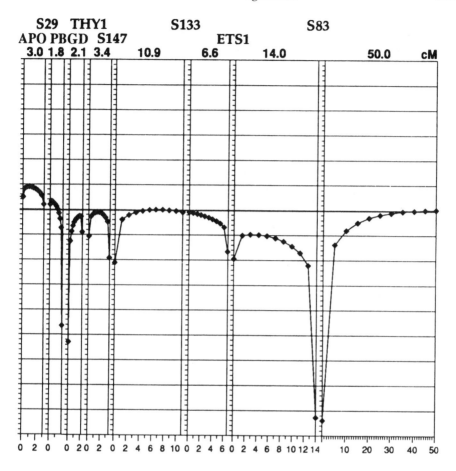

and (c) continuing linkage studies on A–T families known to have informative recombinants. New A–T families are now quickly screened for potentially informative recombinants by using a combination of multiplexed restriction fragment length polymorphisms (RFLPs) and (CA)n repeat microsatellite markers.

The fine map of the ATA/ATC region can be arbitrarily divided into five subregions defined by six markers: STMY, CJ193(S384), CRYA2 (M. James, personal communication), CJ77(S424), S132, and DRD2 (Figure 10.3). Although the Monte Carlo simulations convincingly localize an A–T gene between STMY and S132, data simulations on some subsets of families, e.g. the Turkish subset, show a possible third peak just distal to the peak observed when only group A families are analyzed (Figure 10.4) (62). However, these data, by themselves, are not of statistical significance. When recombinant haplotype from individual families are examined, all data are consistent with localizing a single A–T gene between STMY and CJ 77 (i.e. markers 4 and 5 in Figure 10.5).

As an adjunct to linkage mapping, pulsed field gel electrophoresis (PFGE) has yielded important new relationships. In comparison to Southern blots, PFGE blots contain DNA fragments that are about 50-fold larger because the DNA is digested with rare-cutter enzymes. In this technique, anchor probes, i.e. those known to localize within the pertinent regions, are first hybridized to the PFGE blots; the blots are then stripped and a second less well-localized probe is hybridized to the same blot. When two probes detect the same sized fragment, they are presumed to lie within that fragment's length of one another, e.g. a 200 kb fragment that is visualized by two probes would place those probes within 200 kb of one another, possibly closer but not farther away from one another. Such putative relationships are confirmed by testing the same probes again on fragments created by digesting

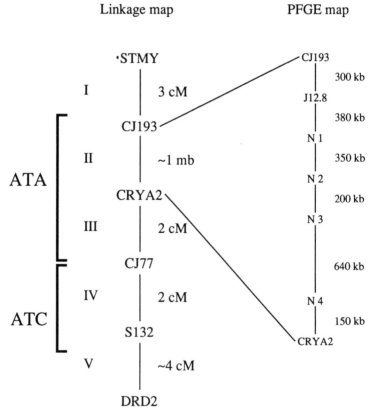

Figure 10.3. Linkage map (left) and pulsed field gel electrophoresis map (right) of ATA/ATC subregions

DNA with other rare-cutter restriction enzymes. The probes we are presently using derive from many collaborating laboratories, including those of P. Concannon, Y. Nakamura, T. Shows, C. Julier, and M. Taylor, as well as from our own experiments. In addition, probes for genes that are reported to localize to 11q22–23 are also tested.

In this way, Uhrhammer *et al.* (63) have so far screened about 50 probes, using more than 40 PFGE blots made with different restriction enzymes. Recently, we were successful in overlapping a set of eight probes that span the region from CJ77 to CRYA2 (Figure 10.3). The sizes of the overlapping fragments total about 2 megabases (Mb). Considering that each common fragment represents only the maximum possible distance between two probes, the actual size of the contiguous segment could be considerably smaller than 2 Mb. Most exciting about establishing a region of contiguous fragments, i.e. a new "contig" region, is that it definitively establishes the order of those probes with respect to one another and allows these probes to be used to recover much larger yeast artificial chromosomes (YAC) clones, thereby recovering all of the DNA within region II. This represents a significant step toward isolating the ATA gene. YAC contig maps of the ATA/ATC region are also being prepared in the laboratories of M. James and M. Taylor (personal communication).

Another approach to further localizing the A–T genes is to develop new polymorphic markers at appropriate places within the map so that these can be tested on A–T families known from previous work to contain informative recombinants. Almost all of the early location scores were generated with biallelic RFLP markers. The most efficient biallelic markers are only informative in one-third of families. Thus, many families were previously studied with markers that did not yield any additional information, greatly slowing progress. Unfortunately, until now, none of the highly polymorphic variable number tandem repeat (VNTR)-type markers has been localized to the A–T region.

Recently, with the discovery of short tandem repeat (STR) sequence polymorphisms (64, 65), linkage analysis has become much more efficient. These markers detect genomic regions containing CA repeats, for example, CACACACACA . . . For reasons unknown, such STRs are not genetically stable and generate multiple new alleles that are composed of differing numbers of repeats of the STR. Most individuals will have two different alleles. This allows the segregation of paternal and maternal haplotypes to be followed. The technology is also simpler and faster than Southern blotting in that (a) less DNA is needed from each family member, because the DNA is amplified by PCR within a few hours, and (b) the annealed DNA strands of differing sizes can be detected without radioisotopes, drying gels, or autoradiograms (66, 67). The PCR product is electrophoresed in a polyacrylamide gel of appropriate concentration to detect 2 bp increments in

216

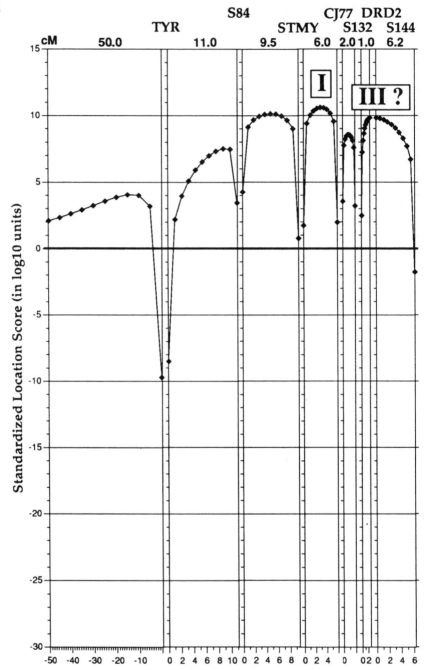

Figure 10.4. Standardized location score estimates, derived by Monte Carlo simula-
perhaps representing group C. Reprinted from Sanal *et al.* (62) by permission of

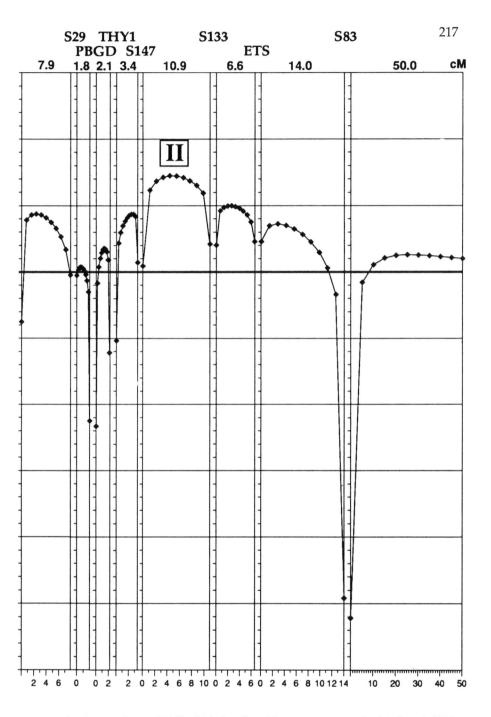

tions and using a subset of 14 Turkish families. Note suggestion of a third peak (III?),
FASCB Journal

218

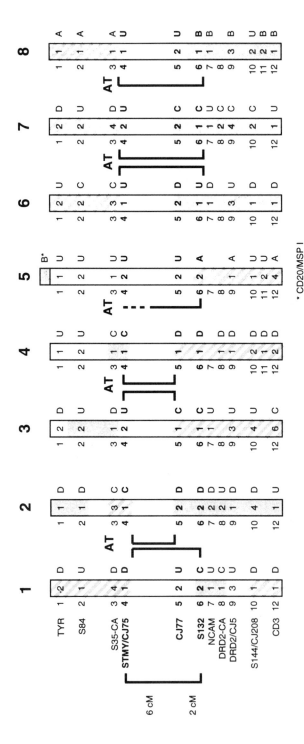

* CD20/MSP I

Figure 10.5. Composite of some informative recombinant haplotypes. The shaded areas contain the A–T gene. Hatched areas represent the other parental chromosome. White areas remain uncommitted. U = Uninformative with regard to segregation of parental haplotypes (A or B; C or D). These data are consistent with the localization of a single A–T gene between markers 4 and 5

fragment sizes that are dictated by the length of the repeat, ranging from 50 bp to 200 bp. Ethidium bromide is used to visualize the double-stranded DNA fragments; a photograph of the gel becomes the permanent record. By mixing DNAs from selected heterozygotes, a control "ladder of alleles" can be established and included as a reference standard in each experiment (Figure 10.6). Several laboratories, including our own, are presently developing new STR markers within the ATA/ATC region.

VARIANTS

Although early genetic studies emphasized the uniformity of the A–T syndrome, variants do exist (25, 68–85). It is presently unclear how to interpret these from a genetic perspective. A 1977 report by Hecht *et al.* (68) described this variability as "genetic heterogeneity". Do variants represent other A–T genes, or other genes? Most of the answers to such questions will come with the isolation of the ATA, ATC and ATD genes, comparing these sequences to the DNA of variants. No doubt compound heteriozygotes will also be identified.

Meanwhile, A–T variants can be categorized in several ways, including both clinical and laboratory variations. Some of the variable clinical parameters are listed in Table 10.1. To those, some laboratory variations can be added (Table 10.2).

Occasional A–T patients do not manifest well-defined telangiectasia (74–78). Conversely, at least three families have been identified in whom some members have classical A–T while others have only severe telangiectasia,

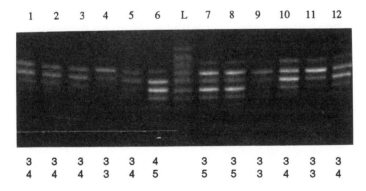

Figure 10.6. Polyacrylamide gel (8%) showing ethidium bromide-stained double-stranded 78–88 bp PCR fragments of the polymorphic DRD2 marker for 12 individuals. By using an "allelic ladder" as the standard (lane L), all alleles are easily recognized (indicated below gel). Lightly staining bands are thought to represent heterodimers (above) or dimers of incorrectly copied "ghost" fragments (below). Photo courtesy of J. Novik

Table 10.1   Clinical variations of A–T

Age of onset of ataxia
Presence or absence of telangiectasia
Presence or absence of immunodeficiency
Severity of immunodeficiency
Associations with other disorders:
   Diabetes
   Cardiac anomalies
   Endocrine defects
   Gastric cancer
   Epilepsy
   Nystagmus
   Clubbing

Table 10.2   Laboratory variations of A–T

Serum alfafetoprotein—abnormal in >95%
Radioresistant DNA synthesis—abnormal in >95%
Chromosomal aberrations—abnormal in >75%
Cell survival after *in vitro* irradiation
Cell survival after *in vitro* exposure to radiomimetic agents

without ataxia (unpublished data). Further, the relationships between the other radiosensitivity syndromes and A–T must eventually be clarified. Are the A–T genes involved in other DNA repair or chromosomal instability syndromes? Some patients have been described with classical clinical features of A–T but with little or no increased radiosensitivity, as measured by either radioresistant DNA synthesis (RDS) or colony survival. This presents a serious issue with regard to complementation grouping since such patients can never be assigned to a complementation group. Perhaps these are the "experiments of nature" that will help us recognize other genes in a more extensive "A–T gene family". But they probably will not account for more than 5% of A–T patients. It seems conservative at the time of writing to estimate that > 95% of "A–T patients" will link their A–T genes to the 11q22–23 region. We also have some preliminary data that suggest a linkage of NBS to 11q22–23 region markers, although the latter syndrome is not as well defined as the A–T syndrome and is more difficult to study.

   Table 10.3 attempts to summarize some of these issues. Generally speaking, four generic categories could be operationally used to classify A–T patients and variants: (a) classical A–T patients, with the minimal criteria of (i) familial, (ii) progressive, early-onset cerebellar ataxia, (iii) radiosensitivity, and (iv) ocular apraxia; (b) patients in complementation group V1 (for reasons discussed above), and others, with radiosensitivity and progres-

Table 10.3 Ataxia–telengiectasia syndromes

	A	T	Radio-sens.	Familial	Chrom. aberr.	AFP	Apraxia	CA	Immune defect	MR	Micro-ceph.	Ref.
Classic A–T												
Generic	+	(+)	+	+	(+)	(+)	(+)	(+)	(+)	−	−	
"A–T variants"												
Generic	(+)	(+)	+	+	+	(+)	(+)	(+)	(+)	+	+	
Curry (V1)	+	+	+	+	+	+	+	−	−	+	+	26
Nijmegen (V1)	−	−	+	+	+	−	−	−	+	+	+	23
Seemanova #7 (V1)	−	−	?	+	+	?	−	−	−	−	+	79
Junker	+	(+)	?	+	(−)	+	+	+	−	−	−	80
Byrne	+	−	?	+	(−)	−	+	+	+	+	?	76
Fiorilli #6	+	−	?	−	+	+	+	?	−	+	?	81
"A–T-like disorders"												
Generic	+	(+)	−	+	−	−	(+)	−	−	(+)	−	
Other radiation hypersensitivity/chromosome breakage syndromes[b]												
Generic	−	−	+	+	+	−	−	(+)	(+)	(+)	+	
Conley (V2)[a]	−	−	+	−	+	−	?	−	+	+	+	82
Wegner (V2)	−	−	+	+	+	−	−	−	+	+	+	83
Seemanova #5	−	−	?	+	?	?	−	+	−	−	+	79

[a]Letter in parentheses denotes A–T complementation group assignment.
[b]Despite the absence of ataxia or telangiectasia, these could also become "A–T variants" if an A–T complementation group assignment were made.
(+), usually positive.
(−), usually negative.

sive cerebellar ataxia that could eventually be tested for complementation of one of the five A–T groups; (c) patients with ataxia who do not manifest radiosensitivity, for whom it will be very difficult to establish whether they are A–T mutations or mutations in other genes until the A–T genes have been isolated, and (d) patients with other radiosensitivity syndromes, without ataxia or telangiectasia. It will be interesting to learn eventually whether any of the latter patients are also A–T mutants.

A–T HETEROZYGOTES

The incidence of A–T heterozygotes in the general population has been estimated between 0.07% and 7% (86). As a rule of thumb, most investigators use 1% as a working model (7).

Many attempts have been made to identify A–T heterozygotes ("het id") since this is important in (a) genetic counselling of A–T families, (b) assessing potential risk for sequelae to radiotherapy, and (c) assessing cancer susceptibility. The unreliability of all "het id" assays has been reviewed at each of the five international A–T workshops (87–91). Paterson *et al.* provided a good overview of "het id" testing in 1985 (88). Paterson was selected for this task because his assay of chronic low-dose gamma radiation was considered the most reliable at that time. A subsequent large study allowed his results to be compared to the actual genotyping for a defective A–T gene in a group A family of 61 members (the same Amish–Mennonite family used in the linkage analyses). The conclusions drawn from this study were that whereas populations of heterozygotes can be clearly distinguished from populations of normals or affecteds, assignments of A–T heterozygosity to individuals, based even on replicate testing by this method, was only accurate in 80–90% of the cases (92). This most likely reflects either the influence of other non-A–T genes on the outcome of these assays or, the need to synchronize cell growth during the assay.

Another assay that has received considerable attention is that described by Parshad *et al.* (93). This assay is based on the chromosomal radiosensitivity of cells during G2 of the cell cycle. Although the assay appeared to distinguish A–T heterozygotes from normals in earlier trials, abnormal results were also described for patients carrying other defective genes such as retinoblastoma, Fanconi anemia, Bloom's syndrome and xeroderma pigmentosum (94). Recently, Scott *et al.* have attempted to use a modified version of the Parshad and Sanford assay to identify A–T heterozygotes, after unsuccessful efforts to repeat the earlier work; they may now be approaching a reliable G2 radiosensitivity assay (95).

The issue of breast cancer risk in A–T heterozygotes has recently received much attention. From epidemiological studies of American families, Swift *et al.* (96) estimate a fivefold increased risk of breast cancer in female A–T heterozygotes. Some argue that because A–T heterozygotes are also more sensitive to ionizing radiation than normals, and such exposure may be expected to increase cancer risk, they should not receive mammograms, relying instead on careful physical examinations. Others retort that the increased sensitivity to radiation is so minimal that it would only increase the incidence of breast CA from 10 000/100 000 to 10 001/100 000 (97). Thus, it is presently recommended that female A–T heterozygotes follow the normal guidelines for mammography examinations. On the other hand, some newer mammography equipment is more efficient than older equipment, reducing exposure rates to half that of older machines. While this difference may be of little importance to the general population, it may be important for A–T heterozygotes. It has been estimated that as many as one in every six women with breast cancer in the USA may be an A–T heterozygote (96).

SUMMARY

How defects in a single gene can lead to such seemingly unrelated biological phenomena as Purkinje cell degeneration, thymic dystrophy, chromosomal instability, radiosensitivity, and telangiectasia, will most likely remain a mystery until the A–T gene(s) is cloned and characterized. How many A–T genes exist also remains unknown at the time of writing. While the complementation groups suggest five genetic defects, these defects need not involve five distinct genes. Linkage studies of > 150 families fail to provide convincing evidence for more than one A–T gene.

Linkage analysis clearly localizes the ATA gene to a 3 cM region of chromosome 11q22–23. A presumptive ATC gene also links to this region. A presumptive ATD gene localizes 30 cM distal to the ATA/ATC gene(s), but still within the 11q22–23 region. A candidate ATD gene (ATDC) has been isolated by Kapp *et al.*; independently it has been mapped to the same region as that indicated by linkage analyses. Despite this, at least two caveats challenge the existence of an ATD gene: (a) no mutations of the ATDC gene have been found in three group D A–T patients, at the time of writing; and (b) formal tests for genetic heterogeneity are not statistically significant.

Several laboratories have established YAC contigs of the ATA/ATC region and are attempting positional cloning. Other laboratories are attempting to use transfection/complementation experiments to isolate the A–T gene(s).

A–T variants exist but have been excluded from linkage analyses. While A–T patients are extremely cancer prone, A–T heterozygotes are also at an increased risk of cancer, especially breast cancer, and manifest an intermediate level of radiosensitivity. The A–T carrier frequency may be as high as 1 per 100 in the general population, thereby constituting a significant public health problem. A reliable carrier identification assay is not yet available.

ACKNOWLEDGEMENTS

This research was supported by the US Department of Energy, the A–T Medical Research Foundation, and the Thomas Appeal A–T Medical Research Trust.

REFERENCES

1. Gatti, R.A. and Vinters, H.V. (1985) Cerebellar pathology in ataxia–telangiectasia: The significance of basket cells. In Gatti, R.A. and Swift, M. (eds) *Ataxia–Telangiectasia: Genetics, Neuropathology, and Immunology of a Degenerative Disease of Childhood.* Liss, New York, pp. 225–232.
2. Vinters, H.V., Gatti, R.A. and Rakic, P. (1985) Sequence of cellular events in cerebellar ontogeny relevant to expression of neuronal abnormalities in ataxia–telangiectasia. In Gatti, R.A. and Swift, M. (eds) *Ataxia–Telangiectasia: Genetics, Neuropathology, and Immunology of a Degenerative Disease of Childhood.* Liss, New York, pp. 233–255.
3. Morrell, D., Cromartie, E. and Swift, M. (1986) Mortality and cancer incidence in 263 patients with ataxia–telangiectasia. *J. Nat. Cancer Inst.,* **77**, 89–92.
4. Boder, E. and Sedgwick, R.P. (1958) Ataxia–telangiectasia: A familial syndrome of progressive cerebellar ataxia, oculocutaneous telangiectasia and frequent pulmonary infection. *Pediatrics,* **21**, 526–554.
5. Boder, E. and Sedgwick, R.P. (1963) Ataxia–telangiectasia: A review of 101 cases. In Walsh, G. (ed.) *Little Club Clinics in Developmental Medicine,* No. 8. Heinemann, London, pp. 110–118.
6. Boder, E. (1985) Ataxia–telangiectasia: An overview. In Gatti, R.A. and Swift, M. (eds) *Ataxia–Telangiectasia: Genetics, Neuropathology, and Immunology of a Degenerative Disease of Childhood.* Liss, New York, pp. 1–63.
7. Gatti, R.A., Boder, E., Vinters, H.V., Sparkes, R.S., Norman, A. and Lange, K. (1991) Ataxia–telangiectasia: An interdisciplinary approach to pathogenesis. *Medicine,* **70**, 99–117.
8. Sedgwick, R.P. and Boder, E. (1991) Ataxia–telangiectasia: In de Jong, J.M.B.V. (ed.) *Handbook of Clinical Neurology Vol. 16: Hereditary Neuropathies and Spinocerebellar Atrophies.* Elsevier, Amsterdam, pp. 347–423.
9. Gatti, R.A. and Hall, K. (1983) Ataxia–telangiectasia: Search for a central hypothesis. In German, J. (ed.) *Chromosome Mutation and Neoplasia.* Liss, New York, pp. 23–41.
10. Gatti, R.A. (1991) Speculations on the ataxia–telangiectasia defect. *Clin. Immunol. Immunopathol.,* **61**, S10–S15.
11. Waldmann, T.A., Misiti, J., Nelson, D.L. and Kraemer, K.H. (1983) Ataxia–telangiectasia: A multisystem hereditary disease with immunodeficiency, impaired organ maturation, X-ray hypersensitivity, and a high incidence of neoplasia. Clinical Conference. *Ann. Intern. Med.,* **99**, 367–379.
12. Thieffry, S., Arthuis, M., Aicardi, J. and Lyon, G. (1961) L'ataxie-telangiectasie. *Rev. Neurol.,* **105**, 390–405.
13. Hecht, F., Koler, R.D., Rigas, D.A., Dahnke, G.S., Case, M.P., Tisdale, V. and Miller, R.W. (1966) Leukaemia and lymphocytes in ataxia–telangiectasia. *Lancet,* **ii**, 1193.
14. Gatti, R.A. and Good, R.A. (1971) Occurrence of malignancy in immunodeficiency diseases. *Cancer,* **28**, 89–98.
15. Waldmann, T.A. and McIntire, K.R. (1972) Serum alpha-fetoprotein levels in patients with ataxia–telangiectasia. *Lancet,* **ii**, 112–115.

16. Gotoff, S.P., Amirmokri, E. and Liebner, E.J. (1967) Ataxia telangiectasia: Neoplasia, untoward response to x-irradiation, and tuberous sclerosis. *Am. J. Dis. Child.*, **114**, 617–625.

17. Taylor, A.M.R., Harnden, D.G., Arlett, C.F., Harcourt, S.A., Lehmann, A.R., Stevens, S. and Bridges, B.A. (1975) Ataxia–telangiectasia: A human mutation with abnormal radiation sensitivity. *Nature*, **258**, 427–429.

18. Cox, R., Hosking, G.P. and Wilson, J. (1978) Ataxia–telangiectasia: Evaluation of radiosensitivity in cultured fibroblasts as a diagnostic test. *Arch. Dis. Child.*, **53**, 386–390.

19. Chen, P.C., Lavin, M.F., Kidson, C. and Moss, D. (1978) Identification of ataxia–telangiectasia heterozygotes: A cancer prone population. *Nature*, **274**, 484–486.

20. Murnane, J.P. and Painter, R.B. (1982) Complementation of the defects in DNA synthesis in irradiated and unirradiated ataxia–telangiectasia cells. *Proc. Nat. Acad. Sci. USA*, **79**, 1960–1963.

21. Jaspers, N.G.J. and Bootsma, D. (1982) Genetic heterogeneity in ataxia–telangiectasia studies by cell fusion. *Proc. Nat. Acad. Sci. USA*, **79**, 2641–2644.

22. Jaspers, N.G.J., Gatti, R.A., Baan, C., Linssen, P.C.M.L. and Bootsma, D. (1988) Genetic complementation analysis of ataxia telangiectasia and Nijmegen breakage syndrome: A survey of 50 patients. *Cytogenet. Cell Genet.*, **49**, 259–263.

23. Weemaes, C.M.R., Hustinx, T.W.J., Scheres, J.M.J.C., Van Munster, P.J.J., Bakkeren, J.A.J.M. and Taalman, R.D.F.M. (1981) A new chromosomal instability disorder: the Nijmegen breakage syndrome. *Acta Paediatr. Scand.*, **70**, 557–562.

24. Jaspers, N.G.J., Painter, R.B., Paterson, M.C., Kidson, C. and Inoue, T. (1985) Complementation analysis of ataxia–telangiectasia. In Gatti, R.A. and Swift, M. (eds) *Ataxia–Telangiectasia: Genetics, Neuropathology, and Immunology of a Degenerative Disease of Childhood.* Liss, New York, pp. 147–162.

25. Jaspers, N.G.J., Taalman, R.D.F.M. and Baan, C. (1988) Patients with an inherited syndrome characterized by immunodeficiency, microcephaly, and chromosomal instability: Genetic relation to ataxia–telangiectasia. *Am. J. Hum. Genet.*, **42**, 66–73.

26. Curry, C.J.R., O'Lague, P., Tsai, J., Hutchinson, H.T., Jaspers, N.G.J., Wara, D. and Gatti, R.A. (1989) AT$_{Fresno}$: A phenotype linking ataxia–telangiectasia with the Nijmegen breakage syndrome. *Amer. J. Hum. Genet.*, **45**, 270–275.

27. Rivat-Peran, L., Buriot, D., Salier, J.-P., Rivat, C., Dumitresco, S.-M. and Griscelli, C. (1981) Immunoglobulins in ataxia–telangiectasia: Evidence for IgG4 and IgA2 subclass deficiencies. *Clin. Immunol. Immunopathol.*, **20**, 99–110.

28. Oxelius, V.-A., Berkel, A.I. and Hanson, L.A. (1982) IgG2 deficiency in ataxia–telangiectasia. *N. Engl. J. Med.*, **306**, 515–520.

29. Gatti, R.A., Bick, M.B., Tam, C.F., Medici, M.A., Oxelius, V.-A., Holland, M., Goldstein, A.L. and Boder, E. (1982) Ataxia–telangiectasia: A multiparameter analysis of eight families. *Clin. Immunol. Immunopathol.*, **23**, 501–516.

30. Ammann, A.J., Cain, W.A., Ishizaka, K., Hong, R. and Good, R.A. (1969) Immunoglobulin E deficiency in ataxia–telangiectasia. *N. Engl. J. Med.*, **281**, 469–474.

31. Roifman, C.M. and Gelfand, E.W. (1985) Heterogeneity of the immunological deficiency in ataxia–telangiectasia: Absence of a clinical–pathological correlation. In Gatti, R.A. and Swift, M. (eds) *Ataxia–telangiectasia: Genetics, Neuropathology, and Immunology of a Degenerative Disease of Childhood.* Liss, New York, pp. 273–285.

32. Eisen, A.H., Karpati, G., Laszlo, T., Andermann, F., Robb, J.P. and Bacal, H.L. (1965) Immunologic deficiency in ataxia–telangiectasia. *N. Engl. J. Med.*, **272**, 18–24.

33. Trompeter, R.S., Layward, L. and Hayward, A.R. (1978) Primary and secondary abnormalities of T cell subpopulations. *Clin. Exp. Immunol.*, **34**, 388–392.
34. Gupta, S. and Good, R.A. (1978) Subpopulations of human T lymphocytes. V. T lymphocytes with receptors for immunoglobulin M or G in patients with primary immunodeficiency disorders. *Clin. Immunol. Immunopathol.*, **11**, 292–296.
35. Weaver, M. and Gatti, R.A. (1985) Lymphocyte subpopulations in ataxia-telangiectasia. In Gatti, R.A. and Swift, M. (eds) *Ataxia–Telangiectasia: Genetics, Neuropathology, and Immunology of a Degenerative Disease of Childhood*. Liss, New York, pp. 309–314.
36. Levis, W.R., Dattner, A.M. and Shaw, S. (1978) Selective defects in T cell function in ataxia–telangiectasia. *Clin. Exp. Immunol.*, **37**, 44–49.
37. Yarchoan, R., Kurman, C.C. and Nelson, D.L. (1985) Defective specific anti-influenza virus antibody production *in vitro* by lymphocytes from patients with ataxia–telangiectasia. In Gatti, R.A. and Swift, M. (eds) *Ataxia–Telangiectasia: Genetics, Neuropathology, and Immunology of a Degenerative Disease of Childhood*. Liss, New York, pp. 315–329.
38. Peter, H.H. (1983) The origin of human NK cells an ontogenic model derived from studies in patients with immunodeficiencies. *Blut*, **46**, 239–248.
39. McCaw, B.K., Hecht, F., Harnden, D.G. and Teplitz, R.L. (1975) Somatic rearrangement of chromosome 14 in human lymphocytes. *Proc. Nat. Acad. Sci. USA*, **72**, 2071–2075.
40. Kojis, T.L., Schreck, R.R., Gatti, R.A. and Sparkes, R.S. (1989) Tissue specificity of chromosomal rearrangements in ataxia–telangiectasia. *Hum. Genet.*, **83**, 347–352.
41. Concannon, P., Gatti, R.A. and Hood, L.E. (1987) Human T cell receptor V_β gene polymorphism. *J. Exp. Med.*, **165**, 1130–1140.
42. Gatti, R.A., Boehnke, M., Crist, M. and Sparkes, R.S. (1985) Genetic linkage studies in ataxia–telangiectasia. In Gatti, R.A. and Swift, M. (eds) *Ataxia–telangiectasia: Genetics, Neuropathology, and Immunology of a Degenerative Disease of Childhood*. Liss, New York, pp. 163–172.
43. Hodge, S.E., Berkel, A.I., Gatti, R.A., Boder, E. and Spence, M.A. (1980) Ataxia-telangiectasia and xeroderma pigmentosum: No evidence of linkage to HLA. *Tissue Antigens*, **15**, 313–317.
44. Ginter, D.N. and Tallapragada, R. (1978) Ataxia–telangiectasia. In McKusick, V. (ed.) *Medical Genetic Studies of the Amish*. Johns Hopkins University Press, Baltimore, pp. 144–145.
45. Gatti, R.A., Berkel, I., Boder, E., Braedt, G., Charmley, P., Concannon, P., Ersoy, F., Foroud, T., Jaspers, N.G.J., Lange, K., Lathrop, G.M., Leppert, M., Nakamura, Y., O'Connell, P., Paterson, M., Salser, W., Sanal, O., Silver, J., Sparkes, R.S., Susi, E., Weeks, D.E., Wei, S., White, R. and Yoder, F. (1988) Localization of an ataxia-telangiectasia gene to chromosome 11q22–23. *Nature*, **336**, 577–580.
46. Gatti, R.A., Shaked, R., Wei, S., Koyama, M., Salser, W. and Silver, J. (1988) DNA polymorphism in the human THY-1 gene. *Hum. Immunol.*, **22**, 145–150.
47. Charmley, P., Foroud, T., Wei, S., Malhotra, U., Concannon, P., Weeks, D.E., Lange, D. and Gatti, R.A. (1990) A primary linkage map of the human chromosome 11q22–23 region. *Genomics*, **6**, 316–323.
48. Julier, C., Nakamura, Y., Lathrop, M., O'Connell, P., Leppert, M., Litt, M., Mohandas, T., Lalouel, J.-M. and White, R. (1990) Detailed map of the long arm of chromosome 11. *Genomics*, **7**, 335–345.
49. Dausset, J., Cann, H., Cohen, D., Lathrop, M., Lalouel, J.-M. and White, R. (1990) Centre d'Etude du Polymorphisme Humain (CEPH): Collaborative genetic mapping of the human genome. *Genomics*, **6**, 575–577.

50. Maslen, C.L., Jones, C., Glaser, T., Magenis, R.E., Sheehy, R., Kellogg, J. and Litt, M. (1988) Seven polymorphic loci mapping to human chromosomal region 11q22–qter. *Genomics,* **2**, 66–75.
51. Budarf, M., Sellinger, B., Griffin, C. and Emanuel, B.S. (1989) Comparative mapping of the constitutional and tumor-associated 11;22 translocations. *Am. J. Hum. Genet.,* **45**, 128–139.
52. Sanal, O., Wei, S., Foroud, T., Malhotra, U., Concannon, P., Charmley, P., Salser, W., Lange, K. and Gatti, R.A. (1990) Further mapping of an ataxia–telangiectasia locus to the chromosome 11q23 region. *Am. J. Hum. Genet.,* **47**, 860–868.
53. McConville, C., Woods, C.G., Farrall, M., Metcalfe, J.A. and Taylor, A.M.R. (1990) Analysis of 7 polymorphic markers at chromosome 11q22–23 in 35 ataxia telangiectasia families: Further evidence of linkage. *Hum. Genet.,* **85**, 215–220.
54. McConville, C.M., Formstone, C.J., Hernandez, D., Thick, J. and Taylor, A.M.R. (1990) Fine mapping of the chromosome 11q22–23 region using PFGE, linkage and haplotype analysis: Localization of the gene for ataxia telangiectasia to a 5 cM region flanked by NCAM/DRD2 and STMY/CJ52.75, ph2.22. *Nucl. Acids Res.,* **18**, 4334–4343.
55. Ziv, Y., Rotman, G., Frydman, M., Dagan, J., Cohen, T., Foroud, T., Gatti, R.A. and Shiloh, Y. (1991) The ATC (ataxia–telangiectasia Group C) locus localizes to chromosome 11q22–q23. *Genomics,* **9**, 373–375.
56. Lange, K. and Sobel, E. (1991) A random walk method for computing genetic location scores. *Amer. J. Hum. Genet.,* **49**, 1320–1334.
57. Foroud, T., Wei, S., Ziv, Y., Sobel, E., Lange, E., Chao, A., Goradia, T., Huo, Y., Tolun, A., Chessa, L., Charmley, P., Sanal, O., Salman, N., Julier, C., Lathrop, G.M., Concannon, P., McConville, C., Taylor, M., Shiloh, Y., Lange, K. and Gatti, R.A. (1991) Localization of an ataxia–telangiectasia locus to a 4 cM interval on chromosome 11q23 by linkage analyses of an international consortium of 111 families. *Am. J. Hum. Genet.,* **49**, 1263–1279.
58. Sobel, E., Lange, E., Jaspers, N.G.J., Chessa, L., Sanal, O., Shiloh, Y., Taylor, A.M.R., Weemaes, C.M.A., Lange, K. and Gatti, R.A. (1992) Ataxia–telangiectasia: Linkage evidence for genetic heterogeneity. *Am. J. Hum. Genet.,* **50**, 1343–1348.
59. Charmley, P., Nguyen, J., Wei, S. and Gatti, R.A. (1991) Genetic linkage analysis and homology of syntenic relationships of genes located on human chromosome 11q. *Genomics,* **10**, 608–617.
60. Kapp, L.N. and Painter, R.B. (1989) Stable radioresistance in ataxia–telangiectasia cells containing DNA from normal human cells. *Int. J. Radiat. Biol.,* **56**, 667–675.
61. Kapp, L.N., Painter, R.B., Yu, L.-C., van Loon, N., Richard, C.W., James, M.R., Cox, D.R. and Murnane, J.P. (1992) Cloning of a candidate gene for ataxia–telangiectasia group D. *Am. J. Hum. Genet.,* **51**, 45–54.
62. Sanal, O., Lange, E., Telatar, M., Sobel, E., Salazar-Novak, J., Ersoy, F., Concannon, P., Tolun, A. and Gatti, R.A. (1992) Ataxia–telangiectasia-linkage analysis of chromosome 11q22–23 markers in Turkish families. *FASEB J.,* **6**, 2848–2852.
63. Uhrhammer, N., Huo, Y. and Gatti, R.A. (in preparation) A contiguous DNA segment at 11q22–23 defined by pulsed field gel electropheresis.
64. Weber, J.L. and May, P.E. (1989) Abundant class of human DNA polymorphisms which can be typed using the polymerase chain reaction. *Am. J. Hum. Genet.,* **44**, 388–396.
65. Edwards, A., Civitello, A., Hammond, H.A. and Caskey, C.T. (1991) DNA typing and genetic mapping with trimeric and tetrameric tandem repeats. *Am. J. Hum. Genet.,* **49**, 746–756.

66. Oudet, C., Heilig, R., Hanauer, A. and Mandel, J.-L. (1991) Nonradioactive assay for new microsatellite polymorphisms at the 5' end of the dystrophin gene, and estimation of intragenic recombination. *Am. J. Hum. Genet.*, **49**, 311–319.
67. Telatar, M., Salazar-Novik, J., Gatti, R.A. and Tolun, A. (submitted) Non-radioactive analysis of (CA)n repeat sequence length polymorphisms. *BioRad. J.*
68. Hecht, F. and McCaw, B.K. (1977) Chromosome instability syndromes. In Mulvihill, J.J., Miller, R.W. and Fraumeni, J.F. (eds) *Genetics of Human Cancer.* Raven Press, New York, pp. 105–123.
69. Taylor, A.M.R., Flude, E., Laher, B., Stacer, M., McKay, E., Watt, J., Green, S.H. and Harding, A.E. (1987) Variant forms of ataxia–telangiectasia. *J. Med. Genet.*, **24**, 669–677.
70. Chessa, L., Fiorilli, M. and Bastianon, V. (1993) Cardiac anomalies in ataxia–telangiectasia. In Gatti, R.A. and Painter, R.B. (eds) *Fifth International Workshop on Ataxia–Telangiectasia.* Springer-Verlag, Heidelberg.
71. Porras, O., Arguedas, O., Gonzalez, L. and Saenz, E. (1993) Epidemiology of ataxia–telangiectasia in Costa Rica. In Gatti, R.A. and Painter, R.B. (eds) *Fifth International Workshop on Ataxia–Telangiectasia.* Springer-Verlag, Heidelberg, pp. xxx–xxx.
72. Sanal, O., Ersoy, F. and Berkel, I. (1993) Epidemiology of ataxia–telangiectasia in Turkey. In Gatti, R.A. and Painter, R.B. (eds) *Fifth International Workshop on Ataxia–Telangiectasia.* Springer-Verlag, Heidelberg.
73. Taylor, A.M.R. and Woods, G. (1993) Variant forms of ataxia–telangiectasia. In Gatti, R.A. and Painter, R.B. (eds) *Fifth International Workshop on Ataxia–Telangiectasia.* Springer-Verlag, Heidelberg.
74. Willems, P.J., van Roy, B.C., Kleijer, W.J. van der Kraan, M., Leroy, J.G. and Martin, J.-J. (1992) Atypical clinical presentation of ataxia–telangiectasia. *J. Med. Genet.*, **31**.
75. Ying, K.L. and Decoteau, W.E. (1981) Cytogenetic anomalies in a patient with ataxia, immune deficiency and high alpha-fetoprotein in the absence of telangiectasia. *Cancer Genet. Cytogenet.*, **4**, 311–317.
76. Byrne, E., Hallpike, J.F., Manson, J.I., Sutherland, G.R. and Thong, Y.H. (1984) Progressive multisystem degeneration with IgE deficiency and chromosomal instability. *J. Neurol. Sci.*, **66**, 307–317.
77. Maserati, E., Ottoline, A., Veggiatti, P., Lanzi, G. and Pasquali, F. (1988) Ataxia without telangiectasia in two sisters with rearrangements of chromosomes 7 and 14. *Clin. Genet.*, **34**, 283–287.
78. Aicardi, J., Barbosas, C., Andermann, E., Andermann, F., Morcos, R., Ghanem, Q., Fukuyama, Y., Awaya, Y. and Moe, P. (1988) Ataxia–ocular motor apraxia: A syndrome mimicking ataxia–telangiectasia. *Ann. Neurol.*, **24**, 497–502.
79. Seemanova, E., Passarge, E., Beneskova, D., Houstek, J., Kasal, P. and Sevcikova, M. (1985) Familial microcephal with normal intelligence, immunodeficiency, and risk for lymphoreticular malignancies: A new autosomal recessive disorder. *Am. J. Med. Genet.*, **20**, 639–648.
80. Junker, A., Teasdale, J.M. and Dunn, H.G. Personal communication.
81. Fiorilli, M., Businco, L., Pandolfi, F., Paganelli, R., Russo, G. and Aiuti, F. (1983) Heterogeneity of immunological abnormalities in ataxia–telangiectasia. *J. Clin. Immunol.*, **3**, 135–141.
82. Conley, M.E., Spinner, M.B., Emanuel, B.S., Nowell, P.C. and Nichols, W.W. (1986) A chromosome breakage syndrome with profound immunodeficiency. *Blood*, **67**, 1251–1256.

83. Wegner, R.D., Metzger, M., Hanefield, N.G., Jaspers, J., Baan, C., Magdorf, K., Kunze, J. and Sperling, K. (1988) A new chromosomal instability disorder confirmed by complementation studies. *Clin. Genet.*, **33**, 20–32.
84. Ziv, Y., Amiel, A., Jaspers, N.G.J., Berkel, A.I. and Shiloh, Y. (1989) Ataxia-telangiectasia: A variant with altered *in vitro* phenotype of fibroblast cells. *Mutat. Res.*, **210**, 211–219.
85. Ziv, Y., Frydman, M., Lange, E., Zelnik, N., Rotman, G., Julier, C., Jaspers, N.G.J., Dagan, Y., Abeliovicz, D., Dar, H., Borochowitz, Z., Lanthrop, M., Gatti, R.A. and Shiloh, Y. (1992) Ataxia–telangiectasia: Linkage analysis in highly inbred Arab and Druze families and differentiation from an ataxia–microcephaly–cataract syndrome. *Hum. Genet.*, **88**, 619–626.
86. Swift, M., Morrell, D., Cromartie, E., Chamberlin, A.R., Skolnick, M.H. and Bishop, D.T. (1986) The incidence and gene frequency of ataxia–telangiectasia in the United States. *Am. J. Hum. Genet.*, **39**, 573–583.
87. Kidson, C., Chen, P. and Imray, P. (1982) Ataxia–telangiectasia heterozygotes: Dominant expression of ionizing radiation sensitive mutants. In Bridges, B.A. and Harnden, D.G. (eds) *Ataxia–Telangiectasia: A Cellular and Molecular Link Between Cancer, Neuropathology, and Immune Deficiency.* Wiley, Chichester, pp. 363–372.
88. Paterson, M.C., MacFarlane, S.J., Gentner, N.E. and Smith, B.P. (1985) Cellular hypersensitivity to chronic gamma-radiation in cultured fibroblasts from ataxia-telangiectasia heterosygotes. In Gatti, R.A. and Swift, M. (eds) *Ataxia–Telangiectasia: Genetics, Neuropathology, and Immunology of a Degenerative Disease of Childhood.* Liss, New York, pp. 73–87.
89. Lehmann, A., Jaspers, N.J.G. and Gatti, R.A. (1987) Ataxia–telangiectasia: Meeting report. *Cancer Res.*, **47**, 4750–4751.
90. Lehmann, A.R., Jaspers, N.G.J. and Gatti, R.A. (1989) Meeting report: Fourth international workshop on ataxia telangiectasia. *Cancer Res.*, **49**, 6162–6163.
91. Taylor, A.M.R., Jaspers, N.G.J. and Gatti, R.A. (submitted) Meeting report: Fifth international workshop on ataxia–telangiectasia. *Cancer Res.*
92. Weeks, D., Paterson, M.C., Lange, K., Andrais, B., Davis, R.C., Yoder, F. and Gatti, R.A. (1991) Assessment of chronic gamma radiosensitivity as an *in vitro* assay for heterozygote identification of ataxia–telangiectasia. *Radiation Res.*, **128**, 90–99.
93. Parshad, R., Sanford, K.K., Jones, G.M. and Tarone, R.E. (1985) G2 chromosomal radiosensitivity of ataxia–telangiectasia heterozygotes. *Cancer Genet. Cytogenet.*, **14**, 163–168.
94. Parshad, R., Sanford, K.K. and Jones, G.M. (1985) Chromosomal radiosensitivity during the G2 cell-cycle period of skin fibroblasts from individuals with familial cancer. *Proc. Nat. Acad. Sci. USA*, **82**, 5400–5403.
95. Scott, D., Jones, L.A., Elyan, S.A.G., Cowan, R. and Ribiero, G. (1993) The radiosensitivity of lymphocytes of A–T heterozygotes and breast cancer patients using cytogenetic and clonogenic assays. In Gatti, R.A. and Painter, R.B. (eds) *Fifth International Workshop on Ataxia–Telangiectasia.* Springer-Verlag, Heidelberg.
96. Swift, A., Morrell, D., Massey, R.B. and Chase, C.L. (1991) Incidence of cancer in 161 families affected by ataxia–telangiectasia. *N. Engl. J. Med.*, **325**, 1831–1836.
97. Withers, H.R. and McBride, W. (1993) Risk–benefit of mammography in A–T women. In Gatti, R.A. and Painter, R.B. (eds) *Fifth International Workshop on Ataxia–Telangiectasia.* Springer-Verlag, Heidelberg.

Chapter 11

Abnormalities of Signal Transduction and T Cell Immunodeficiency

ERWIN W. GELFAND

Division of Basic Sciences, Department of Pediatrics, National Jewish Center for
Immunology and Respiratory Medicine, Denver, Colorado, USA

T cell immunodeficiency encompasses a wide variety of disorders characterized by the failure to generate normal cell-mediated immune responses.
The disorders run the gamut from a complete absence of T cell function such
as may be seen in infants with severe combined immunodeficiency disease
(SCID) to selective defects in cell-mediated immunity, for example in purine
nucleoside phosphorylase deficiency. In addition to these congenital and
genetic disorders of T cell immunity, there is increasing recognition of forms
of acquired T cell immunodeficiency. Here too, the spectrum ranges from
partial to complete absence of T cell-mediated immunity. The most prevalent examples of the acquired disorders include AIDS, post-bone marrow
transplant T cell immunodeficiency, and the deficiencies accompanying
drug therapy such as corticosteroids and cytotoxic agents.

In addition to the designations "genetic" or "acquired", the disorders
may be classified as failures of differentiation, maturation or function. An
attempt at classification according to these criteria is illustrated in Figure
11.1. The assignments are both arbitrary and obviously incomplete but begin
to focus on the pathophysiology of the disorders. This approach may better
define the site of the defect than traditional classifications, as well as un-
masking new options for therapy. Further definition of specific defects affecting T cell function can reveal the importance of specific pathways for T
cell functional maturation in normal individuals. A more recent approach

New Concepts in Immunodeficiency Diseases. Edited by S. Gupta and C. Griscelli
© 1993 John Wiley & Sons Ltd

to the delineation of important signal transduction pathways is the use of "gene-knockout" experiments. These initial studies have confirmed some original biases but have also revealed many surprises.

T LYMPHOCYTE ACTIVATION AND SIGNAL TRANSDUCTION

Signal transduction refers to a series of complex processes in which the binding of ligand to specific receptors at the outer cell surface is perceived by the cell and the signal is transmitted to the nucleus. This is accomplished by an ordered sequence of ionic and biochemical events, and in the nucleus these signals initiate gene transcription and the display of genetically determined T cell differentiative functions.

In many cell types, including T cells, activation is associated with several morphological and metabolic changes. Activated cells increase their cellular volume, exhibit membrane ruffling, form pseudopods and begin to reorganize cytoskeletal proteins. Much attention has been devoted to the biochemical changes which accompany cell activation, especially the rapid increases in phosphatidyl inositol (PI) metabolism and free cytosolic calcium concentrations ($[Ca^{2+}]_i$), changes in cytosolic pH, and tyrosine/serine/threonine phosphorylation of a diverse array of cellular proteins. Many of these changes appear prerequisite for initiation of cell cycle progression and the general increase in protein, lipid and RNA synthesis. The exact relationship between the early metabolic events and the stages of cell cycle progression or acquisition of function in T cells remains unclear. Nevertheless, progression through the cell cycle is accomplished by the induction of increased mRNA levels for a variety of activation-related genes, and many of these genes encode the specific lymphokines and surface receptors necessary for expansion and functional differentiation of activated T cells.

UNIQUE FEATURES OF T CELL ACTIVATION

In many ways the activation of T cells is different from the activation of other cell types. Delineation of specific defects which result in T cell immunodeficiency requires recognition of these unique features if such defects are so restricted to one cell type. There are two possible explanations for emergence of a selective T cell deficiency: (a) only the T cells express a particular protein required for activation, e.g. p56^{lck}; or (b) all cells express the protein but only T cells are absolutely dependent on it, e.g. purine nucleoside phosphorylase.

One of the other distinguishing features of T cell activation is the dependence on cell–cell contact. Activation of T cells by antigen requires accessory or antigen-presenting cells (APC), capable of processing and presenting the appropriate peptide antigen complexed to a major histocompatibility complex (MHC) protein. The ligand for the T cell receptor (TCR) is such a

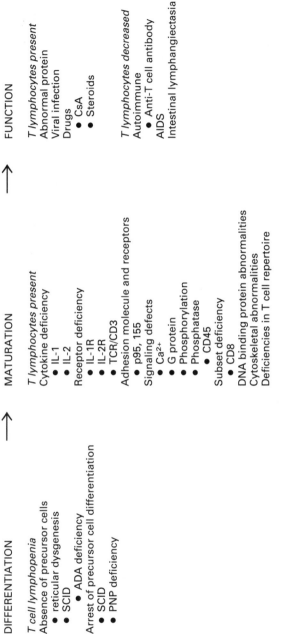

DIFFERENTIATION → MATURATION → FUNCTION

DIFFERENTIATION

T cell lymphopenia
Absence of precursor cells
• reticular dysgenesis
• SCID
  • ADA deficiency
Arrest of precursor cell differentiation
• SCID
• PNP deficiency

MATURATION

T lymphocytes present
Cytokine deficiency
• IL-1
• IL-2
Receptor deficiency
• IL-1R
• IL-2R
• TCR/CD3
Adhesion molecule and receptors
• p95, 155
Signaling defects
• Ca²⁺
• G protein
• Phosphorylation
• Phosphatase
  • CD45
Subset deficiency
  • CD8
DNA binding protein abnormalities
Cytoskeletal abnormalities
Deficiencies in T cell repertoire

FUNCTION

T lymphocytes present
Abnormal protein
Viral infection
Drugs
• CsA
• Steroids

T lymphocytes decreased
Autoimmune
• Anti-T cell antibody
AIDS
Intestinal lymphangiectasia

Figure 11.1. Classification of T cell immunodeficiency disorders

peptide/MHC complex presented by the APC. In the absence of functioning APC, T cells exposed to TCR ligands become unresponsive. In addition to presenting ligands, APC also synthesize important cytokines such as inter-leukin 1 (IL-1).

The key recognition and activation element in the T cell response to anti-gen is a complex receptor composed of: (a) four highly polymorphic sub-units, the α/β, γ/δ chains of the TCR; and (b) the CD3 complex consisting of five distinct invariant polypeptides (1, 2). The TCR and CD3 associate non-covalently to form a functional receptor complex. The α/β heterodimer mediates specific recognition of antigenic peptides complexed to MHC. The CD3 complex is recognized as the signaling moiety of the CD3–TCR com-plex with emphasis on the ζ chain, the only chain with a large cytoplasmic region, including in man seven tyrosine residues that are potential sub-strates for tyrosine protein kinases (TPK) as well as a consensus ATP-binding sequence (3, 4).

Ligand binding to CD3/TCR initiates T cell activation and the expression of activation antigens such as the IL-2 receptor (IL-2R) and IL-4 receptor (IL-4R) and the synthesis/secretion of IL-2 and IL-4. In addition to the CD3/TCR complex, there are other cell surface molecules which play a role in T cell activation. The CD4 and CD8 glycoproteins appear to stabilize and increase the avidity of the interaction between the peptide/MHC complex and CD3/TCR (5). CD4 and CD8 may also transduce an independent signal. The intracellular domains of both proteins are associated with the T cell-specific TPK, p56[lck] (6, 7). Ligation of CD2 can also transduce an indepen-dent signal, initiating T cell activation. The physiological ligand for CD2 is lymphocyte function-associated antigen-3 (LFA-3). CD2–LFA-3 interaction may be important between thymocytes and thymic epithelial cells or be-tween cytotoxic T lymphocytes (CTL) and their targets (8). There are numer-ous other auxiliary receptors on T cells which likely play some role in activation; these include CD28, LFA-1, the inositol-glycan-linked glycopro-teins (e.g. Thy-1, Ly-6), CD43 (sialophorin), and the cell surface tyrosine phosphatase, CD45, described below.

The most downstream events in T cell activation trace the action of the growth-promoting lymphokines IL-2 and IL-4 following binding to their specific receptors. The receptors for these lymphokines have been well char-acterized, but despite this knowledge little is known about the relevant signaling events initiated by binding to the lymphokine-specific receptors.

T CELL METABOLC CHANGES FOLLOWING ACTIVATION

T cell activation and proliferation is thus characterized by three distinct stages or events, each conceivably with its own set of activation signals, metabolic changes, and accessory molecules. Simply stated they are: (a) IL-2 (and IL-4) synthesis and secretion; (b) IL-2R (and IL-4R) expression; and (c) IL-2 (and IL-4)-dependent T cell proliferation.

Interleukin Synthesis and Secretion

The majority of studies have focused on IL-2 production and the metabolic and genetic events regulating induction of this lymphokine. It has been assumed that, to a large extent, IL-4 production is similarly regulated. As with most activation genes, transcriptional regulation accounts for most of the levels of gene expression (9). For IL-2 gene activation, a number of transcription factors respond to signals from the T cell antigen receptor. One of the major transcription factors which binds to the IL-2 enhancer is nuclear factor of activated T cells (NFAT) (10). This protein plays a key role in the inducible control of IL-2 transcription. Although expression of NFAT is somewhat restricted, it is not expressed exclusively in T cells. Other enhancers which are more ubiquitous include NF-κB, AP-1, and Oct-1 (9). If transcriptional regulation of IL-2 gene expression is affected by the enhancing proteins, what controls their expression or initiates their synthesis following CD3/TCR ligation? The prime candidate would be a phosphorylation reaction, a common modification thought to control a number of biologically important processes.

There are at least three consistent early responses to CD3/TCR stimulation (11, 12). The first is increased PI metabolism, hydrolysis resulting in Ca^{2+} mobilization from internal stores secondary to the liberation of inositol trisphosphate (IP3), and activation of protein kinase C (PKC), secondary to production of diacylglycerol. The second early response is the increased tyrosine phosphorylation of several proteins including the CD3 ζ chain. The third response is the major increase in $[Ca^{2+}]_i$ due to transmembrane uptake of Ca^{2+} through ligand-gated Ca^{2+} channels. This response has been linked to the initial two early responses but the data require substantiation.

Our data suggest that increases in IL-2 production and gene transcription are critically dependent on increases in $[Ca^{2+}]_i$ (13, 14). The increases in $[Ca^{2+}]_i$ due to IP3-dependent release of intracellular stores is neither sufficient nor essential (15). What appears essential is transmembrane uptake of Ca^{2+} resulting in sustained increases in $[Ca^{2+}]_i$. The role of APC and MHC determinants in this response have also been characterized, indicating their role in generating the Ca^{2+} signal in T cells (16). The only means for bypassing the role for increased $[Ca^{2+}]_i$ in IL-2 production is by using a phorbol ester as co-mitogen (17). In the absence of extracellular Ca^{2+}, the combination of phorbol ester with co-mitogens such as phytohemagglutinin (PHA) or anti-CD3 can trigger IL-2 production. Calcium uptake across the plasma membrane appears to be through ligand-gated but not voltage-gated Ca^{2+} channels (18). Opening of these channels appears to be regulated at several different levels, including the state of membrane potential at the time of receptor–ligand interaction (19, 20), the level of $[Ca^{2+}]_i$ at the time of ligand binding (21), and possibly by IP3 or a phosphorylated derivative, inositol tetrakisphosphate (IP4) (22, 23). How the Ca^{2+} signal triggers IL-2 production is unclear but it may directly affect NFAT transcription by inducing the nuclear translocation of a cytoplasmic component of NFAT (24).

The activation of PKC and other distinct Ca^{2+}-dependent kinases likely plays major roles in T cell activation. PKC is thought to mediate a variety of later responses, including activation of the Na^+/H^+ exchanger. Surprisingly, inhibition of this exchanger with amiloride analogs does not affect IL-2 production (25).

Phosphorylation of the ζ chain may be essential for IL-2 production. The sequence of events leading to this event are slowly being unraveled and involves a number of different reactions and increases in PTK activity. T cells contain at least three members of the src family of non-receptor PTK genes: lck, fyn and yes (28). The p56[lck] and an isoform of p59[fyn(T)] are found primarily if not exclusively in T lymphocytes (27, 29, 30). p56[lck] is physically associated with CD4 and CD8 (6, 7). Cross-linking of CD4 or CD8 activates lck and the TCR ζ chain is phosphorylated (6). p56[fyn] may physically interact with the CD3 subunits (28), thus serving as a primary signal transduction element of the CD3/TCR complex. Indeed, over-expression of p56[fyn] renders these cells hyper-responsive to protein-tyrosine phosphorylation, Ca^{2+} accumulation, IL-2 production and cell proliferation (31).

Effective coupling of the TCR to the second messenger pathways also requires the presence of CD45. In the absence of CD45—a hematapoietic cell-specific surface glycoprotein with tyrosine phosphatase activity—stimulation of the CD3/TCR fails to result in elevations of $[Ca^{2+}]_i$ (32). These data suggest that CD45 may have an essential role in the control of ζ chain phosphorylation.

The G proteins that transmit information from surface receptors to their intracellular effector systems serve as another level of control of T cell activation. Activation of G proteins often requires their association with the plasma membrane (33). There have been a number of studies attempting to show that phospholipase C activity (which is responsible for PI hydrolysis) is regulated by a G protein coupled to the CD3/TCR. However, in these studies using bacterial toxins or non-hydrolysable GTP analogs, it has been difficult to establish a G protein-mediated coupling between phospholipase C and the TCR (34, 35).

IL-2 Receptor Expression

The high-affinity receptor for IL-2 (IL-2R) is a complex of at least two IL-2 binding molecules (and possibly additional accessory molecules) required for signal transduction (36, 37). Two distinct IL-2 binding proteins have been sequenced and cloned: IL-2Rα (TAC, p55) and IL-2Rβ (p75) (36, 37). IL-2Rα, a low-affinity receptor, crosses the membrane once, has a short intracellular chain and contains no tyrosine residues. This molecule appears simply to function to increase the binding affinity of the receptor complex (36). Cell activation is associated with the increased expression of IL-2Rα mRNA levels and surface protein expression, in a Ca^{2+}-independent manner (13).

In contrast, IL-2Rβ is constitutively expressed on resting T cells. This 75 kDa protein also crosses the membrane once, has a much larger intracellular domain, but nonetheless does not contain intrinsic PTK activity (36, 37).

IL-2-dependent Transmembrane Signaling and Proliferation

Since IL-2 is a potent progression signal to activated T cells, it is likely that the IL-2R is coupled to specific intracellular activation pathways. These pathways clearly differ from those linked to CD3–TCR. Ligation of the IL-2R does not result in PI hydrolysis or increased $[Ca^{2+}]_i$ (38–40). Indeed IL-2-dependent proliferation proceeds in the absence of detectable changes in $[Ca^{2+}]_i$ (38).

Binding of IL-2 to its receptor does lead to an orderly sequence of events, including the tyrosine phosphorylation of a number of proteins (40–43) and the activation of additional kinases such as microtubule-associated protein (MAP-2) kinase (40a) and ribosomal S6 kinase (40). Although phosphorylation of p56^{lck} has been associated with IL-2 binding to its receptor (44, 45), it does not appear essential for cell proliferation (40). In contrast to T cell activation through CD3–TCR, CD45 is also not required for IL-2-dependent proliferation (46). One of the earliest detectable responses to IL-2 is an increase in cytosolic pH, the result of activation of the Na^+/H^+ exchanger. However, this does not appear to be essential for IL-2 signaling (47).

DEFECTIVE SIGNAL TRANSDUCTION AS A CAUSE FOR IMMUNE DEFICIENCY

Although structure–function relationships remain to be established, the unraveling of these complex signal transduction pathways has identified important targets or sites for genetic or acquired T cell dysfunction. A scheme for the role of various critical events in T cell signaling is illustrated in Figure 11.2.

Defects in Antigen Processing and Presentation

Presentation of exogenous protein antigens to helper T cells by APC generally requires that the APC degrade the protein into immunogenic peptides and these peptides bind to an MHC class II molecule. This complex of

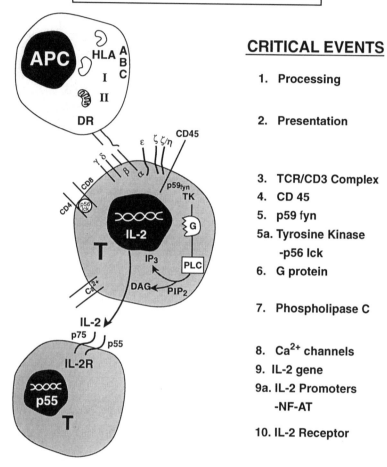

Figure 11.2. T cell signaling pathways

peptide and MHC on the surface of the APC provides the stimulatory ligand for the α/β TCR.

Initiation of T cell signaling therefore requires the generation of the peptide–MHC complex, a mechanism(s) which is poorly understood. Defects in class II molecules would also affect antigen presentation and T cell signaling. A series of mutant APCs have been isolated which were defective in antigen presentation, although their HLA class II genes were normal. These presentation-defective phenotypes include: (a) a deficiency in generating peptides from native proteins; (b) a loss of access of class II molecules to peptides because of abnormal intracellular trafficking of class II molecules; or (c) as a result of as yet undefined steps in antigen processing or presentation (48, 49).

Immunodeficiency syndromes associated with defective expression of HLA class I and II expression have been described by a number of groups (50–52). The clinical presentation has been heterogeneous but often includes normal or near-normal mitogen-induced proliferative responses but absent antigen-induced responses. The defective expression generally affects all circulating cells. It has been shown that the class II-deficient SCID mutation affected a *trans*-acting class II regulatory gene that lies outside the MHC (53). More recently, a factor identified as an HLA class II box binding protein was absent or defective in cells from these patients (54).

Defects in T Lymphocytes that may Manifest as Signaling Abnormalities

TCR/CD3 Complex

The TCR for antigen is a complex consisting of seven polypeptide chains; two form the clonotypic heterodimer which determines antigen specificity (1, 2). The other five constitute the monomorphic CD3 components, thought to be involved in signal transduction. A familial defect in surface expression of the TCR/CD3 complex on otherwise phenotypically normal T lymphocytes has been described (55). As a consequence, impaired activation of T cells was observed with certain antigens and mitogens but not with other TCR-independent stimuli. Both severe and mild phenotypes appear to exist and correlate with differences in the level of TCR surface expression and of T cell function *in vitro*. The biochemical basis of the defect may reside in the impaired association of CD3–ζ chain with other chains of the complex. In view of the multi-subunit nature of the TCR/CD3 complex, it is likely that other biochemical defects in TCR assembly will give rise to immunodeficiency syndromes.

Recently, a T–T hybridoma mutant was described in which the β chain from the antigen-specific α/β heterodimer was substituted with an unselected TCR β chain (56). Surprisingly, the TCR heterodimer of the mutant lost all capacity to be stimulated by specific antigen as well as anti-CD3 antibody. Thus, appropriate pairing of the α/β chains determines not only antigen/MHC specificity, but signaling efficiency of the TCR/CD3 complex itself.

CD45

In T lymphocytes at least four CD45 species can be detected (57). In B cells the major form is a 220 kDa protein, whereas thymocytes express mainly the 180 kDa species (57). All available data suggest that effective coupling of the

TCR to the phosphoinositol second messenger pathway requires the presence of CD45 (32). The important link appears to be between the phosphatase activity of CD45 and the ζ chain of the CD3 complex, which is tyrosine phosphorylated upon T-cell activation. Thus, CD45 may have an essential role in ζ chain phosphorylation. The activity of p56^{lck} may also be modified by the presence or absence of CD45. Down-regulation of CD45 in B cells leads to an impairment of cell signaling as well (58).

Patients deficient in CD45 expression have not been described. A variant pattern of CD45 expression has been found in approximately 8% of normal individuals and is characterized by the persistent expression of CD45RA epitope in T cells (59). Family studies indicate an autosomal mode of inheritance. Memory cell function in these individuals was not altered.

src Family Protein-tyrosine Kinases

The src kinases p56^{lck} and one isoform of p59^{fyn}(T) are fairly well restricted to T cells (27, 29, 30), have been implicated in signal transduction (28) and thus represent important targets for abnormalities associated with immune deficiency. Over-expression of catalytically inactive p59^{fyn} inhibited TCR-mediated activation of otherwise normal thymocytes, suggesting that p59^{fyn} mediates signaling from the TCR complex. Over-expression of p56^{lck} leads to an almost complete loss of CD3 thymocytes, implying that this kinase ordinarily regulates thymocyte development (31).

Both p56^{lck} and p59^{fyn} appear to play major roles in T cell development. Functional deletion of these kinases in transgenic animals resulted in markedly impaired intrathymic development and a profound CD3$^+$ T cell lymphopenia (60, 61).

G Proteins

The G proteins that transmit information from receptors to their intracellular effector systems belong to a large homologous family of trimeric proteins, each with an α subunit that binds guanine nucleotides, and β and γ subunits that are always tightly associated (33). Although several studies indicate that T cells express various G proteins, evidence for the coupling of a G protein to the TCR/CD3 complex is less than compelling and defects in G protein coupling to lymphocyte surface receptors have not been described to date (11, 12, 34, 35).

Phospholipase C

PI-specific phospholipases C (PLC) are present in all cell types studied and have been isolated from lymphocytes as well. At least 5 PI-specific PLC

(PLC$_\alpha$, PLC$_\beta$ (three isoforms), PLC$_{\gamma 1}$, PLC$_{\gamma 2}$ and PLC$_\delta$ (three isoforms)) have been isolated by DNA cloning (62). The variability in the characteristics of PI hydrolysis in different T cell lines may be related to the isozymes of PLC expressed (12). In both T and B lymphocytes, ligation of the TCR/CD3 complex or membrane IgM is associated with tyrosine phosphorylation of PLC$_{\gamma 1}$ (63–66). However, given the ubiquitous expression of the different isoforms of PLC, it seems unlikely that only a single isoform will be tyrosine phosphorylated following lymphocyte surface receptor ligation or that absence of a single isoform would lead to a selective abnormality in lymphocytes alone.

Ca^{2+} Channels

Controlling the permeability of the plasma membrane is one of the main mechanisms by which cells can regulate Ca^{2+} influx and cytosolic Ca^{2+} levels. Since the biophysical properties and pharmacology of Ca^{2+} channels vary in different cell types, Ca^{2+} channels likely represent a heterogeneous group of proteins. In T and B lymphocytes, ligand-gated or mitogen-regulated Ca^{2+} channels have been described (67, 68). Voltage-gated Ca^{2+} channels, common in other cell types, do not appear to be present. In T cells, different types of Ca^{2+} channels based on electrophysical properties have been described and their levels of expression may vary with the stage of development (68). Since the lymphocyte Ca^{2+} channels are sensitive to voltage, i.e. they close when the plasma membrane is depolarized (19, 20), optimal function implies maintenance of a normal resting membrane potential of -60 to -70 mV. Any process which alters the resting potential could interfere with normal Ca^{2+} influx. Most immune deficiencies are characterized by normal Ca^{2+} influx but a failure to initiate, for example, IL-2 gene transcription. There have been some exceptions but delineation of the mechanism underlying the failure of Ca^{2+} mobilization was not defined (69).

Signaling of Gene Transcription

Understanding the control regions of inducible genes and their link to surface receptor-mediated cell signaling has focused on nuclear proteins that may be targets for signals emanating from the antigen receptor. Transcriptional regulation accounts for most of the regulation of T cell activation genes (9). For IL-2, and likely IL-4, gene transcriptional activation, Ca^{2+} influx is associated with activation of NFAT. The influx of Ca^{2+} is perhaps critical for the nuclear shuttling of constitutively expressed cytoplasmic NFAT (24). Together with an inducible nuclear NFAT, the resultant complex positively regulates IL-2 gene activation (9, 70, 71). Drugs such as cyclosporin A and FK-506 interfere with this regulation, inhibiting IL-2 gene activation. Because of its relative restriction to T cells (although it has been described in B cells), abnormalities of NFAT activation or binding could result in immunodeficiency. In a patient with SCID and phenotypically normal numbers of T cells, deficient mRNAs coding for IL-2, IL-3, IL-4 and IL-5 (72) were attributed to an abnormal NFAT nuclear transcription complex (73).

Interleukin-dependent Cell Proliferation

As discussed earlier, whereas the signaling requirements for lymphokine secretion are relatively stringent, the requirements for expression of functional high-affinity IL-2R are less strict and activation of a variety of pathways appears to be stimulated. Isolated defects of interleukin receptor expression have not been described to date except for the possibility of the IL-1R (74).

Ligation of the IL-2R initiates a cascade of events which are shared by many cell types. It is unclear if any downstream events are unique for lymphocytes. Since the immunosuppressant rapamycin interferes with IL-2-dependent proliferation (71, 75), delineation of the target of the drug may reveal an important and unique lymphocyte-specific pathway.

Abnormal Accessory Molecule Expression and Immunodeficiency

CD43, a sialyated molecule found on most leukocytes, has been identified as a major glycoprotein in T cells (76). CD43 has been shown to enhance the antigen-specific activation of T cells, and the intracellular domain, which is hyperphosphorylated during T cell activation, is required for this response (77). Since CD43 is defective in Wiskott–Aldrich syndrome (77), abnormalities of its function may be linked to the pathogenesis of this disorder.

Leukocyte Adhesion Molecules

Leukocyte adhesion deficiency is characterized by mutation in the gene encoding the β subunit shared by three adhesion heterodimers: LFA-1, Mac-1 (CR3), and p150,95. Although presenting primarily as a disorder of phagocytic cell function (due to impaired adherence), T lymphocyte function and adhesion are impaired, especially the response to limiting concentrations of mitogens (78). The consequences are limited because of the redundancy of other T-cell adhesion pathways.

HIV Infection

A number of studies have suggested that HIV or gp120 impairs cell signaling by mitogen or antibody to the TCR/CD3 complex (79). Chronic exposure to the virus or gp120 may lead to persistent elevations of $[Ca^{2+}]_i$, and raised levels of I-P3 and I-P4. It is unclear, however, whether the chronic activation of signal transduction pathways induced by HIV, gp120 or other proteins, for example through CD4, woud impair responses to physiological signals for cell activation, through refractoriness of the relevant pathway.

CONCLUSION

The past few years has resulted in considerable progress in our understanding of the events involved in T and B cell recognition and responses to foreign antigen or other mitogens. A number of surface molecules are involved in the initial recognition events and many proteins, enzymes, ion channels, and nuclear transcription factors play a role in coupling the cell surface response and subsequent signaling events. That these events are exquisitely controlled underscores the potential for abnormalities to develop. Whether genetic or acquired, these abnormalities could manifest as immunodeficiency. Delineation of the hierarchy of events will yield important insight into basic biological processes, definition of new disease mechanisms, and reveal new options for manipulating the immune response.

ACKNOWLEDGEMENTS

I am grateful to all of my colleagues who contributed to the work and evolution of ideas. This work was supported in part by grants AI-26490 and AI-29704 from the NIH.

REFERENCES

1. Samelson, L.E., Harford, J.B. and Klausner, R.D. (1985) Identification of the components of the murine T cell antigen receptor complex. *Cell*, **43**, 223–231.
2. Clevers, H., Alarcon, B., Wileman, T. and Terhorst, C. (1988) The T cell receptor/CD3 complex: A dynamic protein ensemble. *Annu. Rev. Immunol.*, **6**, 629–662.
3. Samelson, L.E., Patel, M.D., Weissman, A.M., Harford, J.B. and Klausner, R.D. (1986) Antigen activation of murine T cells induces tyrosine phosphorylation of a polypeptide associated with the T cell antigen receptor. *Cell*, **46**, 1083–1090.
4. Baniyash, M., Garcia-Morales, P., Luong, E., Samelson, L.E. and Klausner, R.D. (1988) The T cell antigen receptor ζ chain is tyrosine phosphorylated upon activation. *J. Biol. Chem.*, **263**, 18225–18230.
5. Parnes, J.R. (1989) Molecular biology and function of CD4 and CD8. *Adv. Immunol.*, **44**, 265–311.
6. Veillette, A., Bookman, M.A., Horak, E.M., Samelson, L.E. and Bolen, J.B. (1989) Signal transduction through the CD4 receptor involves the activation of the internal membrane tyrosine protein kinase p56[lck]. *Nature*, **338**, 257–259.
7. Barber, E.K., Dasgupta, J.D., Schlossman, S.F., Trevillyan, J.M. and Rudd, C.E. (1989) The CD4 and CD8 antigens are coupled to a protein tyrosine kinase

(p56[lck]) that phosphorylates the CD3 complex. *Proc. Nat. Acad. Sci. USA,* **86,** 3277–3281.

8. Bierer, B.E., Sleckman, B.P., Ratnofsky, S.E. and Burakoff, S.J. (1989) The biologic roles of CD2, CD4 and CD8 in T-cell activation. *Annu. Rev. Immunol.,* **7,** 579–599.

9. Ullman, K.S., Northrop, P., Verweij, C.L. and Crabtree, G.R. (1990) Transmission of signals from the T lymphocyte antigen receptor to the genes responsible for cell proliferation and immune function: The missing link. *Annu. Rev. Immunol.,* **8,** 421–452.

10. Shaw, J.P., Utz, P., Durand, D.B., Toole, J.J., Emmel, E.A. and Crabtree, G.R. (1988) Identification of a putative regulator of early T cell activation genes. *Science,* **241,** 202–205.

11. Altman, A., Mustelin, T. and Coggeshall, K.M. (1990) T lymphocyte activation: A biological model of signal transduction. Crit. Rev. Immunol 1990; **10,** 347–391.

12. Rao, A. (1991) Signaling mechanisms in T cells. *Crit. Rev. Immunol.,* **10,** 495–519.

13. Mills, G.B., Cheung, R.K., Grinstein, S. and Gelfand, E.W. (1985) Increase in cytosolic free calcium concentration is an intracellular messenger for the production of interleukin 2 but not for the expression of the interleukin 2 receptor. *J. Immunol.,* **134,** 1640–1643.

14. Kumagai, N., Benedict, S.H., Mills, G.B. and Gelfand, E.W. (1988) Induction of competence and progression signals in human T lymphocytes by phorbol esters and calcium ionophores. *J. Cell Physiol.,* **137,** 329–336.

15. Gelfand, E.W., Cheung, R.K., Mills, G.B. and Grinstein, S. (1988) Uptake of extracellular Ca^{2+} and not recruitment from internal stores is essential for T-lymphocyte proliferation. *Eur. J. Immunol.,* **18,** 917–922.

16. Nisbet-Brown, E., Cheung, R.K. and Gelfand, E.W. (1985) Antigen-dependent increase in cytosolic free calcium in specific human T lymphocyte clones. *Nature,* **316,** 545–547.

17. Gelfand, E.W., Cheung, R.K., Mills, G.B. and Grinstein, S. (1988) Mitogens trigger a calcium independent signal for proliferation in phorbol ester-treated lymphocytes. *Nature,* **315,** 419–430.

18. Gelfand, E.W., Cheung, R.K. and Grinstein, S. (1986) Mitogen-induced changes in Ca^{2+} permeability are not mediated by voltage-gated K^+ channels. *J. Biol. Chem.,* **261,** 11520–11523.

19. Gelfand, E.W., Cheung, R.K., Mills, G.B. and Grinstein, S. (1987) Role of membrane potential in the response of human T lymphocytes to phytohemagglutinin. *J. Immunol.,* **138,** 527–531.

20. Oettgen, H.C., Terhorst, C., Cantley, L.C. and Rosoff, P.M. (1985) Stimulation of the T3–T cell receptor complex induces a membrane potential-sensitive calcium influx. *Cell,* **40,** 583–590.

21. Gelfand, E.W., MacDougall, S.L., Cheung, R.K. and Grinstein, S. (1989) Independent regulation of Ca^{2+} entry and release from internal stores in activated human B cells. *J. Exp. Med.,* **170,** 315–320.

22. Kuno, M. and Gardner, P. (1987) Ion channels activated by inositol 1,4,5-trisphosphate in plasma membrane of human T lymphocytes. *Nature,* **326,** 301–304.

23. Irvine, R.F. and Moor, R.M. (1986) Microinjection of inositol 1,3,4,5-tetrakisphosphate activates sea urchin eggs by a mechanism dependent on external Ca^{2+}. *Biochem. J.,* **240,** 917–920.

24. Flanagan, W.M., Corthésy, B., Bram, R.J. and Crabtree, G.R. (1991) Nuclear association of a T-cell transcription factor blocked by FK506 and cyclosporin A. *Nature,* **352,** 803–807.

25. Mills, G.B., Cheung, R.K., Cragoe, E.J., Jr, Grinstein, S. and Gelfand, E.W. (1986) Activation of the Na$^+$/H$^+$ antiport is not required for lectin-induced proliferation of human T lymphocytes. *J. Immunol.*, **136**, 1150–1154.

26. Perlmutter, R.M., Marth, J.D., Ziegler, S.F., Garvin, A.M., Pawar, S., Cooke, M.P. and Abraham, K.M. (1988) Specialized protein tyrosine kinase proto-oncogenes in hematopoietic cells. *Biochim. Biophys. Acta*, **948**, 245–262.

27. Cooke, M.P. and Perlmutter, R.M. (1989) Expression of a novel form of the fyn proto-oncogene in hematopoietic cells. *New Biologist*, **1**, 66–74.

28. Samelson, L.E., Phillips, A.F., Loving, E.T. and Klausner, R.D. (1990) Association of the fyn protein tyrosine kinase with the T cell antigen receptor. *Proc. Nat. Acad. Sci. USA*, **87**, 4358–4362.

29. Marth, J.D., Peet, R., Krebs, E.G. and Perlmutter, R.M. (1985) A lymphocyte-specific protein tyrosine kinase is rearranged and overexpressed in the murine T cell lymphoma LSTRA. *Cell*, **43**, 393–404.

30. Voronova, A.F., Adler, H.T. and Sefton, B.M. (1987) Two lck transcripts containing different 5' untranslated regions are present in T cells. *Mol. Cell. Biol.*, **7**, 4407–4413.

31. Cooke, M.P., Abraham, K.M., Forbush, K.A. and Perlmutter, R.M. (1991) Regulation of T cell receptor signaling by a src family protein-tyrosine kinase (p59^{fyn}). *Cell*, **66**, 281–291.

32. Koretzky, G.A., Picus, J., Thomas, M.L. and Weiss, A. (1990) Tyrosine phosphatase CD45 is essential for coupling T-cell antigen receptor to the phosphatidyl inositol pathway. *Nature*, **346**, 66–68.

33. Taylor, C.W. (1990) The role of G proteins in transmembrane signaling. *Biochem. J.*, **272**, 1–13.

34. Gray, L.S., Huber, K.S., Gray, M.C., Hewlett, E.L. and Englehard, V.H. (1989) Pertussis toxin effects on T lymphocytes are mediated through CD3 and not by pertussis toxin catalyzed modification of a G protein. *J. Immunol.*, **142**, 1631–1638.

35. Sasaki, T. and Hasegawa-Sasaki, H. (1987) Activation of polyphosphoinositide phospholipase C by guanosine 5'-O-(3-thio) triphosphate and fluoroaluminate in membrane prepared from a human T cell leukemia line, Jurkat. *FEBS Lett.*, **218**, 87–92.

36. Waldmann, T.A. (1989) The multi-subunit interleukin-2 receptor. *Annu. Rev. Biochem.*, **58**, 875–911.

37. Hatakeyama, M., Tsudo, M., Minamoto, S., Kono, T., Doi, T., Miyata, T., Miyasaka, M. and Taniguchi, T. (1989) Interleukin-2 receptor β chain gene: Generation of three receptor forms by cloned human α and β chain cDNAs. *Science*, **244**, 551–556.

38. Mills, G.B., Cheung, R.K., Grinstein, S. and Gelfand, E.W. (1985) Interleukin 2-induced lymphocyte proliferation is independent of increases in cytosolic free calcium concentrations. *J. Immunol.*, **134**, 2431–2435.

39. Mills, G.B., Stewart, D.J., Mellors, A. and Gelfand, E.W. (1986) Interleukin 2 does not induce phosphatidylinositol hydrolysis in activated T cells. *J. Immunol.*, **136**, 3019–3024.

40. Sawami, H., Terada, N., Franklin, R.A., Okawa, H., Uchiyama, T., Lucas, J.J. and Gelfand, E.W. (1992) Signal transduction by interleukin 2 in human T cells: Activation of tyrosine and ribosomal S6 kinases and cell cycle regulatory genes. *J. Cell Physiol.*, **151**, 367–377.

40a. Terada, N., Lucas, J.J., Szepesi, A., Franklin, R.A., Takase, K. and Gelfand, E.W. (1992) Rapamycin inhibits the phosphorylation of p70 S6 kinase in IL-2 and mitogen-activated human T cells. *Biochem. Biophys. Res. Commun.*, **186**, 1315–1321.

41. Ferris, D.K., Brown, J.W., Ortaldo, J.R. and Farrar, W.L. (1989) IL-2 regulation of tyrosine kinase activity is mediated through the p70–75 β-subunit of the IL-2 receptor. *J. Immunol.*, **143**, 870–876.

42. Saltzman, E.M., White, K. and Casnellie, J.E. (1990) Stimulation of the antigen and interleukin-2 receptors on T lymphocytes activates distinct tyrosine protein kinases. *J. Biol. Chem.*, **265**, 10138–10142.

43. Mills, G.B., May, C., McGill, M., Fung, M., Baker, M., Sutherland, R. and Greene, W.C. (1990) Interleukin 2-induced tyrosine phosphorylation: Interleukin 2 receptor β is tyrosine phosphorylated. *J. Biol. Chem.*, **265**, 3561–3567.

44. Hatakeyama, M., Kono, T., Kobayashi, N., Kawahara, A., Levin, S.D., Perlmutter, R.M. and Taniguchi, T. (1991) Interaction of the IL-2 receptor with the src-family kinase p56[lck]: Identification of a novel intermolecular association. *Science*, **252**, 1523–1528.

45. Horak, I.D., Gress, R.E., Lucas, P.J., Horak, E.M., Waldmann, T.A. and Bolen, J.B. (1991) T-lymphocyte interleukin 2-dependent tyrosine protein kinase signal transduction involves the activation of p56[lck]. *Proc. Nat. Acad. Sci. USA*, **88**, 1996–2000.

46. Pingel, J.T. and Thomas, M.L. (1989) Evidence that the leukocyte-common antigen is required for antigen-induced T lymphocyte proliferation. *Cell*, **58**, 1055–1065.

47. Mills, G.B., Cragoe, E.J., Jr, Gelfand, E.W. and Grinstein, S. (1985) Interleukin 2 induces a rapid increase in intracellular pH through activation of a Na^+/H^+ antiport: Cytoplasmic alkalinization is not required for lymphocyte proliferation. *J. Biol. Chem.*, **260**, 12500–12507.

48. Mellins, E., Smith, L., Arp, B., Cotner, T., Colis, E. and Pious, D. (1990) Defective processing and presentation of exogenous antigens in mutants with normal HLA class II genes. *Nature*, **343**, 71–74.

49. Mellins, E., Arp, B., Singh, D., Carreno, B., Smith, L., Johnson, A.H. and Pious, D. (1990) Point mutations define positions in HLA-DR3 molecules that affect antigen presentation. *Proc. Nat. Acad. Sci. USA*, **87**, 4785–4789.

50. Lisowska-Grospierre, B., Charron, D.J., de Préval, C., Durandy, A., Turmel, P., Griscelli, C. and Mach, B. (1984) Defect of expression of MHC genes responsible for an abnormal HLA class I phenotype and the class II negative phenotype of lymphocytes from patients with combined immunodeficiency. In Albert, E.D., Baur, M.P. and Mayr, W.R. (Eds) *Histocompatibility Testing*. Springer-Verlag, Berlin, pp. 650–655.

51. Niethammer, D., Dopfer, R., Dammer, G., Peter, H., de Préval, C., Mach, B. and Hadam, M.R. (1986) Congenital agammaglobulinemia associated with malabsorption: No expression of MHC-class II antigens due to a regulatory gene defect? In Aiuti, F., Rosen, F.S. and Cooper, M.D. (eds) *Recent Advances in Primary Immunodeficiencies*. Raven Press, New York, pp. 185–193.

52. Fischer, A., Lisowska-Grospierre, B., Anderson, D.C. and Springer, T.A. (1988) Leukocyte adhesion deficiency: Molecular basis and functional consequences. *Immunodef. Rev.*, **1**, 39–54.

53. de Préval, C., Lisowska-Grospierre, B., Loche, M., Griscelli, C. and Mach, B. (1985) A transacting class II regulatory gene unlinked to the MHC controls expression of HLA class II genes. *Nature*, **318**, 291–293.

54. Reith, W., Satola, S., Herrero-Sanchez, C., Amaldi, I., Lisowska-Grospierre, B., Griscelli, C., Hadam, M.R. and Mach, B. (1988) Congenital immunodeficiency

with a regulatory defect in MHC class II gene expression lacks a specific HLA-DR promoter binding protein, RF-X. *Cell*, **53**, 97–906.

55. Alarcon, B., Terhorst, C., Arnaiz-Villena, A., Perez-Aciego, P. and Regueiro, J.R. (1990) Congenital T-cell receptor immunodeficiencies in man. *Immunodef. Rev.*, **2**, 1–16.

56. Reno, T.A., Ley, S., Sugiyama, E., Cantagrel, A., Blumberg, R., Bonventre, J., Terhorst, C. and Yeh, E.T.H. (1990) Defects in signal transduction caused by a T cell receptor β chain substitution. *Eur. J. Immunol.*, **20**, 1417–1422.

57. Thomas, M.L. (1989) The leukocyte common antigen family. *Annu. Rev. Immunol.*, **7**, 339–369.

58. Justement, L.B., Campbell, K.S., Chien, N.C. and Cambier, J.C. (1991) Regulation of B cell antigen receptor signal transduction and phosphorylation by CD45. *Science*, **252**, 1839–1842.

59. Schwinzer, R. and Wonigeit, K. (1990) Genetically determined lack of CD45R–cells in healthy individuals: Evidence for a regulatory polymorphism of CD45 R antigen expression. *J. Exp. Med.*, **171**, 1803–1808.

60. Molina, T.J., Kishihara, K., Siderovski, D.P., van Ewijk, W., Narendran, A., Timms, E., Wakeham, A., Paige, C.J., Hartmann, K.U., Veillette, A., Davidson, D. and Mak, T.W. (1992) Profound block in thymocyte development in mice lacking p56^{lck}. *Nature*, **357**, 161–164.

61. Perlmutter, R.M. Personal communication.

62. Majerus, P.W., Ross, T.S., Cunningham, T.W., Caldwell, K.K., Jefferson, A.B. and Bansal, V.S. (1990) Recent insights in phosphatidylinositol signaling. *Cell*, **63**, 459–465.

63. Park, D.J., Rho, H.W. and Rhee, S.G. (1991) CD3 stimulation causes phosphorylation of phospholipase C-γ_1 on serine and tyrosine residues in a human T-cell line. *Proc. Nat. Acad. Sci. USA*, **88**, 5453–5456.

64. Augustine, J.A., Secrist, J.P., Daniels, J.K., Leibson, P.J. and Abraham, R.T. (1991) Signal transduction through the T cell antigen receptor: Activation of phospholipase C through a G-protein-independent coupling mechanism. *J. Immunol.*, **146**, 2889–2897.

65. Dasgupta, J.D., Granja, C., Druker, B., Lin, L.L., Yunis, E.J. and Relias, V. (1992) Phospholipase C-γ_1 association with CD3 structure in T cells. *J. Exp. Med.*, **175**, 285–288.

66. Carter, R.H., Park, D.J., Rhee, S.G. and Fearon, D.T. (1991) Tyrosine phosphorylation of phospholipase C induced by membrane immunoglobulin in B lymphocytes. *Proc. Nat. Acad. Sci. USA*, **88**, 2745–2749.

67. Gardner, P. (1989) Calcium and lymphocyte activation. *Cell*, **59**, 15–20.

68. Lewis, R.S. and Cahalan, M.D. (1990) Ion channels and signal transduction in lymphocytes. *Annu. Rev. Physiol.*, **52**, 415–430.

69. Chatila, T., Wong, R., Young, M., Miller, R., Terhorst, C. and Geha, R.S. (1989) An immunodeficiency characterized by defective signal transduction in T lymphocytes. *N. Engl. J. Med.*, **320**, 696–702.

70. Emmel, E.A., Verweij, C.L., Durand, D.B., Higgins, K.M., Lacy, E. and Crabtree, G.R. (1989) Cyclosporin A specifically inhibits function of nuclear proteins in T cell activation. *Science*, **246**, 1617–1620.

71. Dumont, F.J., Melino, M.R., Staruch, J.M., Koprak, S.L., Fisher, P.A. and Sigal, N.H. (1990) The immunosuppressive macrolides FK506 and rapamycin act as reciprocal antagonists in murine T cells. *J. Immunol.*, **144**, 1418–1424.

72. Chatila, T., Castigli, E., Pahwa, R., Chirmule, N., Oyaizu, N., Good, R.A. and Geha, R.S. (1990) Primary combined immunodeficiency resulting from defective

transcription of multiple T-cell lymphokine genes. *Proc. Nat. Acad. Sci. USA,* **87,** 10033–10037.

73. Geha, R.S. Personal communication.
74. Chu, E.T., Rosenwasser, L.J., Dinarello, C.A., Rosen, F.S. and Geha, R.S. (1984) Immunodeficiency with defective T-cell response to interleukin 1. *Proc. Nat. Acad. Sci. USA,* **81,** 4945–4949.
75. Terada, N., Lucas, J.J., Szepesi, A., Franklin, R.A., Domenico, J. and Gelfand, E.W. (1993) Rapamycin blocks cell cycle progression of activated T cells prior to events characteristic of the middle to late G_1 phase of the cycle. *J. Cell Physiol.* (in press).
76. Remold-O'Donnell, E., Davis, A.E., Kenney, D., Bhaskar, K.R. and Rosen, F.S. (1986) Purification and chemical composition of gpL115, the human lymphocyte surface sialoglycoprotein that is defective in Wiskott–Aldrich syndrome. *J. Biol. Chem.,* **261,** 7526–7530.
77. Park, J.K., Rosenstein, Y.J., Remold-O'Donnell, E., Bierer, B.E., Rosen, F.S. and Burakoff, S.J. (1991) Enhancement of T-cell activation by the CD43 molecule whose expression is defective in Wiskott–Aldrich syndrome. *Nature,* **350,** 706–709.
78. Fischer, A., Lisowska-Grospierre, B., Anderson, D.C. and Springer, T.A. (1988) Leukocyte adhesion deficiency: Molecular basis and functional consequences. *Immunodef. Rev.,* **1,** 39–54.
79. Pinching, A.J. and Nye, K.E. (1990) Defective signal transduction—A common pathway for cellular dysfunction in HIV infection? *Immunol. Today,* **11,** 256–259.

Chapter 12

The Wiskott–Aldrich Syndrome: An Immunodeficiency Associated with Defects of the CD43 Molecule

YVONNE ROSENSTEIN,[1,3] JOHN K. PARK,[1] BARBARA E. BIERER[1,2] and STEVEN J. BURAKOFF[1,5]

[1]Division of Pediatric Oncology, Dana-Farber Cancer Institute; [2]Hematology–Oncology Division, Brigham and Women's Hospital; [3]Department of Pathology, [4]Medicine, and [5]Pediatrics, Harvard Medical School, Boston, Massachusetts, USA

CD43, also known as sialophorin, leukosialin or large sialoglycoprotein, is a heavily glycosylated, sialic acid-rich protein present on the surface of lymphoid cells. This molecule has been found to be defective in the Wiskott–Aldrich syndrome (WAS), although it is not the primary defect for this X-linked recessive immunodeficiency disorder. This review will focus on the principal features of WAS and on the role of the CD43 molecule as a co-receptor molecule.

THE WISKOTT–ALDRICH SYNDROME

WAS was first described in 1937, when Wiskott reported a family of seven children in which the three brothers had thrombocytopenia, severe eczema, and repeated infections, while the four sisters were healthy (1). The recessive inheritance pattern of this disorder, associated with the X chromosome, was established by Aldrich et al. (2). Immunodeficiency is a

New Concepts in Immunodeficiency Diseases. Edited by S. Gupta and C. Griscelli
© 1993 John Wiley & Sons Ltd

consistent feature of WAS, and the severity of symptoms of this disease tends to increase with the age of the patient (3). In addition to immunodeficiency, thrombocytopenia and eczema, recurrent non-septic arthritis, asthma, bloody diarrhea and nephropathy are also characteristic of this syndrome. Reticular cell hyperplasia in the peripheral lymph nodes and spleen has been observed; tissue eosinophilia, hemophagocytosis, focal fibrosis and progressive depletion of germinal centers have also been described, although less frequently (4).

A variety of therapies have been used with WAS patients. Splenectomy can improve the thrombocytopenia; immunoglobulin replacement therapy, together with prophylactic antibodies, can decrease the incidence of bacterial infections (5, 6). The only curative therapy for the hematological and immunological defects of WAS has been the transplantation of allogeneic histocompatible bone marrow (7–12). Transplantation of children with WAS has been successful in more than 90% of the cases when a histocompatible donor was used (12). Partial engraftment of T cells alone has also resulted in the complete restoration of the immunological functions of WAS patients, strongly suggesting that the immunological problems of these patients are due to a primary T cell defect (7).

The incidence of this disease is four per million live male births (13), and no clustering to a particular geographical area or within a given ethnic group has been found (13). Most affected males do not survive childhood (mean lifespan = 6.5 years). According to a retrospective survey of 301 cases in the USA and Canada, the leading causes of death are infection (59%), bleeding (27%), or lymphoreticular malignancies (12%, of which leukemia and Hodgkin's disease account for 5%) (13).

Molecular genetic studies of WAS patients using restriction fragment length polymorphisms (RFLPs) in conjunction with linkage analysis have localized the WAS locus to the pericentric region of the X chromosome (14, 15). The WAS gene has been localized to the chromosomal region between the TIMP and DXS255 markers, on Xp11.22 (15–18). This information has led to accurate prenatal diagnosis and carrier detection in affected families with greater than 98% confidence (15). Carrier detection has also been attempted using RFLPs in conjunction with methylation pattern analysis of X-linked genes (19, 20).

The severe immunological defects associated with WAS are well characterized on a cellular level, yet the molecular basis is not fully understood. Cellular immune functions are severely compromised in these patients. Lymphocyte counts, normal at birth, appear to decline with age (21–23). T helper (CD4$^+$)/T cytotoxic–suppressor (CD8$^+$) ratios are abnormal with a reduction of T helper cells (24). *In vitro* functional tests have shown that the T cells from WAS patients have a diminished response to antigen-specific and non-specific activation (23, 25, 26). The absence of delayed hypersensitivity reactions on skin testing is also characteristic of WAS (22, 25, 27).

In an attempt to find a defect associated with WAS, a biochemical study of T cells isolated from WAS patients demonstrated that cells from some of the patients lacked the expression of a 115 kDa cell surface glyoprotein, later termed gpL115 (CD43), while others showed decreased levels of this 115 kDa protein. The cells of the latter group, however, expressed on their surface a 135 kDa protein not found on normal non-activated T cells (28, 29). This 135 kDa protein was later identified to be a differentially sialylated form of CD43. These studies provided the first demonstration of a biochemical abnormality associated with T lymphocyte glycoproteins in WAS patients. From a morphological point of view, scanning electron microscopy of T lymphocytes isolated from WAS patients showed that the cells lacked most of the microvillous projections found on normal T cells (30). The biochemistry and function of CD43 will be discussed further below.

Humoral immunity of WAS patients is also impaired. These patients usually have low concentrations of IgM in their serum, while IgA and IgE levels are frequently increased. The levels of IgG are usually normal (21, 22, 27). Antibody titers to blood group antigens and other polysaccharide antigens tend to be extremely low, despite a normal response to protein antigens (22, 27). It has been proposed that the low IgM levels characteristic of these individuals may be a consequence of their inability to respond to polysaccharide antigens (22, 27). A hypercatabolism of immunoglobulins and albumin that has been attributed to the reticulo-endothelial hyperplasia characteristic of WAS patients has also been described (27).

Thrombocytopenia and defective platelet function leading to an increased bleeding tendency are major complications for patients with WAS (31–33). It has been suggested that the thrombocytopenia (platelet counts less than 50×10^9 per liter) may be the result of both decreased production and increased destruction (23, 33, 34). The mean platelet size is reduced, up to two-thirds of normal values (23, 34). In addition, several biochemical and functional abnormalities have been described: impaired aggregation following stimulation with ADP, epinephrine (adrenaline) or collagen (33, 35, 36); hexokinase deficiency (37) and defective mitochondrial carbon dioxide production (35, 37), a consequence of a defect in mitochondrial ATP resynthesis (38).

Following therapeutic splenectomy, prolonged platelet survival results in restoration of size and peripheral platelet counts, suggesting that splenic sequestration of defective platelets may be, in part, responsible for the thrombocytopenia observed in WAS (5, 6). It has also been suggested that the lack or aberrant expression of the 115 kDa protein (CD43) on the surface of T lymphocytes from WAS patients correlated with reduced amounts of glycoprotein GPIb and GPIa on the platelets of some patients (28, 29). These variations were attributed to defects in the *O*-glycosylation of proteins by β-1,6-GlcNAC transferase (26). Abnormalities in the platelet membrane glycoproteins, however, are not a common characteristic of all WAS patients (39).

EXPRESSION AND CHARACTERIZATION OF THE CD43 MOLECULE

A possible link between the immunological and hematological defects of WAS is a defective protein with an M_r of 115 kDa (28). The initial characterization of this protein revealed that it is a sialoglycoprotein and that it is found on a number of different hematopoietic cell lineages. This sialoglycoprotein has been termed gpL115 (28), sialophorin (29), leukocyte large sialoglycoprotein (40) and leukosialin (41, 42). It has been recently shown that they all refer to the same molecule identified by the CD43 cluster of monoclonal antibodies (mAb) (43, 44).

The CD43 Gene

The genes encoding human, rat and murine CD43 have all been cloned and sequenced (42, 45–47). The extracellular, transmembrane and intracellular regions of the polypeptide are all encoded by one exon, suggesting that the different forms of CD43 found within a given species are due to differences in glycosylation. A transmembrane glycoprotein, CD43, appears to be highly conserved in terms of the amino acid sequence of the intracellular and transmembrane regions as well as of the amino acid and carbohydrate composition of the extracellular region. Human CD43 is an integral membrane protein with a 19-amino-acid leader peptide, a 235-amino-acid extracellular domain, a 23-amino acid transmembrane domain and a 123-amino acid intracytoplasmic domain (45, 46). The extracellular domain has several unique characteristics. Consistent with the high levels of O-glycosylation found on this protein, this domain is highly enriched for serines and threonines (39% compared to 12% for average proteins) (46). There is also one potential N-linked glycosylation site in the extracellular domain at residue 220, consistent with previous carbohydrate analyses (41, 48). In mouse CD43 there is also a potential N-linked glycosylation site at position 148 (47). Rat CD43, however, does not contain any potential N-linked glycosylation sites (42). Four significant repeats have been identified in this domain, spanning, in the human, amino acids 127–144, 145–162, 163–180 and 181–198. Comparing the amino acids 163–180 to the other repeats, it was found that 13/18, 15/18, and 13/18 residues were identical, and that 43% of the amino acids were either Ser or Thr. It is likely that the majority of these are glycosylated, considering the extent of glycosylation of this molecule. These repeats may have originated from the duplication of an 18-amino-acid cassette during evolution to generate a highly glycosylated glycoprotein (45). The transmembrane domain, identified by hydrophobicity plots of the predicted sequence, is typical of integral membrane proteins in its length and composition. A 5-amino-acid repeat has been identified (residues 241–246 and 250–255) (45). The intracytoplasmic domain of the human protein has 123 amino acids. It includes a number of potential phosphorylation sites (6 Thr and 11 Ser residues) that might mediate transduction of activation signals (45–47). A potential phosphorylation site for protein kinase C (PKC) has been described at residue 322 (49). The transmembrane and intracellular domains of human, rat, and mouse CD43 are >70% identical; this high degree of structural conservation suggests a physiological function, such as signaling, for this region. *In situ* hybridization techniques have localized the gene for CD43 to chromosome 16 rather than to chromosome X (45, 46). This indicates that a defect in the CD43 structural gene is unlikely to be the primary defect in WAS.

Biochemical Characterization of CD43

The molecular weight of the protein, as determined by sodium dodecyl sulphate–polyacrylamide gel electrophoresis (SDS–PAGE), has been shown to vary for different cell types. Two predominant forms of this molecule can be found on circulating cells of healthy individuals: a 115 kDa form expressed on T lymphocytes, thymocytes and monocytes; and a 135 kDa form found on neutrophils, platelets, and B cells (41, 43, 50). The polypeptide core of both forms of CD43 has a molecular weight of 58 kDa (48, 50, 51). The differences between the two CD43 forms must result from the presence of additional neutral carbohydrates in the higher-molecular-weight species since both forms have approximately 90 O-linked and one N-linked oligosaccharide associated with the polypeptide backbone (41, 52).

The amino acid composition of CD43 is very different from that of the average protein. A low amount of lysine residues (3.3% versus 6.5%) and a high amount of proline (9.9% versus 4.8%), serine (12.5% versus 6.5%) and threonine (12.5% versus 6.5%) are characteristic of the CD43 molecule (47). The relative amounts of proline, glycine and alanine found in CD43 are similar to that of mucin molecules. As a result of this composition, one in every four amino acids is a potential site for O-linked carbohydrate residues (41, 52). This is in accordance with the carbohydrate analysis of CD43. More than 50% of the weight of this protein consists of carbohydrates. Sialic acid, galactose and N-acetyl galactosamine are the predominant polysaccharide residues, with galactose and N-acetyl galactosamine being present in nearly equimolar amounts (25 and 22 residues per 100 amino acids, respectively). One or more sialic acid residues are thought to be linked to each Galβ1-3-GalNAC (41, 48, 52–54), thus resulting in large amounts of sialic acid present on each CD43 molecule. Removal of sialic acid moieties alters the physicochemical properties of this molecule, producing a major shift in the electrophoretic migration of the molecule (115 kDa to 135 kDa) (48, 52).

The particular amino acid and carbohydrate composition of CD43 places the CD43 molecule into a category of heavily glycosylated sialoglycoproteins which includes glycophorin of erythrocytes and GPIb of platelets (41, 52). Rotary shadowing and electron microscopy analyses of purified rat CD43 have shown that the extracellular domain of CD43 has an unfolded rod-like structure that extends to a length of 45 nm (55). This conformation may be the result of the large amount of O-linked sugars present on the CD43 molecule, and/or steric interactions between the peptide-linked GalNAC and adjacent amino acids. This structure is very similar to what has been described for secreted mucin molecules: an expanded structure with oligosaccharide side chains that hydrate and solubilize the relatively insoluble polypeptide core (56, 57). Because of its extended conformation, CD43 is thought to be a surface molecule that enables a cell to establish contact with another cell (55). For human CD43, the mAb L10 has been shown to recognize an epitope within the 78 NH_2-terminal amino acids of the molecule that is not sensitive to neuraminidase treatment of the cells (58). In the rat, while linear protein epitopes can be recognized, the native structure of some of these determinants, as well as their accessibility, can be modified by glycosylation (55).

CD43 is considered to be a major sialic acid bearing protein on the cell surface. The number of CD43 molecules present on the surface of the human lymphoblastoid cell line CEM and on rat thymocytes has been estimated to be approximately 1×10^5 per cell (55).

Cellular and Tissue Expression of CD43

CD43 is expressed on all circulating hematopoietic cells including T cells, thymocytes, B cells, monocytes, granulocytes and platelets, but not on erythrocytes (40, 43, 50, 59). CD43 is expressed early in ontogeny in the bone marrow and therefore may play a role in the regulation of lymphoid maturation (60).

Only 25–30% of the B cells isolated from peripheral blood express CD43, but upon culture with autologous T cells and pokeweed mitogen, 80% of the IgG-producing cells and 30–50% of the IgM-producing cells express CD43. A similar pattern is found in human tonsillar cells (61). The expression of the murine CD43 molecule in B lymphocytes is also upregulated following stimulation with lipopolysaccharide (LPS) (60).

Immunohistochemical localization of CD43 in different tissues has shown that a CD43-like molecule can be found in the rat nervous system. Immunoreactivity with the anti-CD43 mAb W3/13 occurs with structures probably corresponding to neurites and axon terminals in different regions of the central nervous system (62). Other examples of leukocyte antigens (Thy1 and MRC.OX2) have been reported to be present in the central nervous system (63, 64). Even though the biological significance of these observations remains unclear, it is possible that these molecules may play a role in cell–cell interactions and recognition events in both the central nervous system and in the immune system.

CD43-related Defects in WAS

Based on the fact that CD43 in WAS patients has a different electrophoretic mobility and because the gene coding for CD43 does not have introns within the coding sequence, it has been postulated that post-translational modifications may be involved in the altered expression of CD43 in WAS patients. The *O*-linked glycosylation patterns of the CD43 molecule have been analyzed in normal as well as in WAS lymphocytes.

The predominant carbohydrate structure present on lymphocyte CD43 is the tetrasaccharide sialic acid $\alpha2\rightarrow3$Gal$\beta1\rightarrow3$GalNAC6$\leftarrow2\alpha$ sialic acid. It has been proposed that upon activation of T lymphocytes, this structure acquires a higher degree of complexity, through the concerted action of at least five glycosyltransferases, to become the hexasaccharide: sialic acid $\alpha2\rightarrow3$Gal$\beta1\rightarrow3$GalNAC6$\leftarrow1\beta$G1cNAC4$\leftarrow1\beta$Gal3$\leftarrow2\alpha$ sialic acid. This hexasaccharide is also the major oligosaccharide on human neutrophils and platelets (53, 65). Two studies comparing glycosyltransferase activities in hematopoietic cell subpopulations from normal individuals and WAS patients have reported different observations. In both, all glycosyltransferase activities measured, with the exception of $\beta1\rightarrow6$N acetylglucosamine transferase and $\alpha2\rightarrow6$ sialyl transferase, were found to be equivalent in normal individuals and WAS patients. In one, the $\beta1\rightarrow6$N acetylglucosamine transferase activity was found to be decreased in the WAS T lymphocytes (66), providing an explanation for the apparent lack of the CD43 hexasaccharide characteristic of activated T cells. In the other report, however, the activity of $\beta1\rightarrow6$N acetylglucosamine transferase was reported to be greatly enhanced in WAS patients as compared to normal cells. This finding was used to explain the presence on WAS cells of the CD43 isoform that is characteristic of activated T lymphocytes (49, 66). These apparently contradictory results may be explained by the fact that the cell types examined in each study were different (Epstein–Barr virus (EBV) transformed B cells versus resting T cells), and that there were individual variations among the WAS patients studied by the two groups. It has also been observed that under certain conditions the 115 kDa form of CD43 on WAS lymphocytes can be converted into species of both higher and lower molecular weight (67).

Thus, carbohydrate changes may be responsible for the altered forms of the CD43 molecule in WAS patients. Recent studies on expression of CD43 on normal and WAS fibroblasts by transfection also suggest that aberrant glycosylation of CD43 may be restricted to hematopoietic cell lineages, since no difference in the apparent molecular weight of CD43 was observed (68). Taken together these data seem to support the idea that the primary X-linked defect in WAS may affect a gene responsible for the regulation of O-glycosylation.

ANTIGEN RECOGNITION: T CELL RECEPTOR AND CO-RECEPTOR MOLECULES

An effective immune response depends upon regulated interactions of immune cells with antigen-presenting cells or target cells. These interactions are mediated by antigen-specific receptors as well as by adhesion receptors.

The TCR–CD3 Complex

T cell antigen specificity is conferred by the T cell receptor (TCR)–CD3 complex which recognizes foreign antigen bound to major histocompatibility complex (MHC) class I or class II molecules on antigen-presenting cells. The heterodimers $\alpha\beta$ or $\gamma\delta$ that form the TCR are highly polymorphic transmembrane glycoproteins (69–71). The $\alpha\beta$ TCR is expressed on 85–98% of peripheral T cells while the $\gamma\delta$ TCR is expressed only on 2–15% of peripheral T cells. All four polypeptide chains belong to the Ig gene super-family. Similar to the immunoglobulin molecules, their clonal diversity is generated during T cell differentiation through the combinatorial association of their variable (V), diversity (D), joining (J) and constant (C) regions. Their extracellular portions are thought to form domains that are very similar in structure to the Ig domains. Their intracytoplasmic domains comprise only 5–12 amino acids and it is thought that these molecules do not have intrinsic signal-transducing properties. The CD3 complex, which is physically associated with the TCR, may have signal transduction functions.

At least five different non-polymorphic integral membrane proteins constitute the CD3 complex (γ, δ, ε, ζ, and η). They are either non-covalently associated with the $\alpha\beta$ TCR heterodimer or associated with one another (71). The association of the CD3 chain with the TCR is a requirement for the surface expression of the TCR proteins. The very homologous γ, δ and ε chains belong to the Ig gene super-family, while the ζ and η chains, similar to one another, are unrelated to the γ, δ and ε molecules.

Co-receptor Molecules

The TCR–CD3 complex provides the cell with a mechanism for specific antigen (Ag) recognition, and the clonotypic TCR provides Ag specificity to the T cell through recognition of foreign antigen as presented by class I or class II MHC molecules on an antigen-presenting cell (72, 73). Cytotoxic

T lymphocytes (CD8+) usually recognize foreign antigen associated with major histocompatibility complex (MHC) class I molecules, whereas helper cells (CD4+) recognize foreign antigen in the context of MHC class II molecules. Antigen is presented to the TCR in the cleft of MHC molecules formed by two α helices with a β sheet floor. However, even though the signals needed to activate the T cell are transduced to the intracellular environment via the TCR–CD3 complex, additional signals provided via T cell molecules, termed co-receptors, are required for a T cell to commit fully to its functional activity.

Some of those molecules were identified by the use of mAbs that blocked or mimicked the binding of their putative counter-receptors. Co-receptor molecules on T cells are thought to contribute to T cell activation in several ways. By binding to their counter-receptor on the surface of the antigen-presenting cell (or target cell), they stabilize and increase the strength of adhesion between the cells, e.g. LFA-1 (74) and CD2 (75, 76). Some accessory molecules (e.g. CD4, CD8, CD2, CD45) are involved in transducing signals to the intracellular compartment of the T cells, synergizing with TCR–CD3-mediated signals and providing important regulatory functions (75, 77).

THE ROLE OF CD43 IN CELL ACTIVATION

Recent data suggest that, like CD4, CD8, CD2 and CD45, CD43 also functions as a co-receptor molecule. In the absence of any then known physiological ligand(s) for CD43, initial studies on the cellular role of CD43 used monoclonal antibodies.

CD43-mediated Cell Activation

Two anti-CD43 mAbs, B1B6 and E11B, have been used to study the potential role of CD43 in the activation of T cells (78). The B1B6 mAb and the E11B mAb were by themselves poorly mitogenic for peripheral blood T cells, but they did induce the production of IL-2 (78). In addition, both mAbs potently amplified T cell proliferation when the cells were stimulated by phorbol-myristate acetate (PMA), soluble anti-CD3 mAb, concanavalin A (Con A) or phytohemagglutinin (PHA). Whole antibodies were more effective than Fab fragments, suggesting that cross-linking of CD43 molecules is required for efficient signal transduction (78).

In contrast, another anti-CD43 mAb (L10) alone induced the proliferation of peripheral blood T cells at comparable levels to the anti-CD3 mAb OKT3 (59). At optimal concentrations of each mAb, the responses were equal in magnitude and similar in time course. Both mAb-induced responses required the presence of monocytes and both resulted in the expression by T cells of the early activation antigens HLA-DR, IL-2 receptor, and 4F2 (59).

The B1B6 mAb has also been shown to enhance the spontaneous cytotoxic activity of natural killer (NK) cells (79). Pre-incubation of lymphocytes with the B1B6 mAb resulted in increased lysis of the NK-sensitive target cells K562 and Molt-4. Pre-incubation of target cells with the B1B6 mAb, however, had no effect although they also expressed CD43 on their surface, demonstrating that the enhanced killing was not due to a conventional antibody-dependent cellular cytotoxicity (ADCC) reaction. Kinetic analysis of B1B6 mAb-treated and non-treated lymphocytes showed that the cytolytic reaction proceeded at a faster rate in the B1B6 mAb-treated lymphocyte-containing cultures and, for unexplained reasons, the mechanism by which this occurred appeared to be dependent upon the type of target cell. When K562 cells were used, the enhanced killing was due to the recruitment of additional effector cells from the pool of non-binding lymphocytes. When Molt-4 cells were used, the enhanced killing was due to the increased recycling of the already existing effector pool. When tested in the same experimental system, the E11B mAb did not increase NK cell activity. The L10 mAb, which is directed against an epitope on CD43 different from the one recognized by the B1B6 mAb, has been reported to cause only a slight increase in cytotoxic T lymphocytes (CTL)- and NK-mediated cytotoxic activity (59).

B cell activation through the CD43 molecule has also been studied with the B1B6 mAb. Not mitogenic alone, the B1B6 mAb augmented the proliferative response of resting and *in vivo*-activated tonsillar B cells to TPA (12-*O*-tetradecanoyl-phorbol-13-acetate) three- to fivefold. These results were similar to those obtained in studies using antibodies directed against CD22 and CD23. All three of these B cell surface molecules are capable of transducing early activation signals that, in synergy with primary activators of protein kinase C (PKC), are able to induce proliferation (80). B1B6 mAb had no effect on the pokeweed mitogen-induced differentiation of, and the subsequent IgG and IgM production by, peripheral blood and tonsillar B cells (81).

Activation and homotypic adhesion of monocytes has been induced by anti-CD43 mAb. Incubation of monocytes with the L10 mAb for 24–48 hours caused a five- to sevenfold increase in their phorbol ester-induced production of hydrogen peroxide (82).

The function of CD43 on neutrophils has also been investigated. The binding of anti-CD43 polyclonal antibodies to neutrophils selectively inhibited their chemotactic and phagocytic activities. The phagocytosis of both IgG and complement component C3 opsonized particles were equally hindered. The antibodies had no effect, however, on the abilities of the neutrophils to adhere to and spread over substrates. They also had no effect on the enzyme release and superoxide generation capacities of the neutrophils in response to appropriate stimulating agents (83). It was recently shown that upon activation with formyl-Met-Leu-Phe (formyl-leucine-methionylphenylalanine) or with PMA, the CD43 expression decreased on the neutrophil cell surface (84, 85). This was partly explained by the release of CD43+ material with an altered electrophoretic mobility into the culture medium, following activation of the neutrophils (84, 85).

Intracellular Signalling Events Associated with CD43-mediated Activation

Hydrolysis of phosphoinositides leading to the generation of inositol triphosphate (IP3) and diacylglycerol (DAG) and an increase in $[Ca^{2+}]_i$ has been reported to be initiated by the L10 mAb in both peripheral blood T cells and in monocytes (86). To further characterize the intracellular signaling events associated with CD43, the phosphorylation states of the molecule before and after cellular activation were studied. The intracellular domain of CD43 has been found to be constitutively phosphorylated in all cell types expressing the molecule, including erythroid (K562), T lymphoblastoid (HPB-ALL, Jurkat), and myelocytic (HL-60) cell lines, as well as platelets and peripheral blood lymphocytes (49, 87, 88). Finer analysis of the constitutive phosphorylation revealed that there is less than 1 mol of phosphate for every 20 mol of protein and that it occurs only on serine residues (49).

The role of PKC in both the constitutive and inducible phosphorylation of CD43 was examined. Following treatment of cells with PMA, a direct PKC activator, the phosphate content of CD43 increased by 2.5-fold for most cell types (K562, HL-60, Jurkat and platelets) and by 15-fold for peripheral blood lymphocytes (PBL), most of which (85%) are T cells. In K562 and HPB-ALL cells—the most extensively studied cell lines—constitutive and inducible phosphorylation could be selectively inhibited by staurosporine, a potent inhibitor of PKC and cAMP-dependent protein kinases (49, 89). In contrast, HA 1004, a more effective inhibitor of cAMP- and cGMP-dependent protein kinases than of PKC, could not inhibit the constitutive phosphorylation of CD43 in K562 (49). These data, together with the finding that the major phosphorylated peptides before and after PMA-induced hyperphosphorylation were the same, suggested that constitutive as well as inducible phosphorylation of CD43 were most probably catalyzed by PKC. Although a consensus sequence thought to be necessary for the action of PKC has not been identified, a serine residue situated close to basic amino acids has been shown to be a favorable substrate for this enzyme (90). The most likely PKC substrate of CD43 therefore was suggested to be serine-332 (49).

CD43: A Co-stimulatory Molecule

In another approach to investigate the physiological role of CD43, a cDNA encoding the human protein was introduced by electroporation into an antigen-specific murine T cell hybridoma by 155.16 (91). This hybridoma produces IL-2 when the TCR–CD3 complex is stimulated by anti-CD3 mAb or specific antigen. The TCR of the By155.16 hybridoma recognizes the same HLA-DR molecules as those expressed on the human B cell line Daudi. Chosen for these studies was a clone of By155.16 that produced IL-2 only when transfected with genes encoding human T cell accessory molecules such as CD4 (92), CD8 (93), or CD2 (94). The critical dependence on such accessory molecules for activation of the murine hybridoma was exploited to assess the ability of CD43 to function as an accessory or co-stimulatory molecule. Wild-type CD43 or a mutant form of CD43 that lacked the intracytoplasmic portion of the molecule was introduced into the T cell hybridoma (91). Co-expression of TCR–CD3 with CD43 by T cells enhanced the antigen-specific activation of T cells. The inability of the truncated form of the protein to impart responsiveness to the specific antigen recognized by the TCR suggested that the cytoplasmic domain of CD43 is necessary for it to serve as a co-stimulatory molecule (91).

A Ligand for CD43: ICAM-1

In addition to a role in signal transduction, CD43 may be involved in cellular adhesion. The L10 mAb has been shown to induce homotypic adhesion of monocytes (82). This phenomenon was temperature and Mg^+ dependent and was inhibitable by anti-CD18 but not by CD11b mAb, thus demonstrating that there was a partial dependency on LFA-1-mediated aggregation. In neutrophils, cross-linking of CD43 with the anti-CD43 mAb BS-1 induced neutrophil aggregation both in a CD18-dependent and CD18-independent fashion (84).

The role of CD43 in mediating T cell adhesion was further evaluated. The specific interaction of Daudi cells with immobilized immunoaffinity-purified CD43 (94) led to the identification of a ligand on the antigen-presenting cell (Daudi) that interacts with CD43. The binding of Daudi cells to plate-bound immunoaffinity-purified CD43 was shown to be consistently inhibited by anti-ICAM-1 mAbs, suggesting that ICAM-1 could serve as a ligand for CD43. Reciprocal experiments, i.e. the binding of CD43+ cells to plastic-immobilized ICAM-1 were performed, provided further evidence that CD43 is capable of binding to ICAM-1. Additional proof that this interaction is possible came from experiments in which the ability of beads expressing ICAM-1 molecules to form conjugates with beads expressing CD43 was demonstrated (95).

ICAM-1 (CD54), a single-chain glycoprotein of M_r 90–115 kDa, is a member of the Ig-like superfamily. Its structure consists of an extracellular region composed of five Ig-like domains, a transmembrane region, and a cytoplasmic region (96, 97). The expression of ICAM-1 is limited in non-inflamed tissues but is up-regulated on diverse cell types in response to activation or to inflammatory mediators such as bacterial lipopolysaccharide, interleukin 1 (IL-1) and tumor necrosis factor (TNF) (98, 74). ICAM-1 mediates antigen-independent adhesion between leukocytes and their targets. ICAM-1, on the surface of antigen-presenting or target cells, is a counter-receptor for the leukocyte integrins LFA-1 (CD11a/CD18) (98) and Mac-1 (CD11b/CD18) (99). Regulation of ICAM-1/LFA-1 interactions is mediated both by changes in ICAM-1 expression and changes in LFA-1 avidity (98, 100, 101).

Thus, by interacting with ICAM-1, CD43 may favor not only cell–cell adhesion, but also may be involved in mediating signal transduction in T cells, NK cells, B cells and monocytes.

CONCLUSIONS

CD43 appears to have at least two functions in lymphoid cells. Modulation of immune responses may be one function of CD43. The activation of lymphoid cells results from the concerted action of antigen-specific receptors with co-receptor molecules directly involved in strengthening the cell–cell interaction itself and/or facilitating signal transduction through the antigen-specific receptor. By interacting with their counter-receptors on antigen-presenting cells, these co-receptors potentiate the activation signals delivered through the TCR. Activation of lymphoid cells via CD43 has been described in T lymphocytes (59, 78, 94), monocytes (82) and NK cells (79). These data suggest that the CD43 molecule also facilitates signal transduction. In T cells, by interacting with the appropriate counter-receptor(s), CD43 contributes to the generation of an activating signal that will combine with TCR–CD3-transduced signals, ultimately leading to T cell activation.

Based on its abundance on the cell surface, its negative charge and its mucin-like structure, it has also been proposed that CD43 may be involved in regulating cell senescence (29, 30, 102). Other mucin-like proteins are thought to be involved in regulating normal senescence of blood cells: epiglycanin has been described to mask cryptic antigens on a murine mammary tumor cell, controlling its survival (103). Another example of the involvement of mucin-like proteins in regulating cell senescence is provided by glycophorin. Altered expression of this protein plays a role in the accelerated erythrocyte senescence observed in β-thalassemia (104, 105). The CD43 molecules present on the cell surface have been proposed to mask cryptic antigens on the surface of circulating cells. Removal of sialic acid residues from the CD43 molecule increases the sensitivity of this molecule to protease activity (102). *In vivo*, low levels of endogenous sialidase coupled with some protease activity could lead to a modification of the CD43 molecule allowing the subsequent exposure of cryptic antigens on the cell surface, followed by the subsequent removal of cells from circulation.

This possibility is consistent with the progressive decline in T cell number and T cell function characteristic of WAS. Defective glycosylation of CD43 following T cell activation most likely results in the accelerated degradation of the molecule. Secondary to the increased proteolysis of CD43 would be the exposure of the cryptic antigens on T cells as proposed by Remold-O'Donnell and Rosen (102). Another secondary result of abnormal CD43 degradation would be the inability of T cells to use CD43 as a co-receptor molecule. As WAS patients either do not express CD43, or express different forms of it, their immunodeficiency may result from defective T cell adhesion and/or activation.

ACKNOWLEDGEMENT

This work was supported by NIH grant 5RO1 AI31868 (S.J.B.).

REFERENCES

1. Wiskott, A. (1937) Familiarer, angeborener Morbus Werlhofii. *Monatsschr. Kinderheil. Kd.*, **68**, 212–216.
2. Aldrich, R.A., Steinberg, A.G. and Campbell, D.C. (1954) Pedigree demonstrating a sex-linked recessive condition characterized by draining ears, eczematoid dermatitis and bloody diarrhea. *Pediatrics*, **13**, 133–139.
3. Rosen, F.S., Cooper, M.D. and Wedgwood, R.J.P. (1984) The primary immunodeficiencies. *N. Engl. J. Med.*, **311**, 300–310.
4. Snover, D.C., Frizzera, G., Spector, B.D., Perry, G.S., III and Kersey, J.H. (1981) Wiskott–Aldrich syndrome: Histopathologic findings in the lymph nodes and spleens of 15 patients. *Hum. Pathol.*, **12**, 821–831.
5. Lum, L.G., Tubergen, D.G., Corash, L. and Blaese, R.M. (1980) Splenectomy in the management of the thrombocytopenia of the Wiskott–Aldrich syndrome. *N. Engl. J. Med.*, **302**, 892–896.
6. Corash, L., Shafer, B. and Blaese, R.M. (1985) Platelet-associated immunoglobulin, platelet size, and the effect of splenectomy in the Wiskott–Aldrich syndrome. *Blood*, **65**, 1439–1443.
7. Parkman, R., Rappeport, J., Geha, R., Belli, J., Cassady, R., Levey, R., Nathan, D.G. and Rosen, F.S. (1978) Complete correction of the Wiskott–Aldrich syndrome by allogeneic bone-marrow transplantation. *N. Engl. J. Med.*, **298**, 921–927.
8. Kapoor, N., Kirkpatrick, D., Blaese, R.M., Oleske, J., Hilgartner, M.H., Chaganti, R.S., Good, R.A. and O'Reilly, R.J. (1981) Reconstitution of normal megakaryocytopoiesis and immunologic functions in Wiskott–Aldrich syndrome by marrow transplantation following myeloablation and immunosuppression with busulfan and cyclophosphamide. *Blood*, **57**, 692–696.
9. Ochs, H.D., Lum, L.G., Johnson, F.L., Schiffman, G., Wedgwood, R.J. and Storb, R. (1982) Bone marrow transplantation in the Wiskott–Aldrich syndrome: Complete hematological and immunological reconstitution. *Transplantation*, **34**, 284–287.
10. Meuwissen, H.J., Bortin, M.M., Bach, F.H., Porter, I.H., Schreinmachers, D., Harrison, B.A. and Taft, E. (1984) Long-term survival after bone marrow trans-

plantation: A 15-year follow-up report of a patient with Wiskott–Aldrich syndrome. *J. Pediatr.*, **105**, 365–369.

11. Goldsobel, A.B., Ehrlich, R.M., Mendoza, G.R. and Stiehm, E.R. (1985) Bone marrow transplantation for Wiskott–Aldrich syndrome: Report of two cases with use of 2-mercaptoethane sulfonate. *Transplantation*, **39**, 568–570.

12. Rimm, I. and Rappaport, J.M. (1990) Bone marrow transplantation for the Wiskott–Aldrich syndrome: Long-term follow up. *Transplantation*, **50**, 617–620.

13. Perry, G.S., III, Spector, B.D., Schuman, L.M., Mandel, J.S., Anderson, V.E., McHugh, R.B., Hanson, M.R., Fahlstrom, S.M., Krivit, W. and Kersey, J.H. (1980) The Wiskott–Aldrich syndrome in the United States and Canada (1892–1979). *J. Pediatr.*, **97**, 72–78.

14. Peacocke, M. and Siminovitch, K.A. (1987) Linkage of the Wiskott–Aldrich syndrome with polymorphic DNA sequences from the human X chromosome. *Proc. Nat. Acad. Sci. USA*, **84**, 3430–3433.

15. Kwan, S.P., Sandkuyl, L.A., Blaese, M., Kunkel, L.M., Bruns, G., Parmley, R., Skarshaug, S., Page, D.C., Ott, J. and Rosen, F.S. (1988) Genetic mapping of the Wiskott–Aldrich syndrome with two highly-linked polymorphic DNA markers. *Genomics*, **3**, 39–43.

16. Greer, W.L., Mahtani, M.M., Kwong, P.C., Rubin, L.A., Peacocke, M., Willard, H.F. and Siminovitch, K.A. (1989) Linkage studies of the Wiskott–Aldrich syndrome: Polymorphisms at TIMP and the X chromosome centromere are informative markers for genetic prediction. *Hum. Genet.*, **83**, 227–230.

17. de Saint Basile, G., Arveiler, B., Fraser, N.J., Boyd, Y., Graig, I.W., Griscelli, J.C. and Fischer, A. (1989) Close linkage of hypervariable marker DXS255 to disease locus of Wiskott–Aldrich syndrome. *Lancet*, **ii**, 1319–1321.

18. Kwan, S.P., Lahner, T., Haggemann, T., Lu, B., Blaese, M., Ochs, H., Wedgwood, R., Ott, J., Craig, I.W. and Rosen, F.S. (1991) Localization of the gene for the Wiskott–Aldrich syndrome between two flanking markers, TIMP and DXS255 on Xp 11.12–Xp11.3. *Genomics*, **10**, 29–33.

19. Fearon, E.R., Kohn, D.B., Winkelstein, J.A., Vogelstein, B. and Blaese, R.M. (1988) Carrier detection in the Wiskott–Aldrich syndrome. *Blood*, **72**, 1735–1739.

20. Greer, W.L., Kwong, P.C., Peacocke, M., Ip, P., Rubin, L.A. and Siminovitch, K.A. (1989) X-chromosome inactivation in the Wiskott–Aldrich syndrome: A marker for the detection of the carrier state and identification of cell lineages expressing the gene defect. *Genomics*, **4**, 60–67.

21. Wolff, J.A. (1967) Wiskott–Aldrich syndrome: Clinical, immunologic, and pathologic observations. *J. Pediatr.*, **70**, 221–232.

22. Cooper, M.D., Chase, H.P., Lowman, J.T., Krivit, W. and Good, R.A. (1968) Wiskott–Aldrich syndrome: An immunologic deficiency disease involving the afferent limb of immunity. *Am. J. Med.*, **44**, 499–513.

23. Ochs, H.D., Slichter, S.J., Harker, L.A., VonBehrens, W.E., Clark, R.A. and Wedgwood, R.J. (1980) The Wiskott–Aldrich syndrome: Studies of lymphocytes, granulocytes, and platelets. *Blood*, **55**, 243–252.

24. Wade, N.A., Lepont, M.L., Veazey, J. and Mewisson, H.J. (1985) Progressive varicella in three patients with WAS treatment with adenine-arabinoside. *Pediatrics*, **75**, 672–675.

25. Oppenheim, J.J., Blaese, R.M. and Waldmann, T.A. (1970) Defective lymphocyte transformation and delayed hypersensitivity in Wiskott–Aldrich syndrome. *J. Immunol.*, **104**, 835–844.

26. Greer, W.L., Higgins, E., Sutherland, D.R., Novogrodsky, A., Brockhausen, I., Peacocke, M., Rubin, L.A., Baker, M., Dennis, J.W. and Siminovitch, K.A. (1989)

Altered expression of leucocyte sialoglycoprotein in Wiskott–Aldrich syndrome is associated with a specific defect in O-glycosylation. *Biochem. Cell. Biol.*, **67**, 503–509.

27. Blaese, R.M., Strober, W., Brown, R.S. and Waldmann, T.A. (1968) The Wiskott–Aldrich syndrome: A disorder with a possible defect in antigen processing or recognition. *Lancet*, **i**, 1056–1061.

28. Parkman, R., Remold-O'Donnell, E., Kenney, D.M., Perrine, S. and Rosen, F.S. (1981) Surface protein abnormalities in lymphocytes and platelets from patients with Wiskott–Aldrich syndrome. *Lancet*, **ii**, 1387–1389.

29. Remold-O'Donnell, E., Kenney, D.M., Parkman, R., Cairns, L., Savage, B. and Rosen, F.S. (1984) Characterization of a human lymphocyte surface sialoglycoprotein that is defective in Wiskott–Aldrich syndrome. *J. Exp. Med.*, **159**, 1705–1723.

30. Kenney, D., Cairns, L., Remold-O'Donnell, E., Peterson, J., Rosen, F.S. and Parkman, R. (1986) Morphological abnormalities in the lymphocytes of patients with the Wiskott–Aldrich syndrome. *Blood*, **68**, 1329–1332.

31. Pearson, H.A., Shulman, N.R., Oski, F.A. and Eitzman, D.U. (1966) Platelet survival in Wiskott–Aldrich syndrome. *J. Pediatr.*, **68**, 754–760.

32. Krivit, W., Yunis, E. and White, J.G. (1966) Platelet survival studies in the Wiskott–Aldrich syndrome. *Pediatrics*, **37**, 339–342.

33. Grottum, K.A., Hovig, T., Holmsen, H., Foss Abrahamsen, A., Jeremia, M. and Seip, M. (1969) Wiskott–Aldrich syndrome: Qualitative platelet defects and short platelet survival. *Br. J. Haematol.*, **17**, 373–382.

34. Murphy, S., Oski, F.A., Naiman, J.L., Lusch, C.J., Goldberg, S. and Gardner, F.H. (1972) Platelet size and kinetics in hereditary and acquired thrombocytopenia. *N. Engl. J. Med.*, **286**, 499–504.

35. Shapiro, R.S., Gerrard, G.M., Perry, G.S., III, White, J.G., Krivit, W. and Kersey, J.H. (1978) Wiskott–Aldrich syndrome: Detection of carrier state by metabolic stress of platelets. *Lancet*, **i**, 121–124.

36. Kuramoto, A., Steiner, M. and Baldini, M.G. (1970) Lack of platelet response to stimulation in the Wiskott–Aldrich syndrome. *N. Engl. J. Med.*, **282**, 475–479.

37. Baldini, M.G. (1972) Nature of the platelet defect in the Wiskott–Aldrich syndrome. *Ann. NY Acad. Sci.*, **201**, 437–444.

38. Verhoeven, A.J.M., van Oostrum, I.E.A., van Haarlam, H. and Akkerman, J.-W.N. (1989) Impaired energy metabolism in platelets from patients with Wiskott–Aldrich syndrome. *Thromb. Haemost.*, **61**, 10–14.

39. Pidard, D., Didry, D., Le Deist, F., Durandy, A., Griscelli, C., Bellucci, S. and Nurden, A.T. (1988) Analysis of the membrane glycoproteins of platelets in the Wiskott–Aldrich syndrome. *Br. J. Haematol.*, **69**, 529–535.

40. Axelsson, B., Hammarstrom, S., Robertsson, E.-S., Aman, P., Perlmann, P. and Mellstedt, H. (1985) The large sialoglycoprotein of human lymphocytes, I. Distribution on T and B lineage cells as revealed by a monospecific chicken antibody. *Eur. J. Immunol.*, **15**, 417–426.

41. Carlsson, S.R. and Fukuda, M. (1986) Isolation and characterization of leukosialin, a major sialoglycoprotein on human lymphocytes. *J. Biol. Chem.*, **261**, 12779–12786.

42. Killeen, N., Barclay, A.N., Willis, A.C. and Williams, A.F. (1987) The sequence of rat leukosialin (W3/13 antigen) reveals a molecule with O-linked glycosylation of one third of its extracellular amino acids. *EMBO J.*, **6**, 4029–4034.

43. Borche, L., Lozano, F., Vilella, R. and Vives, J. (1987) CD43 monoclonal antibodies recognize the large sialoglycoprotein of human leukocytes. *Eur. J. Immunol.*, **17**, 1523–1526.

44. McMichael, A.J. (ed.) (1987) White cell differentiation antigens. In *Leukocyte Typing III.* Oxford University Press, Oxford, pp. 801–802.

45. Pallant, A., Eskenazi, A., Mattei, M.G., Fournier, R.E., Carlsson, S.R., Fukuda, M. and Frelinger, J.G. (1989) Characterization of cDNAs encoding human leukosialin and localization of the leukosialin gene to chromosome 16. *Proc. Nat. Acad. Sci. USA*, **86**, 1328–1332.

46. Shelley, C.S., Remold-O'Donnell, E., Davis, A.E., Bruns, G.A., Rosen, F.S., Carroll, M.C. and Whitehead, A.S. (1989) Molecular characterization of sialophorin (CD43), the lymphocyte surface sialoglycoprotein defective in Wiskott–Aldrich syndrome. *Proc. Nat. Acad. Sci. USA*, **86**, 2819–2823.

47. Cyster, J., Somoza, C., Killeen, N. and Williams, A.F. (1990) Protein sequence and gene structure for mouse leukosialin (CD43), a T lymphocyte mucin without introns in the coding sequence. *Eur. J. Immunol.*, **20**, 875–881.

48. Fukuda, M., Carlsson, S.R., Klock, J.C. and Dell, A. (1986) Structures of O-linked oligosaccharides isolated from normal granulocytes, chronic myelogenous leukemia cells, and acute myelogenous leukemia cells. *J. Biol. Chem.*, **261**, 12796–12806.

49. Piller, V., Piller, F. and Fukuda, M. (1989) Phosphorylation of the major leukocyte surface sialoglycoprotein, leukosialin, is increased by phorbol 12-myristate 13-acetate. *J. Biol. Chem.*, **264**, 18824–18831.

50. Remold-O'Donnell, E., Zimmerman, C., Kenney, D. and Rosen, F.S. (1987) Expression on blood cells of sialophorin, the surface glycoprotein that is defective in Wiskott–Aldrich syndrome. *Blood*, **70**, 104–109.

51. Axelsson, B., Hammerstrom, S., Finne, J. and Perlmann, P. (1985) The large sialoglycoprotein of human lymphocytes, II. Biochemical features. *Eur. J. Immunol.*, **15**, 427–433.

52. Remold-O'Donnell, E., Davis, A.E., Kenney, D., Bhaskar, K.R. and Rosen, F.S. (1986) Purification and chemical composition of gpL 115, the human lymphocyte surface sialoglycoprotein that is defective in Wiskott–Aldrich syndrome. *J. Biol. Chem.*, **261**, 7526–7530.

53. Carlsson, S.R., Sasaki, H. and Fukuda, M. (1986) Structural variations of O-linked oligosaccharides present in leukosialin isolated from erythroid, myeloid and T lymphoid cells. *J. Biol. Chem.*, **261**, 12787–12795.

54. Piller, F., Weinberg, K., Parkman, R. and Fukuda, M. (1988) Resting T-lymphocytes in Wiskott–Aldrich syndrome carry O-glycans specific for activated normal T-cells. *J. Cell Biol.*, **107**, 191a.

55. Cyster, J., Shotton, D.M. and Williams, A.F. (1991) The dimensions of the T lymphocyte glycoprotein leukosialin and identification of linear protein epitopes that can be modified by glycosylation. *EMBO J.*, **10**, 893–902.

56. Shogren, R., Gerken, T.A. and Jentoft, N. (1989) Role of glycosylation on the conformation and chain dimensions of O-linked glycoproteins: Light scattering studies of ovine submaxillary mucin. *Biochemistry*, **28**, 5525–5536.

57. Jentoft, N. (1990) Why are proteins O-glycosylated? *Trends Biochem. Sci.*, **15**, 291–294.

58. Remold-O'Donnell, E. and Rosen, F.S. (1990) Proteolytic fragmentation of sialophorin (CD43): Localization of the activation-inducing site and examination of the role of sialic acid. *J. Immunol.*, **145**, 3372–3378.

59. Mentzer, S.J., Remold-O'Donnell, E., Crimmins, M.A., Bierer, B.E., Rosen, F.S. and Burakoff, S.J. (1987) Sialophorin, a surface glycoprotein defective in the Wiskott–Aldrich syndrome, is involved in human T lymphocyte proliferation. *J. Exp. Med.*, **165**, 1383–1392.
60. Gulley, M.L., Ogato, L.C., Thorson, J.A., Dailey, M.O. and Kemp, J.D. (1988) Identification of a murine Pan-T cell antigen which is also expressed during the terminal phases of B cell differentiation. *J. Immunol.*, **140**, 3751–3757.
61. Wiken, M., Bjork, P., Axelsson, B. and Perlmann, P. (1988) Induction of CD43 expression during activation and terminal differentiation of human B cells. *Scand. J. Immunol.*, **28**, 457–464.
62. Losy, J., Mahlen, J., Olson, T. and Kristenson, K. (1989) Distribution of leukosialin (W3/13)-like immunoreactivity in the rat nervous central system. *J. Neurocytol.*, **18**, 71–76.
63. Williams, A.F. and Gagnon, J. (1982) Neuronal cell Thy-1 glycoprotein: Homology with immunoglobulin. *Science*, **216**, 693–703.
64. Webb, M. and Barclay, A.N. (1984) Localization of the MRC OX2 glycoprotein on the surface of neurons. *J. Neurochem.*, **43**, 1061–1067.
65. Tsuiji, T., Tsunahisa, S., Watanabe, Y., Yamamoto, K., Tohyama, H. and Osawa, T. (1983) The carbohydrate moiety of human platelet glycocolicin. *J. Biol. Chem.*, **258**, 6335–6339.
66. Piller, F., Piller, V., Fox, R.I. and Fukuda, M. (1988) Human T-lymphocyte activation is associated with changes in O-glycan biosynthesis. *J. Biol. Chem.*, **263**, 15146–15150.
67. Reisinger, D. and Parkman, R. (1987) Molecular heterogeneity of a lymphocyte glycoprotein in immunodeficient patients. *J. Clin. Invest.*, **79**, 595–599.
68. Pallant, A., Fukuda, M. and Frelinger, J.G. (1990) CD43 (leukosialin, sialophorin, large sialoglycoprotein) can be expressed in both normal and Wiskott–Aldrich fibroblasts via transfection of a leukosialin cDNA. *Eur. J. Immunol.*, **20**, 1423–1428.
69. Allison, J.P. and Lanier, L.L. (1987) The structure, function and serology of the T cell receptor complex. *Annu. Rev. Immunol.*, **5**, 503–540.
70. Toyonaga, B. and Mak, T. (1987) Genes of the T cell antigen receptor in normal and malignant cells. *Annu. Rev. Immunol.*, **5**, 585–620.
71. Clevers, H., Alarcon, B., Wileman, T. and Terhorst, C. (1988) The T cell receptor/CD3 complex: A dynamic protein ensemble. *Annu. Rev. Immunol.*, **6**, 629–662.
72. Kappler, J. and Marrack, P. (1987) The T cell receptor. *Science*, **238**, 1073–1079.
73. Davis, M.M. and Bjorkman, P.J. (1988) T cell antigen receptor genes and T cell recognition. *Nature*, **334**, 395–402.
74. Dustin, M.L. and Springer, T.A. (1989) T cell receptor cross-linking transiently stimulates adhesiveness through LFA-1. *Nature*, **341**, 619–624.
75. Bierer, B.E. and Burakoff, S.J. (1989) T-lymphocyte activation: The biology and function of CD2 and CD4. *Immunol. Rev.*, **111**, 267–294.
76. Bierer, B.E., Sleckman, B.P., Ratnofsky, S.E. and Burakoff, S.J. (1989) The biologic roles of CD2, CD4, and CD8 in T-cell activation. *Annu. Rev. Immunol.*, **7**, 579–599.
77. Thomas, M.L. (1989) The leukocyte common antigen family. *Annu. Rev. Immunol.*, **7**, 339–369.
78. Axelsson, B., Youseffi-Etemad, R., Hammerstrom, S. and Perlmann, P. (1988) Induction of aggregation and enhancement of proliferation and IL-2 secretion in human T cells by antibodies to CD43. *J. Immunol.*, **141**, 2912–2917.

79. Vargas-Cortes, M., Axelsson, B., Larsson, A., Berzins, T. and Perlmann, P. (1988) Enhancement of human spontaneous cell-mediated cytotoxicity by a monoclonal antibody against the large sialoglycoprotein (CD43) on peripheral blood lymphocytes. *Scand. J. Immunol.*, **27**, 661–671.

80. Wiken, M., Bjork, P., Axelsson, B. and Perlmann, P. (1989b) Enhancement of human B-cell proliferation by a monoclonal antibody to CD43. *Scand. J. Immunol.*, **29**, 363–370.

81. Wiken, M., Bjork, P., Axelsson, B. and Perlmann, P. (1989a) Studies on the role of CD43 in human B-cell activation and differentiation. *Scand. J. Immunol.*, **29**, 353–361.

82. Nong, Y.-H., Remold-O'Donnell, E., LeBien, T.W. and Remold, H.G. (1989) A monoclonal antibody to sialophorin (CD43) induces homotypic adhesion and activation of human monocytes. *J. Exp. Med.*, **170**, 259–267.

83. Yamamoto, Y., Yamaguchi, T., Sato, K., Nishikawa, Y. and Hiragun, A. (1988) SGP 140: Identification of a novel component on human polymorphonuclear leukocyte cell surface involved in chemotactic and phagocytic activities. *Exp. Hematol.*, **16**, 12–20.

84. Kuijpers, T.W., Hoogerwerf, M., Schwarz, B.R. and Harlan, J. (in press) Crosslinking of sialophorin (CD43) induces neutrophil aggregation in a CD18-dependent and a CD18-independent way. *J. Immunol.*

85. Campanero, M.R., Pulido, R., Alonso, J.L., Pivel, J.P., Pimentel-Munoz, F., Fresno, M. and Sanchez-Madrid, F. (1991) Down regulation by tumor necrosis factor of neutrophil cell surface expression of the sialophorin CD43 and the hyaluronate receptor CD44 through a proteolytic mechanism. *Eur. J. Immunol.*, **21**, 3045–3048.

86. Silverman, L.B., Wong, R.C., Remold-O'Donnell, E., Vercelli, D., Sancho, J., Terhorst, C., Rosen, F., Geha, R. and Chatila, T. (1989) Mechanism of mononuclear cell activation by an anti-CD43 (sialophorin) agonistic antibody. *J. Immunol.*, **142**, 4194–4200.

87. Chatila, T.A. and Geha, R.S. (1988) Phosphorylation of T cell membrane proteins by activators of protein kinase C. *J. Immunol.*, **140**, 4308–4314.

88. Axelsson, B. and Perlmann, P. (1989) Persistent superphosphorylation of leukosialin (CD43) in activated T cells and in tumour cell lines. *Scand. J. Immunol.*, **30**, 539–547.

89. Wong, R.C., Remold-O'Donnell, E., Vercelli, D., Sancho, J., Terhorst, C., Rosen, F., Geha, R. and Chatila, T. (1990) Signal transduction via leukocyte antigen CD43 (sialophorin). Feedback regulation by protein kinase C. *J. Immunol.*, **144**, 1455–1460.

90. Edelman, A.M., Blumenthal, D.K. and Krebs, E.G. (1987) Protein serine/threonine kinases. *Annu. Rev. Biochem.*, **56**, 567–613.

91. Park, J.K., Rosenstein, Y., Remold-O'Donnell, E., Bierer, B.E., Rosen, F.S. and Burakoff, S.J. (1991) Enhancement of T cell activation by the CD43 molecule whose expression is defective in the Wiskott–Aldrich syndrome. *Nature*, **350**, 706–709.

92. Sleckman, B.P., Peterson, A., Jones, W.K., Foran, J.A., Greenstein, J.L., Seed, B. and Burakoff, S.J. (1987) Expression and function of CD4 in a murine T-cell hybridoma. *Nature*, **328**, 351–353.

93. Ratnofsky, S.E., Peterson, A., Greenstein, J.L. and Burakoff, S.J. (1987) Expression and function of CD8 in a murine T cell hybridoma. *J. Exp. Med.*, **166**, 1747–1757.

94. Bierer, B.E., Peterson, A., Gorga, J.C., Herrmann, S.H. and Burakoff, S.J. (1988) Synergistic T cell activation via the physiological ligands for CD2 and the T cell receptor. *J. Exp. Med.*, **168**, 1145–1156.

95. Rosenstein, Y., Park, J.K., Hahn, W.C., Rosen, F.S., Bierer, B.E. and Burakoff, S.J. (1991) CD43, a molecule defective in Wiskott–Aldrich syndrome, binds ICAM-1. *Nature*, **354**, 233–235.

96. Simmons, D., Magkoba, M.W. and Seed, B. (1988) ICAM 1, an adhesion ligand for LFA-1, is homologous to the neural cell adhesion molecule NCAM. *Nature*, **331**, 624–627.

97. Stauton, D.E., Marlin, S.D., Stratowa, C., Dustin, M.L. and Springer, T.A. (1988) Primary structure of intercellular adhesion molecule 1 (ICAM 1) demonstrates interaction between members of the immunoglobulin and integrin supergene families. *Cell*, **52**, 925–933.

98. Rothlein, R., Dustin, M.L., Marlin, S.D. and Springer, T.A. (1986) A human intercellular adhesion molecule (ICAM 1) distinct from LFA-1. *J. Immunol.*, **137**, 1270–1274.

99. Diamond, M.S., Staunton, D.E., Marlin, S.D. and Springer, T.A. (1990) Binding of the integrin MAC-1 (CD11b/cd18) to the third immunoglobulin-like domain of ICAM-1 (CD54) and its regulation by glycosylation. *Cell*, **65**, 961–971.

100. Marlin, S.D. and Springer, T.A. (1987) Purified intercellular adhesion molecule (ICAM-1) is a ligand for lymphocyte function associated antigen-1 (LFA-1). *Cell*, **51**, 813–819.

101. Smith, C.W., Marlin, S.D., Rothlein, R., Toman, C. and Anderson, D.C. (1989) Cooperative interactions of LFA-1 and MAC-1 with intercellular adhesion molecule-1 in facilitating adherence and transendothelial migration of human neutrophils in vitro. *J. Clin. Invest.*, **83**, 2008–2017.

102. Remold-O'Donnell, E. and Rosen, F.S. (1991) Sialophorin (CD43) and the Wiskott–Aldrich syndrome. *Immunodef. Rev.*, **2**, 151–174.

103. Codington, J.F., Cooper, A.G., Miller, D.K., Slayter, H.S., Brown, M.C., Silber, C. and Jeanloz, R.W. (1979) Isolation and partial characterization of an epiglycanin-like glycoprotein from a new non-strain-specific subline of TA3 murine mammary adenocarcinoma. *J. Nat. Cancer Inst.*, **63**, 153–161.

104. Galili, U., Korkesh, A., Kahane, I. and Rachmilewitz, E.A. (1983) Demonstration of a natural antigalactosyl IgG antibody on thalassemic red blood cells. *Blood*, **61**, 1258–1264.

105. Kahane, I., Ben-Chetnit, E., Shifter, A. and Rachmilowitz, E.A. (1980) The erythrocyte membranes in β-thalassemia lower sialic acid levels in glycophorin. *Biochim. Biophys. Acta.*, **596**, 10–17.

Chapter 13

Complement Deficiency: C7, C8 and Properdin

JACOV LEVY* and MENAHEM SCHLESINGER

Soroka Medical Center, Beer-Sheva and Barzilai Hospital, Ashkelon, and Faculty of Medical Sciences, Ben Gurion University of the Negev, Beer-Sheva, Israel

The protein components of the complement systems play a major role in host defences and in the generation of inflammation. Inherited or acquired deficiencies of these proteins are usually associated with increased frequency of either infections or autoimmune inflammatory processes. Activation of the complement system can either be beneficial to the host, as in resistance to invading microorganisms, or it can be detrimental, as in a variety of immunopathologically mediated diseases (1). Most of the severe complement deficiencies are inherited abnormalities associated with either the absence of a protein or the synthesis of a defective molecule. In the last decade, there have been significant developments in the field of complement and even more in complement deficiency states. Studies were conducted on the genetics and epidemiology of terminal complement component deficiencies, on the response to immunization, and on the allotypic determination of patients. Studying patients who have survived meningococcal infections has enlarged the number of patients discovered with terminal complement component deficiencies. We will focus in this chapter on the inherited deficiencies of the late components of the classical pathway, C7 and C8, and of the alternative pathway component, properdin.

---

*Author to whom correspondence should be addressed, at Department of Paediatrics, Soroka Medical Center, PO Box 151, Beer Sheva, Israel 84101.

New Concepts in Immunodeficiency Diseases. Edited by S. Gupta and C. Griscelli

THE FUNCTION OF THE COMPLEMENT SYSTEM

The complement system includes about 30 glycoproteins that interact in a highly regulated fashion in a number of ways, and its activation results in a cascade of interactions among these proteins (see Figure 13.1) (1). The components of the intricate mechanism act together to cause lysis of various microorganisms (2). This task is achieved either by complement components alone or by complement components in cooperation with antibodies and cells that express complement receptors. Thus enzymes, co-factors, receptors and other proteins act in concert to elicit inflammatory and cytocidal reactions in response to foreign antigens (3). In addition, there are several regulatory membrane proteins that protect host cells from accidental complement attack. While complement activation can be triggered by antibody–antigen complexes, it also has its own intrinsic capability for recognizing foreign organisms. Host defence mechanisms that are dependent on or modified by complement activation include opsonization and phagocytosis, recruitment and activation of immunologically active cells at sites of inflammation, processing and clearance of immune complexes, and direct lysis of many types of targets (1). One of the most important functions of complement is to mark microorganisms and other antigens with fragments of C3, thus targeting them to C3 receptor (C3R)-bearing cells, such as phagocytic cells. This in turn causes a significant facilitation of phagocytosis of the foreign antigens—a process termed opsonization. Activation of both the classical or alternative complement pathways leads to the assembly of enzymes (convertases) that cleave the α chain of native C3 between amino acid residues 77 and 78 to yield two fragments. The larger split product, C3b, rapidly undergoes a conformational change, which activates an intramolecular thioester bond on the α chain of C3 that then becomes accessible and forms a covalent linkage with a hydroxyl or amino group on another surface (4, 5). In this fashion, the activated split form of C3, C3b, can bind to a larger number of microorganisms and other antigens. The activation event generates many split products of complement proteins for which specific receptors exist on a variety of inflammatory cells, such as granulocytes, lymphocytes and other cells (6). Binding of these complement-derived products to such receptors results in biological activities such as chemotaxis, vasodilatation and edema, that significantly affect the inflammatory process. The anaphylatoxins C3a, C4a and C5a are biologically active complement-derived split products (see Figure 13.1) that, when injected into animals, induce a response that resembles anaphylaxis (7). They usually promote the secretion of mediators such as histamine and serotonin (5-hydroxy-tryptamine), cause vascular permeability and degranulation of basophils, and induce mucus secretion by tracheal goblet cells and spasmogenic response in smooth muscles (7). In addition, C5a is also strongly chemotactic for phagocytic cells, increases neutrophil adhesiveness and aggregation, triggers lysosomal enzyme release from phagocytes, and stimulates neutrophil oxidative metabolism (8). Complement activation can promote the synthesis and secretion of other inflammatory mediators. Activation of the macrophage by C5a induces the secretion of interleukin 1 (IL-1), which is a potent inflammatory cytokine. IL-1 is also produced and secreted by monocytes triggered by the C3 fragments iC3b and C3b that attach to their respective receptors (9). C5a and other activation products elicit the release of platelet-activating factor (PAF) from many cells and thus affect the arachidonate metabolism via both the lipoxygenase and cycloxygenase pathways (10). The terminal complement components, known together as the membrane attack complex, used in sublytic concentrations were shown to stimulate arachidonate metabolism in cells and platelets and cause the release of prostaglandin E_2, leukotriene B_4 and thromboxane, which contribute to the inflammatory process (11). Complement activation products may interact with substrates of other systems such as the kinin, coagulation and fibrinolytic systems. The terminal complement components that are activated following the deposition of C5b on the cell surface form together the membrane attack complex which causes the death of target cells. This killing activity

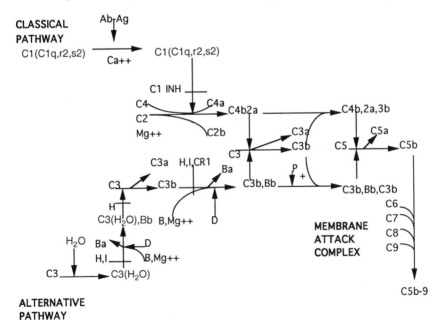

Figure 13.1. Diagram of complement activation cascade. Inhibitors are illustrated by straight, crossing lines. The positive regulatory effect of properdin is shown by an arrow and + sign. Modified from Densen (1991) *Clin. Exp. Immunol.*, **86**, 57–62, by permission of Blackwell Scientific Publications Ltd.

may be directed against viruses, bacteria, fungi, parasites, virus-infected cells and tumor cells. Two theories exist as to the precise mechanism of complement-mediated cytotoxicity: in one model, the polar domains of inserted complement proteins cause local distortion of the phospholipid bilayer, resulting in "leaky patches" (12); the alternative, "pore" model proposes that the polar surfaces of the individual complement components come together to form a hydrophilic channel through the membrane (13).

PATHWAYS OF COMPLEMENT ACTIVATION

Complement activation can occur via two possible pathways—the classical and alternative pathways—both of which lead to the creation of membrane attack (see Figure 13.1). About 30 plasma proteins participate in these pathways, and they can be divided into functional proteins, representing the elements of the various pathways, regulatory proteins with control function and receptors (8). In both the classical and the alternative complement pathways following an initial recognition event, which leads to initiation of the pathway, a proteolytic cascade phase takes place that involves the action of proteases and the recruitment of additional molecules; this is followed by a terminal phase of membrane attack during which the attacked cell dies. The primary function of both the classical and alternative pathways is to form enzymes, termed C3 convertases, that activate and split C3, forming C3b clusters. Concomitant with the formation of C3b clusters, enzymes that activate the fifth component (C5) are generated within the C3b clusters and split C5 into C5a and C5b. C5b initiates a reaction sequence from the sixth component (C6) through to the ninth component (C9), called the terminal pathway, that leads to the formation of a large protein complex termed the membrane attack complex (MAC) (see Figure 13.1). MAC has the ability to damage cell surface membranes, and it can kill certain types of microorganisms (14).

The classical pathway consists of C1, C4, C2 and C3 and is activated by antigen–antibody complexes containing IgM or IgG. Following the binding of C1 to the Fc portion of antibodies that are bound to antigens, C1 becomes an enzyme that can split C4 and C2. The C4 split product C4b binds to the surface of microorganisms and other antigens and becomes an acceptor for C2a, which is the active part of C2. The complex C4b2a thus formed is the C3 convertase of the classical pathway (15).

The alternative pathway can function in the absence of antibodies. There are two possible mechanisms of initiation of the alternative pathway activation (16). One is that it is initiated by hydrolysis of the intramolecular thioester bond of C3, inducing a conformational change in C3 in such a way that it expresses C3b-like conformation and function (1). The other mechanism is that the thioester bond of C3 is directly attacked by a hydroxyl group on the surface, resulting in covalent binding of C3b-like C3 to the surface. Because the product of the alternative pathway C3 convertase is itself a subunit of the enzyme, an amplification loop is generated (1).

Both pathways—the classical and alternative—converge at the point of C3 activity (see Figure 13.1). The C3 convertases of the two pathways are homologous to each other, as are C4 and C3, C4b and C3b, C2 and B, and C2a and Bb (17). Both of the described convertases split C3 in exactly the same way.

The terminal pathway is initiated by C5b—a split product of C5 following the enzymatic action of C5 convertase on C5. C5 convertase is formed following the clustering of C3b on the membrane surface. C4b2a3b in the classical pathway, and C3bBbC3b in the alternative pathway act as efficient convertases. Once C5b is formed, C6 through to C9 bind sequentially to form a large protein complex that contains one molecule each of C5b, C6, C7 and C8, and multiple molecules of C9 (14).

The complement regulatory proteins are of three groups: (a) inhibitors that prevent spontaneous or abortive activation in the fluid phase; (b) regulators that dampen or enhance the normal action of complement against targets; (c) inhibitors that protect host cells from the destructive action of complement (1). Among the well-studied regulatory protein are C1 inhibitor, factor H, factor I and properdin. Properdin has a distinct function of stabilizing the C3 convertase of the alternative pathway (C3bBb), preventing its degradation and potentiating its activity.

DEFICIENCIES OF TERMINAL COMPONENTS AND PROPERDIN

The terminal complement components C5–9 form the cytolytic MAC, and deficiency of any one of these proteins will block MAC formation. The molecular pathology responsible for deficiencies of the human late complement components has in no case yet been fully evaluated. Unlike properdin, no terminal complement gene component has yet been mapped completely, but Southern blot analysis of DNA from C6, C7 and C8β-deficient patients have shown normal-sized gene fragments (18).

Patients with deficiency of C5, C6, C7, C8 and C9 demonstrate a high incidence of neisserial infections and less frequent occurrence of collagen–vascular diseases (19). The reason for the predisposition of the patients to neisserial infections is unknown, but its occurrence suggests a dependence on complement-mediated bacteriolysis for host defence against neisserial species. The collagen–vascular syndromes seen in these patients include discoid lupus, systemic lupus erythematosus (SLE), sclerodactyly, Sjogren's syndrome, nephritis and other immune complex phenomena, rheumatoid arthritis and ankylosing spondylitis (20).

Most of the patients with properdin or late complement component deficiency were discovered following a single or recurrent meningococcal disease. Additional asymptomatic deficient individuals were found when patients' families were subsequently studied. Once patients had been infected they were more susceptible to further infection. The proportionally high incidence of terminal complement protein deficiencies in certain racial groups from different parts of the world suggest that there may be a selective advantage to the heterozygous deficiency state. It has been suggested that the low mortality associated with the meningococcal infections in patients with deficiency of terminal component may be partly due to the absence of the systemic inflammatory consequences of production of the MAC (20).

Some differences between terminal complement components and properdin-deficient patients are shown in Table 13.1.

Table 13.1 Neisserial infections in complement-sufficient versus complement-deficient patients

Parameter	Late complement-sufficient patients	Late complement-deficient patients	Properdin-deficient patients
Frequency of infection (%)	0.0072	60	44
Male : female ratio	1.3 : 1	2.2 : 1	21 : 0
Median age of first infection (years)	3	17	14
Recurrence rate (%)	0.34	41	2
Relapse rate (%)	0.6	7.6	0
Mortality (%)	19	2.9	12[a]

[a]Note: 12% mortality according to ref. 21. Recent works suggest a much lower incidence.

Neisserial infections in patients with late complement components and properdin deficiencies differ from infections in the normal population by various features (Table 13.1). Ross and Densen (20) and Densen (21) comprehensively described a number of interesting observations regarding these infections. Among them are high relapse and recurrence rates but a lower mortality rate in the terminal complement component-deficient patients when compared with complement-sufficient patients undergoing a neisserial infection. The relapse rate was 7.6% in the complement-deficient and 0.6% in normals. The recurrence rate was 41% in the complement-deficient and 0.34% in normals. The mortality, however, was 2.9% in the deficient compared to 19% in the normals. It should be mentioned that data about mortality rates in patients with meningococcal infections were obtained from living survivors who contracted recurrent attacks, and there is no certain way to estimate the number of complement-deficient patients among those who died during their first neisserial infection. Most of the patients who die with fulminant meningococcal infection cannot undergo a complete immunological evaluation, and finding of low CH50 or low individual late complement component level in the sera of the patients can be due to a possible complement component consumption caused by the infection, and does not necessarily show a congenital complement deficiency. The occurrence of complement component deficiency was studied by us in the families of patients who died of neisserial infections and was found to be greater proportionally than its occurrence in the general population (unpublished data), suggesting that the true mortality rate of patients with complement component deficiency is greater than is apparent from examination of the living survivors. Patients with terminal complement component deficiency contract neisserial infection at a mean age of 17 years as compared to normals that have the infection at the mean age of 3 years. Other aspects common to all the terminal component deficiencies include disseminated gonococcal infections and probably a slightly increased incidence of immune complex disease (22–24). This last feature is probably due to the fact that MAC contributes to the elimination of viruses and other microorganisms. No heterozygotes for C3, C5, C6, C7, C8 or C9 have been described with neisserial infection. Subjects with properdin deficiency demonstrate a tendency to neisserial infections that is different than in patients with late complement component deficiency (Table 13.1): relapse and recurrence rates are lower but the mortality rate is higher than in late complement component-deficient patients. There is also a different male : female ratio that stems from the X-linked inheritance of properdin deficiency. Some patients have a fulminant onset of disease with a very high mortality rate (21); however, we and others have described a group of patients with a milder course. We encountered 3 patients with non-fulminant course (25), and Fijen *et al.* reported 9 patients, only one of them with concomitant severe sepsis (26). The past impression that properdin-deficient patients had a fulminant disease with severe outcome stemmed from a report of a single family containing a large number of patients with dysfunctional properdin (27). It seems that two groups of properdin-deficient patients exist, and that they differ from each other according to the severity of their neisserial infection. All properdin-deficient patients described so far did not show a recurrence of their neisserial infection.

C7 DEFICIENCY

C7 is structurally similar to, and genetically linked with, C6 (28). C7 deficiency is quite rare among Caucasians and, in contrast, it is the second most frequent complement deficiency in the Japanese (about 1 in 25 000) (29). In Israel all C7-deficient patients described so far are Sepharadi Jews of either Moroccan or Yemenite origin (25, 30). Deficient individuals may have residual traces of C7, which is presumably dysfunctional.

Hereditary homozygous deficiency of C7 was first reported in 1975 in a 42-year-old woman with CREST syndrome (calcinosis, Raynaud's phenomenon, oesophageal dysfunction, sclerodactyly, telangiectasia) (31) and in a healthy boy (32). Later on, two sisters were described with this defect associated with neisserial infections (33). Since then, about 45 patients with C7 deficiency have been found; most of them were patients surviving from neisserial disease (see Table 13.2). Recently a Japanese adolescent was reported to have C7 deficiency and a persistent haematuria, without evidence of glomerulonephritis or glomerular immunodeposition (34). Three apparently unrelated cases of combined deficiency of C6 and C7 have been reported, reflecting the close genetic linkage of these components (35, 36). One of these patients showed a tendency for *Candida* and *Toxoplasma* infections (36). Patients with complete C7 deficiency display a C7*Q0 silent allele which can be showed using a C7 cDNA probe detecting a TaqI restriction fragment length polymorphism in patients or carriers (37). Three Japanese families showing C7 deficiency were described with an association between the C7 silent allele (C7*Q0) and C6*B (38). Since C6 and C7 loci are closely linked on chromosome 9, the combined deficiencies are likely to be due to a single genetic disorder affecting both genes rather than due to two separate mutations (18, 28). An individual who had meningococcal septicaemia was shown to have a combined deficiency of C7 and C4B (39). Currently a sensitive ELISA assay utilizing a monoclonal antibody directed to native C7 has made it possible to detect and quantitate more accurately patients with complete, partial and functional deficiencies (40). Family studies of patients with C7 deficiency have demonstrated an autosomal co-dominant pattern of inheritance with no evidence of linkage between the A and B loci of the HLA complex and the locus for C7 (41). Some C7-deficient individuals were found to have C7 levels of around 0.3% of the normal mean concentration, which may or may not be functionally active (40). Other C7-deficient subjects presented with C7 levels just above the detection limit of the ELISA (40), which may also be explained by a cross-reactivity of the ELISA antibodies with other plasma constituents.

So far 45 patients with C7 deficiency, most of them discovered following a meningococcal infection, were reported and are described in Table 13.2.

C8 DEFICIENCY

C8 is composed of three polypeptide chains: α, β and γ. The α and γ chains are linked covalently through disulphide bonds to form the α–γ subunit,

Table 13.2 Currently reported C7-deficient patients

Patient no.	Deficiency	Age	Sex	Origin	Infection	Ref.
1	C7	14	M	Japanese	MI	42
2	C7	17	M	Japanese	MI	42
3	C7	15	M	Japanese	MI	42
4	C7	16	M	Japanese	MI	42
5	C7, C6	21	F	White	*Toxopl.*, *Candida*	36
6	C7	3	F	White	MI × 3	43
7	C7	22	M	Swiss	MI	44
8	C7	19	M	Swiss	MI	44
9	C7	16		French	MI × 2	45
10	C7	28	M		MI Carditis	39
11	C7		M			39
12	C7	21	M	Hispanic	MI × 3 IgA defic.	46
13	C7	8	F	Japanese	MI	47
14	C7	19	F		HPM	48
15	C7		M			48
16	C7	40	M	White	Chronic Meningoc., vasculitis	49
17	C7	26	M	Sephardic Jew	Meningitis	30
18	C7	21	F	Sephardic Jew	MI	30
19	C7		M	Sephardic Jew		30
20	C7	5	F	Sephardic Jew	MI	30
21	C7		F	Sephardic Jew		30
22	C7		F	Sephardic Jew		30
23	C7	7	M	Sephardic Jew	MI	30
24	C7	17	F	Sephardic Jew	MI	30
25	C7		F	Sephardic Jew		30
26	C7	10	M	Sephardic Jew	MI × 2	30
27	C7	15	F	Dutch	Meningoc. Toxopl.	26
28	C7	21	M	Dutch	Meningoc. × 2	26
29	C7	4	M	Dutch	Meningoc. × 4	26
30	C7	17	F	White	MI × 3	50
31	C7	20	F	Sephardic Jew	Meningoc.	51
32	C7	25	M	Sephardic Jew	MI	51
33	C7		M	Sephardic Jew		51
34	C7			Danish	MI	52
35	C7	8	M	Japanese		34
36	C7		M	Japanese		34
37	C7		M	Hispanic	MI Recurrent	37
38	C7		M	Hispanic	MI Recurrent	37
39	C7		M	Hispanic		37
40	C7		M	Hispanic		37
41	C7	6	F	Sephardic Jew	MI	25
42	C7	13	M	Sephardic Jew	MI	25
43	C7	21	M	Sephardic Jew	MI	25
44	C7	18	F	Sephardic Jew	MI	25
45	C7	38	M	Sephardic Jew	MI	25

MI, *Neisseria meningitidis* meningitis; Toxopl., toxoplasmosis; Meningoc., meningococcaemia;
HPM, *Haemophilus parainfluenzae* meningitis.

which is highly polymorphic. The β subunit is bound to C8α-γ through non-covalent forces such that the individual chains are present in the intact C8 in an equimolar ratio (53). The β chain possesses a specific recognition site for C5 (54) and the α chain possesses one for C9 (55).

C8 is an important constituent of the lytic MAC, though it paradoxically also prevents membrane damage by binding to the nascent C5b–7 complex in the fluid phase and thus inhibiting its attachment to the nearby membrane surfaces (56).

C8 is a complex molecule, composed of three non-identical chains (α, β and γ), each the product of a distinct gene (57, 58). The structural genes of the distinct C8 chains are closely linked but seem to be differentially expressed. The genes encoding α and β chains are physically linked and situated on chromosome 1, while the genes encoding the γ subunit have been mapped to chromosome 9q (59). The α-γ and β chains are non-covalently linked, while the α and γ chains are held together by disulphide bonds (58). Deficiency of C8 may be the result of a defect in synthesis of either the α-γ unit or of the β unit (60). The first deficiencies of the α-γ chain described presented with functional and immunochemical absence of C8, because the remaining β chain was not detected by conventional antisera (60). Only the C8β defect has been found in Caucasians, whereas defects in the synthesis of C8α-γ predominates in Blacks and Japanese (29). In both forms of deficiency the uninvolved subunit is present in serum at a diminished concentration (61). The admixture of serum from α-γ and β chain-deficient patients permits the reassembly of functional C8 and restores complement activity (60). At present, it is unclear whether the reduction in C8β observed in C8α-γ-deficient subjects reflects the tight 5'–3' linkage between the C8α and C8β loci (62) or is due to a post-translational requirement of C8α-γ for either C8β secretion or protection from intracellular proteolysis (63).

C8 deficiency has a heterogeneous presentation, and dysfunctional C8 subunits have been found in some C8-deficient persons (58). In an analysis of sera of three patients with C8α-γ deficiency it was demonstrated that although they contained minuscule quantities of all three subunit chains, there was an additional dysfunction of C8α-γ, while the β chain was functionally intact despite its low quantity. It is suggested that β chain levels are dependent on the production of α-γ chains but not vice versa (61).

C8 deficiency is the most frequently inherited defect of the late components and, in general, of all the complement components except C2. Analysis of the disease associated with the C8 deficiency reveals a low frequency of autoimmune disease, in contrast to the frequency observed in the abnormalities of the early complement components (64). Most of the patients experience single or repeated episodes of neisserial infections, and they are at increased risk of developing systemic infection with *Neisseria meningitidis* and to a lesser effect with *Neisseria gonorrhoeae* (20).

The increased susceptibility of C8-deficient subjects to neisserial infections has been attributed to the lack of the complement-dependent bactericidal activity in their serum (65). Due to the overlap found between the serum Cγ level in normals and heterozygotes the detection of heterozygotes is not always possible. Tedesco (61) suggested immunoblotting technique in order to overcome this problem. Two families have been identified with antigenically detectable but functionally inactive C8 (66). Individuals with functional C8β deficiency have been shown to express reduced C8β messenger RNA (mRNA), suggesting that their cells produce less C8β-specific mRNA and thus show an abnormality in intracellular events that precede the secretion. The C8β-specific mRNA was detected in the patients using hybridization with radiolabelled C8β probe (67). A transcriptional abnormality was suggested as the cause of this deficiency but the possibility of small deletions or insertions could not be ruled out. A detailed study of a group of C8α-γ-deficient patients revealed that they may present with two types of abnormality: with low level of C8β chain and with a dysfunctional C8α-γ subunit (61). Because the haemolytic activity of the C8α-γ subunit resides in the α chain, it seems likely that a defect in the C8α gene is the basis for C8α-γ deficiency. However, a preliminary report suggests that C8α mRNA is present in normal amounts in fibroblasts from deficient individuals (68). Thus, γ chain deficiency may play a role in this deficiency.

Individuals with C8 deficiency show an absent classical serum haemolytic activity (CH50) similar to patients with other late complement deficiencies, but, because the patients lack either the α-γ or the β subunits, conventional radial immunodiffusion studies often detect the presence of a low quantity of C8 protein (30% of normal in our laboratory). Thus, more sensitive techniques are needed to find heterozygotes, and immunoblotting is usually used (69), utilizing chain-specific monoclonal or polyclonal antibodies (18). The haemolytic activity of the remaining subunit can be assessed by using serum deficient in this subunit. This leads to restoration of haemolytic activity, suggesting that the C8 subunits reassociate in serum (60). The presence of an inhibitor was described in C8β-deficient sera which interfered with full reconstitution. This was thought to be a dysfunctional β chain, interfering with the C8 restoration by competing with the added C8β.

Currently 30 patients were reported with C8 deficiency, and they are shown in Table 13.3.

PROPERDIN DEFICIENCY

Properdin is a regulatory molecule whose task is to stabilize the complex C3bBb of the alternative pathway. Properdin deficiency is the only

Table 13.3 Currently reported C8-deficient patients

Patient	Deficiency	Age	Sex	Origin	Infection	Ref.
1	C8β	12	M	White		66
2	C8β	16	F	White	Bronchitis Sinusitis	66
3	C8	26	M	Sephardic Jew		70
4	C8β	16	M	Sephardic Jew	MI × 4	70
5	C8β	24	M	Sephardic Jew		70
6	C8β	8	M	Sephardic Jew	MI × 2	51
7	C8β		M	Sephardic Jew		30
8	C8β	9	F	Sephardic Jew	Meningitis	30
9	C8β	17	F	Sephardic Jew	Meningitis	30
10	C8β	15	M	Sephardic Jew	MI	30
11	C8α-γ	26	M	Sephardic Jew	MI	30
12	C8β	21	F	Sephardic Jew	MI × 3	30
13	C8β	18	M	Sephardic Jew	MI	30
14	C8	11	M	Dutch	Meningoc. × 2	26
15	C8	30	F	Dutch	Meningoc.	26
16	C8	13	M		MI × 2	71
17	C8	36	F		MI	71
18	C8	6	M		Meningitis	71
19	C8β	13	F	White	MI × 2	71
20	C8β			Danish	MI	52
21	C8	18	M		MI × 3	72
22	C8	10	F	Austrian	Meningoc. × 2	74
23	C8β	27	M	White	TB	74
24	C8				MI	75
25	C8α-γ	20	F	Black	Gonococ.	76
26	C8β	12	M	Sephardic Jew	MI	25
27	C8β		M	Sephardic Jew		25
29	C8β	7	F	Sephardic Jew	MI	25
30	C8β	8	M	Sephardic Jew	MI	25

MI, *Neisseria meningitidis* meningitis; Meningoc., meningococcaemia; TB, tuberculosis; Gonococ., gonococcaemia.

complement component deficiency that demonstrates sex-linked inheritance (77, 78). Properdin synthesis is genetically controlled by a functional gene whose position has been localized by genetic linkage analysis to the proximal part (DXS-255) of the X chromosome short arm, near the centromere, indicating that the deficiency results from an abnormality in the structural gene (79, 62). Recently the complete gene structure of properdin has been described (80).

Although their molecular pathogenesis is not yet clear, three types of properdin deficiency have been described: (a) no detectable activity and extremely low levels of the protein; (b) active and normally structured properdin at about 10% of normal levels; and (c) normal quantities of a dysfunctional protein (81–83). Properdin deficiency has been associated with fulminant and rapidly fatal meningococcal disease in about half of the patients (see Table 13.1). Most of the patients, however, had dysfunctional properdin and were members of one large family. Few recent reports describe a non-fulminant and a favourable outcome to properdin-deficient patients (26, 25). Female carriers may also show an increased risk for overwhelming meningococcal infection (20). The functions of the alternative pathway are invariantly markedly reduced (84). A combination of inherited deficiencies of the complement components properdin and C2 was described in association with recurrent pneumococcal infections (85). In contrast to the patients with late complement component deficiencies who demonstrate an increased frequency of infections but a lower fatality rate than complement-sufficient patients with meningococcal disease, some of the patients with properdin deficiency manifest both increased frequency and severity of infections, with a high fatality rate (78). Recently, however, it has become increasingly clear that, while meningococcal infection is the predominant clinical manifestation, it does not always result in the poor prognosis reported initially (28, 85). We have studied nine properdin-deficient subjects in Israel; two of them had meningococcal infection and one had *Haemophilus influenzae* meningitis, whose course resembled that of late complement component deficiency, rather than the fulminant course previously reported in properdin deficiency. All the individuals were Sephardic Jews who originally immigrated to Israel from Tunisia, which are notorious for their high intermarriage rate. This is in contrast to the very low prevalence of properdin deficiency among Sephardic Jews of Moroccan origin, who show a relatively high prevalence of the late complement components deficiency (30, 25).

The screening for the alternative pathway deficiency states calls for performance of the AP50 test, which in the case of properdin deficiency is very low, albeit not zero, owing to the auxiliary role of properdin in the alternative pathway. The final diagnosis can be established by estimation of properdin serum level. A large overlap exists between the serum properdin level in heterozygotes and in the normal population, which may be accentuated by lyonization and therefore makes the diagnosis of the heterozygotes quite difficult. In our experience the western blot analysis is superior to radial immunodiffusion in the evaluation of this situation. In two Israeli families the genetic study by Southern blot analysis of properdin-deficient sera did not reveal a defect using a DNA probe, suggesting that the defect stems from a point mutation or a regulatory defect rather than a large chromosomal deletion.

In Table 13.4 we present 40 properdin-deficient patients currently reported in the literature.

Table 13.4 Update of properdin-deficient patients

Patient no.	Deficiency	Age (years)	Sex	Origin	Infection	Ref.
1	P	0.1	M	W	Pneu. × 2 Cellulitis Oral *Candida*	86
2	P	15	M	W	MI Death	27
3	P	25	M	W	Meningit. × 2	27
4	P	40	M	W		27
5	P (partial)		M	W	Healthy	87
6	P (partial)		F	W	Healthy	87
7	P	30	M	W	MI Death	77
8	P	18	M	W	MI Death	77
9	P	4	M	W	MI × 2 Measles Death	77
10	P	11	M	Danish	Meningoc. Purpura	88
11	P	20	M	Danish	Meningoc. Sepsis Death	88
12	P	0.11	M	Danish	Meningoc.	88
13	P&C2	9	M	W	Rec. otitis Rec. Pneu. or bacterem.	85
14	P	58	M	Swedish	Healthy	81
15	P	29	M	Swedish	Healthy	81
16	P	16	M	Tunisian Jewish	Meningit.	25
17	P	14	M	Tunisian Jewish	Meningit.	25
18	P		M	Tunisian Jewish	Healthy	25
19	P	47	M	Scottish	Discoid lupus, TB	89
20	P		M	Scottish	Healthy	89
21	P		M	Scottish	Healthy	89
22	P		M	Scottish	Healthy	89
23	P		M	Danish	Chronic meningoc. Low IgG	90
24	P		M	Swedish	Meningoc. Death	91
25	P		M	Swedish	Pneumoc. Pneu. *Borrelia* Meningit.	91
26	P		M	Swedish	Healthy	91
27	P	13	M	W	MI	92

Table 13.4 (*cont.*)

Patient no.	Deficiency	Age (years)	Sex	Origin	Infection	Ref.
28	P	15	M	W	MI	92
29	P	11	M	Dutch	MI	26
30	P	17	M	Dutch	MI	26
31	P	22	M	Dutch	Sepsis Meningoc.	26
32	P	13	M	Dutch	MI	26
33	P	13	M	Dutch	MI	26
34	P	17	M	Dutch	MI	26
35	P	14	M	Dutch	MI ARF	26
36	P	0.1	M	Tunisian Jewish	HIB Meningitis	Not published
37	P	15	M	Tunisian Jewish	Healthy	Not published
38	P	25	M	Tunisian Jewish	Healthy	Not published
39	P	40	M	Tunisian Jewish	Healthy	Not published
40	P		M	Tunisian Jewish	Healthy	Not published

W, White; Pneu., pneumonia; Pneumoc., pneumococcal; Meningoc., meningococcaemia; Meningit., meningitis; MI, *Neisseria meningitidis* meningitis; Rec., recurrent; Bacterem., bacteraemia; TB, tuberculosis; ARF, acute rheumatic fever; HIB, *Haemophilus* influenza group B.

EPIDEMIOLOGY OF TERMINAL COMPLEMENT COMPONENT AND PROPERDIN DEFICIENCIES

All of the complement component deficiencies are inherited in an autosomal recessive manner except properdin deficiency, which is inherited in X-linked fashion. Studies in European and North American populations of patients with late complement component deficiencies suggest that C7 and C8β deficiencies are found predominantly in Caucasians, whereas C8α-γ deficiency is more common in Blacks, Chinese and Hispanics (63). A prevalence of deficiencies of C7, C8 and properdin of approximately 10% has been identified in Sephardic Jews living in Israel presenting with sporadic meningococcal disease (30, 25). In one of the studies (25), 11 individuals with properdin C7 and C8 deficiency were found following meningococcal infections. The patients with C7 and C8 deficiency were all Sephardic Jews originating from Morocco and Yemen, and the patients with properdin deficiency were all Sephardic Jews from Tunisia. Similar observations were made by Zimran *et al.* (30) regarding C7 and C8 deficiencies. A survey done in Holland has found terminal complement-deficiency patients that consisted 21% of 151 survivors of meningococcal diseases (93), while a study from the former USSR showed a 2% likelihood of finding late complement component deficiency among Russian patients who had only one meningococcal infection, and a 40% likelihood among those who had recurrent infections. In this study all the subjects who had recurrent meningococcal disease with proven bacteraemia had complement deficiency (94). It must be emphasized that, because of the infrequent occurrence of complement protein deficiencies, the studies conducted so far involved rather selective populations, usually survivors of neisserial infections, and with the increased selectivity the occurrence of complement component deficiency increases. Fijen has shown an increased selectivity for complement component deficiency in individuals older than 10 years, in those with recurrent neisserial infection and in patients that had infections with meningococcal infection due to uncommon serogroups (26). Densen has pointed out a curious inverse correlation between the prevalence of meningococcal disease in the general population of certain countries and that of meningococcal disease associated with terminal complement component deficiency (21). This inverse incidence may explain the tendency of complement-deficient patients to have infections with strains of *Meningococcus* different from those usually found in their country. It may also suggest that late complement components are particularly important in control of uncommon strains of meningococcus. According to Densen's hypothesis the spread of an epidemic strain among a population in which most individuals are susceptible will affect a proportionally greater number of complement-sufficient than complement-deficient individuals, because the former greatly outnumber the latter. But then, when the number of immune individuals, and, as a consequence, the level of general immunity in that population increases, there is a disproportionately greater decrease in susceptibility to infection in complement-sufficient than in complement-deficient individuals who remain at risk due to their MAC-associated bactericidal defect. Thus, two factors play a major role in the determination of the frequency of meningococcal infection in a given population: one is the incidence of meningococcal disease in the general population of the area, and the other is the prevalence of terminal complement component deficiency in the same population. Similar considerations are justified also in the case of properdin deficiency, in which the alternative complement pathway is compromised due to an impaired stability of the alternative pathway C3-convertase.

BACTERICIDAL EFFECT OF SERUM

A wealth of data support a major role for antibody to subcapsular antigens in protecting normal individuals from meningococcal disease (95, 96). Meningococcal disease caused by a certain serotype confers immunity to other, unrelated serotypes, suggesting the presence of cross-reactive antibodies directed against subcapsular rather than capsular antigens. Although these subcapsular antibodies have also been demonstrated in late-complement-deficient patients, they seem to protect complement-sufficient individuals much better than complement-deficient patients. Antibodies against *Meningococcus* are readily formed in complement-deficient patients, and the immune response to meningococcal disease in these patients is assumed to be similar to that in normal people (21).

Complement-mediated bactericidal activity is one of the mechanisms participating in the immune control of meningococcal infections, and that is severely impaired in patients with late complement component deficiency (97). Neisserial strains can be either serum sensitive or serum resistant (98). Complement-deficient individuals develop infections with serum-sensitive strains of *Neisseria*, but they readily phagocytose and kill these strains (20). Complement-mediated phagocytosis and serum bactericidal killing of 62 strains of *Meningococcus* were studied using C8-depleted and pooled human serum (99). Serogroups B and 29E, but not A, C, Y and W135, were ingested and killed by neutrophils in C8-depleted serum. Group B meningococci were resistant to complement-mediated serum bactericidal activity, whereas group Y were susceptible.

A patient was described with recurrent meningococcal meningitis and a combined deficiency of C8 and antimeningococcal antibody (75).

MANAGEMENT OF PATIENTS WITH PROPERDIN, C7 AND C8 DEFICIENCIES

Specific therapy for the hereditary deficiencies of complement does not presently exist. However, careful clinical supervision and prompt management of infections could make a major impact on the health and survival of the patients. Fever occurring in a patient with properdin, C7 or C8 deficiency dictates an early intervention, like obtaining blood cultures and immediate antibiotic treatment, before the result of the cultures is known. The antibiotic treatment given to the patients with such deficiencies must include antineisserial drugs. Prophylactic administration of antibiotics is not recommended in patients with terminal complement or properdin deficiencies, because of failure of penicillin in the prophylaxis of meningococcal disease (20).

The humoral immune response to meningococcal antigen in persons lacking properdin or one of the terminal complement components has been assumed to be similar to that in normal people. Both natural antibodies and those appearing following meningococcal infection are supposed to supply some degree of protection from recurrent meningococcal infections in prop-

Immunodeficiency Diseases

erdin, C7- or C8-deficient persons as they do in the normal population. But, whereas these antibodies confer significant protection in complement-sufficient individuals, they fail to achieve the same protection in complement-deficient patients. According to Figueroa *et al.* a prior meningococcal disease does not convey protection from subsequent infection in terminal component-deficient individuals, so that the risk of each infection is an independent event and is approximately 39% (63).

Two patients with properdin deficiency were vaccinated with tetravalent meningococcal vaccine and have responded with normal classical pathway-mediated opsonic and bactericidal activities. Their alternative pathway-mediated immune functions have improved moderately (100).

Antibodies against capsular and subcapsular meningococcal antigens have been very efficiently elicited in complement-deficient patients by tetravalent meningococcal vaccine (77, 100). These antibodies were shown to promote the elimination of meningococci in *in vitro* assays that correlate with *in vivo* protection. More studies are necessary in order to clarify the exact mechanism of such elimination. During an acute meningococcal infection there are mainly three immunological mechanisms that participate in the elimination of the bacteria: (a) C3-mediated opsonization; (b) Fc receptor-mediated opsonization; and (c) MAC-mediated bactericidal activity. Obviously, the MAC-mediated action does not exist in late complement component deficiency, while in properdin-deficient patients the classical pathway is usually normal, but there is a significant deficiency in the recruitment of C3 and MAC due to a defective alternate pathway. By induction of antibody response to meningococcal vaccine, a compensatory augmentation of an immune mechanism alternative to the defective complement-mediated (MAC or C3) one is created, which can offer an additional protection to the complement-deficient patients. In fact, a tetravalent (A, C, Y, W135) meningococcal vaccine was given to a properdin-deficient family with a resultant improvement of their *in vitro* anti-*Meningococcus* bactericidal activity (77).

Plasma infusion treatment has been attempted in a variety of patients with complement component deficiency. In several cases, the reversal of clinical and biochemical abnormalities has been of sufficient magnitude and duration to suggest the clinical use of plasma infusion at the onset of an acute infectious event (101, 102). This treatment, however, may be justified only in time of emergency because of the many inconveniences and contraindications involved in a prolonged plasma infusion, which include short *in vivo* half-life of external complement components, transmission of infectious agents, and sensitization.

REFERENCES

1. Kinoshita, T. (1991) Biology of complement: The overture. *Immunol. Today,* **12**, 291–295.
2. Podack, E.R. and Tschopp, J. (1984) Membrane attack by complement. *Mol. Immunol.,* **21**, 589–603.
3. Frank, M.M. and Fries, L.F. (1991) The role of complement in inflammation and phagocytosis. *Immunol. Today,* **12**, 322–326.
4. Levine, R.P. and Dodds, A.W. (1989) The thioester bond of C3. *Curr. Top. Microbiol. Immunol.,* **153**, 73–82.
5. Goldstein, I.M. (1988) Complement: Biologically active products. In Gallin, J.I., Goldstein, I.M. and Sneiderman, R. (eds) *Inflammation: Basic Principles and Clinical Correlates.* Raven Press, New York, pp. 55–74.
6. Ross, G.D. and Medoff, M.E. (1985) Membrane complement receptors specific for bound fragments of C3. *Adv. Immunol.,* **37**, 217–267.
7. Hugli, T.E. and Muller-Eberhard, H.J. (1978) Anaphylatoxins: C3a and C5a. *Adv. Immunol.,* **26**, 1–53.
8. Berger, M. and Frank, M.M. (1989) The serum complement. In Stiehm, E.R. (ed.) *Immunologic Disorders in Infants and Children.* Saunders, Philadelphia, pp. 97–115.
9. Couturier, C., Haeffner-Cavaillon, N., Weiss, L. *et al.* (1990) Induction of cell-associated interleukin 1 through stimulation of the adhesion-promoting proteins LFA-1 and CR3 of human monocytes. *Eur. J. Immunol.,* **20**, 999–1005.
10. Pinckard, R.N., Ludwig, J.C. and McManus, L.M. (1988) Platelet-activating factors. In Gallin, J.I., Goldstein, I.M. and Sneiderman, R. (eds) *Inflammation: Basic Principles and Clinical Correlates.* Raven Press, New York, pp. 139–167.
11. Daniels, R.H., Williams, B.D. and Morgan, B.P. (1990) Stimulation of human rheumatoid synovial cells by non-lethal complement membrane attack. *Immunology,* **71**, 312–316.
12. Esser, A.F. (1991) Big MAC attack: Complement proteins cause leaky patches. *Immunol. Today,* **12**, 316–318.
13. Bhakdi, S. and Tranum-Jensen, J. (1991) Complement lysis: A hole is a hole. *Immunol. Today,* **12**, 318–320.
14. Muller-Eberhard, H.J. (1986) The membrane attack complex of complement. *Annu. Rev. Immunol.,* **4**, 503–528.
15. Ziccardi, R.J. (1981) Activation of the early components of the classical complement pathway under physiologic conditions. *J. Immunol.,* **126**, 1769–1773.
16. Fries, L.F., O'Shea, J.J. and Frank, M.M. (1986) Inherited deficiencies of complement and complement-related proteins. *Clin. Immunol. Immunopathol.,* **40**, 37–49.
17. Campbell, R.D., Law, S.K.A., Reid, K.B.M. *et al.* (1988) Structure, organization and regulation of the complement genes. *Annu. Rev. Immunol.,* **6**, 161–195.
18. Wurzner, R., Orren, A. and Lachmann, P.J. (1992) Inherited deficiencies of the terminal components of human complement. *Immunodef. Rev.,* **3**, 123–147.
19. Johnston, R.B., Jr. (1989) Disorders of the complement system. In Stiehm, E.R. (ed.) *Immunologic Disorders in Infants and Children* (3rd edn.) Saunders, Philadelphia, pp. 384–399.
20. Ross, G.D. and Densen, P. (1984) Complement deficiency states and infection: Epidemiology, pathogenesis and consequences of neisserial and other infections in an immune deficiency. *Medicine,* **63**, 243–273.
21. Densen, P. (1991) Complement deficiencies and meningococcal disease. *Clin. Exp. Immunol.,* **86** (Suppl. 1), 57–62.

22. Breckenridge, R.T., Rosenfeld, S.I., Graff, K.S. *et al.* (1977) Hereditary C5 deficiency in man. Studies of hemostasis and platelet responses to zymosan. *J. Immunol.*, **118**, 12–16.
23. Zeitz, H.J., Miller, G.W., Lint, T.F. *et al.* (1981) Deficiency of C7 with SLE: Solubilization of immune complexes in complement-deficient sera. *Arthritis Rheum.*, **24**, 87–93.
24. Reinitz, E., Lawrence, M., Diamond, B. *et al.* (1986) Arthritis and anti nuclear antibodies with inherited deficiency of the sixth component of complement. *Ann. Rheum. Dis.*, **45**, 431–434.
25. Schlesinger, M., Nave, Y., Levy, J. *et al.* (1990) Prevalence of hereditary properdin, C7 and C8 deficiencies in patients with meningococcal infections. *Clin. Exp. Immunol.*, **81**, 423–427.
26. Fijen, C.A., Kuijper, E.J., Hannema, A.J. *et al.* (1989) Complement deficiencies in patients over ten years old with meningococcal disease due to uncommon serogroups. *Lancet*, **ii**, 585–588.
27. Sjoholm, A.G., Braconier, J.H. and Soderstorm, C. (1982) Properdin deficiency in a family with fulminant meningococcal infections. *Clin. Exp. Immunol.*, **50**, 291–297.
28. Fernie, B.A., Hobart, M.J., DiScipio, R. *et al.* (1991) Molecular characterization of the genes for complement components of C6 and C7. *Complement*, **170** (Abstract 66).
29. Inai, S., Akagaki, Y., Moriyama, T. *et al.* (1989) Inherited deficiencies of the late-acting complement components other than C9 found among healthy blood donors. *Int. Arch. Allergy Appl. Immunol.*, **90**, 274–279.
30. Zimran, A., Rudensky, B., Kramer, M.R. *et al.* (1987) Hereditary complement deficiency in survivors of meningococcal disease: High prevalence of C7/C8 deficiency in Sepharadi Jews. *Q. J. Med.*, **240**, 349–354.
31. Boyer, J.T., Gall, E.P., Normal, M.E. *et al.* (1975) Hereditary deficiency of the seventh component of complement. *J. Clin. Invest.*, **56**, 905–913.
32. Wellek, B. and Opferkuch, W. (1975) A case of deficiency of the seventh component of complement in man. *Clin. Exp. Immunol.*, **19**, 223–235.
33. Lee, T.J., Utsinger, P.D., Snyderman, R. *et al.* (1978) Familial deficiency of the seventh component of complement associated with recurrent bacteremic infections due to *Neisseria*. *J. Infect. Dis.*, **138**, 359–368.
34. Sakano, T., Hamasaki, T., Mori, M. *et al.* (1988) C7 deficiency and persistent hematuria. *Eur. J. Pediatr.*, **147**, 516–517.
35. Lachmann, P.J., Hobart, M.J. and Woo, P. (1978) Combined genetic deficiency of C6 and C7 in man. *Clin. Exp. Immunol.*, **33**, 193–203.
36. Morgan, B.P., Vora, J.P. and Bennett, A.J. (1989) A case of hereditary combined deficiency of complement components C6 and C7 in man. *Clin. Exp. Immunol.*, **75**, 396–401.
37. Coto, E., Martinez-Naves, E., Dominguez, O. *et al.* (1990) DNA polymorphism of the human complement component C7 gene in familial deficiencies. *Hum. Genet.*, **85**, 251–252.
38. Nishimukai, H., Kitamura, H., Takeuchi, Y. *et al.* (1988) Three Japanese families with members carrying C7 silent allele (C7*Q0): Possibility for an association between C7Q0 and C6*B. *Hum. Hered.*, **38**, 246–250.
39. Chapel, H.M., Peto, T.E., Luzzi, G.A. *et al.* (1987) Combined familial C7 and C4B deficiency in an adult with meningococcal disease. *Clin. Exp. Immunol.*, **67**, 55–58.

40. Wurzner, R., Orren, A., Potter, P. *et al.* (1991) Functionally active complement proteins C6 and C7 detected in C6- and C7-deficient individuals. *Clin. Exp. Immunol.*, **83**, 430–437.

41. Lopez-Larrea, C., Dominguez, O., Martinez-Naves, E. *et al.* (1990) Study of genetic polymorphism of seventh complement component in two families with hereditary deficit. *Compl. Inflamm.*, **7**, 90–94.

42. Ngata, M.T., Hara, T., Aoki, Y. *et al.* (1989) Inherited deficiency of ninth component of complement: An increased risk of meningococcal meningitis. *J. Pediatr.*, **114**, 260–264.

43. Nurenberger, W.H., Pietsch, R., Seger, T. *et al.* (1989) Familial deficiency of the seventh component of complement associated with recurrent meningococcal infections. *Eur. J. Pediatr.*, **148**, 758–760.

44. Straub, P.W. and Spath, P.J. (1986) Meningococcal meningitis in isolated familial deficiency of the 7th complement component. *Schweiz. Med. Wochenschr.*, **116**, 699–702.

45. Ragnaud, J.M., Bezian, J.H. and Aubertin, J. (1984) Recurrent *Neisseria meningitidis* meningitis associated with deficiency of the 7th complement component. *Presse Med.*, **13**, 2585.

46. Jimenez-de Diego, L., Fernandez-Ballesteros, A., Varleo-Donoso, C. *et al.* (1982) Deficit de C7 Asociado a meningitis purulenta de repeticion. *Med. Clin. (Barcelona)*, **81**, 347–349.

47. Miyake, T.K., Ohta, K., Kawamori, J. *et al.* (1986) Inherited deficiency of the seventh component of complement associated with meningococcal meningitis. *Microbiol. Immunol.*, **30**, 363–372.

48. Raoult, D.M., Drancourt, H., Gallais, P. *et al.* (1987) *Hemophilus parainfluenzae* meningitis in an adult with an inherited deficiency of the seventh component of complement. *Arch. Intern. Med.*, **147**, 2214.

49. Adams, E.M., Hustead, S., Rubin, P. *et al.* (1983) Absence of the seventh component of complement in a patient with chronic meningococcemia presenting as vasculitis. *Ann. Intern. Med.*, **99**, 35–38.

50. Maitra, S. and Ghosh, S.K. (1989) Recurrent pyogenic meningitis: A retrospective study. *Q. J. Med.*, **73**, 919–929.

51. Molad, Y., Zimran, A., Sidi, Y. *et al.* (1990) Posttraumatic meningococcemia in a patient with deficiency of the C7 complement component. *Isr. J. Med. Sci.*, **26**, 90–92.

52. Nielsen, H.E., Koch, C., Magnussen, P. *et al.* (1989) Congenital deficiencies in selected groups of patients with meningococcal disease. *Scand. J. Infect. Dis.*, **21**, 389–396.

53. Steckel, E.W., York, R.G., Monahan, J.B. *et al.* (1980) The eighth component of human complement: Purification and physicochemical characterization of its unusual subunit structure. *J. Biol. Chem.*, **255**, 11997–12005.

54. Stewart, J.L. and Sodetz, J.M. (1985) Existence of a specific C5 recognition site on the β subunit of human C8. *Complement*, **2**, 76.

55. Stewart, J.L. and Sodetz, J.M. (1985) Analysis of the specific association of the eighth and ninth components of human complement: Identification of a direct role for the α subunit of C8. *Biochemistry*, **24**, 4598–4602.

56. Nemerow, G.R., Yamamoto, K. and Lint, T.F. (1979) Restriction of complement mediated membrane damage by the eighth component of complement: A dual role of C8 in the complement attack sequence. *J. Immunol.*, **123**, 1245–1252.

57. Rao, C.P., Minta, J.O., Laski, B. *et al.* (1985) Inherited C8D subunit deficiency in a patient with recurrent meningococcal infections. *Clin. Exp. Immunol.,* **60**, 183–190.
58. Tedesco, F. (1986) Component deficiencies: The eighth component. *Prog. Allergy,* **39**, 295–306.
59. Snider, J.V., Kaufman, K.M. and Sodetz, J.M. (1990) Chromosomal assignment and physical linkage of the human C8 loci: Implications regarding C8 polymorphism and deficiencies. *Compl. Inflamm.,* **7**, 298–301.
60. Tedesco, F., Densen, P., Villa, M.A. *et al.* (1983) Two types of dysfunctional eighth component of complement molecules in C8 deficiency in man: Reconstitution of normal C8 from the mixture of two abnormal C8 molecules. *J. Clin. Invest.,* **71**, 183–191.
61. Tedesco, F., Roncelli, L., Petersen, B.H. *et al.* (1990) Two distinct abnormalities in patients with C8 α-γ deficiency: Low level of C8 β chain and presence of dysfunctional C8 α-γ subunit. *J. Clin. Invest.,* **86**, 884–888.
62. Goonewardena, P., Sjoholm, A.G., Nilsson, L.A. *et al.* (1988) Linkage analysis of the properdin deficiency gene: Suggestion of a locus in the proximal part of the short arm of the X chromosome. *Genomics,* **2**, 115–118.
63. Figueroa, J.E. and Densen, P. (1991) Infectious diseases associated with complement deficiency. *Clin. Microb. Rev.,* **4**, 359–395.
64. Agnello, V. (1979) Complement deficiency states. *Medicine,* **57**, 1–23.
65. Nicholson, A. and Lepow, H.I. (1979) Host defence against *Neisseria meningitidis* requires a complement-dependent bactericidal activity. *Science,* **205**, 298–299.
66. Tschopp, J., Penea, F., Schifferli, J. *et al.* (1986) Dysfunctional C8 beta chain in patients with C8 deficiency. *Scand. J. Immunol.,* **24**, 715–720.
67. Warnick, P.R. and Densen, P. (1991) Reduced C8 beta messenger RNA expression in families with hereditary C8 beta deficiency. *J. Immunol.,* **146**, 1052–1056.
68. Densen, P.M. and Warnick, P.R. (1989) Molecular basis of C8 deficiency states. *Complement,* **7**, 120–121.
69. Nurenberger, W., Seger, R., Kobler, P. *et al.* (1988) Immunoblot analysis of the eighth component of human complement: Demonstration of subunits and detection of C8 alpha-gamma double and triple bands. *J. Immunol. Methods,* **109**, 257–263.
70. Zimran, A., Kuperman, O., Shemesh, O. *et al.* (1984) Recurrent *Neisseria meningitidis* bacteremia: Association with deficiency of the eighth component of complement in a Sepharadi Jewish family. *Arch. Intern. Med.,* **144**, 1481–1482.
71. Eby, W.M., Irby, W.R., Irby, J.H. *et al.* (1987) Recurrent meningitis with familial C8 deficiency: Case report. *Va. Med.,* **114**, 91–94.
72. Liston, T. (1983) Relapsing *Neisseria meningitidis* infection associated with C8 deficiency. *Clin. Pediatr.,* **22**, 605–607.
73. Kemp, A., Vernon, J., Muller-Eberhard, H.J. *et al.* (1985) Complement C8 deficiency with recurrent meningococcemia: Examination of meningococcal opsonization. *Aust. Pediatr. J.,* **21**, 169–171.
74. Brandslund, I., Teisner, B., Strate, M. *et al.* (1983) The normal occurrence of two molecular forms of the eighth complement component and their concentrations in a family with C8 deficiency. *Eur. J. Clin. Invest.,* **13**, 179–182.
75. Cooke, R.P., Zafar, M. and Haeney, M.R. (1987) Recurrent meningococcal meningitis associated with deficiencies of C8 and anti-meningococcal antibody. *J. Clin. Lab. Immunol.,* **23**, 53–56.

76. Del Rio, C., Stephens, D.S., Knapp, J.S. *et al.* (1989) Comparison of isolates of *Neisseria gonorrheae* causing meningitis and report of gonococcal meningitis in a patient with C8 deficiency. *J. Clin. Microbiol.,* **27,** 1045–1049.
77. Densen, P., Weiler, J., Griffiss, M. *et al.* (1987) Familial properdin deficiency and fatal meningococcemia: Correction of the bactericidal defect by vaccination. *N. Eng. J. Med.,* **316,** 922–926.
78. Goundis, D., Holt, S.M., Boyd, Y. *et al.* (1989) Localization of the properdin structural locus to Xp11.23–Xp21.1. *Genomics,* **5,** 56–60.
79. Nolan, K.F., Willis, A.C., Goundis, D. *et al.* (1991) Gene structure of properdin and expression of a TSR module. *Complement,* **200** (Abstract 199).
80. Morgan, B.P. and Walport, M.J. (1991) Complement deficiency and disease. *Immunol. Today,* **12,** 301–306.
81. Sjoholm, A.G., Soderstrom, C. and Nilsson, L.A. (1988) A second variant of properdin deficiency: The detection of properdin at low concentrations in affected males. *Complement,* **5,** 130–140.
82. Sjoholm, A.G., Kuijper, E.J., Tijssen, C.C. *et al.* (1988) Dysfunctional properdin in a Dutch family with meningococcal disease. *N. Engl. J. Med.,* **319,** 33–37.
83. Anonymous (1988) Properdin deficiency. *Lancet,* **i,** 95–96.
84. Sjoholm, A.G. (1990) Inherited complement deficiency states: Implication for immunity and immunological disease. *APMIS,* **98,** 861–874.
85. Gelfand, E.W., Rao, C.P., Pinta, J.O. *et al.* (1987) Inherited deficiency of properdin and C2 in a patient with recurrent bacteremia. *Am. J. Med.,* **82,** 671–675.
86. Neu, R.L., Stockman, J.A., Spitzer, R.E. *et al.* (1976) 46 XY/46 XY 21q-mosaicism in an infant with neutropenia and properdin deficiency. *J. Med. Genet.,* **13,** 332–334.
87. Davis, C.A. and Forristal, J. (1980) Partial properdin deficiency. *J. Lab. Clin. Med.,* **96,** 633–639.
88. Nielsen, H.A. and Koch, C. (1987) Congenital properdin deficiency and meningococcal infection. *Clin. Immunol. Immunopathol.,* **44,** 134–139.
89. Holme, E.R., Veitch, J., Johnston, A. *et al.* (1989) Familial properdin deficiency associated with chronic discoid lupus erythematosus. *Clin. Exp. Immunol.,* **76,** 76–81.
90. Nielsen, H.E., Koch, C., Mansa, B. *et al.* (1990) Complement and immunoglobulin studies in 15 cases of chronic meningococcemia: properdin deficiency and hypoimmunoglobulinemia. *Scand. J. Infect. Dis.* **22,** 31–36.
91. Soderstrom, C., Sjoholm, A.G., Svensson, R. *et al.* (1989) Another Swedish family with complete properdin deficiency: Association with fulminant meningococcal disease in one male family member. *Scand. J. Infect. Dis.,* **21,** 259–265.
92. Spath, P.J., Tisian, Z., Schaad, U.B. *et al.* (1985) Association of heterozygous C4A and complete factor P deficient conditions. *Complement,* **2,** 74 (Abstract 212).
93. Swart, A.G., Fijen, C.A.P., Kuijper, E.J. *et al.* (1991) Complement deficiencies in infections with *Neisseria meningitidis. Complement,* **227** (Abstract 269).
94. Platonov, A.E. and Beloborodov, V.B. (1991) Late complement deficiency in the USSR: The situation in 1991. *Complement,* **211** (Abstract 229).
95. Goldschneider, I., Gotschlich, E.C. and Artenstein, M.S. (1969) Human immunity to *Meningococcus.* 1. The role of human antibodies. *J. Exp. Med.,* **129,** 1307–1326.
96. Goldschneider, I., Gotschlich, E.C. and Artenstein, M.S. (1969) Human immunity to *Meningococcus.* 2. Development of natural immunity. *J. Exp. Med.,* **129,** 1327–1335.

97. Griffiss, J.M. (1982) Epidemic meningococcal disease: Synthesis of a hypothetical immunoepidemiologic model. *Rev. Infect. Dis.*, **4**, 159–172.
98. Rice, P.A., McCormick, W.M. and Kasper, D.L. (1980) Natural serum bactericidal activity against *Neisseria gonorrheae* isolates from disseminated, locally invasive and uncomplicated disease. *J. Immunol.*, **124**, 2105–2109.
99. Ross, S.C., Rosenthal, P.J., Berberich, H.M. *et al.* (1987) Killing of *Neisseria meningitidis* by human neutrophils: Implication for normal and complement-deficient individuals. *J. Infect. Dis.*, **155**, 1266–1275.
100. Soderstrom, C., Braconier, J.H., Kayhty, H. *et al.* (1989) Immune response to tetravalent meningococcal vaccine: Opsonic and bactericidal functions of normal and properdin deficient sera. *Eur. J. Clin. Microbiol. Infect. Dis.*, **8**, 220–224.
101. Alper, C.A., Abramson, N., Johnston, R.B., Jr. *et al.* (1970) Increased susceptibility to infection associated with abnormalities of complement-mediated functions of the third component of complement. *N. Eng. J. Med.*, **282**, 349–354.
102. Rao, C.P., Minta, J.O., Laski, B. *et al.* (1985) Inherited C8D subunit deficiency in a patient with recurrent meningococcal infections: In vivo functional kinetic analysis of C8. *Clin. Exp. Immunol.*, **60**, 183–190.

Chapter 14

Related Pathogenesis of Immunoglobulin A Deficiency and Common Variable Immunodeficiency

JOHN E. VOLANAKIS[1] and MAX D. COOPER[2]

[1]Division of Clinical Immunology and Rheumatology, Department of Medicine, and [2]Division of Developmental and Clinical Immunology, Department of Pediatrics, Medicine, Microbiology, and Pathology, Comprehensive Cancer Center, University of Alabama at Birmingham and Howard Hughes Medical Institute, Birmingham, Alabama, USA

Immunoglobulin A (IgA) deficiency (IgA-D), usually defined by extremely reduced levels of serum IgA (<5 mg/dl) in the presence of normal IgM and IgG levels, is the most frequently observed primary immunodeficiency (1). The incidence is approximately one in 700 individuals of European descent. While affected individuals are often healthy, clinical manifestations of IgA-D may include recurrent infections, gastrointestinal disorders, autoimmune syndromes, allergic diseases and malignancies (2).

Common variable immunodeficiency (CVI), the second most frequently recognized primary immunodeficiency, is defined by low serum IgG and IgA levels, usually associated with low IgM levels as well (1). The clinical presentation of CVI is characterized by recurrent sinopulmonary, gastrointestinal and systemic infections. Like IgA-D, CVI is not considered a single disease entity, but rather a group of immune disorders having in common a profound defect in antibody production. However, most CVI individuals, and virtually all IgA-D patients, exhibit a distinct phenotype characterized by normal numbers of B cells of all Ig isotypes and of T cells as well. The

New Concepts in Immunodeficiency Diseases. Edited by S. Gupta and C. Griscelli terms IgA-D and CVI refer to these particular subsets of immunodeficient individuals in this review.

Here we examine the pathogenesis of IgA-D and CVI with emphasis on recent evidence supporting a common genetic basis for these two immunodeficiencies (3, 4). This proposal is based on the partially overlapping phenotypes of IgA-D and CVI, their occurrence in members of the same family, their similar B cell maturational defects, and their association with the same major histocompatibility complex (MHC) haplotypes.

CELLULAR BASIS OF IgA-D AND CVI

The apparent proximal cause of IgA-D and CVI is an arrest in the B cell differentiation pathway (5, 6). Both immunodeficiencies are characterized by profound deficits in plasma cells producing the Ig isotypes that are missing in the serum. In IgA-D, the defect almost always involves IgA1- and IgA2-secreting cells and sometimes IgG2- and IgG4-secreting cells as well (7, 8). In CVI, cells secreting the different IgG and IgA isotypes are rare and IgM-secreting cells are decreased to a variable extent. Despite these deficits, IgA-D and CVI individuals have normal numbers of Ig-bearing B cell precursors for all Ig isotypes. However, their circulating B cells appear to be immature, resembling those present in neonates in that most isotype-switched B cells still express IgM (9) (Figure 14.1). Similarity with their neonatal counterparts is supported further by functional analysis. B cells from CVI individuals may respond to pokeweed mitogen stimulation and to Epstein–Barr virus (EBV)-transformation by producing reasonable amounts of IgM, but not IgG and IgA (10, 11). Similarly, stimulation of B cells from IgA-D individuals with either pokeweed mitogen or EBV fails to induce IgA-secreting cells.

Since T cells are important in regulating growth and maturation of B cells, their possible involvement in the pathogenesis of IgA-D and CVI has been investigated extensively. However, few clear demonstrations of T cell defects have emerged. As one possible example, IgA and IgG deficiency are frequent features of ataxia telangiectasia—an autosomal recessive syndrome characterized by variable defects of cellular and humoral immunity (1). Thymic hypoplasia leading to T cell deficiency (12) provides a logical explanation for the Ig deficiency as B cells are produced normally in this syndrome. In a few individuals with IgA-D, evidence favoring selective IgA suppression by T cells has been reported (13, 14), but convincing experimental support for the existence of an isotype-specific suppressor T cell has been difficult to obtain. When T cells from IgA-D or CVI individuals have been examined for their capacity to support the *in vitro* differentiation of Ig+ B cells from normal individuals, they have performed normally in most instances (15, 16). This implies that they are able to provide all the cytokines needed for isotype switching and terminal plasma cell differentiation.

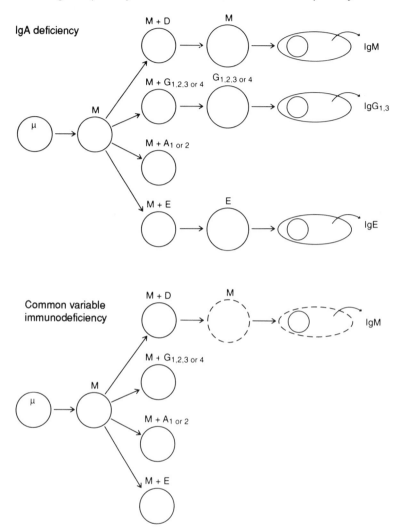

Figure 14.1. Schematic representation of the B cell defects in IgA-D and CVI. Immunoglobulin isotypes expressed on the surface of the cells are indicated by upper-case letters and numbers. Curved arrows indicate secreted immunoglobulins. In IgA-D the IgA-bearing B cells, and in some cases IgG2- and IgG4-bearing B cells, fail to differentiate into antibody-secreting plasma cells. In CVI the differentiation arrest involves more isotypes. The dashed lines indicate that in some cases of CVI the IgM-bearing B cells may undergo terminal differentiation into IgM-secreting plasma cells. From ref. 2. Reproduced by permission of Harwood Academic Publishers GmbH

However, it should be noted that these *in vitro* assays measure the terminal differentiation of relatively mature primed B cells, whereas B cells being sampled in the circulation of IgA-D and CVI individuals appear relatively immature. Therefore, the possibility of a more subtle dysfunction of T cells or other types of auxiliary cells required in the initial maturational steps of the B cell population cannot be excluded. In conclusion, the available data do not pinpoint the nature of the primary functional abnormality underlying IgA-D or CVI. An inherent B cell defect could exist or, alternatively, the signals needed for B cell maturation may not be available.

POSSIBLE GENETIC BASIS FOR IgA-D AND CVI

The molecular defect responsible for the B cell differentiation arrest in IgA-D and CVI patients remains unknown. The vast majority of individuals with IgA-D and CVI have normal Ig genes, including the basic genetic elements necessary for isotype switching as evidenced by the expression of all Ig isotypes on their B cells. Analysis of the Cα genes and their upstream switch regions in a few IgA-D patients supports this conclusion (17). More compelling support comes from the demonstration that silent IgA allotypes of IgA-D individuals may be expressed normally in their offspring (18). The rare cases of homozygous Cα gene deletions have involved either the Cα1 or the Cα2 gene, in contrast to the deficiency of both IgA isotypes in IgA-D individuals (19, 20).

The importance of genetic factors in the pathogenesis of IgA-D and CVI is indicated by several lines of evidence, including the unequal distribution of these immunodeficiencies among racially distinct populations, their familial occurrence, and their association with certain HLA antigens and MHC haplotypes. The incidence of IgA-D differs significantly among different populations. Several studies from Europe and North America indicate that IgA-D is relatively common, being present in one of every 500–700 individuals in these populations (21–24). By contrast, a large study in Japan revealed a 1:18 500 incidence of IgA-D, more than 25-fold lower than that among Europeans (25). A low incidence of IgA-D has also been reported among Malaysians (26). IgA-D also seems to be relatively rare among African Americans. This is suggested by reports of a greater than 20:1 ratio of white to black IgA-D patients in regions of the United States with large African American populations (27, 28). No large population studies have been reported for CVI, but it is also thought to be more frequent among individuals of European descent.

Additional evidence indicating that genetic factors play an important role in the pathogenesis of IgA-D and CVI derives from reports of families with multiple immunodeficient individuals. In fact, several of these families contain both IgA-D and CVI individuals, providing strong support to the hypothesis of a common underlying defect for these syndromes (29). Among 21 families containing 31 IgA-D and CVI individuals described recently, five had more than one immunodeficient member (4). Of these five

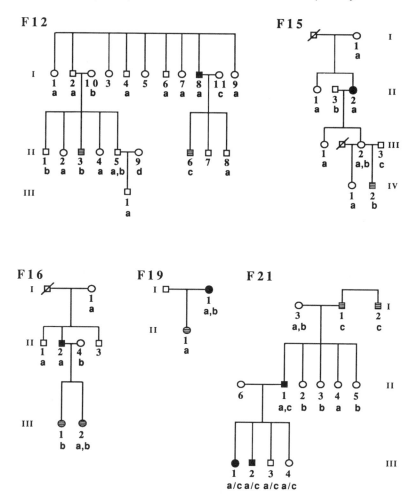

Figure 14.2. Trees of families with two or more IgA-D/CVI members. CVI is indicated by closed symbols and IgA-D by hatched symbols. Dead family members are indicated by a diagonal line through the symbol. Generations are numbered with roman numerals and individuals with arabic numbers. Lower-case letters indicate haplotypes I (HLA-DQB1*0201, -DR3, C4B-Sf, C4A-0, G11-15, Bf-0.4, C2-a, HSP-7.5, TNFα-5, HLA-B8, -A1) or II (HLA-DQB1*0201, -DR7, C4B-S, C4A-L, G11-4.5, Bf-0.6, C2-b, HSP-9, TNFα-9, HLA-B44, -A29) as follows. Family (F) 12: a, b, c, and d haplotype I; F15: a and c, haplotype I, b, haplotype II; F16: a and b, haplotype II; F19: a, haplotype I; F21: a, b, and c, haplotype I; a/c, haplotype I could be either a or c. From ref. 4. Reproduced by permission of the American Society for Clinical Investigation, Inc.

multiplex families, one had five immunodeficient members, two had three each and another two had two each (Figure 14.2). Characteristically, all five of these families included both IgA-D and CVI members.

ASSOCIATIONS WITH MHC CLASS I AND II GENES

Initial studies on possible associations between IgA-D and HLA antigens were prompted by the higher incidence of IgA-D among patients with HLA-associated diseases. Initially, IgA-D in patients with autoimmune and atopic diseases was found to be associated with the HLA-A1, A2, and -B8 antigens (30, 31). Subsequent investigations suggested an association of IgA-D with a number of class I and/or class II HLA antigens, including A1, A28, B8, B14, B40, DR3, and DR7 (32–34), irrespective of associated diseases. An association with the haplotype HLA-A1, B8, DR3 also became evident from these studies. A more recent report has suggested that susceptibility to IgA-D is imparted by MHC class II gene(s) (35). Among 95 IgA-D individuals, this study identified three susceptibility and one protective DR-DQ haplotype. Susceptibility haplotypes had in common HLA-DQ β-chain alleles characterized by a neutral amino acid (valine or alanine) at position 57. The protective allele had a negatively charged aspartyl residue at that position. It is of interest that the same amino acids at the same residue of the HLA-DQ β chain were previously reported to endow susceptibility to or protection from insulin-dependent diabetes mellitus (IDDM) (36, 37). More recent evidence, however, indicates that susceptibility to IDDM can be attributed to MHC loci other than HLA-DQB1 (38–40). It has also been noted that of four MHC haplotypes associated with IDDM, all of which have a neutral alanyl residue of position 57 of the HLA-DQ β chain, only one is associated with IgA-D/CVI (41). Nevertheless, the fact that residue 57 is located in the antigen-peptide-binding groove of the HLA-DQ β chain makes the reported association with IgA-D attractive within the context of a possible defect in T cell/B cell interactions.

MHC CLASS III CANDIDATE GENES

A report from Western Australia (42) first indicated that IgA-D may be associated with a gene (or genes) located within the MHC class III gene cluster in linkage disequilibrium with class I and/or class II alleles. The class III MHC region, occupying about 1100 kb of DNA between the class I and the class II gene clusters, includes at least 36 genes, most of which are expressed in a variety of cell types (43–45). Included are the genes encoding the complement proteins C4A, C4B, C2, and factor B, the P450 enzyme 21-hydroxylase, the major heat-shock protein HSP70, the tumor necrosis factors α and β, the valyl-tRNA synthetase (46) and a small nuclear protein, termed RD (47). The function of the products of the remaining 23 genes mapped in this region is currently unknown.

Studies from our group have also suggested that a gene(s) imparting susceptibility to both IgA-D and CVI is located within the class III region of the MHC (3, 4). These studies, on 12 IgA-D and 19 CVI individuals from 21 families and 79 of their immediate relatives, defined MHC haplotypes by analyzing polymorphic markers for 11 genes or their products between HLA-DQB1 and HLA-A. The most striking finding was the repetitive occurrence of certain MHC haplotypes in the majority of the immunodeficient individuals. Two of these haplotypes, HLA-DQB1*0201, -DR3, C4B-Sf, C4A-0, G11-15, Bf-0.4, C2-a, HSP-7.5, TNFα-5, HLA-B8, -A1 and HLA-DQB1*0201, -DR7, C4B-S, C4A-L, G11-4.5, Bf-0.6, C2-b, HSP-9, TNFα-9, HLA-B44, -A29 (Figure 14.3), were encountered in 24 of the 31 immunodeficient individuals, representing 14 of the 21 families of the study. The first of these haplotypes is the one most frequently observed in IgA-D/CVI (48) and is characterized by a deletion involving the major part of the C4A gene, the entire CYP450-21-hydroxylase A gene and the 5'-most region of the C4B gene (49). The association of this haplotype with IgA-D has been ascertained by two independent surveys of individuals selected on the sole basis of homozygosity for this haplotype, which revealed that 1 of 14 (42) and 2 of 10 (4) such individuals had IgA-D. Conversely, these two haplotypes are rarely seen in Asian populations in which IgA-D is uncommon (41). Finally, there were no differences in the distribution of the haplotypes identified in our studies among IgA-D and CVI individuals, consistent with the idea of a shared defect for these conditions.

   In several immunodeficient individuals, these MHC haplotypes were not conserved in their entirety, a finding that could be explained by past crossover events. Inspection of these partially conserved MHC haplotypes (Figure 14.3) suggests that they all share the MHC class III subregion between the C4B and the C2 genes. This observation has focused our search for a candidate susceptibility gene to this region of chromosome 6. The MHC class III subregion between the C4B and C2 genes occupies about 75 kb of DNA and contains the genes CYP450-21-hydroxylase A, C4A, G11, RD, and Bf (43). Of these, the first is a pseudogene. C4A is currently the most interesting of these genes in the context of antibody deficiency and is discussed in more detail below. The RD gene encodes a 42 kDa nuclear polypeptide characterized by a highly unusual 48-amino acid region composed entirely of the repeating dipeptide Arg-Asp or in a few cases Arg-Glu (47, 50). Based on amino acid sequence homologies, it seems likely that RD constitutes a small nuclear ribonucleoprotein (snRNP). Finally, Bf encodes the complement protein factor B, which provides the catalytic subunit of the C3/C5-convertase of the alternative pathway of complement activation.

POSSIBLE ROLE OF C4A IN B CELL TRIGGERING

The C4A and C4B genes encode the two isotypes of the fourth component of human complement. Comparison of their cDNA sequences has revealed

FAM	ID#	Dx	DQB1	DR	C4B	C4A	G11	BF	C2	HSP	TNF	B	A
					haplotype A								
F08	II.1	CVID	*0201	(4)	Sf	0	15	0.4	a	7.5	5	8	32
F15	II.2	CVID	*0501	1	Sf	0	15	0.4	a	7.5	5	60	24
F10	I.1	CVID	*0201	3	Sf	0	15	0.4	a	7.5	5	8	1
F12	I.8	CVID	*0201	3	Sf	0	15	0.4	a	7.5	5	8	1
F19	I.1	CVID	*0201	3	Sf	0	15	0.4	a	(7.5)	5	8	1
F21	II.1	CVID	(*0201)	3	Sf	0	15	0.4	a	7.5	5	8	1
F21	III.1	CVID	*0201	3	Sf	0	15	0.4	a	7.5	5	8	1
F21	I.1	IgAD	*0201	3	Sf	0	15	0.4	a	7.5	5	8	1
F21	I.2	IgAD	*0201	3	Sf	0	15	0.4	a	7.5	5	8	1
F12	II.3	IgAD	*0201	3	Sf	0	15	0.4	a	7.5	5	8	1
F17	II.1	IgAD	*0201	3	Sf	0	15	0.4	a	7.5	5	8	1
F19	II.1	IgAD	*0201	3	Sf	0	15	0.4	a	(7.5)	5	8	1
F12	II.6	IgAD	*0301	4	L	L	15	0.6	a	7.5	5	8	1
F21	III.2	CVID	*0303	7	S	L	15	0.4	a	9	9	58	2
F01	II.1	CVID	(*0503)	1	L	L	15	0.6	a	9	9	70	1
F09	I.2	CVID	*0302	4	L	L	15	0.4	a	9	9	38	1
F14	II.1	CVID	*0301	6	L	L	15	0.4	a	9	9	18	2
F07	II.1	IgAD	X	8	L	L	15	0.4	a	(7.5)	9	16	X
F02	II.1	CVID	*0503	X	0	L	15	0.4	d	7.5	(9)	X	X
F20	II.2	CVID	*0602	x	L	L	15	0.4	e	9	9	39	2
F03	II.2	CVID	*0501	1	L	L	15	0.4	a	(9)	9	44	2
F16	III.2	IgAD	*0201	7	S	L	15	0.4	a	7.5	9	14	1
F04	I.1	CVID	*0502	2	L	L	15	0.4	a	9	9	61	32
F15	IV.2	IgAD	*0301	4	L	L	15	0.4	d	9	5	60	3
F05	II.2	CVID	*0501	6	L	L	4.5	0.6	b	9	9	44	29
F13	II.1	CVID	*0201	7	S	L	4.5	0.6	a	7.5	9	52	26
F16	II.2	CVID	*0201	7	S	L	4.5	0.6	b	9	9	44	29
F06	II.1	IgAD	*0201	7	S	L	4.5	0.6	b	9	9	44	29
F18	II.2	IgAD	*0201	7	S	L	4.5	0.6	b	9	9	39	x
F16	II.1	IgAD	*0201	7	S	L	4.5	0.6	a	7.5	9	44	28
F11	I.1	CVID	*0501	9	S	L	4.5	0.6	d	(7.5)	5	x	24

Figure 14.3. MHC haplotypes of IgA-D and CVI individuals (4). Alleles of the C4B gene are designated as Sf (short-fused), L (long), S (short) or O (deleted). Alleles of the C4A gene are designated as O (deleted) or L (long); alleles for the G11, Bf, HSP70 and TNFα genes are designated by the length in

greater than 99% homology (51). Of the 14 nucleotide differences, 12 are clustered within the C4d region and cause 9 amino acid substitutions. Despite their striking homology, C4A and C4B have very different reactivities (52, 53). Folowing activation by C$\overline{1s}$, the C4b fragment of C4A preferentially forms amide bonds with free amino ($-NH_2$) groups by a transacylation reaction involving a metastable thiolester bond. In contrast, C4B preferentially forms ester bonds with hydroxyl ($-OH$) groups of sugar residues. Thus, the C4A isotype is involved primarily in the formation of the classical pathway C3 convertase on the surface of antigen–antibody complexes,

DQB1	DR	C4B	C4A	G11	Bf	C2	HSP	TNF	B	A
				haplotype B						
*0301	10	S,S	L	15	0.4	a	7.5	9	14	11
*0302	4	S	L	15	0.6	a	9	9	35	26
*0302	4	L	L	15	0.4	a	9	9	7	3
*0301	4	L	L	4.5	0.6	a	(9)	5	8	1
*0303	9	L	L	4.5	0.6	b	(9)	5	44	26
(*0201)	3	Sf	0	15	0.4	a	7.5	5	8	1
*0302	4	L	L	15	0.4	a	9	9	7	x
*0602	1	L	L	15	0.6	a	7.5	9	38	24
*0501	x	L	L	15	0.4	a	9	9	62	x
*0201	7	S	L	15	0.4	a	7.5	9	14	1
*0602	11	L	L	15	0.4	a	9	5	35	25
*0602	x	S	L	15	0.4	a	(9)	5	8	3
*0201	3	Sf	0	15	0.4	a	7.5	5	8	1
*0201	3	Sf	0	15	0.4	a	7.5	5	8	1
(*0501)	2	L	L	15	0.4	a	9	9	49	3
*0301	11	L	L	15	0.4	a	9	9	51	2
*0302	4	L	L	15	0.4	a	9	9	60	26
*0301	4	L	L	15	0.4	a	(9)	9	x	29
*0303	X	S	L	15	0.4	a	9	(5)	X	X
*0201	7	S	L	15	0.4	a	7.5	9	13	30
*0201	7	S	L	4.5	0.6	a	(7.5)	9	45	1
*0201	7	S	L	4.5	0.6	a	7.5	9	44	28
*0201	3	S	L	4.5	0.6	b	9	9	44	29
*0201	7	S	L	4.5	0.6	b	9	5	8	1
*0502	2	L	L	15	0.4	a	9	9	35	2
*0301	4	L	L	15	0.4	a	9	5	44	28
*0201	7	S	L	15	0.4	a	7.5	9	14	1
*0201	7	S	L	4.5	0.6	b	9	9	44	29
*0303	x	L	L	15	0.4	a	9	5	44	2
*0201	7	S	L	4.5	0.6	b	9	9	44	29
*0302	10	L	L	15	0.6	a	(9)	9	60	2

kilobases of their polymorphic fragments; haplotypes of the C2 gene are designated as a to i. Parentheses indicate deduced assignment of allele; x, unknown allele. Reproduced by permission of the American Society for Clinical Investigation, Inc.

whereas the C4B isotype is responsible mainly for assembly of the C3 convertase on the surface of bacterial cells. The contrasting reactivities of the two isotypes of C4 suggests they may play different roles in the development and maturation of immune responses.

Studies in animals and man indicate that inherited or experimentally induced deficiencies of components of the classical complement pathway, including deficiency of C4, are associated with diminished antibody responses to T-dependent and T-independent antigens (54–57). Complement-deficient animals characteristically exhibit decreased primary and secondary responses with failure or diminution of isotype switching during secondary responses. Recent studies (58) indicate that the defective immune responses of C4-deficient guinea pigs can be normalized by reconstituting the animals with human C4A, but not with human C4B. In addition, humans with inherited deficiencies of C1, C4, C2, or C3 have significantly depressed levels of IgG4, suggesting defective isotype switching (59).

Complement may be involved in the maturation of immune responses through the attachment of C4 and C3 fragments to antigen following binding of IgM antibody and activation of the classical pathway. The presence of C4b and C3b on the antigen facilitates its localization to two cell types involved in the primary antibody response: B lymphocytes, which express the complement receptors CR1 and CR2; and follicular dendritic cells, which express CR1, CR2 and CR3 (60) and are involved more in the development of memory B lymphocytes. Complement receptors on follicular dendritic cells may serve to retain antigen for interaction with germinal center B cells (61), whereas their main function on B cells is thought to be the initiation or facilitation of signal transduction.

Of the two complement receptors on B lymphocytes, CR1 and CR2, the latter may mediate the enhancing effect of complement on the primary antibody response. Monoclonal antibody to murine CR1 suppresses the immune response to T-dependent antigens modestly, whereas an antibody against an epitope shared by murine CR1 and CR2 can be markedly immunosuppressive (62). Similar immunosuppression can be achieved by treating mice with a soluble form of recombinant human CR2 which inhibits competitively ligand binding to CR2 without interacting directly with the cells (63). Human CR2 has binding sites for iC3b and C3dg and also for EBV (64, 65). CR2 probably does not directly transmit signals to the B cell, but is a ligand-binding subunit of two distinct membrane protein complexes: a biomolecular complex of CR2 and CR1 (66); and a CR2–CD19–TAPA1–Leu13 complex (67, 68). The CR2–CR1 complex has not been shown to have signal-transducing capability, although antibody to CR1 may have an augmenting effect on B cell differentiation and antibody production (69). However, the primary purpose of the CR2–CR1 complex may be to capture antigen coated with C3b, process the C3b to iC3b and C3dg, the ligands for CR2, and transfer the antigen–C3dg complex to the CR2 component of the complex, which may then diffuse away to become associated with CD19 (70).

The CR2–CD19–TAPA1–Leu13 complex is probably the critical site at which the complement and immune systems interact. CR2 associates directly with CD19 (67), a member of the Ig super-family that is restricted to cells of the B lineage being expressed from the earliest recognizable stage of B cell development through mature B cells and memory B cells. CD19 associates with TAPA1 (68), a non-lymphocyte-specific molecule which is characterized by four membrane-spanning regions (71, 72). TAPA1 associates with the 16 kDa membrane protein, Leu13 (71). Ligation of the CR2–CD19–TAPA1–Leu13 complex with antibody causes the activation of two B cell enzyme systems: a protein tyrosine kinase (PTK) (73) which is probably distinct from that activated by the surface Ig complex and is required for activation of the second enzyme system, a phospholipase C (PLC) (73, 74). Activation of distinct PTKs and PLCs by the antigen-specific Ig and the antigen-non-specific CR2–CD19–TAPA1–Leu13 complexes, offers a mechanism by which these two complexes may interact synergistically. Cross-linking surface IgM to CR2, as would occur when antigen coated with C3 fragments interacts with a B cell expressing Ig specific for that antigen, lowers by 100-fold the number of surface IgM complexes that need to be ligated to achieve maximal release of intracellular Ca^{2+} and maximal proliferation (75). Thus, the CR2–CD19–TAPA1–Leu13 complex may function as an accessory complex that must be cross-linked to the antigen receptor complex for the B cell to respond to low concentrations of antigen; the co-capping observed of the CR2–CD19–TAPA1–Leu13 complex with the mIg complex on B cells (76) indicates that mechanisms exist that promote this interaction.

These considerations suggest a possible link between the C4A gene deletion characterizing the haplotype most frequently associated with IgA-D/CVI (Figure 14.3) and the resulting susceptibility to immunodeficiency. Two additional facts bear on this discussion. First, there are more than ten allotypes of each C4 isotype (77). Subtle differences among these allotypes were hypothesized to underly autoimmune diseases (78). However, with the exception of the C4A6 allotype, which cannot support the assembly of a C5-convertase (79), no functional differences among C4 allotypes have been reported. Second, substitution of a single Asp for His at position 1106 by site-directed mutagenesis converted C4B to C4A in terms of functional activity (80). It seems possible that similar mutations in the alleles of the C4A gene associated with IgA-D/CVI risk haplotypes could result in attenuated function.

COMBINED ROLE OF GENETIC AND ENVIRONMENTAL FACTORS

Neither our data nor those reported by other investigators provide sufficient information to assign the mode of inheritance of IgA-D and CVI. In a few families an autosomal recessive pattern of inheritance is apparent, but in others an autosomal dominant mode with low penetrance could best explain the data. Moreover, the data demonstrate clearly that members of the same family can be MHC haploidentical but discordant for immunodeficiency. The putative susceptibility gene within the MHC region thus may predispose to both IgA-D and CVI, but does not constitute a sufficient condition for expression of immunodeficiency. Additional environmental and or genetic factors appear necessary for the development of the deficient state. Examples of environmental factors participating in the pathogenesis of IgA-D and CVI are provided by infectious agents and also by certain drugs. Intrauterine infection with rubella virus (81) may result in IgA-D or, less frequently, CVI. Congenital cytomegalovirus or *Toxoplasma gondii* infections can be associated with IgA-D (82), and persistent cytomegalovirus infection is observed in some adults with CVI (83). Phenytoin treatment of patients with seizure disorders may produce a decrease in serum IgA and IgA-D in genetically susceptible individuals (84, 85). Treatment with gold salts, sulfasalazine, antimalarials, and captopril is also reported to induce IgA-D (2). Discontinuance of the drug usually results in return of IgA levels to normal in these individuals. A diverse spectrum of drugs and infectious agents may thus serve as cofactors in the induction of antibody deficiencies, particularly IgA-D, in genetically predisposed individuals.

CONCLUSIONS

Previously thought to be extremely heterogeneous disorders, CVI and IgA-D have proven to be related diseases in many instances. The two immunodeficiency patterns represent polar ends of a disease spectrum ranging from a selective deficiency in the production of IgA antibodies to an inability to produce antibodies of any isotype, and are often seen in several members of the same family. Location of the underlying susceptibility gene(s) to the MHC region of chromosome 6 is suggested by the frequent occurrence of certain MHC haplotypes in both CVI and IgA-D patients. Conversely, these ancestral haplotypes are rare among Asians, in whom IgA-D (and probably CVI) is 25 times less common than in Caucasians. Highly polymorphic, the MHC genes tend to be inherited as a block (the so-called linkage-disequilibrium phenomenon), making precise mapping of the postulated susceptibility gene(s) a difficult task. Two MHC genes are current favorite candidates, one or both of which could serve as susceptibility genes for Ig deficiency. One is the DQ locus, in particular those DQ β chain genes encoding a neutral amino acid at position 57. The other candidate is a class III MHC gene, perhaps the C4A gene which is often deleted in affected patients. While the class II genes are involved in T and B cell interactions, the C4A gene product indirectly enhances antigen triggering of B cells in isotype-switched antibody responses. Adding to the complexity of this genetic puzzle is the fact that individuals with identical MHC haplotypes, even within the same family, may or may not express immunodeficiency. Environmental factors which may serve to tip the balance into Ig deficiency include both infectious agents and drugs.

ACKNOWLEDGEMENTS

We thank our colleagues Drs Z.B. Zhu, F.M. Schaffer, K.J. Macon, J. Palermos, R. Go, R.D. Campbell, and H.W. Schroeder, Jr, for sharing their ideas and efforts on this project. The expert secretarial assistance of Mrs Paula Kiley is gratefully acknowledged. The original research reported here was supported in part by USPHS grants AI30879, AI21067, CA13148, and AR03555. Max D. Cooper is a Howard Hughes Medical Institute investigator.

REFERENCES

1. Eibl, M., Griscelli, C., Seligmann, M., Aiuti, F., Kishimoto, T. *et al.* (1989) Primary immunodeficiency diseases: Report of a WHO Sponsored Meeting. *Immunodef. Rev.*, **1**, 173–205.

2. Schaffer, F.M., Monteiro, R.C., Volanakis, J.E. and Cooper, M.D. (1991) IgA deficiency. *Immunodef. Rev.*, **3**, 15–44.

3. Schaffer, F.M., Palermos, J., Zhu, Z.B., Barger, B.O., Cooper, M.D. and Volanakis, J.E. (1989) Individuals with IgA deficiency and common variable immunodeficiency share polymorphisms of major histocompatibility complex class III genes. *Proc. Nat. Acad. Sci. USA*, **86**, 8015–8019.

4. Volanakis, J.E., Zhu, Z.-B., Schaffer, F.M., Macon, K.J., Palermos, J., Barger, B.O., Go, R., Campbell, R.D., Schroeder, H.W., Jr and Cooper, M.D. (1992) Major histocompatibility complex class III genes and susceptibility to immunoglobulin A deficiency and common variable immunodeficiency. *J. Clin. Invest.*, **89**, 1714–1922.

5. Conley, M.E. and Cooper, M.D. (1981) Immature IgA B cells in IgA-deficient patients. *N. Engl. J. Med.*, **305**, 495–497.

6. Cooper, M.D., Lawton, A.R. and Bockman, D.E. (1971) Agammaglobulinaemia with B lymphocytes: Specific defect of plasma-cell differentiation. *Lancet*, **ii**, 791–794.

7. Oxelius, V.A., Laurell, A.B., Lindquist, B., Golebiowska, H., Axelsson, U., Bjorkander, J. and Hanson, L.A. (1981) IgG subclasses in selective IgA deficiency: Importance of IgG2–IgA deficiency. *N. Engl. J. Med.*, **304**, 1476–1477.

8. Preud'homme, J.L. and Hanson, L.A. (1990) IgG subclass deficiency. *Immunodef. Rev.*, **2**, 129–149.

9. Gathings, W.E., Lawton, A.R. and Cooper, M.D. (1977) Immunofluorescent studies of the development of pre-B cells, B lymphocytes and immunoglobulin isotype diversity in humans. *Eur. J. Immunol.*, **7**, 804–810.

10. Pereira, S., Webster, D. and Platts-Mills, T. (1982) Immature B cells in fetal development and immunodeficiency: Studies of IgM, IgG, IgA, and IgD production in vitro using Epstein–Barr virus activation. *Eur. J. Immunol.*, **12**, 540–546.

11. Haber, P.L., Kubagawa, H. and Cooper, M.D. (1983) Epstein–Barr virus-induced immunoglobulin synthesis by B cells from individuals with late onset pan-hypogammaglobulinemia. *J. Clin. Immunol.*, **3**, 253–259.

12. Peterson, R.D.A., Cooper, M.D. and Good, R.A. (1966) Lymphoid tissue abnormalities associated with ataxia telangiectasia. *Am. J. Med.*, **41**, 342–359.

13. de la Concha, E.G., Oldham, G., Webster, A.D., Asherson, G.L. and Platts-Mills, T.A. (1977) Quantitative measurements of T- and B-cell function in "variable" primary hypogammaglobulinaemia: evidence for a consistent B-cell defect. *Clin. Exp. Immunol.*, **27**, 208–215.

14. Waldmann, T.A., Blaese, R.M., Broder, S. and Krakauer, R.S. (1978) Disorders of suppressor immunoregulatory cells in the pathogenesis of immunodeficiency and autoimmunity. *Ann. Intern. Med.*, **88**, 226–238.
15. Cassidy, J.T., Oldham, G. and Platts-Mills, T.A.E. (1979) Functional assessment of a B cell defect in patients with selective IgA deficiency. *Clin. Exp. Immunol.*, **35**, 296–305.
16. Klemola, T.K., Eskola, J. and Savilnati, E. (1988) T- and B-cell functions in IgA-deficient patients. *Scand. J. Immunol.*, **28**, 301–306.
17. Hammarström, L., Carlsson, B., Smith, C.I.E., Wallin, J. and Wieslander, L. (1985) Detection of IgA heavy chain constant region genes in IgA deficient donors: Evidence against gene deletions. *Clin. Exp. Immunol.*, **60**, 661–664.
18. Hammarström, L., de Lange, G.G. and Smith, C.I.E. (1987) IgA2 allotypes determined by restriction fragment length polymorphism in IgA deficiency: Re-expression of the silent A2m(2) allotype in the children of IgA-deficient patients. *J. Immunogenet.*, **14**, 197–201.
19. Lefranc, M.-P., Lefranc, G. and Rabbitts, T.H. (1982) Inherited deletion of immunoglobulin heavy chain constant region genes in normal human individuals. *Nature*, **300**, 760–762.
20. Engström, P.E., Norhagen, G.E., Bottaro, A., Carbonara, A.O., Lefranc, G., Steinitz, M., Söder, P.O., Smith, C.I.E. and Hammarström, L. (1990) Subclass distribution of antigen-specific IgA antibodies in normal donors and individuals with homozygous Cα1 or Cα2 gene deletions. *J. Immunol.*, **145**, 109–116.
21. Koistinen, J. (1975) Selective IgA deficiency in blood donors. *Vox Sang.*, **29**, 192–202.
22. Frommel, D., Moullec, J., Lambin, P. and Fine, J.M. (1973) Selective serum IgA deficiency: Frequency among 15,200 French blood donors. *Vox Sang.*, **25**, 513–518.
23. Cassidy, J.T. and Nordby, G.L. (1975) Human serum immunoglobulin concentrations: Prevalence of immunoglobulin deficiencies. *J. Allergy Clin. Immunol.*, **55**, 35–48.
24. Clark, J.A., Callicoat, P.A., Brenner, N.A., Bradley, C.A. and Smith, D.M. (1983) Selective IgA deficiency in blood donors. *Am. J. Clin. Pathol.*, **80**, 210–213.
25. Kanoh, T., Mizumoto, T., Yasuda, N., Koya, M., Ohno, Y., Uchino, H., Yoshimura, K., Ohkubo, Y. and Yamaguchi, H. (1986) Selective IgA deficiency in Japanese blood donors: Frequency and statistical analysis. *Vox Sang.*, **50**, 81–86.
26. Yadav, M. and Iyngkaran, N. (1979) Low incidence of selective IgA deficiency in normal Malaysians. *Med. J. Malaysia*, **34**, 145–148.
27. Lawton, A.R., Royal, S.A., Self, K.S. and Cooper, M.D. (1972) IgA determinants on B-lymphocytes in patients with deficiency of circulating IgA. *J. Lab. Clin. Med.*, **80**, 26–33.
28. Buckley, R.H. (1975) Clinical and immunologic features of selective IgA deficiency. *Birth Defects: Original Article Series*, **XI**, 134–141.
29. Wollheim, F.A., Williams, R.C. Jr (1965) Immunoglobulin studies in six kindreds of patients with adult hypogammaglobulinemia. *J. Lab. Clin. Med.*, **66**, 433–445.
30. Ambrus, M., Hernadi, E. and Bajtai, G. (1977) Prevalence of HLA-A1 and HLA-B8 antigens in selective IgA deficiency. *Clin. Immunol. Immunopathol.*, **7**, 311–314.
31. Østergaard, P.A. and Eriksen, J. (1979) Association between HLA-A1 B8 in children with extrinsic asthma and IgA deficiency. *Eur. J. Pediatr.*, **131**, 263–270.
32. Oen, K., Petty, R.E. and Schroeder, M.L. (1982) Immunoglobulin A deficiency: Genetic studies. *Tissue Antigens*, **19**, 174–182.
33. Hammarström, L. and Smith, C.I.E. (1983) HLA-A, B, C and DR antigens in immunoglobulin A deficiency. *Tissue Antigens*, **21**, 75–79.

34. Hammarström, L., Axelsson, U., Björkander, J., Hanson, L.A., Möller, E. and Smith, C.I.E. (1984) HLA antigens in selective IgA deficiency: Distribution in healthy donors and patients with recurrent respiratory tract infections. *Tissue Antigens*, **24**, 35–39.

35. Olerup, O., Smith, C.I.E. and Hammarström, L. (1990) Different amino acids at position 57 of the HLA-DQβ chain associated with susceptibility and resistance to IgA deficiency. *Nature (Lond.)*, **347**, 289–290.

36. Todd, J.A., Bell, J.I. and McDevitt, H.O. (1987) HLA-DQβ gene contributes to susceptibility and resistance to insulin-dependent diabetes mellitus. *Nature (Lond.)*, **329**, 599–604.

37. Morel, P.A., Dorman, J.S., Todd, J.A., McDevitt, H.O. and Trucco, M. (1988) Aspartic acid at position 57 of the HLA-DQβ chain protects against type 1 diabetes: A family study. *Proc. Nat. Acad. Sci. USA*, **85**, 8111–8115.

38. Todd, J.A. (1990) Genetic control of autoimmunity in type 1 diabetes. *Immunol. Today*, **11**, 122–129.

39. Segall, M. and Bach, F.H. (1990) HLA and disease: The perils of simplification. *N. Engl. J. Med.*, **322**, 1879–1881.

40. Faustman, D., Li, X., Lin, H.Y., Fu, Y., Eisenbarth, G., Avruch, J. and Guo, J. (1991) Linkage of faulty major histocompatibility complex class I to autoimmune diabetes. *Science*, **254**, 1756–1761.

41. French, M., Dawkins, R., Christiansen, F.T., Zhang, W., Degli-Esposti, M.A. and Saueracker, G. (1991) Reply. *Immunol. Today*, **12**, 135–136.

42. Wilton, A.N., Cobain, T.J. and Dawkins, R.L. (1985) Family studies in IgA deficiency. *Immunogenetics*, **21**, 333–342.

43. Sargent, C.A., Dunham, I. and Campbell, R.D. (1989) Identification of multiple HTF-island associated genes in the human major histocompatibility complex class III region. *EMBO J.*, **8**, 2305–2312.

44. Spies, T., Blanck, G., Bresnahan, M., Sands, J. and Strominger, J.L. (1989) A new cluster of genes within the human major histocompatibility complex. *Science*, **243**, 214–217.

45. Kendall, E., Sargent, C.A. and Campbell, R.D. (1990) Human major histocompatibility complex contains a new cluster of genes between the HLA-D and complement C4 loci. *Nucleic Acids Res.*, **18**, 7251–7257.

46. Hsieh, S.L. and Campbell, R.D. (1991) Evidence that gene G7a in the human major histocompatibility complex encodes valyl-tRNA synthetase. *Biochem. J.*, **278**, 809–816.

47. Cheng, J., Macon, K.J. and Volanakis, J.E. (submitted) Characterization of the protein encoded by gene RD in the human MHC class III region.

48. French, M.A.H. and Dawkins, R.L. (1990) Central MHC genes, IgA deficiency and autoimmune diseases. *Immunol. Today*, **11**, 271–274.

49. Carroll, M.C., Palsdottir, A., Belt, K.T. and Porter, R.R. (1985) Deletion of complement C4 and steroid 21-hydroxylase genes in the HLA class III region. *EMBO J.*, **4**, 2547–2552.

50. Lévi-Strauss, M., Carroll, M.C., Steinmetz, M. and Meo, T. (1988) A previously undetected MHC gene with an unusual periodic structure. *Science*, **240**, 201–204.

51. Yu, C.Y., Belt, K.T., Giles, C.M., Campbell, R.D. and Porter, R.R. (1986) Structural basis of the polymorphism of human complement components C4A and C4B: Gene size, reactivity and antigenicity. *EMBO J.*, **5**, 2873–2881.

52. Isenman, D.E. and Young, J.R. (1984) The molecular basis for the difference in immune hemolysis activity of the Chido and Rodgers isotypes of human complement C4. *J. Immunol.*, **132**, 3019–3027.

53. Law, S.K.A., Dodds, A.W. and Porter, R.R. (1984) A comparison of the properties of two classes, C4A and C4B, of the human complement component C4. *EMBO J.*, **3**, 1819–1823.

54. Böttger, E.C., Hoffman, T., Hadding, U. and Bitter-Suermann, D. (1985) Influence of genetically inherited complement deficiencies on humoral immune response in guinea pigs. *J. Immunol.*, **135**, 4100–4107.

55. O'Neil, K.M., Ochs, H.D., Heller, S.R., Cork, L.C., Morris, J.M. and Winkelstein, J.A. (1988) Role of C3 in humoral immunity: Defective antibody production in C3-deficient dogs. *J. Immunol.*, **140**, 1939–1945.

56. Böttger, E.C. and Bitter-Suermann, D. (1987) Complement and the regulation of humoral immune responses. *Immunol. Today*, **8**, 261–264.

57. Jackson, C.G., Ochs, H.D. and Wedgwood, R.J. (1979) Immune response of a patient with deficiency of the fourth component of complement and systemic lupus erythematosus. *N. Engl. J. Med.*, **300**, 1124–1129.

58. Finco, O., Li, S., Cuccia, M., Rosen, F.S. and Carroll, M.C. (1992) Structural differences between the two human complement C4 isotypes affect the humoral immune response. *J. Exp. Med.*, **175**, 537–543.

59. Bird, P. and Lachmann, P.J. (1988) The regulation of IgG subclass production in man: Low serum IgG4 in inherited deficiencies of the classical pathway of C3 activation. *Eur. J. Immunol.*, **18**, 1217–1222.

60. Ahearn, J.M. and Fearon, D.T. (1989) Structure and function of the complement receptors CR1 (CD35) and CR2 (CD21). *Adv. Immunol.*, **46**, 183–219.

61. Liu, Y.J., Johnson, G.D., Gordon, J. and MacLennan, I.C.M. (1992) Germinal centres in T-cell-dependent antibody responses. *Immunol. Today*, **13**, 17–21.

62. Heyman, B., Wiersma, E.J. and Kinoshita, T. (1990) In vivo inhibition of the antibody response by a complement receptor-specific monclonal antibody. *J. Exp. Med.*, **172**, 665–668.

63. Hebell, T., Ahearn, J.M. and Fearon, D.T. (1991) Suppression of the immune response by a soluble complement receptor of B lymphocytes. *Science*, **254**, 102–105.

64. Martin, D.R., Yuryev, A., Kalli, K.R., Fearon, D.T. and Ahearn, J.M. (1991) Determination of the structural basis for selective binding of Epstein–Barr virus to human complement receptor type 2. *J. Exp. Med.*, **174**, 1299–1311.

65. Carel, J.C., Myones, B.L., Frazier, B. and Holers, V.M. (1990) Structural requirements for C3dg/Epstein–Barr virus receptor (CR2/CD21) ligand binding, internalization and viral infection. *J. Biol. Chem.*, **265**, 12293–12299.

66. Tuveson, D.A., Ahearn, J.M., Matsumoto, A.K. and Fearon, D.T. (1991) Molecular interactions of complement receptors on B lymphocytes: A CR1/CR2 complex distinct from the CR2/CD19 complex. *J. Exp. Med.*, **173**, 1083–1089.

67. Matsumoto, A.K., Kopicky-Burd, J., Carter, R.H., Tuveson, D.A., Tedder, T.F. and Fearon, D.T. (1991) Intersection of the complement and immune systems: A signal transduction complex of the B lymphocyte-containing complement receptor type 2 and CD19. *J. Exp. Med.*, **173**, 55–64.

68. Bradbury, L., Kansas, G., Levy, S., Evans, R.L. and Tedder, T.F. (1991) CD19 is a component of a signal transducing complex on the surface of B cells that includes CD21, TAPA-1 and LEU-13. *FASEB J.*, **5**, A611.

69. Daha, M.R., Bloem, A.C. and Baillieux, R.E. (1984) Immunoglobulin production by human peripheral lymphocytes induced by anti-C3 receptor antibodies. *J. Immunol.*, **132**, 1197–1201.

70. Volanakis, J.E. and Fearon, D.T. (1993) The molecular biology of the complement system. In McCarty, D.J. and Koopman, W.J. (eds) *Arthritis and Allied Conditions: A Textbook of Rheumatology*, 12th edn. Lea & Febiger, Philadelphia, pp. 455–67.
71. Takahashi, S., Doss, C., Levy, S. and Levy, R. (1990) TAPA-1, the target of an antiproliferative antibody, is associated on the cell surface with the Leu-13 antigen. *J. Immunol.*, **145**, 2207–2213.
72. Oren, R., Takahashi, S., Doss, C., Levy, R. and Levy, S. (1990) TAPA-1, the target of an antiproliferative antibody, defines a new family of transmembrane proteins. *Mol. Cell. Biol.*, **10**, 4007–4015.
73. Carter, R.H., Tuveson, D.A., Park, D.J., Rhee, S.G. and Fearon, D.T. (1991) The CD19 complex of B lymphocytes. *J. Immunol.*, **147**, 3663–3671.
74. Pezzutto, A., Dörken, B., Rabinovitch, P.S., Ledbetter, J.A., Moldenhauer, G. and Clark, E.A. (1987) CD19 monoclonal antibody HD37 inhibits anti-immunoglobulin-induced B cell activation and proliferation. *J. Immunol.*, **138**, 2793–2799.
75. Carter, R.H., Spycher, M.O., Ng, Y.C., Hoffman, R. and Fearon, D.T. (1988) Synergistic interaction between complement receptor type 2 and membrane IgM on B lymphocytes. *J. Immunol.*, **141**, 457–463.
76. Pesando, J.M., Bouchard, L.S. and McMaster, B.E. (1989) CD19 is functionally and physically associated with surface immunoglobulin. *J. Exp. Med.*, **170**, 2159–2164.
77. Mauff, G., Alper, C.A., Awdeh, Z., Batchelor, J.R., Bertrams, J. *et al.* (1983) Statement on the nomenclature of human C4 allotypes. *Immunobiology*, **164**, 184–191.
78. Porter, R.R. (1983) Complement polymorphism, the major histocompatibility complex and associated diseases: A speculation. *Mol. Biol. Med.*, **1**, 161–168.
79. Dodds, A.W., Law, S.K. and Porter, R.R. (1985) The origin of the very variable haemolytic activities of the common human complement component C4 alotypes including C4-A6. *EMBO J.*, **4**, 2239–2244.
80. Carroll, M.C., Fathallah, D.M., Bergamaschini, L., Alicot, E.M. and Isenman, D.E. (1990) Substitution of a single amino acid (aspartic acid for histidine) converts the functional activity of human complement C4B to C4A. *Proc. Nat. Acad. Sci. USA*, **87**, 6868–6872.
81. Soothill, J.F., Hayes, K. and Dudgeon, J.A. (1966) The immunoglobulin in congenital rubella. *Lancet*, **i**, 1385–1388.
82. Rosen, F.S. (1980) Immune deficiencies: An overview. In Gelfand, E.W. and Dosch, H.M. (eds) *Biological Basis of Immunodeficiency*. Raven Press, New York, pp. 1–14.
83. Döcke, W.D., Simon, H.U., Fietze, E., Prösch, S., Diener, C. *et al.* (1991) Cytomegalovirus infection and common variable immunodeficiency. *Lancet*, **338**, 1957.
84. Aarli, J.A. (1976) Drug-induced IgA deficiency in epileptic patients. *Arch. Neurol.*, **33**, 296–299.
85. Shakir, R.A., Behan, P.O., Dick, H. and Lambie, D.G. (1978) Metabolism of immunoglobulin A, lymphocyte function, and histocompatibility antigens in patients on anticonvulsants. *J. Neurol. Neurosurg. Psychiatry*, **41**, 307–311.

Chapter 15

The Molecular Basis of Chronic Granulomatous Disease

DIRK ROOS

Central Laboratory of The Netherlands Red Cross Blood Transfusion Service and
Laboratory of Experimental and Clinical Immunology of the University of
Amsterdam, The Netherlands

Chronic granulomatous disease (CGD) is a clinical syndrome characterized by recurrent bacterial and fungal infections that are very difficult to treat (1–3). CGD is a rare disease, with an estimated incidence between 1 : 250 000 and 1 : 1 000 000. The disease usually manifests itself in early childhood and is predominantly found in boys. The most common sites of infection are the subcutaneous tissues, the lungs and the lymph nodes, and occasionally the liver and the bones. Most infections are caused by *Staphylococcus aureus* and Gram-negative enteric bacteria. *Aspergillus* pneumonia is a serious problem in these patients. Unless treated with intracellularly active antibiotics, CGD may be fatal at an early age. A special feature that has given its name to the disease is the development of chronic inflammations and multiple granulomas composed of giant cells and lipid-filled histiocytes. These granulomas may obstruct gastrointestinal or genitourinary tracts.

Specific immunity (antibody mediated and T cell mediated) develops normally in CGD patients, and levels of complement components are normal. Phagocytes (neutrophils, eosinophils and monocytes) are present in the circulation of CGD patients in normal numbers, and these cells move to infected areas and ingest microorganisms in a normal fashion (2). The release of microbicidal proteins from the granules into the phagosomes that contain the ingested microorganisms is also normal (2), but the release of reactive oxygen-derived products in the phagosomes is absent (4) due to a defect in the enzyme NADPH:O_2 oxidoreductase (NADPH oxidase) (5–7). This leads to the failure of CGD phagocytes to kill ingested microorganisms and

New Concepts in Immunodeficiency Diseases. Edited by S. Gupta and C. Griscelli
© 1993 John Wiley & Sons Ltd

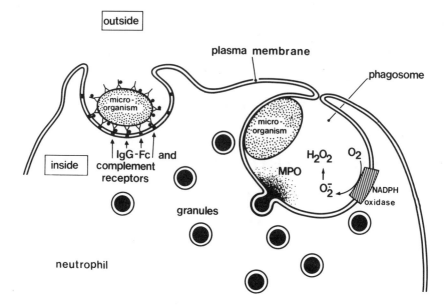

Figure 15.1. Schematic representation of phagocytosis, degranulation and generation of oxygen radicals. Microorganisms opsonized with specific IgG antibodies and complement fragments C3b/iC3b (asterisks) attach to Fc-γ receptors and complement receptors, respectively. This attachment induces phagocytosis, fusion of intracellular granules with the phagosome membrane and activation of the NADPH oxidase. Superoxide generated by the NADPH oxidase is spontaneously dismuted into hydrogen peroxide (H_2O_2). One of the enzymes released into the phagosome is myeloperoxidase (MPO), which catalyses the formation of hypochlorous acid from hydrogen peroxide and chloride ions. Reproduced from D. Roos (1991) The respiratory burst of phagocytic leukocytes. *Drug Invest.* (Suppl. 2) **3**, 48–53, by permission of Adis International

illustrates the importance of oxygen radicals in our defence against bacteria and fungi (Figure 15.1).

In this chapter, the present knowledge on the composition of the NADPH oxidase will be briefly reviewed. In addition, recent data will be presented on the mutations in this enzyme that lead to CGD. Finally, improved methods for prenatal diagnosis and advances in therapy will be described.

NADPH OXIDASE

General Properties

NADPH oxidase catalyses the reduction of molecular oxygen to superoxide ($O_2^{\overline{.}}$) (5). The reducing equivalents for this reaction, obtained from NADPH in the cytosol, are transferred to O_2 on the other side of the membrane (Figure 15.1). The overall reaction is as follows:

$$\text{NADPH} + 2O_2 \xrightarrow{\text{NADPH oxidase}} \text{NADP}^+ + 2O_2^{\bar{}} + H^+$$

NADPH oxidase is dormant in resting phagocytes and becomes activated upon adherence of microorganisms to these cells. Activation of NADPH oxidase results in increased oxygen uptake by the phagocytes, a process called the "respiratory burst".

Simultaneously with the generation of superoxide, hydrogen peroxide (H_2O_2) is also formed by the phagocytes (8). This is a secondary product, derived from superoxide in a spontaneous or superoxide dismutase (SOD)-catalysed reaction (9, 10):

$$2O_2^{\bar{}} + 2H^+ \xrightarrow[\text{or by SOD}]{\text{spontaneous}} H_2O_2 + O_2$$

In principle, $O_2^{\bar{}}$ and H_2O_2 might give rise to the formation of other, more reactive agents, such as hydroxyl radicals ($\cdot$OH) and singlet oxygen ($^1O_2$). However, the idea that phagocytes produce $\cdot$OH radicals has not been supported by convincing experimental evidence (11–13). Formation of hydroxyl radicals remains possible in a Fenton-type reaction inside target cells (14). Generation of $^1O_2$ has been shown to occur in eosinophils, but to a minor extent (15).

Superoxide is only weakly bactericidal, but H_2O_2 is more powerful in this respect. Moreover, H_2O_2 is converted by the haem enzyme myeloperoxidase into potent microbicidal hypohalites, such as hypochlorous acid (HOCl) (16). Myeloperoxidase is present in the azurophil granules of neutrophils and in the granules of monocytes, and is released into the phagocytic vacuole (Figure 15.1). Thus, in the phagolysosome, HOCl is formed. Interestingly, eosinophils contain another peroxidase, called eosinophilic peroxidase, which prefers bromide over chloride as a substrate (17), thus generating hypobromous acid (HOBr). HOCl and HOBr react with taurine and other β amino acids to form stable, microbicidal N-chloramines and N-bromamines (18, 19).

Cytochrome b_{558}

Studies of CGD families have shown that different genetic patterns of transmission of this disease exist: X-linked as well as autosomal (20–23). This indicated that the NADPH oxidase consists of more than one component, encoded by genes located either at the X chromosome or at an autosome. Subsequently, it was discovered that the X-linked form of CGD corresponds to the absence of a haem protein, called cytochrome b_{558}, in the phagocytes from these patients (24–27). This protein has a low redox potential (28) and is therefore considered to be the terminal NADPH oxidase component that donates electrons directly to molecular oxygen. The idea emerged that cytochrome b_{558} is the X chromosome-encoded component of the NADPH oxidase and that one or more other components might be autosome encoded. The truth proved to be more complicated.

First, several patients were reported with X-linked inheritance of CGD and decreased but measurable levels of cytochrome b_{558} in their phagocytes (29). However, recent experiments in our laboratory with cells from five of such X-linked variant CGD patients have shown that this subgroup of CGD belongs to the same complementation group as X-linked cytochrome b_{558}-negative CGD (29). Indeed, the mutations identified in the X-linked variant CGD patients and in the X-linked cytochrome b_{558}-negative CGD patients are located in the same NADPH oxidase component, encoded by an X-linked gene (30).

In addition, we discovered a family in which CGD was apparently transmitted in an autosomal fashion, although the cells from the three affected children (one boy, two girls) were practically devoid of cytochrome b_{558} (31). Fusion of monocytes from these patients with those of CGD patients with the X-linked, cytochrome b_{558}-negative form of the disease or with those of autosomal, cytochrome b_{558}-positive CGD patients resulted in heterokaryons with restored NADPH oxidase activity. Monocytes from the latter two groups fused with each other also showed this NADPH oxidase complementation (32). These studies proved that at least three different gene products are involved in NADPH oxidase activity.

The apparent discrepancy of both autosomal and X-linked cytochrome b_{558} deficiency was resolved by the discovery that this protein is composed of two subunits (33, 34), one of which is encoded by an X-linked gene and the other by an autosomal gene (35, 36). As expected, autosomal cytochrome b_{558}-negative CGD is caused by mutations in the autosome-encoded α subunit of cytochrome b_{558} (p22-*phox*) and X-linked cytochrome b_{558}-negative CGD by mutations in the X chromosome-encoded β subunit of cytochrome b_{558} (gp91-*phox*) (35, 36).* The fact that both subunits of cytochrome b_{558} are missing in either form of CGD (33, 34, 37, 38) is probably due to decreased stability of single subunits as compared to the $\alpha\beta$ heterodimer.

Both p22-*phox* (39) and gp91-*phox* (35, 40, 41) have been cloned, and the cDNA nucleotide sequence has been determined. P22-*phox* consists of 195 amino acids, with three or four hydrophobic regions that could serve as membrane-anchoring regions (42). There are no glycosylation sites in this protein. Stable mRNA for p22-*phox* is found not only in phagocytes but also in all other cell types that have been investigated (39). The subunit gp91-*phox*

---

*The following abbreviations have been internationally agreed among investigators of NADPH oxidase: p22-*phox*, α subunit of cytochrome b_{558} (molecular mass = 22 kDa); gp91-*phox*, β subunit of cytochrome b_{558} (molecular mass = 91 kDa); p47-*phox*, 47 kDa cytosolic component of the NADPH oxidase; p67-*phox*, 67 kDa cytosolic component of the NADPH oxidase; p = protein, gp = glycoprotein, *phox* = phagocyte oxidase.

consists of 570 amino acids, with five or six hydrophobic regions that could represent transmembrane domains. In addition, five potential N-glycosylation sites are present, three of which are located on a segment that might protrude at the extracellular side of the plasma membrane (35, 40, 42). Indeed, gp91-*phox* has been identified as a glycoprotein, with an M^r of 76 000 to 92 000 (33, 34, 38, 43, 44). In the various types of phagocytes, the glycosylation appears to be different. Glycosylation does not appear to be necessary for functional activity of cytochrome b_{558} (44). The C-terminus of gp91-*phox* has been found to be located intracellularly, and to function as a "docking site" for cytoplasmic components of the NADPH oxidase (42, 45). Stable mRNA for gp91-*phox* is found exclusively in phagocytes, the only cell type that expresses NADPH oxidase activity (35).

Cytochrome b_{558} contains two haem groups per molecule (34). The attachment sites for the haems were originally supposed to be located on p22-*phox*, based on haem-binding motifs in the amino acid sequence of this peptide (38, 39) and on radiation-inactivation analysis (46). More recent evidence suggests, however, that one haem is bound to gp91-*phox* and that the other haem is shared between the two subunits (47). Electron paramagnetic resonance (EPR) data indicate that both haem groups may contain a six-coordinate ion (48). This indicates that oxygen cannot directly react with the haem groups, in accord with the slow and slight shift in the optical spectrum of cytochrome b_{558} after reaction with carbon monoxide (28, 49, 50). Instead, oxygen may be reduced to superoxide at an extracellular site of the protein. Whether other intrinsic redox groups are involved in this reaction is not known.

Cell-free Activation System

The "cell-free" activation system of NADPH oxidase has provided further insight into the composition of this enzyme. In this system, phagocyte plasma membranes are mixed with phagocyte cytosol, NADPH, GTP, Mg^{2+} ions, and an anionic amphiphilic agent to "activate" the NADPH oxidase (usually a low concentration of sodium dodecyl sulphate (SDS) or arachidonic acid) (51–55). The superoxide generated in this system is truly dependent on NADPH oxidase activity, because fractions from CGD phagocytes are inactive in this assay (54) (Figure 15.2). Under optimal conditions, close to 100% of the $O_2^{\text{‒}}$ production by intact cells can be recovered in the cell-free system.

The necessity of both membranes and cytosol in this system indicates that either the enzyme is located in the membrane and needs one or more cytosolic factors for its activation, or the enzyme consists of both membrane-bound and cytosolic components, which cooperate for $O_2^{\text{‒}}$ generation. This last model implicates translocation of cytosolic component(s) of the NADPH oxidase to the plasma membrane, because the $O_2^{\text{‒}}$ generation—after activa-

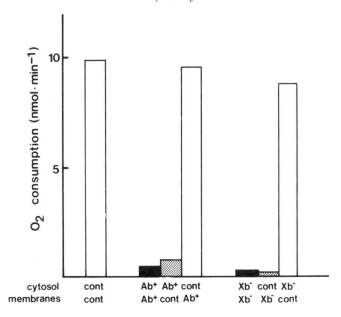

Ab+ = aut. cytochrome b₅₅₈ positive CGD

Xb⁻ = X-linked cyt. b₅₅₈ negative CGD

Figure 15.2. NADPH oxidase activity in the cell-free activation system. A mixture of neutrophil membranes (2×10^6 cell equivalents), neutrophil cytosol (2×10^6 cell equivalents), SDS (100 µM), NADPH (200 µM) and GTP-γ-S (10 µM) was incubated at 27 °C, and the oxygen consumption was measured. Membranes and cytosol were obtained from neutrophils of either healthy individuals (cont), A47⁰ CGD patients or X91⁰ CGD patients. Similar results to those shown with X91⁰ CGD neutrophil fraction were obtained with neutrophil fractions from A22⁰ CGD patients. Reproduced with permission from A.J. Verhoeven, B.G.J.M. Bolscher and D. Roos (1991), The superoxide-generating enzyme in phagocytes: physiology, protein composition and mechanism of activation. In C. Vigo-Pelfrey (ed.) *Membrane Lipid Oxidation*, Vol. II. CRC Press, Boca Raton, FL, pp. 41–63

tion of intact cells or in the cell-free system—is confined to the membrane fraction (56–62), and the cytosol loses activating potential (62, 63). Indeed, both in the cell-free system and in intact neutrophils, translocation of cytosolic components to the plasma membrane upon NADPH oxidase activation has been observed (63–66). Moreover, the NADPH oxidase activity generated in the cell-free system is enhanced with increasing amounts of cytosol, whereas the rate of activation of this process is independent of the cytosol concentration (55, 67). This, too, indicates that the cytosol contains one or more structural components of the NADPH oxidase.

When either membrane or cytosol fractions from CGD cells were mixed in the cell-free activation system with their normal counterparts, this revealed that cytochrome b_{558}-negative CGD cells (from either X-linked or autosomal patients) contain defective membranes and normal cytosol (54, 58) (Figure 15.2). This confirmed the membrane localization of cytochrome b_{558}. Interestingly, the reverse was found with cytochrome b_{558}-positive cells, viz. defective cytosol and normal membranes (68, 69) (Figure 15.2). Indeed, by mixing the normal cytosol from cytochrome b_{558}-negative CGD cells with the normal membranes from cytochrome b_{558}-positive CGD cells, complementation was also found in the cell-free activation system (70).

Cytosolic Components

However, the cell-free activation system proved to be a real breakthrough in NADPH oxidase research when it was applied to testing various cytosol fractions for the presence of an NADPH oxidase component. Several groups discovered that neutrophil cytosol contains three, or maybe even four, different proteins involved in NADPH oxidase activity (55, 71–74). At present, two cytosolic proteins have definitely been identified as NADPH oxidase components, because CGD patients with defects in these proteins are now known (71, 72, 75). These proteins have been cloned and sequenced (76–78), and found to have molecular masses of 47 and 67 kDa. For this reason, they are indicated as p47-*phox* and p67-*phox*, respectively. Unfortunately, the amino acid sequence of these proteins does not clarify their function.

However, both p47-*phox* and p67-*phox* carry two regions that are 18–40% homologous with so-called SH3 regions of non-receptor tyrosine kinases, of which *src* is the classical example. Similar regions are present in non-erythroid α spectrin, phospholipase C γ, GTPase-activating proteins and myosin I of yeast (78). Because all of these proteins are cytosolic proteins that move to the plasma membrane or cytoskeleton upon cell activation, these regions are supposed to be important for binding of p47-*phox* and p67-*phox* to structural cell proteins upon cell activation. The cytosolic C-terminus of gp91-*phox* is required for this translocation (45). In addition, the presence of p47-*phox* is required for translocation of p67-*phox*, but p47-*phox* will also translocate without p67-*phox* (66). Therefore, p47-*phox* and p67-*phox* probably integrate with cytochrome b_{558} in the formation of an active NADPH oxidase complex. It is not known whether p47-*phox* and/or p67-*phox* possess GTPase-activating properties for any GTP-binding proteins.

Additional Proteins

Several additional NADPH oxidase components have been suggested, but their identification is far from complete. First, experiments with reagents

Table 15.1 Properties of NADPH oxidase components

		p22-*phox*	gp91-*phox*	p47-*phox*	p67-*phox*
Gene	Locus	CYBA	CYBB	NCF1	NCF2
	Chrom. location	16q24	Xp21.1	7q11.23	1q25
	Size	8.5 kb	30 kb	17–18 kb	25–30 kb
	Exons	6	13	9	?
mRNA	Size	0.8 kb	5 kb	1.4 kb	2.4 kb
Protein	Amino acids	195	570	390	526
	Mol. wt predicted	20.9 kDa	65 kDa	44.6 kDa	60.9 kDa
	Mol. wt SDS–PAGE	22	76–92	47	67
	pI	10.0	9.7	10	6
	Location in resting phagocyte	Membrane	Membrane	Cytoplasm	Cytoplasm
	Post-translational modification	Phosphorylated	N-linked carbohydrates; Phosphorylated	Phosphorylated during oxidase activation	–

that block NADPH binding sites have provided evidence that the NADPH-binding component of the oxidase may be located in the cytosol of non-activated neutrophils, and that this component may translocate to the plasma membrane upon activation in the cell-free system (79). Labelling experiments with an NADPH analogue have indicated that this may be a protein of 32 kDa (80). On the other hand, Kakinuma *et al.* (81) have shown that a flavoprotein exists in neutrophil plasma membranes that forms a semiquinone radical after cell activation, with a redox potential between that of $NADPH/NADP^+$ and O_2/O_2^-. Thus, this flavoprotein may be involved in electron transfer from NADPH to oxygen, but the protein has not been identified.

Recently, Segal *et al.* (82) have proposed that cytochrome b_{558} itself may be an FAD-containing flavoprotein that binds NADPH. This suggestion was based on the low FAD content of neutrophil membranes from cytochrome b_{558}-negative CGD patients (also noted by other investigators, but to a variable degree; 26, 27, 83, 84), on sequence homology between gp91-*phox* and the ferridoxin NADP⁺ reductase family of reductases in the putative NADPH and FAD binding sites, and on (weak) labelling of purified cytochrome b_{558} with an NADPH analogue. Segal *et al.* (82) suggested that the membrane-bound flavoprotein investigated by Kakinuma *et al.* (81) might be identical to cytochrome b_{558}. If so, this would be the first flavocytochrome identified in higher eukaryotic cells.

Another cytosolic protein required for NADPH oxidase activity in the cell-free system has been called neutrophil cytosolic factor 3 (NCF-3) (72), soluble oxidase component I (SOC-I) (55, 74) or sigma 1 (85). This protein needs GTP for its translocation to the plasma membrane (74). Recently, sigma 1 has been purified and identified as the 22 kDa GTP-binding protein *rac-1* (86, 87). In contrast, Knaus *et al.* (88) found the closely related G-protein *rac-2* to regulate NADPH oxidase activity. Probably, these proteins are involved in promoting the formation of an active NADPH oxidase complex at the plasma membrane. Malech and colleagues have partly purified a cytosolic protein of 28 kDa that proved to be sufficient for reconstituting NADPH oxidase activity in a system with neutrophil membranes, recombinant p47-*phox* and recombinant p67-*phox* (89). Whether this 28 kDa protein is identical to a *rac* protein is not known. Also unknown is the function of *rap-1*, a small GTP-binding protein associated with cytochrome b_{558} in the membrane (90).

The problem with these additional proteins needed for NADPH oxidase activity is that CGD patients with a deficiency in any of these proteins have not been identified. In fact, such patients may never be found, because Clark *et al.* (75), in a survey of 94 CGD patients, was able to localize the defect in these patients either in the cytochrome b_{558} α or β subunit, in p47-*phox* or in p67-*phox*. It may well be that the additional protein(s) is (are) not specific for the NADPH oxidase but instead possess more general properties needed for activation/translocation of various cellular proteins. Lesions in such vital "activating" proteins might be lethal before or shortly after birth.

It must also be realized that activation of NADPH oxidase in the cell-free system may proceed via a mechanism totally different from that involved in the intact phagocyte. The respiratory burst is initiated in an intact phagocyte by ligand binding to cell surface receptors (e.g. Fc regions of opsonic immunoglobulins to Fc receptors, opsonic fragments of complement component C3 to complement receptors or high doses of chemotaxins to chemotaxin receptors). These receptors then undergo a conformational change and couple to tyrosine kinases or to membrane-bound GTP-binding proteins, which in their turn activate phospholipases and/or other protein kinases. In this chain of events, intracellular second messengers such as Ca^{2+} ions, inositol phosphates, leukotrienes, phosphatidic acid and diglycerides play an essential role. It is assumed that protein phosphorylation and/or protein acylation is required for the ultimate NADPH oxidase assembly. Indeed, phosphorylation of p47-*phox* is known to occur in the intact cell, at two serine residues in the cytosol and at six additional serine residues after translocation to the plasma membrane (91–94). This process will diminish the positive charge of p47-*phox* and thus facilitate interaction of this protein with the membrane. However, in the cell-free system, ATP is not required for either the translocation of p47-*phox* or for the induction of NADPH oxidase activity (55, 58, 95). Thus, proteins recognized in the cell-free activation system as required for NADPH oxidase activity do not necessarily play an identical role in the intact cell.

Model

Taking these data together, Figure 15.3 shows a tentative model of the NADPH oxidase. In the resting phagocyte, the two subunits of cytochrome b_{558} are located in the plasma membrane. The cytosol of resting phagocytes contains p47-*phox* and p67-*phox*. P47-*phox* is phosphorylated and translocates to cytochrome b_{558} upon activation. Depending on this process, p67-*phox* also translocates. As previously discussed, other proteins may also be involved in the assembly of the active NADPH oxidase complex, such as an NADPH-binding protein, and one or more regulatory proteins. Probably p47-*phox* and p67-*phox* are needed to induce a comformational change in cytochrome b_{558}, but do not take part in electron transfer themselves. The small G proteins may have similar activity-inducing properties. If Segal's

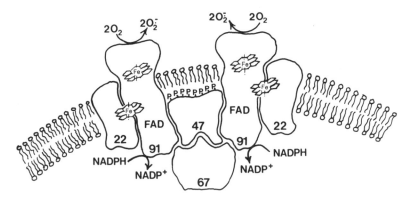

Figure 15.3. Schematic model of the phagocyte NADPH oxidase. In resting cells, p47-*phox* (47) and p67-*phox* (67) are located in the cytosol. After NADPH oxidase activation, these components translocate to the plasma membrane and integrate with the membrane-bound components gp91-*phox* (91) and p22-*phox* (22). Activating proteins (e.g. *rac-1*) may also translocate to the membrane. This results in formation of an active NADPH oxidase complex, which accepts two electrons from each NADPH molecule at the NADPH binding site on gp91-*phox* and transmits these through FAD and the haems to two molecules of oxygen at the other side of the plasma membrane, thus generating superoxide

concept (82) is true, electron flow may proceed from the NADPH binding site on gp91-*phox* via the flavin and the haems to oxygen. In this complex, the two electrons derived from each NADPH molecule must be delivered to two separate oxygen molecules. This may be achieved consecutively at the same place or simultaneously at two different places on the two cytochrome b_{558} molecules that are probably located within each NADPH oxidase structure (96).

BIOCHEMICAL LESIONS IN CGD

Lesions in p22-*phox*

The CYBA gene encoding p22-*phox* is located on the long arm of chromosome 16 and contains six exons (36). Mutations in this gene that inactivate p22-*phox* lead to an autosomal form of CGD. This type of CGD is rare, probably accounting for less than 5% of all CGD patients. Seven of these so-called A22 patients* have been studied in detail (36, 97, 98).

Table 15.3 shows that in all but one of these patients mRNA of apparently normal size was present in normal amounts on northern blots. In the one patient without detectable mRNA for p22-*phox*, southern blot analysis of genomic DNA after treatment with restriction enzymes revealed a homozygous deletion in the p22-*phox* gene that removed all but the extreme 5' coding sequence of the gene. Patients 2, 3, 5 and 6 were shown to suffer from A22⁰ CGD due to point mutations in the open reading frame. Patient 2 is a compound heterozygote for two mutations that predict a frame shift and a non-conservative amino acid replacement, respectively. The same Arg-90→Gln replacement was found in homozygous form in three patients from one family (no. 5 in Table 15.3). Patients 3 and 6 are homozygous for other missense mutations, resulting in other non-conservative amino acid changes.

Patient 4 is unusual, because she is a homozygote for a mutation that leads to cytochrome b_{558} inactivation but not to loss of cytochrome b_{558} protein or haem (97). Thus, the patient suffers from A22⁺ CGD. The Pro-156→Gln substitution found in this patient was shown to occur in a cytoplasmic region of p22-*phox*.

Finally, we have recently identified an A22⁰ CGD patient who is homozygous for a deletion of exon 4 in the p22-*phox* mRNA (patient 7, Table 15.3). Polymerase chain reaction (PCR)-amplified genomic DNA of this region had a normal size, indicating that the absence of exon 4 was not due to

---

*The new classification of CGD is shown in Table 15.2. Deficiency of p22-*phox* leads to (autosomal) A22 CGD. When no p22-*phox* protein is detectable, the superscript 0 is added; with diminished p22-*phox* protein, the superscript − is added; and with normal p22-*phox* protein levels, the superscript + is added (A22⁰ CGD, A22⁻ CGD, A22⁺ CGD). Similarly, deficiency in gp91-*phox* leads to X91⁰ CGD, X91⁻ CGD or X91⁺ CGD; deficiency in p47-*phox* to A47⁰ CGD, A47⁻ CGD or A47⁺ CGD; and deficiency in p67-*phox* to A67⁰ CGD, A67⁻ CGD or A67⁺ CGD.

322

Table 15.2 Classification of CGD

Subtype of CGD	Frequency (% of cases)	Component affected	Haem spectrum	gp91-phox protein (blot)	p22-phox protein (blot)	p47-phox protein (blot)	p67-phox protein (blot)	Defect in cell-free system	Oxidase activity (% of normal)
X91^0	~60	gp91-phox	Absent	Absent	Strongly diminished	Normal	Normal	Membrane	0
X91$^-$	<5	gp91-phox	Diminished	Diminished	Diminished	Normal	Normal	Membrane	10–30
X91$^+$	<1	gp91-phox	Normal	Normal	Normal	Normal	Normal	Membrane	2–5
A22^0	<5	p22-phox	Absent	Absent	Absent	Normal	Normal	Membrane	2–3
A22$^+$	<1	p22-phox	Normal	Normal	Normal	Normal	Normal	Membrane	0
A47^0	~30	p47-phox	Normal	Normal	Normal	Absent	Diminished	Cytosol	0–2
A67^0	<5	p67-phox	Normal	Normal	Normal	Normal	Absent	Cytosol	0–2

Table 15.3 Mutations in p22-*phox* in A22 CGD patients

Patient (Sex)	Initials	CGD subtype	Mutation	p22-*phox* mRNA	p22-*phox* protein and haem	Nucleotide change	Amino acid change	Ref.
1. (♀)	L.N.	A22⁰	>10 kb deletion (homozygous)	Absent	Absent	NA	NA	36
2. (♂)	G.S.	A22⁰	(a) Point deletion	Present	Absent	C272 deletion	Frameshift	36
			(b) Missense	Present	Absent	G297→A	Arg-90→Gln	
3. (♀)	O.P.	A22⁰	Missense (homozygous)	Present	Absent	C382→A	Ser-118→Arg	36
4. (♀)	I.L.	A22⁺	Missense (homozygous)	Present	Normal	C495→A	Pro-156→Gln	97
5. (2♀, 1♂)	fam. S.	A22⁰	Missense (homozygous)	Present	Absent	G297→A	Arg-90→Gln	98
6. (♀)	A.G.	A22⁰	Missense (homozygous)	Present	Absent	A309→G	His-94→Arg	98
7. (♂)	W.d.S.	A22⁰	Missense (homozygous)	Present	Absent	Intron 4 donor splice site G(+1)→A	Deletion exon 4	98

NA, not applicable. Patients 5 are two sisters and one brother.

a deletion in the gene. The flanking intron sequence of exon 4 revealed a single point mutation in the consensus donor splice site sequence (Table 15.3). Thus, in this patient, an mRNA splicing defect occurs that leads to skipping of exon 4. Because this is an in-frame deletion, a shortened polypeptide will be synthesized.

In three additional patients suspected to suffer from A22[0] CGD, no mutations were found in the coding sequence of the p22-*phox* cDNA, despite the appearance of ostensibly normal mRNA on northern blots (M. de Boer, Amsterdam, personal communication; J.P. Hossle, Zürich, personal communication).

Figure 15.4 shows a simplified structure of p22-*phox* and the small mutations in this polypeptide found so far. Mutations in the N-terminal, hydrophobic half of the protein all result in loss of cytochrome b_{558} expression. Apparently, such mutations either result in intrinsically unstable p22-*phox* protein or in p22-*phox* that is unable to form a stable heterodimer with gp91-*phox*. Of special interest is the His-94→Arg substitution in patient 6 (Table 15.3). This mutation removes the histidine that is probably involved in haem binding (36, 47). Although p22-*phox* contains two histidines, the His-72 is polymorphic and may be replaced by Tyr-72 without consequences

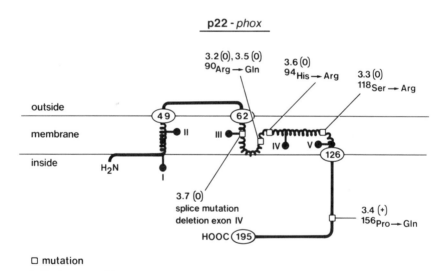

Figure 15.4. Schematic representation of p22-*phox*. Indicated are the possible orientation of the peptide in the membrane (42), the N- and C-terminal, the intron positions (roman numbers) and the small mutations in the A22 CGD patients: (0) indicates A22[0], (+) indicates A22[+] CGD. Patient numbers refer to tables in the text. Adapted from an idea of Dr J. Curnutte, with permission. Mutations leading to frameshifts have not been included

for NADPH oxidase activity (36). However, because the neutrophils from patient 6 did not contain measurable amounts of cytochrome b_{558} subunits on western blot either, the His-94 substitution affects the stability and/or the association of p22-*phox* with gp91-*phox* as well.

The Pro-156→Gln mutation in the hydrophilic C-terminal part of p22-*phox* leaves the haem and the association with gp91-*phox* intact. Perhaps this amino acid substitution interferes with the interaction of cytochrome b_{558} with other NADPH oxidase components, and in this way causes NADPH oxidase inactivation. Altogether, seven mutations have been found in seven A22 CGD families, indicating that this type of CGD is very heterogeneous in nature. Moreover, only four polymorphisms have been recognized in the reading frame of p22-*phox* so far (36, 98). Apparently, small changes in the structure of p22-*phox* already lead to instability and/or loss of function of this protein.

Lesions in gp91-*phox*

The CYBB gene encoding gp91-*phox* is located on the short arm of the X chromosome (35, 99) and contains 13 exons (99a). Mutations in this gene account for all cases of X-linked CGD. This type of CGD is the most common one encountered (50–60% of all patients).

Several X91⁰ patients are known with large deletions in the Xp21 area, sometimes causing other clinical syndromes in addition to CGD (35, 99–101). When the genomic organization shows no large deletions, mRNA analysis may give an indication as to the defect within the gene. In contrast to early evidence (35, 40), we found detectable mRNA for p91-*phox* in the large majority of X91⁰ patients. However, sometimes the amount or the size of the mRNA is subnormal.

Table 15.4 shows a survey of ten patients with apparently normal gp91-*phox* mRNA. In three patients, no gp91-*phox* protein or haem was detectable. In these patients, we found two point mutations that predict non-conservative amino acid replacements and one point mutation that leads to a premature termination codon (30). In three other patients, a 70–90% decrease in gp91-*phox* (and p22-*phox*) protein and haem was observed, as well as a similar decrease in NADPH oxidase activity of intact neutrophils and in the cell-free activation system (29, 30). Sequence analysis of the gp91-*phox* cDNA revealed single point mutations predicting incorporation of different amino acids. Two additional X91⁻ patients (maternal cousins) analysed in the laboratory of Dr John Curnutte showed a similar single amino acid replacement (patients 7.1 and 7.2, Table 15.4).

Occasionally, CGD patients present with phagocytes of the X91⁺ subtype: X-linked inheritance of the disease, inactive NADPH oxidase, but normal cytochrome b_{558} protein and haem levels. Two of such patients have been

Table 15.4 Mutations in gp91-*phox* in X91 CGD patients with normal gp91-*phox* mRNA

Patient	Initials	CGD subtype	Mutation	gp91-*phox* mRNA	gp91-*phox* protein and/or haem	Nucleotide change	Amino acid change	Ref.
1. (♂)	P.B.	X91⁰	Missense	Normal	Absent	C637→T	His-209→Tyr	30
2. (♂)	B.C.	X91⁰	Missense	Normal	Absent	C229→T	Arg-73→stop	30
3. (♀)	E.P.	X91⁰	Missense	Normal	Absent	A314→G	His-101→Arg	30
4. (♂)	F.B.	X91⁻	Missense	Normal	Decreased	G1178→C	Gly-389→Ala	30
5. (♂)	J.L.	X91⁻	Missense	Normal	Decreased	G734→C	Cys-244→Ser	30
6. (♂)	R.L.	X91⁻	Missense	Normal	Decreased	G478→A	Ala-156→Thr	30
7.1 (♂)	D.H.	X91⁻	Missense	Normal?	Decreased	?	Glu-309→Lys	–
7.2 (♂)	T.C.	X91⁻	Missense	Normal?	Decreased	?	Glu-309→Lys	–
8. (2♂)	R.C./D.C.	X91⁺	Missense	Normal	Normal	C1256→A	Pro-415→His	102
9. (♂)	M.G.	X91⁺	Missense	Normal	Normal	Intron 11 acceptor splice site A(−1)→G	Deletion amino acids 488–497 in exon 12	103

Patient 3 is a female carrier with extreme lyonization (2–5% positive cells in the NBT test). In this patient, the control sequence of gp91-*phox* cDNA was found as well. Patients 7.1 and 7.2 are maternal first cousins. Patients 8 are two brothers.

Table 15.5 Mutations in gp91-*phox* in X91 patients with decreased gp91-*phox* mRNA

Patient (Sex)	Initials	CGD subtype	Mutation	gp91-*phox* mRNA	gp91-*phox* protein and/or haem	Nucleotide change	Amino acid change	Ref.
1. (♂)	G.Q.	X91⁰	Single bp deletion	Decreased	Absent	T134 deletion	Frameshift	104
2. (♂)	T.F.	X91⁰	Single bp deletion	Decreased	Absent	T59 deletion	Frameshift	–
3. (♂)	J.W.	X91⁰	120 bp deletion	Decreased	Absent	?	Deletion amino acids 530–570	35, 105
4.1 (♂)	T.W.	X91⁰	~3 kb deletion	Decreased	Absent	?	Deletion exon 5, frameshift	–
4.2 (♂)	N.W.	X91⁰	~3.5 kb deletion	Decreased	Absent	?	Deletion exon 6 + 7	–
5. (♂)	T.S.	X91⁰	14 kb deletion	Decreased?	Absent	?	Deletion exon 4–9, frameshift	–
6. (♂)	P.E.	X91⁰	40 bp insertion	Decreased?	Absent	Insert between G702 and C703	13 amino acids extra after Gly-230, frameshift	–
7. (♂)	C.B.	X91⁰	Missense	Decreased	Absent	Intron 7 donor splice site T(+2)→A	Deletion exon 7, frameshift	104, 106
8. (♂)	D.D.	X91⁰	Missense	Decreased, smaller	Absent	Intron 5 donor splice site A(+3)→T	Deletion exon 5, frameshift	104, 106
9. (♂)	R.W.	X91⁰	Missense	Decreased	Absent	Intron 3 donor splice site G(+5)→A	Deletion exon 3	106
10. (♂)	E.Zw.	X91⁰	Missense	Decreased	Absent	Intron 1 acceptor splice site G(−1)→A	Deletion exon 2	106
11. (♂)	R.H.	X91⁰	Missense	Decreased	Absent	C633→A	Deletion Trp-206–end	106

Patients 4.1 and 4.2 are two brothers.

analysed for the mutation in the gp91-*phox* gene. In family 8 (with two affected brothers), a single nucleotide substitution was found, leading to a Pro→His substitution at position 415 (102). In patient 9, an elderly man who was recognized as a CGD patient at the age of 69 years, an acceptor splice site mutation was found that apparently activates a cryptic splice site in exon 12 (103). As a result, a 30-nucleotide stretch of this exon is skipped during gp91-*phox* mRNA splicing, and the gp91-*phox* peptide is predicted to lack ten amino acids near its C-terminus.

Table 15.5 shows the mutations found in X91⁰ patients with decreased amounts of gp91-*phox* mRNA. Here, the diversity of mutations is even larger. Two patients showed single base-pair deletions, leading to frame-shifts and premature stop codons downstream of the mutations (104, de Boer and Roos, unpublished). Four other patients were found to have larger deletions in their gp91-*phox* cDNA (105). Remarkably, patients 4.1 and 4.2 (Table 15.5), who are brothers, present with two different deletions (de Boer and Roos, unpublished). Analysis of the genomic DNA with restriction enzymes confirmed the size analysis of the PCR-amplified cDNA. Moreover, the mother of these patients was found to carry both of these deletions in her genomic DNA, as well as the normal composition. This family is now studied in more detail (cDNA sequencing and karyotyping).

One patient (no. 6, Table 15.5) was found with a 40 bp insertion at the intron 6/exon 7 boundary (de Boer and Roos, unpublished). This proved to be a 40 bp repeat, probably caused by unequal crossing-over. As a result, 13 additional amino acids are predicted to be incorporated, followed by 23 different amino acids and a premature termination of peptide synthesis due to a frameshift.

Five patients were identified with deletions in the mRNA for gp91-*phox* due to splicing errors (104, 106). All of these patients had decreased levels of gp91-*phox*, but in only one case was the smaller size of the mRNA already detectable on a northern blot. In patients 7, 8 and 9 (Table 15.5), exon skipping appeared to be due to single nucleotide substitutions in the donor splice sites of the relevant exons, i.e. in the first five nucleotides of the introns succeeding these exons. In patient 10, a missense mutation was found in the acceptor splice site of exon 2, i.e. in the last two nucleotides of intron 1. This leads to skipping of exon 2 during mRNA splicing. Thus, exons 2, 3, 5 and 7 are skipped entirely in these patients. Apparently, these exons do not contain cryptic splice sites that are activated when the normal donor or acceptor splice sites are mutated (as happened in exon 12 of patient 9, Table 15.4). However, the reverse occurred in patient 11 of Table 15.5. In this patient, a mutation in exon 6 apparently created a new splice site that was preferred over the normal donor splice site of this exon. The reason for this preference is not known, but might be due to the upstream (5') position of the new splice site, or to a better fit with the nucleotide sequence of the splicing enzyme. It is also not known why these last five patients had decreased levels of gp91-*phox* mRNA, in contrast to patient 9 of Table 15.4. Perhaps the downstream (3') position of the mutation in the mRNA of this last patient, or the small size of the deletion (30 nucleotides), led to a more stable mRNA species than in the other five patients.

Finally, in five additional patients suspected of suffering from X91⁰ CGD, gp91-*phox* mRNA was undetectable on northern blot. Nevertheless, treatment with reverse transcriptase of the mRNA from these patients and amplification by PCR with primers specific for gp91-*phox* mRNA yielded fragments of the expected size, and enough for sequence analysis. However, the composition of these products were normal (de Boer and Roos, unpublished). Therefore, in these patients, the disease may be due to the formation of unstable gp91-*phox* mRNA, for instance caused by mutations in the 3' non-coding region. Alternatively, mutations in a promoter region may have led to decreased formation of gp91-*phox* mRNA. However, caution should be taken when interpreting these results. First, in two of these patients, the X-linked nature of the disease was not proven (e.g. by a mosaic in the nitroblue-tetrazolium dye (NBT) test from an obligate carrier or by monocyte hybridization). Second, contamination of the PCR reaction with normal cDNA for gp91-*phox* can never be excluded. Identification of the mutation in these last five patients awaits further analysis.

This list of different mutations leading to X91 CGD clearly illustrates the very heterogeneous nature of these lesions. Because polymorphisms within the coding region of the CYBB gene are not known, it appears that the gp91-*phox* polypeptide is extremely sensitive to mutations.

Figure 15.5 shows a simplified structure of gp91-*phox* and the small mutations in this polypeptide found so far. As in the p22-*phox* subunit, mutations in the N-terminal half of gp91-*phox*, which contains most of the hydrophobic stretches that might serve as membrane-spanning regions, lead to loss of stability and/or loss of haem moieties. Especially the mutations found in patients 1 and 3 (Table 15.4), which remove histidyl residues, may have direct consequences for haem binding. Other mutations in this part of gp91-*phox* may weaken the secondary structure of the protein. In contrast, mutations in the C-terminal, hydrophilic part of gp91-*phox*, of which at least the extreme C-terminus is located in the cytosol (45), lead to loss of function, but not to loss of stability or haem binding. According to Segal *et al.* (82), the Pro-415 (mutated in patients 8, Table 15.4) may be involved in NADPH binding to cytochrome b_{558}. Loss of gp91-*phox* protein in patient 5.3 may be due to decreased mRNA stability, because the 3' untranslated region belongs to exon 13. Probably, this whole exon is missing in this patient.

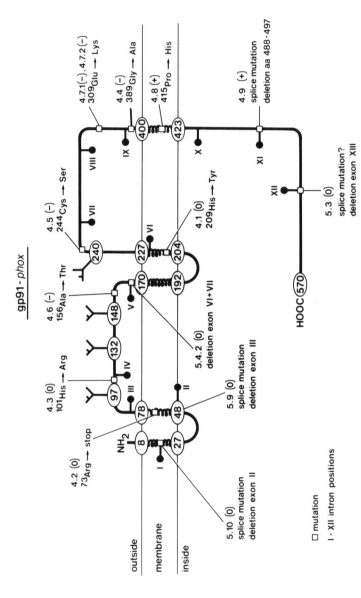

Figure 15.5. Schematic representation of gp91-*phox*. Indicated are the possible orientation of the peptide in the membrane (42), the N- and C-terminal, the intron positions (roman numbers), the possible glycosylation sites (Y) and the small mutations in the X91 CGD patients: (0) indicates X91⁰, (–) indicates X91⁻, (+) indicates X91⁺ CGD patients. Patient numbers refer to tables in the text. Mutations leading to frameshifts have not been included. Adapted from ref. 168

Lesions in p47-*phox* or p67-*phox*

The NCF1 gene encoding p47-*phox* is located on the long arm of chromosome 7, and the NCF2 gene encoding p67-*phox* on the long arm of chromosome 1 (107). The structures of these genes are not yet known. Defects in these genes lead to the autosomal A47 and A67 types of CGD. A47 CGD is quite common (about one-third of all CGD patients), but A67 CGD is rare (probably less than 5% of all CGD patients). In CGD patients who lack western blot-detectable p47-*phox* or p67-*phox*, mRNA for these proteins was present in apparently normal amounts and with a normal size, as judged from northern blots with RNA isolated from mononuclear leucocytes (77, 78, 108, 109).

In a number of unrelated CGD patients with p47-*phox* deficiency, the genetic defect has been characterized. A dinucleotide deletion at a GTGT tandem repeat, corresponding to the acceptor site of the intron 1/exon 2 junction, was reported to cause this type of CGD (108, 109). Some patients have a homozygous GT deletion; others are compound heterozygotes for this deletion in combination with missense mutations leading to Lys→Glu or Thr→Ala substitutions (109). It is remarkable that this type of CGD is apparently much less heterogeneous than the A22 and X91 types. One preliminary report has appeared on the mutation in a A67⁰ CGD patient (110). An insertion of about 100 bp was found to be located between codons 212 and 324 of the 526-residue coding region. The precise mutation has not yet been reported.

Other Lesions

Defects in the NADPH oxidase may be caused, in principle, by lesions in structural components, in activating components or in substrate provision. Defects in the four proteins described in the previous paragraphs all concern mutations in genes of structural oxidase components. Two defects in activating components and one in substrate provision are known, leading to clinical syndromes that sometimes resemble CGD.

Leucocyte Adhesion Deficiency

Defects in the β subunit of the LeuCAM (leucocyte cell adhesion molecules), also called β2 integrins, cause the well-known syndrome of leucocyte adhesion deficiency (LAD). This family of adhesion proteins consists of three members: the leucocyte function-associated antigen-1 (LFA-1; CD18/11a), the complement receptor type 3 (CR3; CD18/11b) and the glycoprotein gp150,95 (CD18/11c). The β2 subunit (CD18) is identical for each family member; the α subunit is different. A deficiency in β2 results in the lack of all three adhesion proteins in the cells. Several mutations in β2 have been shown to cause LAD (111).

In general, the β2 proteins are involved in the ability of the leucocytes to reach their destination in the tissues. For instance, phagocyte diapedesis depends on the proper adhesion of these cells to and movement through the endothelial cells of the blood vessels. This diapedesis phenomenon is mediated by binding of CR3 on the phagocytes to its "counter-structure" or "addressin" on the endothelial cells. LAD is therefore characterized by the inability of the phagocytes to leave the circulation and reach the site of an infection in the tissues. As a result, LAD patients suffer from very serious, non-purulent bacterial infections and impaired wound healing.

However, because CR3 is also a receptor for the iC3b fragment of complement component C3, and as such involved in the activation of the phagocyte bactericidal mechanisms by iC3b-opsonized microorganisms, LAD phagocytes are also unable to activate the NADPH oxidase through iC3b-opsonized particles (112–114) (see Figure 15.1). Although other opsonins exist (IgG antibodies, C3b fragments) that activate phagocytes through other receptors (Fc-γ receptors, CR1), these back-up mechanisms may fail. For instance, IgG antibodies that have bound complement fragments may not be able to contact Fc-γ receptors any more, because the binding region for these receptors is sterically hindered by the complement fragments. Moreover, many microorganisms bind iC3b rather than C3b fragments (114). Thus, bacterial killing by LAD cells may also be disturbed.

Besides the direct function of CR3 in the activation of the NADPH oxidase by iC3b-coated particles, CR3 is also involved in oxidase activation by other agents. For example, phorbol-myristate acetate (PMA) activation of the respiratory burst is sometimes severely depressed in LAD cells (113–115). This can be mimicked by normal neutrophils in the presence of certain anti-CR3 antibodies (Roos *et al.* unpublished). The mechanism of this phenomenon is unknown.

Glycogen Storage Disease Type Ib

Glycogen storage disease type I is a metabolic disease caused by a defect in the activity of glucose 6-phosphatase (G6Pase), normally present in liver, kidney and intestinal mucosa cells. This enzyme activity is dependent on the coupling of three integral microsomal membrane components: (a) a glucose 6-phosphate (G6P)-specific translocase that shuttles G6P across the membrane; (b) the enzyme G6Pase, a non-specific phosphohydrolase; and (c) a phosphate translocase that mediates the efflux of inorganic phosphate. Glycogen storage disease type I may be caused by a deficiency of hepatic G6Pase (type Ia) or by a deficiency of the hepatic G6P translocase (type Ib). Both defects prevent the conversion of G6P to glucose, resulting in hypoglycaemia during fasting. The clinical features of these deficiencies are indistinguishable, except that patients with type Ib are often neutropenic and prone to recurrent infections whereas patients with type Ia are not. Respiratory burst activity is greatly reduced in glycogen storage disease type Ib neutrophils and monocytes (116–120).

It is not clear what the relation is between the hepatic microsomal G6P translocase defect and the deficiency in phagocyte respiratory burst, nor how a defect in G6P translocase can produce alterations in phagocytic cell function while the absence of G6Pase does not. Bashan *et al.* (119) found a strongly impaired uptake of glucose in type Ib neutrophils (but not in type Ib lymphocytes) and hypothesized that this might account for the metabolic defect in these cells. However, Kilpatrick *et al.* (120) noted that diminished respiratory burst activity of type Ib phagocytes remains in the absence of glucose. In addition, NADPH oxidase and hexose monophosphate shunt activity were found to be normal in type Ib neutrophil *lysates* (117, 119). Therefore, the impaired respiratory burst activity in the intact phagocytes of these patients might be related to NADPH oxidase *activation* rather than in NADPH oxidase components or substrate provision. Indeed, Kilpatrick *et al* (120) found decreased calcium storage in these cells and a decreased ability to mobilize this calcium. However, the cause of this signalling defect remains to be established.

Leucocyte Glucose 6-phosphate Dehydrogenase Deficiency

Another defect is known to cause a shortage of NADPH in phagocytes, thus indirectly causing a deficiency of the NADPH oxidase. This extremely rare condition is caused by a deficiency of glucose 6-phosphate dehydrogenase (G6PD) in the leucocytes (usually G6PD deficiency is limited to the erythrocytes). In resting G6PD-deficient phagocytes, the NADPH concentration can be maintained at a sufficiently high level for the cell function, but during phagocytosis the NADPH demand of the oxidase cannot be met. Thus, superoxide production is very low, and a clinical syndrome indistinguishable from CGD results (121–124).

Glutathione Peroxidase Deficiency

In 1970, Holmes *et al.* (125) described a partial deficiency of glutathione peroxidase in the leucocytes of two unrelated, female CGD patients. The CGD brother of one of these patients (126), as well as an unrelated, male CGD patient (127), showed similar depressed activities of this enzyme in their leucocytes. The causal relation between glutathione peroxidase deficiency and failure of superoxide generation has never been explained satisfactorily (128).

Recently, two of these patients have been reexamined by Curnutte *et al.* (129). Purified neutrophils from these patients contained normal glutathione peroxidase activity and mRNA, but were devoid of cytochrome b_{558}. In one patient, this was due to a lack of gp91-*phox* mRNA; in the other, it was due to mutations in the two alleles of the p22-*phox* gene. Thus, it appears that mutations involving either the large or the small subunit of cytochrome b_{558}, and not glutathione peroxidase deficiency, are responsible in these patients for the CGD phenotype.

DIAGNOSIS OF CGD

In a patient with clinical symptoms suggestive of CGD, the following laboratory tests should be performed. In the plasma or serum, the levels of immunoglobulins and complement components should be normal, as well as the opsonizing capacity for various microorganisms. Lymphocyte reactivity in all aspects should also be normal. Phagocyte reactivity (usually tested with neutrophils purified from blood) should be normal, except for parameters of the respiratory burst (see below) and the killing of certain microorganisms by the phagocytes. Cultures made from infected areas in CGD usually show catalase-positive bacteria (*Staphylococcus aureus*, *Escherichia coli*, pneumococci) or catalase-positive fungi (*Candida albicans*), and the phagocytes of the patients fail to kill catalase-positive microorganisms *in vitro* (1–3). This is caused by the fact that catalase-negative microorganisms excrete hydrogen peroxide, which aids in the intracellular destruction of these organisms by CGD cells.

Recognition of Patients

Parameters of the respiratory burst frequently used for the identification of CGD patients are the following. Oxygen consumption in response to particulate or soluble stimuli is generally measured with an oxygen electrode (130). For this purpose, purified neutrophils, total leucocytes (130), or even full blood (Roos *et al.*, unpublished) are mixed with pre-opsonized bacteria, yeast or zymosan particles (extracted yeast membranes). Alternatively, these microorganisms are mixed with the phagocytes in the presence of about 10% human serum. For soluble stimuli the protein kinase C (PKC) activator PMA and the chemotaxin formyl-methionyl-leucyl-phenylalanine (FMLP) are frequently used, but other agents, such as cytochalasin E, arachidonic acid, other free fatty acids or membrane-perturbing agents are also active. All of these agents induce a sharp increase in oxygen consumption (and formation of oxidase products) by phagocytes from normal individuals, but not by those from CGD patients. Depending on the genetic subgroup of CGD, and in some rare variants, a weak reaction is sometimes detectable (29, 131, 132).

Generation of the primary product of the NADPH oxidase reaction, superoxide, can also be used for the detection of CGD patients. Several assays for O_2^- are available; the best known are the reduction of ferri-cytochrome c, the chemiluminescence reaction and the NBT test. Reduction of ferri-cytochrome c is usually measured spectrophotometrically at 550 nm against a reference cuvette containing SOD (133). To avoid non-specific reduction, acetylated cytochrome c is sometimes used. To avoid oxidation of the ferro-cytochrome c, catalase should be added. Chemiluminescence is measured in a luminometer. It is a sensitive assay, which is rendered even more sensitive by amplification of the signal with lucigenin or luminol. The signal with lucigenin is O_2^- specific, i.e. completely quenched by SOD. The signal with luminol is partly dependent on O_2^- and partly on H_2O_2 (catalase sensitive). Moreover, with luminol the signal is also dependent on the presence of a peroxidase, either from the cells or added to the assay mixture. Thus, luminol-enhanced chemiluminescence is deficient in CGD but also in myelo-peroxidase deficiency.

The NBT test can be used for quantification of the amount of O_2^- produced (after extraction of its reduction product formazan with pyridine) as well as in a qualitative microscopic test for evaluation of the ability of individual cells to produce O_2^- (134). The latter test is also known as the NBT slide test, and is based on the formation of insoluble, black deposits within each O_2^--forming cell (Figure 15.6). This test is very useful for the distinction of cells with an active NADPH oxidase from those without, but cannot be very well used for the quantification of the oxidase activity of individual cells. In a semi-quantitative NBT slide test, CGD subgroups may be distinguished (135).

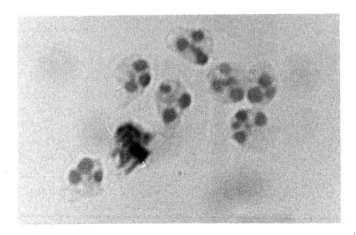

Figure 15.6. NBT slide test with neutrophils from an X91[0] carrier. The cells were incubated with nitroblue tetrazolium (NBT), stimulated with PMA and stained with nuclear fast red as described in ref. 130. Normal cells produce O_2^-, which reduces NBT to black formazan precipitates in these cells; cells deficient in NADPH oxidase activity do not show this reaction. One normal and seven deficient cells are visible

The formation of H_2O_2 is another parameter of the respiratory burst that can be used for the recognition of CGD patients. This product can be measured with an H_2O_2 electrode (136) or fluorimetrically by oxidation of scopoletin (137) or homovanillic acid (138). A recent development is the measurement of a fluorescent oxidation product (accumulated) in a large number of individual cells by flow cytometry; this method quantifies both the fraction of active cells and the oxidase activity per cell (139). However, because cell samples have to be fixed before analysis, kinetic experiments cannot be performed on-line.

Carrier Detection

Due to the lyonization phenomenon, carriers of X-linked diseases can be recognized by assays at the single-cell level. During early embryonic development, one of the X chromosomes in each female cell is inactivated. This is a random process that may affect either a "normal" X chromosome or an X chromosome that carries a mutation. If this process takes place at a stage when already several cells have been formed that will give rise to a certain organ or tissue (e.g. the bone marrow), then the completely developed organ or tissue will contain a mixture of normal and mutated cells. At the single-cell level, this is detectable as a mosaic of functional and non-functional cells. In X-linked CGD, the NBT slide test with activated phagocytes (usually with PMA) is used for this purpose, and shows a mixture of O_2^- forming cells (with black formazan deposits) and inactive cells (without these deposits). An example is shown in Figure 15.6. Thus, mothers and maternal grandmothers of CGD patients with the X-linked form of the disease (obligate heterozygotes) and about half of the sisters and maternal aunts of these patients often show a mosaic in the NBT slide test. However, about one-third of all X-linked defects arise from new mutations. Thus, "obligate" carriers are often normal. Moreover, extreme lyonization toward the normal phenotype may obscure the detection of carriers. A less sensitive test for the detection of carriers of X-linked CGD is measurement of the respiratory burst by the phagocytes of these individuals.

Carriers of the autosomal types of CGD are less easy to recognize. Even in phagocytes from the parents of such patients, who are obligate heterozygotes, no abnormalities in any of the respiratory burst parameters can be detected. Recently, however, we have found that this problem may be overcome by careful analysis of these reactions with a combination of agents (140). Oxygen consumption with PMA, but not with FMLP or with serum-treated zymosan (STZ), is significantly lower in autosomal CGD carriers than in normal individuals. This can be clearly demonstrated when FMLP or STZ is added in succession to PMA to the cells: an increase of more than 100% in the rate of oxygen consumption is then observed with neutrophils from carriers of autosomal CGD, whereas those of normal individuals show an increase of only about 40%. Thus, the gene-dose effect is apparent with the relatively weak stimulus PMA, but not with the stronger stimuli FMLP or STZ. This may be due to the PKC activation induced by PMA and the additional activation pathways induced by FMLP and STZ (141).

With the introduction of the cell-free activation system with arachidonic acid or SDS, it has also become possible to recognize autosomal CGD carriers in this way. Cytosol from carrier neutrophils mixed with plasma membranes from normal cells often shows intermediate O_2^- production between normal values and patient values (68).

Until now, these assays have only been performed with cells from carriers of autosomal, cytochrome *b*-positive CGD, and distinction between A47 and A67 CGD has not yet been made. Perhaps assays for heterozygote detection based on reaction with antisera against NADPH oxidase components will become available in future. However, the ultimate test for carrier detection, be it X linked or autosomal, has to be based on gene analysis.

Genetic Classification

As mentioned earlier in this chapter, complementation analysis of monocyte heterokaryons from CGD patients has proved the existence of three genetic subgroups of the disease (31, 32). In this way, X91, A22 and A47 CGD have been differentiated. Complementation analysis is also possible in the cell-free activation system (70). In this way, the fourth subgroup of A67 CGD was discovered (72). Later, antibodies against p47-*phox* and against p67-*phox* have made the distinction between A47⁻ and A67⁻ CGD very easy (75). In case of X91⁰ and A22⁰ CGD, however, both cytochrome b_{558} subunits turned out to be absent in both types of CGD (33, 34, 37, 38). Therefore, distinction between these two types of CGD has to be made by other means.

Complementation between X91 and A22 CGD in the cell-free system does not occur (70), also because both subunits of cytochrome b_{558} are absent in both types of CGD. Thus, in case of CGD patients with a cytochrome b_{558} deficiency, from uninformative families, distinction between X91⁰ and A22⁰ CGD is still difficult. Although this distinction is not important for treatment of the patients, and although the answer will be known once the mutation has been identified, it may sometimes be convenient to make the distinction in an early phase of the investigations, e.g. to know in which gene to expect a mutation. In that case, monocyte fusions may still be indicated (29).

Prenatal Diagnosis

Before the NADPH oxidase components had been cloned, prenatal diagnosis of CGD could only be performed by analysis of umbilical blood, e.g.

with the NBT slide test or with a whole-blood oxygen consumption assay (142). However, fetal blood samples cannot be obtained before 16–18 weeks gestation. This means second-trimester abortions for carriers of affected fetuses. In an attempt to accelerate the diagnosis, Nakamura *et al.* (143) suggested the use of monoclonal antibodies to detect cytochrome b_{558} in macrophages of chorionic villi obtained at 7–8 weeks gestation. This technique did indeed succeed in normal tissue but was not yet tested on fetuses with CGD. Therefore, its value remains to be established.

With the availability of molecular reagents, phagocytic cells are no longer required for the detection of genetic defects in NADPH oxidase components. Either restriction fragment length polymorphisms (RFLPs) or detection of specific gene defects in fetal DNA obtained by chorionic villus biopsy or amniocentesis can provide the means for a definite diagnosis for families at risk. Most efforts in this respect have been directed towards X91 CGD, because sons from carriers of this disease have a 50% chance of being a patient, irrespective of the husband of the carrier.

In case of a complete or partial gene deletion, simple southern blot analysis will suffice to recognize patients. Indeed, in the family of patient 3 (Table 15.5), this technique has been employed to demonstrate that a subsequent male fetus was unaffected (105). However, most families at risk for X91 CGD do not have DNA abnormalities that are detectable in this manner. Fortunately, two RFLPs within the CYBB gene after digestion with the restriction enzyme *Nsi*I have now been recognized (101, 144–146), increasing to about 50% the proportion of families to whom first-trimester prenatal diagnosis can be offered. Moreover, three regions with a variable number of tandem repeats (VNTRs) are present in the CYBB gene (147). It is to be expected that polymorphism at this region, due to allelic differences in the number of repeats, can be used for further increasing the reliability of RFLP-based X91 CGD detection (148).

Of course, if the specific, family-based mutation can be identified, prenatal diagnosis becomes relatively simple. Recently (149), we have demonstrated in this way the CGD status of a subsequent male fetus in the family of patient 9 (Table 15.5). Linkage studies with RFLPs around the CYBB locus confirmed this diagnosis with >98% reliability. On request of the family, the pregnancy was terminated at week 15. The diagnosis was confirmed on fetal blood cells by lack of oxygen consumption and a negative NBT slide test. Subsequently, this method of prenatal diagnosis was used in two additional cases (de Boer and Roos, unpublished). In both families, the mutation was first established as point mutations in the coding sequence of CYBB (patient 2, Table 15.4, and patient 2, Table 15.5). Subsequently, the chorionic DNA was analysed, checked for fetal origin and found to be normal in both cases. Linkage studies confirmed these diagnoses.

Within the NCF2 gene, one RFLP has been discovered after digestion with

*Hind*III (150). This has been used to analyse a fetus in a family in which a patient with A67⁰ CGD had previously been born. This proband patient and her mother were homozygous for this RFLP; the father was heterozygous. Fetal DNA, obtained from amnionic fibroblasts taken at 12 weeks gestation and grown for 3 weeks, showed the fetus to be a heterozygote for this RFLP as well, indicating that the fetus had received a normal allele from the father. The baby was carried to term, and a boy was born after a normal delivery. Cord blood samples showed normal oxidative function by NBT slide test and chemiluminescence.

TREATMENT OF CGD

CGD manifests itself as a very heterogeneous syndrome, not only in the type of infectious microorganisms and in the different infected tissues, but also in the age at which the patients present with the infections and in the frequency of the infectious episodes. This is understandable, given the heterogeneity in the molecular pathogenesis of the disease. Several investigators have noted that, in general, those patients with the cytochrome b_{558}-deficient forms of CGD follow a more severe clinical course than those with defects in cytosolic NADPH oxidase components (1, 68, 151). There is, however, no correlation between the amount of superoxide generated by the patients' phagocytes and the severity of the clinical course: patients with the X91⁻ subtype of CGD, who may have neutrophils that generate 10–30% of the normal amount of O_2^-, suffer from infections as severe as patients without any NADPH oxidase capacity (29). In contrast, carriers of X91⁰ CGD with only a few per cent of normal neutrophils due to non-random X chromosome inactivation may be completely healthy (152). Perhaps it is more beneficial for the host to possess a few neutrophils with full bactericidal capacity than to possess a large number of neutrophils with low bactericidal capacity.

Until recently, the major approach to treatment of CGD patients was aimed at prevention and aggressive treatment of infections. Prevention includes routine immunizations, prompt cleaning and antiseptic treatment of skin wounds, careful anal and dental hygiene, abstinence from smoking and avoidance of contact with decaying plant material that may contain *Aspergillus* spores (153). The use of prophylactic antibiotics, especially sulphamethoxazole–trimethoprim, is very effective (154–157). Treatment includes prompt surgical drainage of abscesses and early and prolonged use of systemic antimicrobials. The use of daily white blood cell transfusions in life-threatening situations has also been advised (155). Allogeneic bone marrow transplantation has been attempted, but with little success due to severe transplantation complications (158, 159).

The latest development in the treatment of CGD has been the use of interferon-γ (IFNγ). (A detailed description of IFNγ treatment is given in

Chapter 17.) First, it was proved that addition of IFNγ *in vitro* enhanced both the superoxide production and the level of mRNA for gp91-*phox* of normal phagocytes (160, 161). Thereafter, neutrophils and monocytes from X91⁰, X91⁻ and A47⁰ CGD patients were treated with IFNγ *in vitro*. Cells from X91⁰ CGD patients did not respond, but those from X91⁻ and A47⁰ CGD patients did (131, 162, 163). Based on these findings, two small groups of CGD patients were treated with subcutaneous injections of IFNγ (163, 164). In general, the same phenomena were noted: a large increase in O_2^- generating capacity and killing of *Staphylococcus aureus in vitro*, and modest increase in haem signal and mRNA for gp91-*phox* in Xb⁻ patients. All A47⁰ patients responded, but to a limited degree. Of the X91⁰ patients, only a few responded with a partial restoration of functions. Given the fact that many of the X91⁰ patients will suffer from gene deletions and translation termination mutations, this last result is not surprising.

However, these limited studies did not involve enough patients to evaluate any clinical benefits of IFNγ. Therefore, a large multi-centre study has been carried out, in which 128 CGD patients were enrolled (165). The patients were randomized according to sex, use of prophylactic antibiotics, genetic background of their disease and treatment centre. The study was placebo controlled and double blind. The results showed that recombinant human IFNγ, given in a dose of 0.05 mg/m² subcutaneously three times a week, caused a 70% reduction in the incidence of serious infections (requiring hospitalization and the use of parenteral antibiotics), regardless of the type of CGD. In contrast to the earlier reports, however, most patients in this larger study showed no significant improvement in O_2^- production or bacterial killing by their neutrophils *in vitro*. Thus, recombinant human IFNγ appears to boost host defence by other mechanisms, e.g. by augmentation of macrophage NADPH oxidase, non-oxidative mechanisms and/or improvement of diapedesis and locomotion.

Finally, because CGD is a disorder of marrow-derived cells with well-defined genetic defects, transfer of the correct gene for the defective NADPH oxidase component into pluripotent haematopoietic stem cells would, in principle, constitute definitive therapy. The genetically engineered stem cells can then be returned to the bone marrow of a patient, with subsequent production of corrected mature phagocytes. Carriers for X91⁰ CGD with less than 10% of normal cells may have a normal phenotype (152), suggesting that correction of only a small percentage of the cells in CGD patients will result in a clinical improvement or cure. Stable production of p47-*phox* protein by retrovirally transfected B lymphocytes from A47⁰ CGD patients has been reported (166). However, transcription of DNA sequences in mature phagocytes requires *cis* elements and *trans* factors that have not yet been fully elucidated (99a). Experimental problems in this field of investigation are the low transfection efficiency of transformed myelomonocytic cell lines and the lack of immortalized, deficient phagocytic cells. Transgenic animals are now being used to avoid these problems (167). Hopefully, this will result in the not too distant future in gene therapy to effect a true cure for CGD patients.

ACKNOWLEDGEMENTS

I thank Martin de Boer, Rob van Zwieten, Ben Bolscher and Angelique de Klein for their experimental work, John Curnutte, Tony Segal, Jed Gorlin and Steve Chanock for sharing unpublished results, and Ron Weening and Arthur Verhoeven for critical remarks. The experimental work from our group reported in this study was financially supported by grant no. 900-503-110 from The Netherlands Organization for Scientific Research.

REFERENCES

1. Tauber, A.I., Borregaard, N., Simons, E. and Wright, J. (1983) Chronic granulomatous disease: A syndrome of phagocyte oxidase deficiencies. *Medicine*, **62**, 286–309.
2. Curnutte, J.T. and Babior, B.M. (1987) Chronic granulomatous disease. In Harris, H. and Hirschhorn, K. (eds) *Advances in Human Genetics*. Plenum Press, New York, pp. 229–297 and 474–476.
3. Forrest, C.B., Forehand, J.R., Axtell, R.A., Roberts, R.L. and Johnston, R.B. (1988) Clinical features and current management of chronic granulomatous disease. *Hematol. Oncol. Clin. N. Am.*, **2**, 253–267.
4. Holmes, B., Page, A.R. and Good, R.A. (1967) Studies of the metabolic activity of leukocytes from patients with a genetic abnormality of phagocyte function. *J. Clin. Invest.*, **46**, 1422–1432.
5. Curnutte, J.T., Kipnes, R.S. and Babior, B.M. (1974) Defect in pyridine nucleotide dependent superoxide production by a particulate fraction from the granulocytes of patients with chronic granulomatous disease. *N. Engl. J. Med.*, **290**, 593–597.
6. Hohn, D.C. and Lehrer, R.I. (1975) NADPH oxidase deficiency in X-linked chronic granulomatous disease. *J. Clin. Invest.*, **55**, 707–713.
7. De Chatelet, L.R., McPhail, L.C., Mullikin, D. and McCall, C.E. (1975) An isotopic assay for NADPH oxidase activity and some characteristics of the enzyme from human polymorphonuclear leukocytes. *J. Clin. Invest.*, **55**, 714–721.
8. Iyer, G.Y.N., Islam, M.F. and Quastel, J.H. (1961) Biochemical aspects of phagocytosis. *Nature*, **192**, 535–541.
9. Weening, R.S., Wever, R. and Roos, D. (1975) Quantification of the production of superoxide radicals by phagocytizing human granulocytes. *J. Lab. Clin. Med.*, **85**, 245–252.
10. Root, R.K. and Metcalf, J.A. (1977) H_2O_2 release from human granulocytes during phagocytosis. Relationship to superoxide anion formation and cellular catabolism of H_2O_2: Studies with normal and cytochalasin B-treated cells. *J. Clin. Invest.*, **60**, 1266–1279.
11. Britigan, B.E., Rosen, G.M., Chai, Y. and Cohen, M.S. (1986) Do human neutrophils make hydroxyl radical? Determination of free radicals generated by

human neutrophils activated with a soluble or a particulate stimulus using electron paramagnetic resonance. *J. Biol. Chem.*, **261**, 4426–4431.

12.	Samuni, A., Black, C.D.V., Krishna, C.M., Malech, H.L., Bernstein, E.F. and Russo, A. (1988) Hydroxyl radical production by stimulated neutrophils reappraised. *J. Biol. Chem.*, **263**, 13797–13801.

13.	Britigan, B.E., Coffman, T.J. and Buettner, G.R. (1990) Spin trapping evidence for the lack of significant hydroxyl radical production during the respiration burst of human phagocytes using a spin adduct resistant to superoxide-mediated destruction. *J. Biol. Chem.*, **265**, 2650–2656.

14.	Warren, J.S., Ward, P.A. and Johnson, K.J. (1988) The respiratory burst and mechanisms of oxygen-radical mediated tissue injury. In Sbarra, A.J. and Strauss, R.R. (eds) *The Respiratory Burst and Its Physiological Significance*. Plenum Press, New York, pp. 299–314.

15.	Kanofsky, J.R., Hoogland, H., Wever, R. and Weiss, S.J. (1988) Singlet oxygen production by human eosinophils. *J. Biol. Chem.*, **263**, 9692–9696.

16.	Weiss, S.J., Klein, R. and Slivka, A. (1982) Chlorination of taurine by human neutrophils: Evidence for hypochlorous acid generation. *J. Clin. Invest.*, **70**, 598–607.

17.	Weiss, S.J., Test, S.T., Eckmann, C.M., Roos, D. and Regiani, S. (1986) Brominating oxidants generated by human eosinophils. *Science*, **234**, 200–203.

18.	Weiss, S.J., Lampert, M.B. and Test, S.T. (1983) Long-lived oxidants generated by human neutrophils: Characterization and bioactivity. *Science*, **222**, 625–628.

19.	Yazdanbakhsh, M., Eckmann, C.M. and Roos, D. (1987) Killing of schistosomula by taurine chloramine and taurine bromamine. *Am. J. Trop. Med. Hyg.*, **37**, 106–110.

20.	Windhorst, D.B., Page, A.R., Holmes, B., Quie, P.G. and Good, R.A. (1968) The pattern of genetic transmission of the leukocyte defect in fatal granulomatous disease of childhood. *J. Clin. Invest.*, **47**, 1026–1034.

21.	Azimi, P.H., Bodenberger, J.G., Hintz, R.L. and Kontras, S.B. (1968) Chronic granulomatous disease in three female siblings. *J. Am. Med. Assoc.*, **206**, 2865–2870.

22.	Quie, P.G., Kaplan, E.L., Page, A.R., Gruskay, F.L. and Malawista, S.E. (1968) Defective polymorphonuclear leukocyte function and chronic granulomatous disease in two female children. *N. Engl. J. Med.*, **278**, 976–980.

23.	Baehner, R.L. and Nathan, D.G. (1968) Quantitative nitroblue tetrazolium test in chronic granulomatous disease. *N. Engl. J. Med.*, **278**, 971–976.

24.	Segal, A.W., Jones, O.T.G., Webster, D. and Allison, A.C. (1978) Absence of a newly described cytochrome *b* from neutrophils of patients with chronic granulomatous disease. *Lancet*, **ii**, 446–449.

25.	Segal, A.W., Cross, A.R., Garcia, R.C., Borregaard, N., Valerius, N., Soothill, J.F. and Jones, O.T.G. (1983) Absence of cytochrome b_{245} in chronic granulomatous disease: A multicenter European evaluation of its incidence and relevance. *N. Engl. J. Med.*, **308**, 245–251.

26.	Bohler, M.C., Seger, R.A., Mouy, R., Vilmer, E., Fischer, A. and Griscelli, C. (1986) A study of 25 patients with chronic granulomatous disease: A new classification by correlating respiratory burst, cytochrome *b* and flavoprotein. *J. Clin. Immunol.*, **6**, 136–145.

27.	Ohno, Y., Buescher, E.S., Roberts, R., Metcalf, J. and Gallin, J.I. (1986) Re-evaluation of cytochrome *b* and flavin adenine dinucleotide in neutrophils from patients with chronic granulomatous disease and description of a family with probable autosomal recessive inheritance of cytochrome *b* deficiency. *Blood*, **67**, 1132–1138.

28. Cross, A.R., Jones, O.T.G., Harper, A.M. and Segal, A.W. (1981) Oxidation–reduction properties of the cytochrome *b* found in the plasma membrane fraction of human neutrophils: A possible oxidase in the respiratory burst. *Biochem. J.*, **194**, 599–606.

29. Roos, D., De Boer, M., Borregaard, N., Bjerrum, O.W., Valerius, N.H., Seger, R.A., Mühlebach, T., Belohradsky, B.H. and Weening, R.S. (1992) Chronic granulomatous disease with partial deficiency of cytochrome b_{558} and incomplete respiratory burst: Variants of the X-linked, cytochrome b_{558}-negative form of the disease. *J. Leukocyte. Biol.*, **51**, 164–171.

30. Bolscher, B.G.J.M., De Boer, M., De Klein, A., Weening, R.S. and Roos, D. (1991) Point mutations in the β-subunit of cytochrome b_{558} leading to X-linked chronic granulomatous disease. *Blood*, **77**, 2482–2487.

31. Weening, R.S., Corbeel, L., De Boer, M., Lutter, R., Van Zwieten, R., Hamers, M.N. and Roos, D. (1985) Cytochrome *b* deficiency in an autosomal form of chronic granulomatous disease: A third form of chronic granulomatous disease recognized by monocyte hybridization. *J. Clin. Invest.*, **75**, 915–920.

32. Hamers, M.N., De Boer, M., Meerhof, L.J., Weening, R.S. and Roos, D. (1984) Complementation in monocyte hybrids revealing genetic heterogeneity in chronic granulomatous disease. *Nature*, **307**, 553–555.

33. Segal, A.W. (1987) Absence of both cytochrome b_{245} subunits from neutrophils in X-linked chronic granulomatous disease. *Nature*, **326**, 88–91.

34. Parkos, C.A., Allen, R.A., Cochrane, C.G. and Jesaitis, A.J. (1987) Purified cytochrome *b* from human granulocyte plasma membrane is comprised of two polypeptides with relative molecular weights of 91,000 and 22,000. *J. Clin. Invest.*, **80**, 732–742.

35. Royer-Pokora, B., Kunkel, L.M., Monaco, A.P., Goff, S.C., Newburger, P.E., Baehner, R.L., Cole, F.S., Curnutte, J.T. and Orkin, S.H. (1986) Cloning the gene for an inherited human disorder—chronic granulomatous disease—on the basis of its chromosomal location. *Nature*, **322**, 32–38.

36. Dinauer, M.C., Pierce, E.A., Bruns, G.A.P., Curnutte, J.T. and Orkin, S.H. (1990) Human neutrophil cytochrome-*b* light chain (p22-*phox*): Gene structure, chromosomal location, and mutations in cytochrome negative autosomal recessive chronic granulomatous disease. *J. Clin. Invest.*, **86**, 1729–1737.

37. Parkos, C.A., Dinauer, M.C., Jesaitis, A.J., Orkin, S.H. and Curnutte, J.T. (1989) Absence of both 91 kD and 22 kD subunits of human neutrophil cytochrome *b* in two genetic forms of chronic granulomatous disease. *Blood*, **73**, 1416–1420.

38. Verhoeven, A.J., Bolscher, B.G.J.M., Meerhof, L.J., van Zwieten, R., Keijer, J., Weening, R.S. and Roos, D. (1989) Characterization of two monoclonal antibodies against cytochrome b_{558} of human neutrophils. *Blood*, **73**, 1686–1694.

39. Parkos, C.A., Dinauer, M.C., Walker, L.E., Allen, R.A., Jesaitis, A.J. and Orkin, S.H. (1988) Primary structure and unique expression of the 22 kilodalton light chain of human neutrophil cytochrome *b*. *Proc. Nat. Acad. Sci. USA*, **85**, 3319–3323.

40. Dinauer, M.C., Orkin, S.H., Brown, R., Jesaitis, A.J. and Parkos, C.A. (1987) The glycoprotein encoded by the X-linked chronic granulomatous disease locus is a component of the neutrophil cytochrome b complex. *Nature*, **327**, 717–720.

41. Teahan, C., Rowe, P., Parker, P., Totty, N. and Segal, A.W. (1987) The X-linked chronic granulomatous disease gene codes for the beta chain of cytochrome b_{245}. *Nature*, **327**, 720–721.

42. Imajoh-Ohmi, S., Tokita, K., Ochiai, H., Nakamura, M. and Kanegasaki, S. (1992) Topology of cytochrome b_{558} in neutrophil membrane analyzed by anti-peptide antibodies and proteolysis. *J. Biol. Chem.*, **267**, 180–184.

43. Harper, A.M., Chaplin, M.F. and Segal, A.W. (1985) Cytochrome b_{245} from human neutrophils is a glycoprotein. *Biochem. J.*, **227**, 783–788.

44. Kleinberg, M.E., Rotrosen, D. and Malech, H.L. (1989) Asparagine-linked glycosylation of cytochrome b_{558} large subunit varies in different human phagocytic cells. *J. Immunol.*, **143**, 4152–4157.

45. Rotrosen, D., Kleinberg, M.E., Nunoi, H., Leto, T., Gallin, J.L. and Malech, H.L. (1990) Evidence for a functional domain of phagocyte oxidase cytochrome b_{558}. *J. Biol. Chem.*, **265**, 8745–8750.

46. Nugent, J.H., Gratzer, W. and Segal, A.W. (1989) Identification of the haem-binding subunit of cytochrome b_{245}. *Biochem. J.*, **264**, 921–924.

47. Quinn, M.T., Mullen, M.L. and Jesaitis, A.J. (1991) Evidence for two hemes in the neutrophil cytochrome *b* structure. *Clin. Res.*, **39**, 353a.

48. Hurst, J.K., Loehr, T.M., Curnutte, J.T. and Rosen, H. (1991) Resonance Raman and electron paramagnetic resonance structural investigations of neutrophil cytochrome b_{558}. *J. Biol. Chem.*, **266**, 1627–1634.

49. Morel, F. and Vignais, P.V. (1984) Examination of the oxidase function of the *b*-type cytochrome in human polymorphonuclear leukocytes. *Biochim. Biophys. Acta*, **764**, 213–225.

50. Lutter, R., Van Schaik, M.L.J., Van Zwieten, R., Wever, R., Roos, D. and Hamers, M.N. (1985) Purification and partial characterization of the *b*-type cytochrome from human polymorphonuclear leukocytes. *J. Biol. Chem.*, **260**, 2237–2244.

51. Heyneman, R.A. and Vercauteren, R.E. (1984) Activation of a NADPH oxidase from horse polymorphonuclear leukocytes in a cell-free system. *J. Leukocyte Biol.*, **36**, 751–759.

52. Bromberg, Y. and Pick, E. (1984) Unsaturated fatty acids stimulate NADPH-dependent superoxide production by a cell-free system derived from macrophages. *Cell. Immunol.*, **88**, 213–221.

53. McPhail, L.C., Shirley, P.S., Clayton, C.C. and Snyderman, R. (1985) Activation of the respiratory burst enzyme from human neutrophils in a cell-free system: Evidence for a soluble cofactor. *J. Clin. Invest.*, **75**, 1735–1739.

54. Curnutte, J.T. (1985) Activation of human neutrophil nicotinamide adenine dinucleotide phosphate, reduced (triphosphopyridine nucleotide, reduced) oxidase by arachidonic acid in a cell-free system. *J. Clin. Invest.*, **75**, 1740–1743.

55. Bolscher, B.G.J.M., van Zwieten, R., Kramer, I.J.M., Weening, R.S., Verhoeven, A.J. and Roos, D. (1989) A phosphoprotein of M_r 47,000, defective in autosomal chronic granulomatous disease, copurifies with one of two soluble components required for NADPH:O_2 oxidoreductase activity in human neutrophils. *J. Clin. Invest.*, **83**, 757–763.

56. Tauber, A.I. and Goetzl, E.J. (1979) Structural and catalytic properties of the solubilized superoxide-generating activity of human polymorphonuclear leukocytes: Solubilization, stabilization in solution and partial characterization. *Biochemistry*, **18**, 5576–5584.

57. Gabig, T.G. and Babior, B.M. (1979) The O_2^--forming oxidase responsible for the respiratory burst in human neutrophils: Properties of the solubilized enzyme. *J. Biol. Chem.*, **254**, 9070–9074.

58. Curnutte, J.T., Kuver, R. and Scott, P.J. (1987) Activation of neutrophil NADPH oxidase in a cell-free system: Partial purification of components and characterization of the activation process. *J. Biol. Chem.*, **262**, 5563–5569.

59. Clark, R.A., Leidal, K.G., Pearson, D.W. and Nauseef, W.M. (1987) NADPH oxidase of human neutrophils: Subcellular localization and characterization of an arachidonate-activatable superoxide-generating system. *J. Biol. Chem.*, **262**, 4065–4074.

60. Fujita, I., Takeshige, K. and Minakami, S. (1987) Characterization of the NADPH-dependent superoxide production activated by sodium dodecyl sulfate in a cell-free system of pig neutrophils. *Biochim. Biophys. Acta*, **931**, 41–48.

61. Gabig, T.G., English, D., Akard, L.P. and Schnell, M.J. (1987) Regulation of neutrophil NADPH oxidase activation of a cell-free system by guanine nucleotides and fluoride: Evidence for participation of a pertussis and cholera toxin-insensitive G protein. *J. Biol. Chem.*, **262**, 1685–1690.

62. Tanaka, T., Makino, R., Iizuka, T., Ishimura, Y. and Kanegasaki, S. (1988) Activation by saturated and monounsaturated fatty acids of the O_2^--generating system in a cell-free preparation from neutrophils. *J. Biol. Chem.*, **263**, 13670–13676.

63. Ambruso, D.R., Bolscher, B.G.J.M., Stokman, P.M., Verhoeven, A.J. and Roos, D. (1991) Assembly and activation of the NADPH:O_2 oxidoreductase in human neutrophils after stimulation with phorbol-myristate acetate. *J. Biol. Chem.*, **265**, 924–930. Correction: *J. Biol. Chem.*, **265**, 19370–19371.

64. Clark, R.A., Volpp, B.D., Leidal, K.G. and Nauseef, W.M. (1990) Two cytosolic components of the human neutrophil respiratory burst oxidase translocate to the plasma membrane during cell activation. *J. Clin. Invest.*, **85**, 714–721.

65. Doussière, J., Pilloud, M.-C. and Vignais, P.V. (1990) Cytosolic factor in bovine neutrophil oxidase activation: Partial purification and demonstration of translocation to a membrane fraction. *Biochemistry*, **29**, 2225–2232.

66. Heyworth, P.G., Curnutte, J.T., Nauseef, W.M., Volpp, B.D., Pearson, D.W., Rosen, H. and Clark, R.A. (1991) Neutrophil nicotinamide adenine dinucleotide phosphate (reduced form) oxidase assembly: Translocation of p47-*phox* and p67-*phox* requires interaction between p47-*phox* and cytochrome b_{558}. *J. Clin. Invest.*, **87**, 352–356.

67. Babior, B.M., Kuver, R. and Curnutte, J.T. (1988) Kinetics of activation of the respiratory burst oxidase in a fully soluble system from human neutrophils. *J. Biol. Chem.*, **263**, 1713–1718.

68. Curnutte, J.T., Berkow, R.L., Roberts, R.L., Shurin, S.B. and Scott, S.J. (1988) Chronic granulomatous disease due to a defect in the cytosolic factor required for nicotinamide adenine dinucleotide phosphate oxidase activation. *J. Clin. Invest.*, **82**, 606–610.

69. Caldwell, S.E., McCall, C.E., Hendricks, C.L., Leone, P.A., Bass, D.A. and McPhail, L.C. (1988) Coregulation of NADPH oxidase activation and phosphorylation of a 48-kD protein(s) by a cytosolic factor defective in autosomal recessive chronic granulomatous disease. *J. Clin. Invest.*, **82**, 1485–1496.

70. Curnutte, J.T. (1992) Molecular basis of the autosomal recessive forms of chronic granulomatous disease. *Immunodef. Rev.*, **3**, 149–172.

71. Volpp, B.D., Nauseef, W.M. and Clark, R.A. (1988) Two cytosolic neutrophil oxidase components absent in autosomal chronic granulomatous disease. *Science*, **242**, 1295–1297.

72. Nunoi, H., Rotrosen, D., Gallin, J.I. and Malech, H.L. (1988) Two forms of autosomal chronic granulomatous disease lack distinct neutrophil cytosol factors. *Science*, **242**, 1298–1301.

73. Curnutte, J.T., Scott, P.J. and Mayo, L.A. (1989) The cytosolic components of the respiratory burst oxidase: Resolution of four components, two of which are missing in complementing forms of chronic granulomatous disease. *Proc. Nat. Acad. Sci. USA*, **86**, 825–829.

74. Bolscher, B.G.J.M., Denis, S.W., Verhoeven, A.J. and Roos, D. (1990) The activity of one soluble component of the cell-free NADPH:O_2 oxidoreductase of human neutrophils depends on guanosine 5'-O-(3-thio)-triphosphate. *J. Biol. Chem.*, **265**, 15782–15787.

75. Clark, R.A., Malech, H.L., Gallin, J.I., Nunoi, H., Volpp, B.D., Pearson, D.W., Nauseef, W.M. and Curnutte, J.T. (1989) Genetic variants of chronic granulomatous disease: Prevalence of deficiencies of two cytosolic components of the NADPH oxidase system. *N. Engl. J. Med.*, **321**, 647–652.

76. Volpp, B.D., Nauseef, W.M., Donelson, J.E., Moser, D.R. and Clark, R.A. (1989) Cloning of the cDNA and functional expression of the 47-kilodalton cytosolic component of human neutrophil respiratory burst oxidase. *Proc. Nat. Acad. Sci. USA*, **86**, 7195–7199 (Erratum: *Proc. Nat. Acad. Sci. USA*, **86**, 9563).

77. Lomax, K.R., Leto, T.L., Nunoi, H., Gallin, J.I. and Malech, H.L. (1989) Recombinant 47-kilodalton cytosol factor restores NADPH oxidase in chronic granulomatous disease. *Science*, **245**, 409–412 (Erratum: *Science*, **246**, 987).

78. Leto, T.L., Lomax, K.J., Volpp, B.D., Nunoi, H., Sechler, J.M.G., Nauseef, W.M., Clark, R.A., Gallin, J.I. and Malech, H.L. (1990) Cloning of a 67-kD neutrophil oxidase factor with similarity to a non-catalytic region of $p60_{c\text{-}src}$. *Science*, **248**, 727–730.

79. Smith, R.M., Curnutte, J.T. and Babior, B.M. (1989) Affinity labeling of the cytosolic and membrane components of the respiratory burst oxidase by the 2',3'-dialdehyde derivative of NADPH: Evidence for a cytosolic location of the nucleotide binding site in the resting cell. *J. Biol. Chem.*, **265**, 1958–1962.

80. Umei, T., Babior, B.M., Curnutte, J.T. and Smith, R.M. (1991) Identification of the NADPH-binding subunit of the respiratory burst oxidase. *J. Biol. Chem.*, **266**, 6019–6022.

81. Kakinuma, K., Kaneda, M., Chiba, T. and Ohnishi, T. (1986) Electron spin resonance studies on a flavoprotein in neutrophil plasma membranes: Redox potentials of the flavin and its participation in NADPH oxidase. *J. Biol. Chem.*, **261**, 9426–9432.

82. Segal, A.W., West, I., Wientjes, F., Nugent, J.H.A., Chavan, A.J., Haley, B., Garcia, R.C., Rosen, H. and Scrace, G. (1992) Cytochrome b_{245} is a flavocytochrome containing FAD and the NADPH binding site of the microbicidal oxidase of phagocytes. *Biochem. J.*, **284**, 781–88.

83. Cross, A.R., Jones, O.T.G., Garcia, R. and Segal, A.W. (1982) The association of FAD with the cytochrome-b_{245} of human neutrophils. *Biochem. J.*, **208**, 759–763.

84. Gabig, T.G. and Lefker, B.A. (1984) Deficient flavoprotein component of the NADPH dependent O_2^--generating oxidase in the neutrophils from three male patients with chronic granulomatous disease. *J. Clin. Invest.*, **73**, 701–705.

85. Pick, E., Kroizman, T. and Abo, A. (1989) Activation of the superoxide-forming NADPH oxidase of macrophages requires two cytosolic components—one of them is also present in certain nonphagocytic cells. *J. Immunol.*, **143**, 4180–4187.

86. Abo, A., Pick, E., Hall, A., Totty, N., Teahan, C.G. and Segal, A.W. (1992) Activation of the NADPH oxidase involves the small GTP-binding protein p21rac1. *Nature*, **353**, 668–670.

87. Pick, E. and Gorzalczany, Y. (1992) Further studies on the third cytosolic component of the phagocyte NADPH oxidase (Sigma 1). *Eur. J. Clin. Invest.*, **22**, A40.

88. Knaus, U.G., Heyworth, P.G., Evans, T., Curnutte, J.G. and Bokoch, G.M. (1991) Regulation of phagocyte oxygen radical production by the GTP-binding protein Rac 2. *Science*, **254**, 1512–1515.

89. Kwong, C.H., Malech, H.L. and Leto, T.L. (1991) Three cytosolic proteins are necessary and sufficient for reconstituting NADPH oxidase in neutrophil membrane. *Clin. Res.*, **39**, 273A.

90. Quinn, M.T., Parkos, C.A., Walker, L.E., Orkin, S.H., Dinauer, M.C. and Jesaitis, A.J. (1989) Association of a *ras*-related protein with cytochrome *b* of human neutrophils. *Nature*, **342**, 198–200.

91. Okamura, N., Curnutte, J.T., Roberts, R.L. and Babior, B.M. (1988) Relationship of protein phosphorylation to the activation of the respiratory burst in human neutrophils: Defects in the phosphorylation of a group closely related 48-kDa proteins in two forms of chronic granulomatous disease. *J. Biol. Chem.*, **263**, 6777–6782.

92. Okamura, N., Malawista, S.E., Roberts, R.L., Rosen, H., Ochs, H.D., Babior, B.M. and Curnutte, J.T. (1988) Phosphorylation of the oxidase-related 48K phosphoprotein family in the unusual autosomal cytochrome-negative and X-linked cytochrome-positive types of chronic granulomatous disease. *Blood*, **72**, 8811–8816.

93. Heyworth, P.G., Shrimpton, C.F. and Segal, A.W. (1989) Localization of the 47kDa phosphoprotein involved in the respiratory-burst NADPH oxidase of phagocytic cells. *Biochem. J.*, **260**, 243–248.

94. Rotrosen, D. and Leto, T.L. (1990) Phosphorylation of neutrophil 47-kDa cytosolic oxidase factor: Translocation to membrane is associated with distinct phosphorylation events. *J. Biol. Chem.*, **265**, 19910–19915.

95. Ligeti, E., Doussière, J. and Vignais, P. (1988) Activation of the O_2^--generating oxidase in plasma membrane from bovine polymorphonuclear neutrophils by arachidonic acid, a cytosolic factor of protein nature, and nonhydrolyzable analogues of GTP. *Biochemistry*, **27**, 193–200.

96. Quinn, M.T., Parkos, C.A. and Jesaitis, A.J. (1989) The lateral organization of components of the membrane skeleton and superoxide generation in the plasma membrane of stimulated human neutrophils. *Biochim. Biophys. Acta*, **987**, 83–94.

97. Dinauer, M.C., Pierce, E.A., Erickson, R.W., Mühlebach, T.J., Messner, H., Orkin, S.H., Seger, R.A. and Curnutte, J.T. (1991) Point mutation in the cytoplasmic domain of the neutrophil p22-phox cytochrome *b* subunit is associated with a nonfunctional NADPH oxidase and chronic granulomatous disease. *Proc. Nat. Acad. Sci. USA*, **88**, 11231–11235.

98. De Boer, M., De Klein, A., Hossle, J.-P. Seger, R., Corbeel, L., Weening, R.S. and Roos, D. (1992) Cytochrome b_{558}-negative, autosomal recessive chronic granulomatous disease: Two new mutations in the cytochrome b_{558} light chain of the NADPH oxidase (p22-*phox*). *Am. J. Hum. Genet.*, **51**, 1127–1135.

99. Baehner, R.L., Kunkel, L.M., Monaco, A.P., Haines, J.L., Courneally, P.M., Palmer, C., Heerema, N. and Orkin, S.H. (1986) DNA linkage analysis of

X-chromosome-linked chronic granulomatous disease. *Proc. Nat. Acad. Sci. USA*, **83**, 3398–3401.

99a. Skalnik, D.G., Strauss, E.C. and Orkin, S.H. (1991) CCAAT displacement protein as a repressor of the myelomonocytic-specific gp91-phox gene promoter. *J. Biol. Chem.*, **266**, 16736–16744.

100. Frey, D., Mächner, M., Seger, R.A., Schmid, W. and Orkin, S.H. (1988) Gene deletion in a patient with chronic granulomatous disease and McLeod syndrome: Fine mapping of the X^k gene locus. *Blood*, **71**, 252–255.

101. Pelham, A., O'Reilly, M.-A., Malcolm, S., Levinsky, R.J. and Kinnon, C. (1990) RFLP and deletion analysis for X-linked chronic granulomatous disease using the cDNA probe: Potential for improved prenatal diagnosis and carrier determination. *Blood*, **76**, 820–824.

102. Dinauer, M.C., Curnutte, J.C., Rosen, H. and Orkin, S.A. (1989) A missense mutation in the neutrophil cytochrome *b* heavy chain in cytochrome-positive X-linked chronic granulomatous disease. *J. Clin. Invest.*, **84**, 2012–2016.

103. Schapiro, B.L., Newburger, P.E., Klempner, M.S. and Dinauer, M.C. (1991) Chronic granulomatous disease presenting in a 69-year-old man. *N. Engl. J. Med.*, **325**, 1786–1790.

104. Roos, D., Bolscher, B.G.J.M. and De Boer, M. (1992) Generation of reactive oxygen species by phagocytes. In van Furth, R. (ed.) *Biology of Monocytes and Macrophages*, Kluwer, Dordrecht, pp. 243–253.

105. Orkin, S.H. (1989) Molecular genetics of chronic granulomatous disease. *Annu. Rev. Immunol.*, **7**, 227–307.

106. De Boer, M., Bolscher, B.G.J.M., Dinauer, M.C., Orkin, S.H., Smith, C.I.E., Ahlin, Å., Weening, R.S. and Roos, D. (1992) Splice site mutations are a common cause of X-linked chronic granulomatous disease. *Blood.*, **80**, 1553–1558.

107. Francke, U., Hsieh, C.-L., Foellmer, B.E., Lomax, K.J., Malech, H.L. and Leto, T.L. (1990) Genes for two autosomal recessive forms of chronic granulomatous disease assigned to 1q25 (*NCF2*) and 7q11.23 (*NCF1*). *Am. J. Hum. Genet.*, **47**, 483–492.

108. Casimir, C.M., Bu-Ghanim, H., Rodaway, A.R., Bentley, D.L., Rowe, P. and Segal, A.W. (1991) Autosomal recessive chronic granulomatous disease caused by deletion at a dinucleotide repeat. *Proc. Nat. Acad. Sci. USA*, **88**, 2753–2757.

109. Chanock, S.J., Barrett, D.M., Curnutte, J.C. and Orkin, S.H. (1991) Gene structure of the cytolosic component, *phox*-47 and mutations in autosomal recessive chronic granulomatous disease. *Blood*, **78**, 165a.

110. Kenney, R.T., Malech, H.L., Gallin, J.I. and Leto, T.L. (1990) Amplification mapping of p67[phox] deficient chronic granulomatous disease. *Clin. Res.*, **38**, 434A.

111. Kishimoto, T.K., Hollander, N., Roberts, T.M., Anderson, D.C. and Springer, T.A. (1987) Heterogeneous mutations in the beta subunit common to LFA-1, Mac-1 and p150,95 glycoproteins cause leukocyte adhesion deficiency. *Cell*, **50**, 193–202.

112. Anderson, D.C., Schmalsteig, F.C., Arnaout, M.A., Kohl, S., Tosi, M.F., Dana, N., Buffone, G.J., Hughes, B.J., Brinkley, B.R., Dickey, W.D., Abramson, J.S., Springer, T., Boxer, L.A., Hollers, J.M. and Smith, C.W. (1984) Abnormalities of polymorphonuclear leukocyte function associated with a heritable deficiency of high molecular weight surface glycoproteins (GP 138): Common relationship to diminished cell adherence. *J. Clin. Invest.*, **74**, 536–551.

113. Weisman, S.J., Berkow, R.L., Plantz, G., Torres, M., McGuire, W.A., Coates, T.D., Haak, R.A., Floyd, A., Jersild, R. and Baehner, R.L. (1985) Glycopro-

tein-180 deficiency: Genetics and abnormal neutrophil activation. *Blood*, **65**, 696–704.

114. Hoogerwerf, M., Weening, R.S., Hack, C.E. and Roos, D. (1990) Complement fragments C3b and iC3b coupled to latex induce a respiratory burst in human neutrophils. *Mol. Immunol.*, **27**, 159–167.

115. Nauseef, W.M., De Alarcon, P., Bale, J.F. and Clark, R.A. (1986) Aberrant activation and regulation of the oxidative burst in neutrophils with Mo1 glycoprotein deficiency. *J. Immunol.*, **137**, 636–642.

116. Narisawa, K., Ishizawa, S., Okumura, H., Tada, K. and Kuzuya, T. (1986) Neutrophil metabolic dysfunction in genetically heterogeneous patients with glycogen storage disease type 1b. *J. Inherited Metab. Dis.*, **9**, 297–300.

117. Seger, R., Steinmann, B., Tiefenauer, L., Matsunaga, T. and Gitzelmann, R. (1984) Glycogenosis 1b: Neutrophil microbicidal defects due to impaired hexose monophosphate shunt. *Pediatr. Res.*, **18**, 297–299.

118. Gahr, M. and Heyne, K. (1983) Impaired metabolic function of polymorphonuclear leukocytes in glycogen storage disease 1b. *Eur. J. Pediatr.*, **140**, 329–330.

119. Bashan, N., Hagai, Y., Potashnik, R. and Moses, S.W. (1988) Impaired carbohydrate metabolism of polymorphonuclear leukocytes in glycogen storage disease 1b. *J. Clin. Invest.*, **81**, 1317–1322.

120. Kilpatrick, L., Garty, B.-Z., Lundquist, F., Hunter, K., Stanley, C.A., Baker, L., Douglas, S.D. and Korchak, H.M. (1990) Impaired metabolic function and signaling defects in phagocytic cells in glycogen storage disease type 1b. *J. Clin. Invest.*, **86**, 196–202.

121. Cooper, M.R., DeChatelet, L.R., McCall, C.E., La Via, M., Spurr, C.L. and Baehner, R.L. (1972) Complete deficiency of leukocyte glucose-6-phosphate dehydrogenase with defective bactericidal activity. *J. Clin. Invest.*, **51**, 769–778.

122. Baehner, R.L., Johnston, R.B. and Nathan, D.C. (1972) Comparative study of the metabolic and bactericidal characteristics of severely glucose-6-phosphate dehydrogenase deficient polymorphonuclear leukocytes and leukocytes from children with chronic granulomatous disease. *J. Reticuloendothel. Soc.*, **12**, 150–169.

123. Gray, G.R., Klebanoff, S.J., Stamatayannopoulos, G., Austin, T., Naiman, S.C., Yoshida, A., Kliman, M.R. and Robinson, G.C. (1973) Neutrophil dysfunction, chronic granulomatous disease and non-spherocytic haemolytic anaemia caused by complete deficiency of glucose-6-phosphate dehydrogenase. *Lancet*, **ii**, 530–534.

124. Vives Corrons, J.L., Feliu, E., Pujades, M.A., Cardellach, F., Rozman, C., Carreras, A., Jou, J.M., Vallespi, M.T. and Zuazu, F.J. (1982) Severe glucose-6-phosphate dehydrogenase (G6PD) deficiency associated with chronic hemolytic anemia, granulocyte dysfunction, and increased susceptibility to infections: Description of a new molecular variant (G6PD Barcelona). *Blood*, **59**, 428–434.

125. Holmes, B., Park, B.H., Malawista, S.E., Quie, P.G., Nelson, D.L. and Good, R.A. (1970) Chronic granulomatous disease in females: A deficiency of leukocyte glutathione peroxidase. *N. Engl. J. Med.*, **283**, 217–221.

126. Malawista, S.E. and Gifford, R.H. (1975) Chronic granulomatous disease of childhood with leukocyte glutathione peroxidase deficiency in a brother and a sister: A likely autosomal recessive inheritance. *Clin. Res.*, **23**, 416 (Abstract).

127. Matsuda, I., Oka, Y., Taniguchi, N., Furuyama, M., Kodama, S., Arashima, S. and Mitsuyama, T. (1976) Leukocyte glutathione peroxidase deficiency in a male patient with chronic granulomatous disease. *J. Pediatr.*, **88**, 581–583.

128. Roos, D., Weening, R.S. and Loos, J.A. (1979) The protective role of glutathione: The effect of congenital defects of glutathione metabolism on the function of erythrocytes, eye lens cells, and phagocytic leukocytes. A review and some personal observations. In Güttler, F., Seakins, J.W.T. and Harkness, R.A. (eds) *Inborn Errors of Immunity and Phyagocytosis.* MTP Press, Lancaster, pp. 261–286.

129. Curnutte, J.T., Dinauer, M.C., Gelbart, T., Woodman, R.C., Orkin, S.H., Quie, P.G., Newburger, P.E. and Malawista, S.E. (1990) Rare variant forms of chronic granulomatous disease: Neutrophil glutathione peroxidase deficiency revisited. *Clin. Res.*, **38**, 350A.

130. Weening, R.S., Roos, D. and Loos, J.A. (1974) Oxygen consumption of phagocytizing cells in human leukocyte and granulocyte preparations: A comparative study. *J. Lab. Clin. Med.*, **83**, 570–576.

131. Weening, R.S., Frenkel, J., Hoogerwerf, M., Van Lier, R. and Roos, D. (1989) Effect in vivo and in vitro of recombinant interferon-gamma on cellular and clinical parameters in severe leukocyte adherence deficiency. *Eur. J. Clin. Invest.*, **19**, A58.

132. Bemiller, L.S., Rost, J.R., Ku-Balai, T.L. and Curnutte, T.L. (1991) The production of intracellular oxidants by stimulated neutrophils correlates with the clinical severity of chronic granulomatous disease (CGD). *Blood*, **78**, 377a.

133. Weening, R.S., Wever, R. and Roos, D. (1975) Quantitative aspects of the production of superoxide radicals by phagocytizing human granulocytes. *J. Lab. Clin. Med.*, **85**, 245–252.

134. Segal, A.W. (1974) Nitroblue tetrazolium tests. *Lancet*, **ii**, 1248–1252.

135. Meerhof, L.J. and Roos, D. (1986) Heterogeneity in chronic granulomatous disease detected with an improved nitroblue tetrazolium slide test. *J. Leukocyte Biol.*, **39**, 699–711.

136. Test, S.T. and Weiss, S.J. (1984) Quantitative and temporal characterization of the extracellular H_2O_2 pool generated by human neutrophils. *J. Biol. Chem.*, **259**, 399–405.

137. Root, R.K., Metcalf, J., Oshino, N. and Chance, B. (1975) H_2O_2 release from human granulocytes during phagocytosis. I. Documentation, quantitation, and some regulating factors. *J. Clin. Invest.*, **55**, 945–955.

138. Roos, D., Voetman, A.A. and Meerhof, L.J. (1983) Functional activity of enucleated human polymorphonuclear leukocytes. *J. Cell Biol.*, **97**, 368–377.

139. Rothe, G., Emmendörffer, A., Oser, A., Roesler, J. and Valet, G. (1991) Flow cytometric measurement of the respiratory burst activity of phagocytes using dihydrorhodamine 123. *J. Immunol. Methods*, **138**, 133–135.

140. Verhoeven, A.J., Van Schaik, M.L.J., Roos, D. and Weening, R.S. (1988) Detection of carriers of the autosomal form of chronic granulomatous disease. *Blood*, **71**, 505–507.

141. Koenderman, L., Tool, A., Roos, D. and Verhoeven, A.J. (1989) 1,2-Diacylglycerol accumulation in human neutrophils does not correlate with respiratory burst activation. *FEBS Lett.*, **243**, 399–403.

142. Newburger, P.E., Cohen, H.J., Rothchild, S.B., Hobbins, J.C., Malawista, S.E. and Mahoney, M.J. (1979) Prenatal diagnosis of chronic granulomatous disease. *N. Engl. J. Med.*, **300**, 178–181.

143. Nakamura, M., Imajoh-Ohmi, S., Kanegasaki, S., Kurozumi, H., Sato, K., Kato, S. and Miyazaki, Y. (1990) Prenatal diagnosis of cytochrome-deficient chronic granulomatous disease. *Lancet*, **336**, 118–119.

144. Battat, L. and Francke, U. (1989) NsiI RFLP at the X-linked chronic granulomatous disease locus (CYBB). *Nucleic Acids Res.*, **17**, 3619.

145. Mühlebach, T.J., Robinson, W., Seger, R.A. and Mächler, M. (1990) A second NsiI RFLP at the CYBB locus. *Nucleic Acids Res.*, **18**, 4966.
146. Francke, U., Ochs, H.D., Darras, B.T. and Swaroop, A. (1990) Origin of mutations in two families with X-linked chronic granulomatous disease. *Blood*, **76**, 602–606.
147. Gorlin, J. (1991) Identification of $(CA/GT)_n$ polymorphisms within the X-linked chronic granulomatous disease (X-CGD) gene: Utility for prenatal diagnosis. *Blood*, **78**, 433a.
148. Ugozzoli, L., Yam, P., Petz, L.D., Ferrara, G.B., Champlin, R.E., Forman, S.J., Koyal, D. and Wallace, R.B. (1991) Amplification by the polymerase chain reaction of hypervariable regions of the human genome for evaluation of chimerism after bone marrow transplantation. *Blood*, **77**, 1607–1615.
149. De Boer, M., Bolscher, B.G.J.M., Sijmons, R.H., Scheffer, H., Weening, R.S. and Roos, D. (1992) Prenatal diagnosis in a family with X-linked chronic granulomatous disease with the use of the polymerase chain reaction. *Prenat. Diag.*, **12**, 773–777.
150. Kenney, R.T., Malech, H.L., Roberts, R.L., Gallin, J.L. and Leto, T.L. (1991) Amniocentesis diagnosis of a normal fetus in a family with p67phox deficient chronic granulomatous disease using a polymorphic gene marker. *Clin. Res.*, **39**, 274A.
151. Weening, R.S., Adriaansz, L.H., Weemaes, C.M.R., Lutter, R. and Roos, D. (1985) Clinical differences in chronic granulomatous disease in patients with cytochrome *b*-negative or cytochrome *b*-positive neutrophils. *J. Pediatr.*, **107**, 102–104.
152. Roos, D., Weening, R.S., De Boer, M. and Meerhof, L.J. (1986) Heterogeneity in chronic granulomatous disease. In Vossen, J. and Griscelli, C. (eds) *Progress in Immunodeficiency Research and Therapy II*. Elsevier, Amsterdam, pp. 139–146.
153. Smith, R.M. and Curnutte, J.T. (1991) Molecular basis of chronic granulomatous disease. *Blood*, **77**, 673–686.
154. Weening, R.S., Kabel, P., Pijman, P. and Roos, D. (1983) Continuous therapy with sulfamethoxazole–trimethoprim in patients with chronic granulomatous disease. *J. Pediatr.*, **103**, 127–130.
155. Gallin, J.I., Buescher, E.S., Seligmann, B.E., Nath, J., Gaither, T. and Katz, P. (1983) Recent advances in chronic granulomatous disease. *Ann. Intern. Med.*, **99**, 657–674.
156. Mouy, R., Fischer, A., Vilmer, E., Seger, R. and Griscelli, C. (1989) Incidence, severity, and prevention of infections in chronic granulomatous disease. *J. Pediatr.*, **114**, 555–560.
157. Margolis, D.M., Melnick, D.A., Alling, D.W. and Gallin, J.I. (1990) Trimethoprim–sulfamethoxazole in the management of chronic granulomatous disease. *Clin. Res.*, **38**, 558A.
158. Rappeport, J.M., Newburger, P.E., Goldblum, R.M., Golman, A.S., Nathan, D.G. and Parkman, R. (1982) Allogeneic bone marrow transplantation for chronic granulomatous disease. *J. Pediatr.*, **101**, 952–958.
159. Kamani, N., August, C.S., Campbell, D.E., Hassan, N.F. and Douglas, S.D. (1988) Marrow transplantation in chronic granulomatous disease: An update, with 6-year follow-up. *J. Pediatr.*, **113**, 697–700.
160. Cassatella, M.A., Della Bianca, V., Berton, G. and Rossi, F. (1985) Activation by gamma interferon of human macrophage capability to produce toxic oxygen molecules is accompanied by decreased K_m of the superoxide-generating NADPH oxidase. *Biochem. Biophys. Res. Commun.*, **132**, 908–914.

161. Berton, G., Zeni, L., Cassatella, M.A. and Rossi, F. (1986) Gamma interferon is able to enhance the oxidative metabolism of human neutrophils. *Biochem. Biophys. Res. Commun.*, **138**, 1276–1282.
162. Ezekowitz, R.A.B., Orkin, S.H. and Newburger, P.E. (1987) Recombinant interferon gamma augments phagocyte superoxide production and X-chronic granulomatous disease gene expression in X-linked variant chronic granulomatous disease. *J. Clin. Invest.*, **80**, 1009–1016.
163. Sechler, J.M.G., Malech, H.L., White, C.J. and Gallin, J.I. (1988) Recombinant human interferon-γ reconstitutes defective phagocyte function in patients with chronic granulomatous disease of childhood. *Proc. Nat. Acad. Sci. USA*, **85**, 4874–4878.
164. Ezekowitz, R.A.B., Dinauer, M.C., Jaffe, H.S., Orkin, S.H. and Newburger, P.E. (1988) Partial correction of the phagocyte defect in patients with X-linked chronic granulomatous disease by subcutaneous interferon gamma. *N. Engl. J. Med.*, **319**, 146–151.
165. International Chronic Granulomatous Disease Cooperative Study Group (1991) A controlled trial of interferon gamma to prevent infection in chronic granulomatous disease. *N. Engl. J. Med.*, **324**, 509–516.
166. Cobbs, C.S., Malech, H.L., Leto, T.L., Freeman, S.M., Blaese, R.M., Gallin, J.I. and Lomax, K.J. (1992) Retroviral expression of recombinant p47^{phox} protein by Epstein–Barr virus-transformed B lymphocytes from a patient with autosomal chronic granulomatous disease. *Blood*, **79**, 1829–1835.
167. Skalnik, D.G., Dorfman, D.M., Perkins, A.S., Jenkins, N.A., Copeland, N.G. and Orkin, S.H. (1991) Targeting of transgene expression to monocyte/macrophages by the gp91-phox promoter and consequent histiocytic malignancies. *Proc. Nat. Acad. Sci. USA*, **88**, 8505–8509.
168. Hopkins, P.J., Bemiller, L.S. and Curnutte, J.T. (1992) Chronic granulomatous disease: Diagnosis and classification at the molecular level. *Clin. Lab. Med.*, **12**, 277–304.

Part C

THERAPY

Chapter 16

Effects of Granulocyte Colony-stimulating Factor in Patients with Severe Chronic Neutropenia

KARL WELTE, CORNELIA ZEIDLER, ALFRED REITER and
HANSJÖRG RIEHM
Paediatric Haematology and Oncology, Medical School Hannover, Germany

Neutrophils are qualitatively and quantitatively the most important phagocytic cells defending the human body against acute bacterial infections (1). Therefore, diseases associated with severe chronic neutropenia are characterized by a high susceptibility to bacterial infections such as septicaemia, pneumonia, skin abscesses, otitis media, stomatitis, gingivitis, perianal abscesses, etc. The most common organisms responsible for these infections are *Staphylococcus aureus* and Gram-negative bacteria. The generation of neutrophils by proliferation and differentiation of granulocyte precursor cells is under the control of a family of haematopoietic growth factors such as interleukin 3 (IL-3), granulocyte–macrophage colony-stimulating factor (GM-CSF), and granulocyte colony-stimulating factor (G-CSF) (2). IL-3, GM-CSF and G-CSF have been shown to increase neutrophilic granulocytes *in vivo* in preclinical studies and in phase I–III clinical studies (3, 4). The most promising haematopoietic growth factor for treatment of severe chronic neutropenia states is G-CSF because it acts on neutrophilic progenitor and precursor cells only and demonstrates only minor adverse affects. Therefore, in this chapter we will focus mainly on the impact of G-CSF in the treatment of severe chronic neutropenia states.

G-CSF is a glycoprotein with a molecular weight of 19 600 (glycosylated)

New Concepts in Immunodeficiency Diseases. Edited by S. Gupta and C. Griscelli
© 1993 John Wiley & Sons Ltd

or 18,800 (unglycosylated) and consists of 174 amino acids (5, 6). It is produced by endothelial cells, fibroblasts and monocytes/macrophages and stimulates proliferation and differentiation of myeloid progenitor cells such as colony forming unit-granulocyte macrophage (CFU-GM) myeloblasts and promyelocytes up to the mature neutrophils (7). G-CSF exerts its biological activities through binding to a G-CSF-specific, high-affinity receptor (8, 9). The G-CSF receptor is a single polypeptide chain with 759 or 812 amino acids (two forms of G-CSF receptors due to alternative splicing) respectively, and consists of extracellular fibronectin-like and immunoglobulin-like domains, a transmembrane domain and an intraplasmatic domain (10). The signal transduction mechanisms activated by binding of G-CSF to its receptor are poorly understood.

Preclinical studies with recombinant human G-CSF (rhG-CSF) demonstrated its potent *in vivo* activities by stimulating dose-dependent neutrophilic granulopoiesis (11). The clinical trials with rhG-CSF in adults, mainly in patients with chemotherapy-induced neutropenia, have been reviewed by a variety of authors (3, 4). Because G-CSF was identified as growth and differentiation factor of cells of the neutrophilic lineage, the effects of G-CSF in haematological disorders involving the granulocytic progenitors or precursor cells are of considerable interest for both basic researchers and clinicians. In the following, the benefit of rhG-CSF treatment in patients with severe chronic neutropenia will be discussed. RhG-CSF was provided by Amgen (Thousand Oaks, California). It was expressed in *Escherichia coli* and purified to homogeneity (6). The rhG-CSF had a specific activity of approximately 10^8 U/mg protein, and was endotoxin free. The phase II clinical trials in patients with severe chronic neutropenia were approved by the Ethical Committee on the Use of Human Subjects in Research at the Medizinische Hochschule Hannover, Germany, and informed consent was obtained before entry into the studies.

SEVERE CONGENITAL NEUTROPENIA

Severe congenital neutropenia (SCN) or Kostmann's syndrome is a congenital disorder characterized by persistent severe absolute neutropenia (500 neutrophils per microlitre or less) usually detected in the first months of life which is associated with a maturational arrest of neutrophil precursors at the promyelocyte/myelocyte stage (12–15). In early infancy these children experience the onset of bacterial infections, particularly otitis media, pneumonia, gingivitis, urinary tract infections and abscess formations. Progression of local infection to severe septicaemia, meningitis, peritonitis, or severe enteritis accounts for the high morbidity and mortality seen in early childhood in this disease. In the past, investigators attempted to stimulate neutrophil production in these patients with infusions of fresh plasma, leucocyte transfusions, administration of steroids, testosterone, cysteine, vitamin E6, or lithium. None of these treatment modalities have altered the severity of the neutropenia. Bone marrow transplantation has been shown to correct this usually lethal disorder by replacing the patient's marrow with marrow from a normal sibling (16). However, the availability of an HLA-compatible sibling donor for only 25–30% of patients limits its therapeutic application.

Bonilla and co-workers reported in 1989 initial results of G-CSF treatment in five patients with severe congenital neutropenia (17). All five patients achieved a complete response. Responses were achieved with bolus injections of 10 µg/kg per day in two patients, and continuous infusions of 10, 30 or 60 µg/kg per day in three patients. Responses could be maintained with daily subcutaneous injections of 3, 6 or 18 µg/kg per day. The number of infection episodes was reduced in all patients.

In our clinic, 32 patients (18 male, 14 female; age: 0–23 years) with the confirmed diagnosis of SCN were entered into the study (18). The diagnosis of SCN was established on the basis of a peripheral blood absolute neutropenia (less than 200 cells per microlitre), bone marrow with a maturational arrest at the promyelocyte/myelocyte level, and the clinical onset of recurrent bacterial infections within the first year of life. The bone marrow was normo- or hyper-cellular with normal erythroid, lymphoid and megakaryocytic lineages. This patient population also exhibited a compensatory eosinophila, monocytosis, and hypergammaglobulinaemia. No evidence of anti-neutrophil antibodies was present. Seven patients received 1–3 months prior to rhG-CSF treatment with rhGM-CSF without neutrophil response (6 of 7 patients) (18).

All patients were initially treated with 3 µg/kg per day subcutaneously (s.c.) for 14 days. In patients who had no response within this time, the dose was escalated to 10 µg/kg per day for another 14 days, then in case of no response in 2-week intervals to 20, 30, up to 120 µg/kg per day until the absolute neutrophil count (ANC) was above 1000/µl. Patients with complete responses (ANC > 1000/µl) at any dose level were eligible for enrolment into a maintenance therapy. As mentioned above, the dose for maintenance treatment was based on that dose level inducing a complete neutrophil response of 1000 cells per microlitre or greater and was between 3 and 60 µg/kg per day s.c. or 120 µg/kg per day continuous intravenously.

Effects of rhG-CSF on Blood Cells

The effects of rhG-CSF on blood neutrophil counts of all responders are shown in Figure 16.1. RhG-CSF administration led in 30 of 32 patients to an increase in ANC to levels above 1000/µl (Figure 16.1). The dosages needed to achieve an ANC of 1000/µl were between 3 µg/kg per day and 120 µg/kg per day. The course of ANCs from three patients, who responded at different doses of rhG-CSF (5, 20, and 50 µg/kg per day, respectively), are

358 *Therapy*

shown in detail in Figure 16.2. Patients 9 and 31 showed no or only a minor response even at the highest doses (60 µg/kg per day s.c. or 120 µg/kg per day as continuous infusion) with an increase in ANC from 0 to about 200/µl. The dose regimen required to maintain an ANC of above 1000/µl varied from patient to patient and was between 3 and 60 µg/kg per day. Seventeen patients required rhG-CSF dosages between 3 and 10 µg/kg per day, nine patients between 10 and 20 µg/kg per day, and four patients between 40 and 60 µg/kg per day. The mean and standard deviation of all patients at approximately 1, 3, 6, 12, and 24 months of rhG-CSF treatment are shown in Figure 16.1. Due to the daily oscillation of neutrophil counts observed in all patients (see also Figure 16.2), the standard deviation at a given point in time is high. However, this oscillation did not affect the beneficial clinical responses. The neutrophils showed normal functions as judged by phagocytosis, intracellular killing of staphylococci, and reactive oxygen production (19). Chemotaxis towards formyl-methionyl-leucyl-phenylalanine

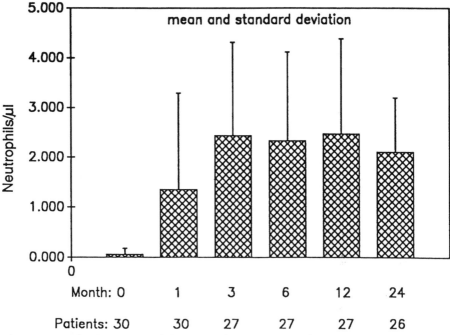

Figure 16.1. Absolute neutrophil counts of 30 patients with severe congenital neutropenia. (1) Thirty-two patients from Austria, Belgium, Germany, Greece, Great Britain, France, Italy, Israel and Switzerland were enrolled to the rhG-CSF treatment study in Hannover. Two patients did not respond to rhG-CSF therapy. (2) The high standard deviation is due to the high day-to-day oscillation of ANCs

Figure 16.2. (opposite) Dose heterogeneity of response to rhG-CSF

SEVERE CONGENITAL NEUTROPENIA

rhG—CSF treatment

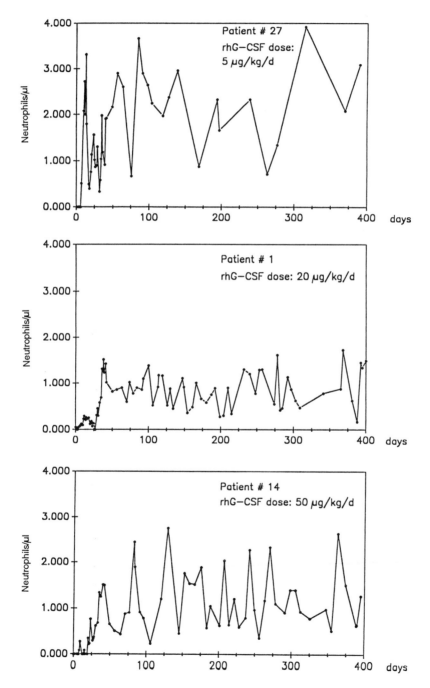

(FMLP) and other chemoattractants (interleukin 8 (IL-8), C5a, leukotriene B_4 (LTB$_4$), platelet-activating factor (PAF)), however, was reduced (20). The absolute eosinophil counts (AEoC) did not change significantly during rhG-CSF therapy in all patients. The absolute monocyte counts (AMC) increased twofold to eightfold in the majority of patients during rhG-CSF treatment. The most dramatic increase in AMC has been seen in patient number 3. However, this patient started the rhG-CSF treatment with an AMC which was already excessively high (3438/μl), and this increased further up to 24800/μl during the first 6 weeks of treatment. The number of CFU-GMs, myeloblasts and promyelocytes in the bone marrow during rhG-CSF treatment did not change significantly during rhG-CSF maintenance treatment.

Clinical Responses

In all patients, the number and severity of bacterial infections decreased significantly, which could also be documented by a significant reduction in the use of intravenous antibiotics when the first 4 weeks of treatment were compared with any other time interval of the rhG-CSF treatment thereafter. Four children suffered from severe bacterial or fungal infections on initiation of rhG-CSF treatment. During rhG-CSF treatment, lung infiltrates in patient number 1 caused by peptostreptococcus were dramatically resolved within 6 weeks of therapy. During the 6 weeks prior to rhG-CSF treatment, this patient suffered from septic temperatures and respiratory problems, and received combinations of various intravenous antibiotics. During the first 6 weeks of rhG-CSF treatment, her pulmonary situation resolved to a degree that the intravenous antibiotics could be discontinued. This resolution appeared in association with the increase in neutrophils. In the following 4 years, no severe bacterial infections have developed in this patient. Patient number 11 suffered from severe infiltrates within the entire left lung prior to the response to rhG-CSF. This patient responded at a dose of 120 μg/kg per day as continuous infusion; the destroyed left lung was removed, and she recovered from the pneumonectomy without problems. Subsequently, the dose of rhG-CSF for maintenance treatment could be reduced to 60 μg/kg per day s.c., and an ANC of above 1000/μl has been maintained since then. She has now been without severe infection for 2 years. In patient number 12, a severe anal abscess and anal fistula, which had persisted for about 1 year prior to rhG-CSF treatment, in spite of surgical intervention and antibiotic treatment, resolved within 3 months during rhG-CSF therapy. Patient number 13 had suffered for more than 2 of the 3 years of his life from fungal liver abscesses. As soon as the neutrophils increased, the liver abscesses shrank and were no longer detectable at an exploratory laparotomy on day 90 of rhG-CSF treatment.

Adverse Events

The adverse events leading to a temporary discontinuation of rhG-CSF treatment included necrotizing cutaneous vasculitis (patient number 5), generalized severe vasculitis (patient number 17) and mesangioproliferative glomerulonephritis (patient number 22), and were all associated with a prompt increase in ANC and not with the dose of rhG-CSF. All three patients suffered from these side effects at the lowest dose of rhG-CSF (3 μg/kg per day). Patient number 5 now receives rhG-CSF at a dose of 0.8 μg/kg per day. At this dose, this patient has an ANC of 500–1000/μl without further recurrence of the vasculitis. In patient number 22, rhG-CSF was continued 1 year later without recurrence of the glomerulonephritis. Of the total population of 32 patients, 10 patients suffered from mild osteopenia and 2 patients from severe osteoporosis. This adverse event is most likely linked to the underlying disease, since 5 of the 12 patients suffered from this side effect prior to rhG-CSF therapy. It cannot be excluded, however, that rhG-CSF treatment worsened the decalcification of bones by increasing the number of osteoclasts. This was supported by recently published data on bone modulation by CSFs: G-CSF-treated mice showed a significant increase in osteoclast numbers with reduction of bone thickness (21). About one-third of the patients demonstrated splenomegaly (approx. 1–3 cm below the costal margin). Patient number 6 developed myelodysplastic syndrome after 2 years of G-CSF treatment with monosomy 7 of the myeloid cells and transition into an acute myeloid leukaemia. Patient number 17 developed acute monoblastic leukaemia 6 months after discontinuation of rhG-CSF therapy. The development of leukaemia in two patients in this small group of patients is worrying. However, the predisposition of patients with severe congenital neutropenia for acute myeloid leukaemias has already been reported prior to the G-CSF treatment era (22, 23). These data suggest that severe congenital neutropenia is a pre-malignant disease. The adverse events of all patients treated with rhG-CSF in our clinic, including idiopathic neutropenia and cyclic neutropenia patients, are summarized in Table 16.1.

Conclusion

In 30 of 32 patients with severe congenital neutropenia, rhG-CSF induced an increase of blood neutrophils to above 1000/μl. The dose necessary to reach and maintain an ANC of above 1000/μl varied from patient to patient and ranged between 3 and 60 μl/kg per day. The neutrophils in the rhG-CSF-treated patients had normal functional activities as judged by *in vitro* functions and by clinical parameters. In four patients, there was a resolution of severe bacterial infections (pneumonitis, liver abscess, anal abscess) which had been resistant to intravenous antibiotic treatment prior to rhG-CSF

Table 16.1   Adverse events in patients with chronic neutropenia (all patients, n = 50) during rhG-CSF treatment

	n	Severity	Relationship to rhG-CSF therapy	Outcome
Osteopenia	10	Mild/moderate	Possibly	Still exists
Splenomegaly	6	Mild/moderate	Possibly	Still exists
Hepatosplenomegaly	4	Mild/moderate	Possibly	Still exists
Thrombocytopenia	3	Moderate	Probably	Still exists
Osteoporosis	2	Severe	Possibly	Still exists
Vasculitis	2	Moderate	Probably	No residual defect
Glomerulonephritis	2	Severe	Probably	No residual defect
Anaemia	2	Moderate	Probably	Still exists
Myelodysplasia (MDS)	1	Severe	Unlikely	Still exists
Leukaemia	1	Severe	Unlikely	Still exists

1. The adverse events vasculitis and glomerulonephritis are related to an abrupt increase in blood neutrophils and, therefore, are most likely caused by activated neutrophils
2. All other adverse events are most likely linked to the underlying disease. Osteoporosis, splenomegaly, anaemia, MDS and leukaemia were reported to be seen in severe congenital neutropenia patients prior to the G-CSF era, However, it cannot be excluded that rhG-CSF had an influence on these events

therapy. The maintenance treatment did not lead to an exhaustion of myelopoiesis: all patients have now been treated for at least 12 months. The ANC of all patients was stable during the maintenance treatment and no increases in the dose have been necessary to maintain the ANC during long-term treatment. The number and severity of infections decreased significantly in all patients during rhG-CSF treatment, as compared with a similar time period prior to therapy.

Although rhG-CSF treatment changed the life of these children dramatically, the pathogenesis of the underlying disease is still not known. Hypotheses for the genetic disposition affecting these patients include defective production of G-CSF or defective response of neutrophil precursors to G-CSF or other haematopoietic growth factors. Defective G-CSF production does not seem likely in light of new data which show that the serum from these patients contains normal or elevated levels of G-CSF as judged by Western blot analysis and *in vitro* bioassays (24, 25). Defective G-CSF response by reduced binding affinity of G-CSF to its receptor or low G-CSF receptor numbers can also be excluded by data showing that binding of G-CSF to its receptor, as judged by Scatchard analysis, is normal and the receptor numbers on neutrophils from patients with severe congenital neutropenia are rather elevated (26). The different mutations in intracellular events following binding of G-CSF to its receptor, however, could explain the variations from patient to patient in response to rhG-CSF and the dose needed (3–60 µg/kg per day) to achieve an ANC of 1000/µl.

In summary, these findings demonstrate that rhG-CSF is the most promising of all available treatments for severe congenital neutropenia. The correction of neutropenia with resultant improvement of clinical status can dramatically change the high morbidity and, therefore, the quality of life in these patients.

CYCLIC NEUTROPENIA

Cyclic neutropenia (or cyclic haematopoiesis) is a rare blood disease characterized by regular cyclic fluctuations in the numbers of blood neutrophils, platelets, and reticulocytes (27, 28). Patients with this disease typically have regularly recurring symptoms of fever and mucosal ulcers during periods of neutropenia.

Cyclic neutropenia has been attributed to a regulatory abnormality affecting blood cell formation at the stem cell level, but the precise defect in these cells is not yet known. Marrow transplantation from a child with cyclic neutropenia to a sibling with leukaemia resulted in the transfer of the disease, suggesting a defect within the pluripotent stem cell compartment. Most patients with cyclic neutropenia are given the diagnosis in childhood, but its onset in some patients later in life suggests that it may also be an acquired disorder. Only a few patients, almost exclusively adults, have been reported to respond to any therapy, including corticosteroids, androgens, splenectomy, and plasmapheresis.

In a study reported by Hammond and co-workers in 1989, six patients with cyclic neutropenia were treated with rhG-CSF (29). All had a history of recurrent aphthous stomatitis, pharyngitis, lymphadenopathy, fever, and numerous infections during periods of neutropenia. Serial blood cell counts, findings on bone marrow examination and signs and symptoms were evaluated before and during the daily administration of G-CSF (3–10 µg/kg per day), either intravenously or subcutaneously.

Recombinant human G-CSF increased the mean (±SEM) neutrophil counts from 717±171 per microlitre to 9814±2198 per microlitre. In five of the six patients, the cycling of blood cell counts continued, but the length of the period decreased from 21 to 14 days. The number of days of severe neutropenia was reduced significantly. Neutrophil turnover increased almost fourfold, whereas neutrophil migration to a skin chamber was normal. G-CSF therapy reduced the frequency of oropharyngeal inflammation, fever, and infections in these patients. During the first 40 months of treatment, no typical mouth ulcers or bacterial infections occurred; recurrent gingivitis improved (29).

We have treated four patients with cyclic neutropenia with rhG-CSF (30). After an observation period of one cycle, patients were started with 3 µg/kg per day s.c. for 42 days, after which the dose was adjusted to 1, 3 or 5 µg/kg per day for maintenance therapy depending on the median ANC. All four patients responded to a dose between 1 and 3 µg/kg per day. The time course of neutrophils in one of the patients is shown in Figure 16.3. Before treatment with rhG-CSF, all four patients had a history of recurrent bacterial infections. During rhG-CSF therapy, the number and severity of infections decreased significantly.

Conclusion

The studies by Hammond *et al.* (29) and by us demonstrate that the effect of G-CSF on neutrophil counts translates into clinical benefits: the reduction in the frequency of infectious episodes and the reduction in the severity of the symptoms of infection and inflammation. The clinical improvement in these patients is as dramatic as in patients with severe congenital neutropenia. The benefit of rhG-CSF treatment can be achieved by very low dosages (1–3 µg/kg per day). Hammond *et al.* (29) reported splenic enlargement and mild bone pain. In our patients we have not observed any adverse event. From these data we conclude that G-CSF is the best available therapy of cyclic neutropenia.

ACQUIRED CHRONIC NEUTROPENIA

Acquired chronic neutropenia can be classified depending on the pathomechanisms responsible for the neutropenia:

- Postinfectious.
- Drug-induced.
- Immune-neutropenia.
- Neutropenia associated with T or B cell abnormalities.
- Neutropenia associated with metabolic abnormalities.

We have treated so far one 17-year-old patient with chronic neutropenia persisting 10 years after infectious mononucleosis. This patient responded to rhG-CSF at a dose of 3 µg/kg per day with an increase of neutrophils to above 1000/µl. He has been receiving rhG-CSF treatment for more than 2 years, without any recurrence of severe infections.

A 14-year-old boy with severe neutropenia associated with hyper-IgM syndrome and agammaglobulinaemia responded well to rhG-CSF at a dose of 3 µg/kg per day. The combination of rhG-CSF treatment and regular immunoglobulin substitution led to a dramatic improvement in the quality of his life. However, the IgM levels remain to be elevated.

Two children with glycogen storage disease type Ib associated with numerous recurrent bacterial infections (31) as a result of neutropenia and neutrophil dysfunction (32) (defective H_2O_2 generation, decreased calcium

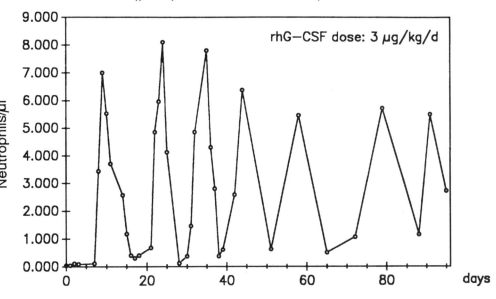

Figure 16.3. Response pattern to rhG-CSF of a patient with severe cyclic neutropenia. Prior to rhG-CSF therapy, the absolute neutrophil counts in this patient cycled with maximum neutrophil counts of approximately 500/μl

mobilization, defective chemotaxis) were treated with rhG-CSF. RhG-CSF at doses of 3 μg/kg per day increased the average neutrophil counts from less than 300 cells per microlitre to more than 1200 cells per microlitre (33). Two subpopulations of neutrophils could be identified by their capacity to produce H_2O_2: one subpopulation generated H_2O_2 normally and a second was defective in H_2O_2 production. The doses of rhG-CSF effectively enhanced and maintained that subpopulation of neutrophils which produced normal amounts of H_2O_2. Moreover, these CSF-induced neutrophils demonstrated effective phagocytosis of zymosan particles and killing of staphylococci. Chemotaxis was decreased and could not be normalized by treatment with rhG-CSF. We conclude that maintenance treatment with rhG-CSF improved the quality of life in both patients: the number and severity of bacterial infections decreased markedly during treatment. Long-term treatment with rhG-CSF (24 and 22 months, respectively) was well tolerated, and no adverse clinical events were observed. Glycogen storage-related side effects, such as hepatomegaly and acidosis, however, were not influenced by rhG-CSF treatment (33).

Severe neutropenia can also be associated with Schwachman's syndrome, a rare multi-organ disease characterized by chondrodysplasia, dwarfism, and exocrine pancreas insufficiency (34, 35). The degree of neutropenia is variable. In a patient with Schwachman's syndrome, rhG-CSF treatment (10 µg/kg per day) has been shown to correct neutropenia and associated infections (Zeidler *et al.*, manuscript in preparation).

Immune neutropenia occurs commonly in infants (36, 37). Since this disease is benign and self-limiting within the first 2 years of life in most of the patients, G-CSF therapy is not indicated.

CHRONIC IDIOPATHIC NEUTROPENIA

The onset of chronic idiopathic neutropenia can occur at any age from infancy to adulthood. Neutrophil counts are commonly below 500/µl, and the bone marrow examination reveals normal numbers of myeloid progenitors with an arrest of neutrophilic granulopoiesis at a late stage of maturation. The pathomechanisms involved in idiopathic neutropenia are not known. Patients with chronic idiopathic neutropenia suffer from frequent episodes of severe bacterial infections similar to children with congenital neutropenia (see above). Recently, rhG-CSF has been used effectively to treat an adult patient with idiopathic neutropenia (38).

We have treated 12 patients with idiopathic neutropenia with rhG-CSF according to a protocol identical to that for treatment of severe congenital neutropenia (see treatment plan of severe congenital neutropenia). Of these patients, ten responded to rhG-CSF (Freund and Welte, manuscript in preparation). The doses needed to achieve neutrophil counts above 1000/µl varied between 1 µg/kg per day and 3.6 µg/kg per day s.c. In all patients who responded to rhG-CSF, the number and severity of infections decreased dramatically. The two patients who did not respond to rhG-CSF subsequently developed within 1 year aplastic anaemia. In these two patients, our hypothesis is that the severe neutropenia was the first sign of the later development of general aplasia of bone marrow cells.

SUMMARY

In children with all types of severe chronic neutropenia the development of rhG-CSF for therapeutic use changed the quality of their life dramatically. Lacking the most important cells in the defence against bacterial infections— the neutrophilic granulocytes—these patients suffered from episodes of severe, often life-threatening bacterial infections. They spent numerous days in hospital, requiring intravenous antibiotic treatment. Recurrence of bacterial infections at the same site led to irreversible tissue damage, for example in the lung, requiring often disabling surgical interventions.

In most patients, rhG-CSF treatment induced an increase of blood and tissue neutrophils to a level high enough to guarantee a normal defence against bacterial infections. The quality of life improved substantially in these children. The fact that they have to inject themselves daily does not cause any problems.

However, it is still too early to be sure about all side effects of this chronic treatment. Development of leukaemia in a few patients with congenital neutropenia is most likely due to pathomechanisms of the underlying disease. Osteopenia or osteoporosis could be explained by effects of the high levels of endogenous G-CSF or rhG-CSF on the number and activation of osteoclasts (21). The longer life expectancy of these patients might reveal symptoms of the underlying disease which have not been recognized prior to the rhG-CSF treatment era.

Overall, taken in consideration all possible adverse events during our short observation period, all patients who responded to rhG-CSF benefited from this treatment to a degree never considered to be possible before.

ACKNOWLEDGEMENT

Supported in part by grants from the Deutsche Forschungsgemeinschaft (We 942/2-1).

REFERENCES

1. Curnutte, J.T. and Boxer, L.A. (1987) Disorders of granulopoiesis and granulocyte functions. In Nathan, D.G. and Oski, F.A. (eds) *Hematology of Infancy and Childhood*. Saunders, Philadelphia, pp. 797–847.
2. Metcalf, D. (1989) The molecular control of cell division, differentiation commitment and maturation in haemopoietic cells. *Nature*, **339**, 27.
3. Andreef, M. and Welte, K. (1989) Hematopoietic colony-stimulating factors. *Semin. Oncol.*, **16**, 211–229.
4. Groopman, J.E. (1990) Status of colony-stimulating factors in cancer and AIDS. *Semin. Oncol.*, **17**, 31.
5. Welte, K., Platzer, E., Lu, L., Gabrilove, J., Levi, E., Mertelsmann, R. and Moore, M.A.S. (1985) Purification and biochemical characterization of human pluripotent hematopoietic colony stimulating factor. *Proc. Nat. Acad. Sci. USA*, **82**, 1526.
6. Souza, L.M., Boone, T.C., Gabrilove, J., Lai, P.H., Zsebo, K.M., Murdock, D.C., Chazin, V.R., Burszewski, J., Lu, H., Chen, K.K., Barendt, J., Platzer, E., Moore, M.A.S., Mertelsmann, R. and Welte, K. (1986) Recombinant human granulocyte colony stimulating factor: Effects on normal and leukemic myeloid cells. *Science*, **232**, 61.
7. Demetri, G.D. and Griffin, J.D. (1991) Granulocyte colony-stimulating factor and its receptor. *Blood*, **78**, 2791–2808.
8. Fukunaga, R., Ishizaka-Ikeda, E., Seta, Y. and Nagata, S. (1990) Expression cloning of a receptor for murine granulocyte colony-stimulating factor. *Cell*, **61**, 341.
9. Fukunaga, R., Seto, Y., Mizushima, S. and Nagata, S. (1990) Three different mRNAs encoding human granulocyte colony-stimulating factor receptor. *Proc. Nat. Acad. Sci. USA*, **87**, 8702.
10. Larson, A., Davis, T., Curtis, B.M., Gimpel, S., Cosman, D., Park, L., Sorensen, E., March, C. and Smith, C.A. (1990) Expression cloning of a human G-CSF receptor:

A structural mosaic of hematopoietin receptor, immunoglobulin and fibronectin domains. *J. Exp. Med.*, **172**, 1559.

11. Welte, K., Bonilla, M.A., Gillio, A.P., Boone, T.C., Potter, G.K., Gabrilove, J.L., Moore, M.A.S., O'Reilly, R.J. and Souza, L.M. (1987) Recombinant human granulocyte colony stimulating factor: Effects on hematopoiesis in normal and cyclophosphamide-treated primates. *J. Exp. Med.*, **165**, 941.

12. Kostmann, R. (1956) Infantile genetic agranulocytosis. *Acta. Paediatr. Scand.*, **45**, (Suppl. 105): 1.

13. Kostmann, R. (1975) Infantile genetic agranulocytosis: A review with presentation of ten new cases. *Acta. Paediatr. Scand.*, **64**, 362.

14. Wriedt, K., Kauder, E. *et al.* (1970) Defective myelopoiesis in congenital neutropenia. *N. Engl. J. Med.*, **283**, 1072.

15. Amato, D., Freedman, M.H. and Saunders, E.F. (1976) Granulopoiesis in severe congenital neutropenia. *Blood*, **47**, 531.

16. Rappeport, J.M., Parkman, R. *et al.* (1980) Correction of infantile agranulocytosis by allogeneic bone marrow transplantation. *Am. J. Med.*, **68**, 605.

17. Bonilla, M.A., Gillio, A.P., Ruggeiro, M., Kernan, N.A., Brochstein, J.A., Abboud, M., Fumagalli, L., Vincent, M., Gabrilove, J.L., Welte, K., Souza, L.M. and O'Reilly, R.J. (1989) Effects of recombinant human granulocyte colony-stimulating factor on neutropenia in patients with congenital agranulocytosis. *N. Engl. J. Med.*, **320**, 1574–1580.

18. Welte, K., Zeidler, C., Reiter, A., Müller, W., Odenwald, E., Souza, L. and Riehm, H. (1990) Differential effects of granulocyte–macrophage colony-stimulating factor and granulocyte colony-stimulating factor in children with severe congenital neutropenia. *Blood*, **75**, 1056–1063.

19. Roesler, J., Emmendörffer, A., Elsner, J., Zeidler, C., Lohmann-Matthes, M.L. and Welte, K. (1991) In vitro functions of neutrophils induced by treatment with rhG-CSF in severe congenital neutropenia. *Eur. J. Haematol.*, **46**, 112–118.

20. Elsner, J., Roesler, J., Emmendörffer, A., Zeidler, C., Lohmann-Matthes, M.L. and Welte, K. (1992) Altered function and surface marker expression of neutrophils induced rhG-CSF treatment in severe congenital neutropenia. *Eur. J. Haematol.*, **48**, 10–19.

21. Lee, M.Y., Fukunaga, R., Lee, T.J., Lottsfeldt, J.L. and Nagata, S. (1991) Bone modulation in sustained hematopoietic stimulation in mice. *Blood*, **77**, 2135–2141.

22. Gilman, P.A., Jackson, D.P. *et al.* (1970) Congenital agranulocytosis: Prolonged survival and terminal acute leukemia. *Blood*, **36**, 576.

23. Rosen, R.B. and Kang, S.J. (1979) Congenital agranulocytosis terminating in acute myelomonocytic leukaemia. *J. Pediatr.*, **94**, 406.

24. Pietsch, T., Bührer, C., Mempel, K., Menzel, T., Steffens, U., Schrader, C., Santos, F., Zeidler, C. and Welte, K. (1991) Blood mononuclear cells from patients with severe congenital neutropenia are capable of producing granulocyte colony-stimulating factor. *Blood*, **77**, 1234–1237.

25. Mempel, K., Pietsch, T., Menzel, T., Zeidler, C. and Welte, K. (1991) Increased serum levels of granulocyte colony-stimulating factor (G-CSF) in patients with severe congenital neutropenia. *Blood*, **77**, 1919–1922.

26. Kyas, U., Pietsch, T. and Welte, K. (1992) Expression of receptors for granulocyte colony stimulating factor on neutrophils from patients with severe congenital neutropenia. *Blood*, **79**, 1144–1147.

27. Wright, D.G., Dale, D.C. *et al.* (1981) Human cyclic neutropenia: Clinical review and long-term follow-up of patients. *Medicine*, **60**, 1.

28. Dale, D.C. and Hammond, W.P., IV (1988) Cyclic neutropenia: A clinical review. *Blood* (Rev. 2), 178–185.
29. Hammond, W.P., IV, Price, T.H., Souza, L.M. and Dale, D.C. (1989) Treatment of cyclic neutropenia with granulocyte colony-stimulating factor. *N. Engl. J. Med.*, **320**, 1306–1311.
30. Freund, M., Luft, S., Schöber, C., Heussner, P., Schrezenmaier, H., Porzolt, F. and Welte, K. (1990) Differential effect of GM-CSF and G-CSF in cyclic neutropenia. *Lancet*, **336**, 313.
31. Schaub, J. and Heyne, K. (1983) Glycogen storage disease type Ib. *Eur. J. Pediatr.*, **140**, 283–288.
32. DiRocco, M., Borrone, C., Dallegri, F. *et al.* (1984) Neutropenia and impaired neutrophil function in glycogenosis type Ib. *J. Inherited Metab. Dis.*, **7**, 151–154.
33. Schroten, H., Roesler, J., Breidenbach, T. *et al.* (1991) Granulocyte and granulocyte–macrophage colony-stimulating factors for treatment of neutropenia in glycogen storage disease type Ib. *J. Pediatr.*, **119**, 748–754.
34. Schwachman, H., Diamond, L.K. *et al.* (1964) The syndrome of pancreatic insufficiency and bone marrow dysfunction. *J. Pediatr.*, **65**, 645.
35. Aggett, P.J., Cavanagh, N.P.C. *et al.* (1980) Schwachman's syndrome. *Arch. Dis. Child.*, **55**, 331.
36. Lalezari, P., Jiang, A. *et al.* (1975) Chronic autoimmune neutropenia due to anti-NA2 antibody. *N. Engl. J. Med.*, **293**, 744.
37. Boxer, L.A. (1981) Immune neutropenias: Clinical and biological implications. *Am. J. Pediatr. Hematol. Oncol.*, **3**, 89.
38. Jakubowski, A.A., Souza, L., Kelly, F. *et al.* (1989) Effects of human granulocyte colony-stimulating factor in a patient with idiopathic neutropenia. *N. Engl. J. Med.*, **320**, 38.

Chapter 17

Interferon γ in Chronic Granulomatous Diseases of Childhood

JOHN I. GALLIN

Laboratory of Host Defenses, National Institute of Allergy and Infectious Diseases, National Institutes of Health, Bethesda, Maryland, USA

The chronic granulomatous diseases of childhood (CGD) are a group of disorders of oxidative metabolism with a phenotype characterized by abnormal hydrogen peroxide formation. The biochemistry of these diseases has been the subject of recent reviews (1–3), including an article by Roos (chapter 15, this volume). CGD is characterized clinically by recurrent life-threatening infections with catalase-positive microorganisms such as *Staphylococcus aureus* and *Aspergillus* spp. (1) and increased granuloma formation. The granulomas can occlude vital structures such as the esophagus and ureter and thereby be life threatening. Until recently management has been largely supportive. Aggressive surgery for deep-seated infections and prolonged use of antibiotics have been central to therapy (1). In some centers white blood cell transfusions have also been used for treatment of life-threatening infections. Steroids have an important role in managing the granulomatous complications of CGD (4). Low-dose prednisone can reverse life-threatening granulomas obstructing vital structures.

Despite aggressive medical management the incidence of life-threatening infections is a significant threat to patients. Prophylactic antibiotics, particularly with trimethoprim–sulfamethoxazole, has prolonged the interval between infections from about once every 9 months to once every 4 years without changing the prevalence of fungal infections (5). Recently, new hope for CGD patients has become available through the use of interferon γ (IFNγ) as adjunct therapy.

New Concepts in Immunodeficiency Diseases. Edited by S. Gupta and C. Griscelli
© 1993 John Wiley & Sons Ltd

PROPERTIES OF IFNγ

IFNγ is a member of a group of proteins that are related by their ability to *interfere* with viral infection. IFNs have been classified as IFNα, -β, and -γ (6–8). IFNα was originally known as leukocyte IFN because it was produced by peripheral blood mononuclear cells and was also called type I IFN. IFNβ, known originally as fibroblast IFN because of its cell of origin, was also called type I IFN. IFNα and -β are the classical IFNs induced by viral infection. Over 20 IFNα genes have been described, and the reason for the complexity of this gene system is unknown. There is only a single IFNβ gene known. IFNβ is antigenically distinct from IFNα although IFNα and -β display 15–30% amino acid sequence homology. Nevertheless, both forms of type I IFN bind to the same receptor on the surface of target cells, indicating that the binding site of these two molecules has been conserved.

IFNγ, also called immune IFN or type II IFN, is molecularly and functionally distinct from the type I IFNs (9–11). IFNγ is induced by unique stimuli and to date is known to be produced by only T lymphocytes and by natural killer (NK) cells (12). Viral infection of these cells does not induce IFNγ production. Moreover, although IFNγ has the biological activities ascribed to IFNα and -β, it has one to two logs lower specific antiviral activity. On the other hand, IFNγ is 100–10 000 times more active as an immune-modulator compared with the other classes of IFNs. This has led to the observation that whereas IFNα and -β have primarily antiviral activity with some immune-modulatory activity, IFNγ is primarily an immune-modulator that can also exert some antiviral activity (7).

The gene for human IFN-γ is 6 kb in size and contains four exons and three introns (9–11). The human IFNγ gene is localized to the long arm of chromosome 12 (12q24.1), and activation of the gene leads to the generation of a 1.2 kb mRNA that encodes a 166-amino acid polypeptide (13, 14). Human IFNγ contains two N-linked glycosylation sites. Differential glycosylation leads to heterogeneity of the molecular weight of the molecule (17–50 kDa). Glycosylation is not important for expression of IFNγ activity although it appears to influence the circulatory half-life of the molecule (15–17).

Although the functionally important regions of the IFNγ molecule have not been precisely identified, current data indicate that both the amino and carboxy termini play critical roles in maintaining an active conformation of the protein. The X-ray crystallographic structure of human IFNγ established a dimeric nature of the protein (18). The molecule is primarily helical (62%) and lacks β sheet structure. Each subunit consists of six α helices held together by short non-helical regions. The model predicts that both the amino and carboxy termini are exposed and therefore may play important functional roles in mediating receptor binding.

CELLULAR SOURCES OF IFNγ

The T lymphocyte is the major source of IFNγ, with both CD8 T cells and certain subsets of CD4 T cells capable of active synthesis (7, 8). In the mouse the CD4 T cell subset, T_H1, produces interleukin 2 (IL-2), IFNγ, lymphotoxin and high levels of tumor necrosis factor (TNF), while T_H2 T cells do not produce the first three but instead produce limited amounts of TNF as well as IL-4, IL-5, IL-6 and IL-10, which are not produced by T_H1 cells. Both T_H1 and T_H2 cells produce the cytokines IL-3 and granulocyte–macrophage colony-stimulating factor (GM-CSF). Because IL-2 IFNγ, and lymphotoxin are important in promoting cytotoxic T lymphocyte and macrophage effector functions, T_H1 cells are thought to be primarily involved in cell-mediated immunity. In contrast, because IL-4, IL-5, IL-6 and IL-10 have important roles in regulating B lymphocyte growth and development, the T_H2 cells are thought to be responsible for humoral immunity.

IFNγ is produced by T cells primarily by stimulation with antigen in the context of either major histocompatibility (MHC) class II antigens (Ia antigen for CD4 lymphocytes) or MHC class 1 (for CD8 T cells). *In vitro*, IFNγ can be induced by either direct stimulation of the T cell receptor/CD3 complex with antibodies such as anti-CD3, T cell mitogens such as concanavalin A or phytohemagglutinin, or pharmacological stimuli such as phorbol-myristate acetate (PMA) plus calcium ionophores (e.g. ionomycin). IFNγ production is amplified by products of T cells and macrophages such as IL-2, hydrogen peroxide and the leukotrienes LTB_4, LTC_4 and LTD_4 (19–24).

IFNγ is also produced by NK cells (12, 22, 25). Although mitogen can induce NK cells to produce IFNγ, particularly if the cells are exposed to IL-2, NK cells are especially prone to produce IFNγ when exposed to bacteria or microbial products (25–28). As a consequence it has been suggested that IFNγ produced by NK cells represents the host's first line of defense against microbial pathogens that are susceptible to killing by activated macrophages.

BIOLOGICAL FUNCTIONS INDUCED BY IFNγ

A wide array of biological functions are induced by IFNγ. One of the most important functions is the regulation of MHC class I and class II expression on a variety of immunologically important cells (29–31). These include endothelial cells, epithelial cells, and the mononuclear phagocytes (32, 33). It is of interest that although IFNγ stimulates MHC class expression in most cells, in B cells it inhibits MHC class II expression (34). IFNγ up-regulation of MHC gene expression is probably important for antigen presentation (35, 36).

The mononuclear phagocyte is one of the prime targets for IFNγ which regulates differentiation and function of these cells (7, 8). For example, IFNγ promotes differentiation of monocyte–myeloid precursor cells in the bone marrow and promotes antigen-presenting activity of macrophages through both MHC class II expression and increasing several intracellular enzymes thought to be important in antigen presentation. IFNγ also enhances macrophage IL-1 production and expression of the intercellular adhesion molecule 1 (ICAM-1). IFNγ also stimulates macrophage TNFα production, Fc receptor expression, complement genes C2 and factor B, phagocytosis, and macrophage production of hydrogen peroxide, nitrogen oxides, tryptophan degradation and synthesis of antimicrobial granule proteins (8, 36–39). IFNγ also stimulates oxidative metabolism in neutrophils (40).

IFNγ affects other elements of the immune system. In mice and in humans IFNγ regulates immunoglobulin (Ig) isotope selection, with class-specific IgG enhancement and inhibition of IgE production (41, 42). On T cells, IFNγ exerts an antiproliferative effect on the T_H2 subset of CD4 T cells and thereby influences the production of a number of cytokines (43, 44) as described above. Thus, IFNγ has the capacity to regulate both the cellular and humoral limbs of immunity through its actions on T and B lymphocytes as well as on endothelial cells, epithelial cells and mononuclear phagocytes. Through this multitude of actions IFNγ has the potential to be an important therapeutic agent for enhancing host defenses. This potential has been dramatically demonstrated in the group of patients with CGD (44).

INITIAL STUDIES OF IFNγ WITH CGD PHAGOCYTES

In 1988 Sechler *et al.* and Ezekowitz *et al.* (40, 45) published independently that IFNγ could stimulate macrophages from certain patients with CGD to reduce nitroblue tetrazolium dye (NBT), produce superoxide anion and to kill *Staphylococcus aureus*. The dose–response curve for IFNγ indicated that the 50% maximal response was obtained with approximately 100 units/ml and required 2–3 days of macrophage exposure to IFNγ.

Sechler *et al.* (40) showed that IFNγ partially corrected the defect in neutrophils and monocytes from patients with CGD. For example, monocytes obtained from 19 of 30 patients with CGD treated with IFNγ *in vivo* were found to produce superoxide when stimulated with PMA *in vitro*. Monocytes from 15 of 16 patients with cytochrome *b*-positive CGD and from 4 of 14 patients with cytochrome *b*-negative CGD also responded. Western blot studies of cells obtained from one CGD patient who received IFNγ *in vivo* indicated that increased superoxide production correlated with an increase in the 91 kDa chain of membrane-bound cytochrome b_{558}. The effects of IFNγ on monocyte function persisted for greater than a week after therapy was concluded.

Ezekowitz *et al.* (45) reported that when IFNγ was administered to nine CGD patients, the phagocyte respiratory burst was stimulated only in those patients with X-linked CGD and unusually mild clinical manifestations of the disease. Two patients who responded were brothers whose neutrophils prior to treatment produced 10% and 18% of normal superoxide. Ezekowitz *et al.* showed an increase in mRNA for the 91 kDa subunit of cytochrome b_{558} and the authors suggested that the X-linked type of CGD whose phagocytes retain the ability to produce some superoxide have a defect in the regulation of synthesis of the 91 kDa subunit of cytochrome b_{558}. They also suggested that IFNγ stimulates expression of the 91 kDa subunit gene, thereby compensating to some extent for the defect in these patients. In related studies with normal cells, Abramson *et al.* (46) have shown that IFNγ induces the 47 kDa cytosolic protein and 91 kDa membrane component of cytochrome b_{558} of phagocytes. Furthermore, the induction of these proteins in cells from certain patients probably accounts for at least a portion of increased host defenses in these patients.

Sechler *et al.* (40) pointed out that phagocytes obtained from some CGD patients given IFNγ responded with increased bactericidal activity, although enhancement of superoxide generation was not observed. These data suggested that *in vivo* IFNγ simulates not only the oxidative metabolism but also non-oxidative bactericidal mechanisms. Based on these observations, the suggestion that therapy with IFNγ could benefit patients even without simulation of the respiratory burst was reasonable (40, 45).

MULTI-CENTER CLINICAL TRIAL OF IFNγ IN CGD

The studies published in 1988 (40, 45) indicated that subcutaneous IFNγ was readily tolerated and enhanced phagocyte bactericidal capacity in CGD. As an extension of these preliminary studies an international, multi-center, placebo-controlled, randomized, double-blind study was undertaken (44). One hundred and twenty-eight patients were randomized to receive placebo or IFNγ. Patient groups were matched for age and stratified by presence or absence of antibiotics. The mean age was 14.3 years for the IFNγ group and 15.0 years for the placebo group. There were 12 females (19%) and 51 males (81%). In the group of patients receiving IFNγ, 45 (71%) had X-linked CGD and 18 (29%) had the autosomal recessive form of CGD; in the placebo group, 41 patients (63%) had X-linked CGD and 24 (37%) had the autosomal recessive form. The dose of IFNγ was 50 µg/m². The primary end-point was denoted as the length of time before a serious infection occurred. Serious infection was defined as that which required hospitalization and treatment with parenteral antibiotics; the secondary end-points were defined as the effects on the patient's existing condition, the number of serious infections, and the duration of hospitalization. Of the patients in the control and treatment groups, 85% and 89%, respectively, were receiving antibiotics prophylactically and 3% and 2%, respectively, were receiving steroids. The duration of the study was projected as 1 year, but the study was discontinued after an interim analysis was conducted at the 9-month point.

The results of the study were dramatic and indicated that the number of infections that occurred in the CGD patients receiving IFNγ were reduced significantly compared with the patients receiving placebo. Infections were reduced at all anatomical locations. Recombinant IFNγ-treated patients experienced a 72% reduction in the relative risk of serious infection compared to control patients. In addition, there was a significant reduction in the duration of hospitalization for an infection in CGD patients receiving IFN-γ.

The collaborative study failed to demonstrate that IFNγ had a significant effect on neutrophilic bactericidal activity against *Staphylococcus aureus*; in this respect the study differed from previous studies in which a beneficial effect on phagocyte function was observed (40, 45). The differences between the collaborative study and prior publications probably reflect variation in technique among the various centers in which the studies were performed. It is of interest that in parallel with the collaborative studies *in vitro*, studies performed with neutrophils from patients from the NIH receiving IFNγ demonstrated improved *in vitro* damage to *Aspergillus conidia* by their neutrophils compared with cells from NIH patients receiving placebo (47). Furthermore, a review of the frequency of fungal infections in 70 patients with CGD followed at NIH from 1988 to 1990 indicated reduced fungal infections in CGD patients receiving IFNγ (48).

Subgroup analysis demonstrated that IFNγ was of benefit regardless of the use of prophylactic antibiotics or the pattern of inheritance of CGD. Young patients, less than 10 years of age, derived particular benefit. No patients developed antibody against IFNγ during the study.

There were minimal toxic reactions in patients receiving IFNγ. Symptoms of toxicity included fever, chills, myalgias, rashes, and mild erythema at the injection site. All of these adverse effects were alleviated by acetaminophen. Adverse effects were more apparent in patients greater than 10 years of age, although even in these older patients the drug was well tolerated. No patients developed antibodies against IFNγ, and the adverse consequences of granuloma formation, which theoretically could have been aggravated (49), did not worsen with its use. Based on these studies IFNγ was licensed by the US Food and Drug Administration for patients with CGD in December 1990—less than 3 years after the initial *in vitro* studies suggesting IFNγ might be useful in CGD. It is now recommended that prophylactic antibiotics and IFNγ be used for treatment of children with CGD. The non-specific enhancement of host defenses by IFNγ suggests it may have broad applicability as a therapeutic agent in compromised hosts. The possible use of IFNγ in many patients with compromised host defenses is intriguing and under evaluation in several laboratories.

REFERENCES

1. Gallin, J.I. and Malech, H.L. (1990) Update on chronic granulomatous disease of childhood: Immunotherapy and potential for gene therapy. *JAMA,* **263,** 1533–1537.

2. Gallin, J.I., Leto, T.L., Rotrosen, R., Kwong, C.H. and Malech, H.L. (1992) Delineation of the phagocyte NADPH oxidase through studies of chronic granulomatous diseases of childhood. *Curr. Opinion Immunol.,* **4,** 53–56.

3. Roos, R. (1993) Molecular basis of chronic granulomatous disease. Chapter 15, this volume.

4. Chin, T.W., Stiehm, E.R., Falloon, J. and Gallin, J.I. (1987) Corticosteroids in the treatment of obstructive lesions of chronic granulomatous disease. *J. Pediatr.,* **111,** 349–352.

5. Margolis, D.H., Melnick, D.A., Alling, D.W. and Gallin, J.I. (1990) Trimethoprim–sulfamethoxazole prophylaxis in the management of chronic granulomatous disease. *J. Infect. Dis.,* **162,** 723–726.

6. Petska, S., Langer, J.A., Zoon, K.C. and Samuel, C.E. (1987) Interferons and their actions. *Annu. Rev. Biochem.,* **56,** 727–777.

7. Sheehan, K.C. and Schreiber, R.D. (1992) The synergy and antagonism of interferon-γ and TNF. In Beutler, B. (ed.) *Tumor Necrosis Factors: The Molecules and their Emerging Role in Medicine.* Raven Press, New York, pp. 145–178.

8. Nathan, C. (1992) Interferon and inflammation. In Gallin, J.I., Goldstein, I.M. and Snyderman, R. (eds) *Inflammation: Basic Principles and Clinical Correlates* (2nd edn). Raven Press, New York, pp. 265–290.

9. Gray, P.W., Leung, D.W., Pennica, D. *et al.* (1982) Expression of human immune interferon cDNA in *E. coli* and monkey cells. *Nature,* **295,** 503–508.

10. Gray, P.W. and Goeddel, D.V. (1982) Structure of the human immune interferon gene. *Nature,* **298,** 859–863.

11. Gray, P.W. and Goeddel, D.V. (1983) Cloning and expression of murine immune interferon cDNA. *Proc. Nat. Acad. Sci. USA,* **80,** 5842–5846.

12. Trinchieri, G., Matsumoto-Kobayashi, M., Clark, S.V., London, L. and Perussia, B. (1984) Response of resting human peripheral blood natural killer cells to interleukin 2. *J. Exp. Med.,* **160,** 1147–1169.

13. Trent, J.M., Olson, S. and Lawn, R.M. (1982) Chromosomal localization of human leukocyte, fibroblast, and immune interferon genes by means of in situ hybridization. *Proc. Nat. Acad. Sci. USA,* **79,** 7809–7813.

14. Naylor, S.L., Sakaguchi, A.Y., Shows, T.B., Law, M.L., Goeddel, D.V. and Gray, P.W. (1983) Human immune interferon gene is located on chromosome 12. *J. Exp. Med.,* **157,** 1020–1027.

15. Kelker, H.C., Yip, Y.K., Anderson, P. and Vilcek, J. (1983) Effects of glycosidase treatment on the physiochemical properties and biological activity of human interferon-gamma. *J. Biol. Chem.,* **258,** 8010–8013.

16. Rutenfranz, I. and Kirchner, H. (1988) Pharmacokinetics of recombinant murine interferon-gamma in mice. *J. Interferon Res.,* **8,** 573–580.

17. Cantell, K., Schellekens, H., Pyhala, L., Hirvonen, S., Van der Meide, P.H. and DeReus, A. (1986) Pharmacokinetic studies with human and rat interferon-gamma in different species. *J. Interferon Res.,* **6,** 671–675.

18. Ealick, S.E., Cook, W.J., Vijay-Kumar, S. *et al.* (1991) Three-dimensional structure of recombinant human interferon-gamma. *Science,* **252,** 698–702.

19. Kasahara, T., Hooks, J.J., Dougherty, S.F. and Oppenheim, J.J. (1983) Interleukin 2-mediated immune interferon (IFN-gamma) production by human T cells subsets. *J. Immunol.*, **130**, 1784–1789.
20. Vilcek, J., Henriksen-DeStafano, D., Siegel, D., Klion, A., Robb, R.J. and Le, J. (1985) Regulation of IFN-gamma induction in human peripheral blood cells by exogenous and endogenously produce interleukin 2. *J. Immunol.*, **135**, 1851–1856.
21. Farrar, W.L, Birchenall-Sparks, M.C. and Young, H.B. (1986) Interleukin 2 induction of interferon-gamma mRNA synthesis. *J. Immunol.*, **137**, 3836–3840.
22. Munakata, T., Semba, U., Shibuya, Y., Kuwano, K., Akagi, M. and Arai, S. (1985) Induction of interferon-gamma production by human natural killer cells stimulated by hydrogen peroxide. *J. Immunol.*, **134**, 2449–2455.
23. Johnson, H.M. and Torres, B.A. (1984) Leukotrienes: Positive signals for regulation of gamma-interferon production. *J. Immunol.*, **132**, 413–416.
24. Johnson, H.M., Russell, J.K. and Torres, B.A. (1986) Second messenger role of arachidonic acid and its metabolites in interferon-gamma production. *J. Immunol.*, **137**, 3053–3056.
25. Handa, K., Suzuki, R., Matsui, H., Shimizu, Y. and Kumagai, K. (1983) Natural killer (NK) cells as a responder to interleukin 2 (IL 2). II. IL 2-induced interferon gamma production. *J. Immunol.*, **130**, 988–992.
26. Bancroft, G.J., Schreiber, R.D., Bosma, G.C., Bosma, M.J. and Unanue, E.R. (1987) A T cell-independent mechanism of macrophage activation by interferon-gamma. *J. Immunol.*, **139**, 1104–1107.
27. Bancroft, G.J., Sheehan, K.C., Schreiber, R.D. and Unanue, E.R. (1989) Tumor necrosis factor is involved in the T cell-independent pathway of macrophage activation in scid mice. *J. Immunol.*, **143**, 127–130.
28. Wherry, J.C., Schreiber, R.D. and Unanue, E.R. (1991) Regulation of gamma interferon production by natural killer cells in scid mice: Roles of tumor necrosis factor and bacterial stimuli. *Infect. Immun.*, **59**, 1709–1715.
29. Wherry, J.C., Schreiber, R.D. and Unanue, E.R. (1990) Mechanism of interferon-γ production by natural killer cells in scid mice. *FASEB J.*, **4**, A1701.
30. Basham, T.Y. and Merigan, T.C. (1983) Recombinant interferon-gamma increases HLA-DR synthesis and expression. *J. Immunol.*, **130**, 1492–1494.
31. King, D.P. and Jones, P.P. (1983) Induction of Ia and H-2 antigen on a macrophage cell line by immune interferon. *J. Immunol.*, **131**, 315–318.
32. Basham, T.Y., Nickoloff, B.J., Merigan, T.C. and Morhenn, V.B. (1985) Recombinant gamma interferon differentially regulates class II antigen expression and biosynthesis on cultured normal human keratinocytes. *J. Interferon Res.*, **5**, 23–32.
33. Boss, J.M. and Strominger, J.L. (1986) Regulation of a transfected human class II major histocompatibility complex gene in human fibroblasts. *Proc. Nat. Acad. Sci. USA*, **83**, 9139–9143.
34. Mond, J.J., Carman, J., Sarma, C., Ohara, J. and Finkelman, F.D. (1986) Interferon-gamma suppresses B cell stimulation factor (BSF-1) induction of class II MHC determinants on B cells. *J. Immunol.*, **137**, 3534–3537.
35. Stone-Wolff, D.S., Yip, Y.K., Kelker, H.C. *et al.* (1984) Interrelationships of human interferon-gamma with lymphotoxin and monocyte cytotoxin. *J. Exp. Med.*, **159**, 828–843.
36. Hart, P.H., Whitty, G.A., Piccoli, D.S. and Hamilton, J.A. (1989) Control by IFN-gamma and PGE2 of TNF alpha and IL-1 production by human monocytes. *Immunology*, **66**, 376–383.
37. Green, S.J., Crawford, R.M., Hockmeyer, J.T., Meltzer, M.S. and Nacy, C.A. (1990) *Leishmania major* amastigotes initiate the L-arginine-dependent killing mechanism

in IFN-gamma-stimulated macrophages by induction of tumor necrosis factor-alpha. *J. Immunol.*, **145**, 4920–4927.

38. Erbe, D.V., Collins, J.E., Shen, L., Graziano, R.F. and Fanger, M.W. (1990) The effects of cytokines on the expression and function of Fc receptors for IgG on human myeloid cells. *Mol. Immunol.*, **27**, 57–67.

39. Strunk, R.C., Cole, F.S., Perlmutter, D.H. and Colten, H.R. (1985) Gamma-interferon increases expression of class III complement genes C2 and factor B in human monocytes and in murine fibroblasts transfected with human C2 and factor B genes. *J. Biol. Chem.*, **260**, 15280–15285.

40. Sechler, J.M.G., Malech, H.L., White, C.J. and Gallin, J.I. (1988) Recombinant human interferon-gamma reconstitutes defective phagocyte function in patients with chronic granulomatous disease of childhood. *Proc. Nat. Acad. Sci. USA*, **85**, 4874–4878.

41. Finkelman, F.D., Holmes, J., Katona, I.M. *et al.* (1990) Lymphokine control of in vivo immunoglobin isotype selection. *Annu. Rev. Immunol.*, **8**, 303–333.

42. King, C.L., Gallin, J.I., Malech, H.L., Abramson, S.L. and Nutman, T.B. (1989) Regulation of immunoglobin production in hyperimmunoglobin E recurrent-infection syndrome by interferon-γ. *Proc. Nat. Acad. Sci. USA*, **86**, 10085–10089.

43. Mosmann, T.R. and Coffman, R.L. (1989) TH1 and TH2 cells: Different patterns of lymphokine secretion lead to different functional properties. *Annu. Rev. Immunol.*, **7**, 145–173.

44. Gallin, J.I., Malech, H.L., Melnick, D.A. *et al.* (1991) The International Chronic Granulomatous Disease Cooperative Study Group. A phase III study establishing efficacy of recombinant human interferon gamma for infection prophylaxis in chronic granulomatous disease. *N. Engl. J. Med.*, **324**, 509–516.

45. Ezekowitz, R.A., Dinaur, M.C., Jaffe, H.S., Orkin, S.H. and Newburger, P.E. (1988) Partial correction of the phagocyte defect in patients with X-linked chronic granulomatous disease by subcutaneous interferon gamma. *N. Engl. J. Med.*, **319**, 146–151.

46. Abramson, S.L., Lomax, K.J., Malech, H.L. and Gallin, J.I. (1990) Recombinant human interferon-gamma and interlukin-4 regulate gene expression of several phagocyte oxidase components. *Clin. Res.*, **38**, 236A (Abstract).

47. Rex, J.H., Bennett, J.E., Gallin, J.I., Malech, H.L., DeCarlo, E.S. and Melnick, D.A. (1991) In vivo interferon gamma therapy augments the in vitro ability of chronic granulomatous disease neutrophils to damage *Aspergillus* hyphae. *J. Infect. Dis.*, **163**, 849–852.

48. Gallin, J.I. (1991) Interferon-γ in the management of chronic granulomatous disease. *Rev. Infect. Dis.*, **13**, 973–978.

49. Weinberg, J.B., Hobbs, M.M. and Misukonis, M.A. (1985) Phenotypic characterization of gamma interferon-induced human monocyte polykaryons. *Blood*, **66**, 1241–1246.

Chapter 18

Peripheral Stem Cell Transplantation

ANNE KESSINGER

Internal Medicine Department, University of Nebraska Medical Center, Omaha, Nebraska, USA

Hematopoietic progenitors are a constant subpopulation of the circulating mononuclear cells in the peripheral blood of laboratory animals (1–3). About 20 years ago, they were found in the human circulation as well (4). This discovery was soon followed by studies which compared and contrasted the characteristics of human circulating progenitors with their counterparts in the bone marrow (5). Perhaps the most clinically important characteristic that the two populations of progenitors were found to share is their ability to restore marrow function (6, 7). Thus, after administration of marrow-lethal irradiation and/or high-dose cytotoxic chemotherapy, either bone marrow or peripheral stem cells can be transplanted to provide hematological recovery.

BLOOD AND MARROW STEM CELL COLLECTION

Because hematopoietic progenitors (and presumably pluripotent stem cells) are less abundant in peripheral blood than in bone marrow (8), collecting sufficient numbers for transplantation from peripheral blood is more tedious and time consuming than collecting them from marrow. Collecting bone marrow for transplantation generally can be accomplished in about an hour (9), but collection of peripheral stem cells for transplantation requires approximately three to six apheresis procedures over at least as many days (10). After harvesting an autologous bone marrow product, the cells are cryopreserved and stored, usually in liquid nitrogen, until the time of

New Concepts in Immunodeficiency Diseases. Edited by S. Gupta and C. Griscelli
© 1993 John Wiley & Sons Ltd

reinfusion. The entire cryopreservation process routinely requires several hours to complete. The several peripheral stem cell collections necessary for one patient's transplant must each be cryopreserved and stored daily, resulting in a much more labor-intensive undertaking. Bone marrow is commonly harvested in an operating suite while the patient receives general anesthesia. In contrast, patients who have peripheral stem cells collected avoid the discomfort associated with multiple bone marrow aspirations from the posterior iliac crests and the collections are done without anesthesia in an outpatient setting. Thus there are both advantages and disadvantages to collection of stem cells from either peripheral blood or bone marrow, and neither procedure is clearly preferable to the other.

ADVANTAGES OF AUTOLOGOUS PERIPHERAL STEM CELL TRANSPLANTATION

The demonstrated advantages of autologous peripheral stem cell transplantation as compared with autologous bone marrow transplantation are essentially two. First, peripheral stem cells can be used as an alternative graft product source for patients who are candidates for high-dose (marrow-ablative) therapy and autologous hematopoietic stem cell rescue for underlying malignancies but have bone marrow abnormalities that preclude marrow transplantation. The most common abnormalities of an unfit marrow graft product are hypocellularity and contamination with malignant cells. Hypocellularity in traditional marrow harvest sites can result from prior pelvic irradiation or other therapy for the underlying malignancy. Peripheral stem cells have worked well, providing hematopoietic rescue for patients with hypocellular marrow (11). Lymphoma patients with histopathological evidence of bone marrow metastases at the time of stem cell harvesting who have received high-dose therapy and autologous peripheral stem cell transplant have experienced complete remission and long-term event-free survival (12). In fact, the outcome of these patients is at least as good as that of lymphoma patients with normal bone marrow who have been treated with high-dose therapy and autologous bone marrow transplantation.

The second reason peripheral blood-derived stem cells may be preferable to bone marrow-derived stem cells for autografting is that hematopoietic recovery following transplantation is accelerated for some patients. If the transplanted peripheral stem cells are collected at a time when their numbers are deliberately expanded in the circulation (i.e. mobilized), the recovery of marrow function after autografting occurs approximately a week sooner than if autologous bone marrow or non-mobilized peripheral stem cells are transplanted (13). The most common methods currently used to mobilize stem cells from extravascular sites into the circulation include administration of myelosuppressive chemotherapy (14) and administration of hematopoietic growth factors (15). Unfortunately, not all patients respond to mobilization attempts. Those at greatest risk to fail appear to be patients who have already been treated with multiple courses of combination therapy and those who have bone marrow metastases (16, 17). Successful mobilization is not required to collect peripheral stem cells, and transplanted non-mobilized cells will restore bone marrow function (12). If, however, the transplanted cells are successfully mobilized, marrow function recovers more rapidly (13).

CIRCULATING PLURIPOTENT HEMATOPOIETIC STEM CELLS

While there is general agreement that infused autologous peripheral stem cells will re-establish marrow function that was ablated with high doses of anti-cancer therapy, some doubt exists about the capability of these cells to sustain hematopoiesis. Sustained hematopoiesis requires the presence of pluripotent hematopoietic stem cells, and to date there is no conclusive evidence that such a cell exists in the human circulation. Admittedly, sustained hematopoiesis has been observed following high-dose chemotherapy plus total body irradiation and autologous peripheral stem cell infusion (12). That observation, however, does not prove that pluripotent stem cells were transplanted since there was no means to distinguish the progeny of autologous peripheral stem cells from the progeny of autologous bone marrow stem cells to confirm that the long-term hematopoiesis was a result of transplanted pluripotent peripheral cells. If the human peripheral stem cell population consists solely of committed progenitors incapable of indefinite self-renewal, autologous transplantation of those cells could have restored marrow function long enough to permit recovery of severely damaged resident pluripotent stem cells in the bone marrow. When the transplanted committed progenitors had completed their differentiation to mature blood cells, recovered bone marrow pluripotent cells were able to sustain hematopoiesis.

There are at least four pieces of presumptive evidence to suggest that the human pluripotent hematopoietic stem cell does circulate. First, newer culture assay techniques designed to detect long-term culture-initiating cells (cells more primitive than CFU-GM progenitors) have verified the presence of these cells in the human circulation (18). Second, as mentioned above, long-term hematopoiesis has resulted from autologous peripheral stem cell transplantation following high-dose therapy and total body irradiation (12), and reports of engraftment followed by aplasia in patients who have received peripheral stem cell transplantation are essentially non-existent. Third, pluripotent hematopoietic stem cells are known to circulate in murine (19) and canine (20, 21) peripheral blood because transplanted allogenic peripheral stem cells from a donor of different sex than the recipient have successfully restored long-term marrow function following marrow-ablative irradiation that was demonstrated to be of donor origin. Fourth, although the situation is not directly comparable to human peripheral stem cells, pluripotent stem cells are known to circulate in human cord blood. This was first proved when the cord blood from a newborn female was transplanted to her HLA-identical male sibling who had been treated for Fanconi's anemia with marrow-ablative radio/chemotherapy (22). After the transplant, cytogenetic studies of aspirated bone marrow and peripheral blood of the recipient demonstrated a 46,XX chromosomal complement. Marrow recovery for this patient has been sustained with no evidence of male cells, demonstrating that pluripotent stem cells were indeed transplanted.

At least three different strategies could be used to prove the pluripotent stem cell circulates in humans. First, conclusive proof could be provided if an established assay for the human pluripotent stem cell were available. Second, performance of a successful human allogenic peripheral stem cell transplant where donor progeny could be distinguished from the recipient would also provide sufficient evidence. One such attempt has been reported (23). A patient with acute lymphocytic leukemia in third complete remission was advised to consider an allogeneic bone marrow transplant. An HLA-identical sibling was identified. The potential donor preferred not to have his bone marrow harvested, but he was a willing peripheral stem cell donor. A chromosomal marker present in the donor was lacking in the recipient, providing a means to identify the origin of subsequent recipient hematopoiesis. Since the majority of circulating mononuclear cells are T lymphocytes (24), the apheresis products were T cell depleted to the number that would ordinarily be found in a routine allogeneic bone marrow product. The depletion was done (25) in an attempt to reduce any increased risk of developing graft-versus-host disease (GVHD) above the risk inherent in an allogeneic bone marrow transplant. Following high-dose radio/chemotherapy, the cryopreserved allogeneic cells were thawed and infused. Reappearance of circulating granulocytes occurred 8 days after transplantation, and by the seventh day 1.1×10^9 granulocytes per liter were present. Only donor hematopoietic cells were identified in the blood or the bone marrow after the transplant. Because the patient died of fungal sepsis 32 days after transplant, sustained hematopoiesis of donor origin could not be verified.

A third method of confirming the presence of pluripotent hematopoietic stem cells in the human circulation would make use of the now available technique of retroviral marking (26). A viral genetic marker could be inserted in autologous cells collected from peripheral blood prior to transplantation. If pluripotent stem cells were present and were marked, the inserted gene should be detectable indefinitely in the recovered hematopoietic cells, but if only committed progenitors were marked the patient's hematopoietic cells would, over time, revert to an unmarked status.

CIRCULATING ALLOGENEIC CELLS AND IMMUNODEFICIENCY DISORDERS

Allogeneic bone marrow transplantation is the therapy of choice for severe combined immunodeficiency disease (SCID) (27). Allogeneic peripheral stem cell transplants, administered with an intent to restore all hematopoietic lineages of the patient, as yet have not been used because human hematopoietic stem cells have not been definitively identified in the circulation. However, allogeneic peripheral blood mononuclear cells have been used as a therapy for SCID.

In 1980, the first report describing immunoreconstitution of a patient with SCID after infusion of allogeneic blood-derived leukocytes appeared in the literature (28). The patient was a 10-month-old male whose only relative suitable to serve as an HLA-identical allogeneic donor was his father. The father, for personal reasons, refused to serve as a bone marrow donor, but consented to a leukapheresis procedure. The patient received 5×10^8 mononuclear cells per kilogram body weight intravenously without prior marrow-ablative therapy. Methotrexate was administered to the patient in an effort to prevent GVHD. No GVHD was encountered, with the possible exception of a mild skin rash that resolved without therapy. Improvement of both cellular and humoral immune functions was documented soon after the allogeneic infusion, but no evidence of engraftment of erythropoietic or granulocytic precursors in the bone marrow was found. The improvement in immune function resulted in an improved clinical course with disappearance of chronic infections that plagued the child prior to the leukocyte infusion. He continued free of significant illnesses for the 12-month follow-up period described in the report.

In 1986, a second case was reported (29). This patient was a 7-month-old female with SCID whose 64-year-old grandfather was the only suitable related HLA-identical potential donor she had. He refused to donate bone marrow but consented to donate circulating mononuclear cells, which were collected with a single apheresis procedure. No marrow-ablative therapy was administered prior to the leukocyte infusion and she received 18.8×10^8 mononuclear cells per kilogram body weight intravenously. No attempt to prevent GVHD was made in this instance, and approximately 1 month later she developed neutropenia and elevated liver function studies. A liver biopsy confirmed GVHD. Treatment with a short course of prednisone eliminated the symptoms. For the 5 years she was followed after the infusion, she remained free of significant infections. Her immune function measured by a variety of parameters became normal, but only her peripheral blood lymphocytes were of the XY (donor) karyotype. Granulocyte antigens were all of recipient type (XX) and spontaneously dividing bone marrow cells were also exclusively XX.

These two case reports contain some interesting points to consider. Although the first patient received at least one log fewer mononuclear cells than are present in the graft products of most autologous non-mobilized peripheral stem cell transplants, the second patient received more blood-derived mononuclear cells than are usually infused to restore tri-lineage hematopoiesis in the bone marrow (12). Yet neither of these patients had evidence of bone marrow engraftment. Only circulating lymphocytes were found to be of donor origin, and these persisted for as long as 54 months (the longest follow-up reported) after the infusion. Perhaps the lack of marrow-suppressive therapy prior to either infusion was an important factor in this result. Since the marrow space was not "emptied" with myeloablative therapy, the infused mononuclear cells (which presumably contained hematopoietic progenitors) may have been presented with an environment that was unsuitable for the establishment of proliferation. When immunodeficient patients receive marrow-toxic therapy prior to allogeneic bone marrow transplantation, sustained engraftment with donor cells occurs in the bone marrow (30).

Since bone marrow engraftment did not occur in the two patients who received allogeneic peripheral blood mononuclear cells, a different mechanism was responsible for the observed immunological reconstitution. Some have suggested that proliferation of long-lived peripheral blood lymphocytes was responsible (29)—a mechanism which may also explain the immune reconstitution that was observed in other SCID patients who received unfractionated (i.e. lymphocyte-replete) allogeneic bone marrow transplants but failed to exhibit evidence of bone marrow engraftment (31). Patients with immunodeficiency diseases who received either marrow-ablative therapy prior to allogeneic bone marrow transplant or fractionated (T cell-depleted) allogeneic bone marrow transplants have demonstrated immune reconstitution as well as bone marrow engraftment. These patients likely recovered immune function via a second mechanism: engraftment of lymphopoietic stem cells.

The lack of development of significant GVHD in the two patients who received peripheral blood leukocytes is intriguing. GVHD has been reported in a limited number of patients with solid tumors and (more often) hematological malignancies and in patients with immunodeficient states following transfusion of normal allogeneic blood products (32). Once established, this disease is resistant to therapy and is usually fatal. The lymphocytes in just one unit of packed red blood cells have been sufficient to cause the disease (33). Recently fatal transfusion-related GVHD also has been reported in immunocompetent patients who received normal blood products from relatives with similar HLA types (34). However, the two patients with SCID who received HLA-identical immunocompetent T lymphocytes from related donors developed either no GVHD or mild GVHD that was easily managed with minimal therapy. Certainly not every immunodeficient patient develops GVHD following transfusion of allogeneic blood products; no patient with AIDS has yet developed transfusion-related GVHD. Because the failure of the two patients to develop severe transfusion-related GVHD is not understood, GVHD remains an issue when considering allogeneic HLA-matched leukocyte infusions to treat patients with SCID. Perhaps, for the present, this approach should be reserved for patients with no other therapeutic option.

REFERENCES

1. Goodman, J.W. and Hodgson, G.S. (1962) Evidence for stem cells in the peripheral blood of mice. *Blood*, **19**, 702–715.
2. Cavins, J.A., Scheer, S.C., Thomas, E.D. and Feerebee, J.W. (1964) The recovery of lethally irradiated dogs given infusions of autologous leukocytes preserved at 80°C. *Blood*, **23**, 38–42.
3. Storb, R., Graham, R.C., Epstein, R.B., Sale, G.E. and Thomas, E.D. (1977) Demonstration of hemopoietic stem cells in the peripheral blood of baboons by cross circulation. *Blood*, **50**, 537–547.
4. McCredie, K.B., Hersh, E.M. and Freireich, E.J. (1971) Cells capable of colony formation in the peripheral blood of man. *Science*, **171**, 293–294.
5. Verma, D.S., Spitzer, G., Zander, A.R., Fisher, R., McCredie, K.B. and Dicke, K. (1980) The myeloid progenitor cell: A parallel study of subpopulations in human marrow and peripheral blood. *Exp. Hematol.*, **8**, 32–43.
6. Korbling, M., Dorken, B., Ho, A.D., Pezzutto, A., Hunstein, W. and Fliedner, T.M. (1986) Autologous transplantation of blood-derived hemopoietic stem cells after myeloablative therapy in a patient with Burkitt's lymphoma. *Blood*, **67**, 529–532.
7. Appelbaum, F.R., Sullivan, K.M., Buckner, C.D., Clift, R.A., Deeg, H.J., Fefer, A., Hill, R., Mortimer, J., Nieman, P.E., Sanders, J.E., Singer, J., Stewart, P., Storb, R. and Thomas, E.D. (1987) Treatment of malignant lymphoma in 100 patients with chemotherapy, total body irradiation, and marrow transplantation. *J. Clin. Oncol.*, **5**, 1340–1347.
8. McCarthy, D.M. and Goldman, J.M. (1984) Transfusion of circulating stem cells. *CRC Crit. Rev. Clin. Lab. Sci.*, **20**, 1–24.
9. Kessinger, A. and Armitage, J.O. (1987) Harvesting marrow for autologous transplantation from patients with malignancies. *Bone Marrow Transplant.*, **2**, 15–18.
10. Lasky, L.C., Hurd, D.D., Smith, J.A. and Haake, R. (1989) Peripheral blood stem cell collection and use in Hodgkin's disease: Comparison with marrow in autologous transplantation. *Transfusion*, **29**, 323–327.
11. Korbling, M., Holle, R., Haas, R., Knaouf, W., Dorken, B., Ho, A.D., Kuse, R., Pralle, H., Fliedner, T.M. and Hunstein, W. (1990) Autologous blood stem-cell transplantation in patients with advanced Hodgkin's disease and prior radiation to the pelvic site. *J. Clin. Oncol.*, **8**, 978–985.
12. Kessinger, A., Vose, J.M., Bierman, P.J. and Armitage, J.O. (1991) High dose therapy and autologous peripheral stem cell transplantation for patients with bone marrow metastases and relapsed lymphoma: An alternative to bone marrow purging. *Exp. Hematol.*, **19**, 1013–1016.
13. Kessinger, A. and Armitage, J.O. (1991) The evolving role of peripheral stem cell transplantation following high-dose therapy for malignancies. *Blood*, **77**, 211–213.

14. To, L.B., Shepperd, K.M., Haylock, D.N., Dyson, P.G., Charles, P., Thorp, D.L., Dale, B.M., Dart, G.W., Roberts, M.M., Sage, R.E. and Juttner, C.A. (1990) Single high doses of cyclophosphamide enable the collection of high numbers of hemopoietic stem cells from the peripheral blood. *Exp. Hematol.*, **18**, 442–447.

15. Haas, R., Ho., A.D., Bredthauer, U., Cayeux, S., Egerer, G., Knouf, W. and Hunstein, W. (1990) Successful autologous transplantation of blood stem cells mobilized with recombinant human granulocyte–macrophage colony-stimulating factor. *Exp. Hematol.*, **18**, 94–98.

16. Korbling, M. and Martin, H. (1988) Transplantation of hemapheresis-derived hemopoietic stem cells: A new concept in the treatment of patients with malignant lymphohemopoietic disorders. *Plasma Ther. Transfus. Technol.*, **9**, 119–132.

17. Cantin, G., Marchand-Laroche, D., Bouchard, M.M. and Leblond, P.F. (1989) Blood-derived stem cell collection in acute nonlymphoblastic leukemia: Predictive factors for a good yield. *Exp. Hematol.*, **17**, 991–996.

18. Dooley, D.C. and Law, P. (1992) Detection and quantitation of long-term culture-initiating cells in normal human peripheral blood. *Exp. Hematol.*, **20**, 156–160.

19. Goodman, J.W. and Hodgson, G.S. (1962) Evidence of stem cells in the peripheral blood of mice. *Blood*, **19**, 702–714.

20. Korbling, M., Fliedner, T.M., Calvo, W., Ross, W.M., Nothdurft, W. and Steinbach, I. (1979) Albumin density gradient purification of canine hemopoietic blood stem cells (HBSC): Long-term allogeneic engraftment without GVH-reaction. *Exp. Hematol.*, **7**, 277–288.

21. Gerhartz, H.H., Nothdurft, W., Carbonell, F. and Fliedner, T.M. (1985) Allogeneic transplantation of blood stem cells concentrated by density gradients. *Exp. Hematol.*, **13**, 136–142.

22. Gluckman, E., Broxmeyer, H.E., Auerbach, A.D., Friedman, H.S., Douglas, G.W., Deveragie, A., Esperou, H., Thierry, D., Socie, G., Lehn, P., Cooper, S., English, D., Kurtzberg, J., Bard, J. and Boyse, E.A. (1989) Hematopoietic reconstitution in a patient with Fanconi's anemia by means of umbilical-cord blood from an HLA-identical sibling. *N. Engl. J. Med.*, **321**, 1174–1178.

23. Kessinger, A., Smith, D.M., Strandjord, S.E., Landmark, J.D., Dooley, D.C., Law, P., Coccia, P.F., Warkentin, P.I., Weisenburger, D.D. and Armitage, J.O. (1989) Allogeneic transplantation of blood-derived, T cell-depleted hemopoietic stem cells after myeloablative treatment in a patient with acute lymphoblastic leukemia. *Bone Marrow Transplant.*, **4**, 643–646.

24. Ohta, Y., Fujiwara, K., Nishi, T. and Oka, H. (1986) Normal values of peripheral lymphocytes and T cell subsets at a fixed time of day: A flow cytometric analysis with monoclonal antibodies in 210 healthy adults. *Clin. Exp. Immunol.*, **64**, 146–149.

25. Dooley, D.C., Law, P. and Alsop, P. (1987) A new density-gradient for the separation of large quantities of rosette-positive and rosette-negative cells. *Exp. Hematol.*, **15**, 296–303.

26. Bayever, E., Haines, K., Duprey, S., Rappaport, E., Douglas, S.D. and Surrey, S. (1988) Neomycin resistance of human bone marrow in long-term culture following retroviral gene transfer. *Exp. Cell Res.*, **179**, 168–180.

27. Bortin, M.M. and Rimm, A.A. (1977) Severe combined immunodeficiency disease: Characterization of the disease and results of transplantation. *JAMA*, **238**, 591–600.

28. Rich, K.C., Richman, C.M., Mejias, E. and Daddona, P. (1980) Immunoreconstitution by peripheral blood leukocytes in adenosine deaminase-deficient severe combined immunodeficiency. *J. Clin. Invest.*, **66**, 389–395.

29. Polmar, S.H., Schacter, B.Z. and Sorensen, R.U. (1986) Long-term immunological reconstitution by peripheral blood leucocytes in severe combined immune deficiency disease: Implications for the role of mature lymphocytes in histocompatible bone marrow transplantation. *Clin. Exp. Immunol.*, **64**, 518–525.
30. O'Reilly, R.J., Kapoor, N., Kirkpatrick, D., Cunningham-Rundels, S., Pollack, M.S., Dupont, B., Hodes, M.Z., Good, R.A. and Reisner, Y. (1983) Transplantation for severe combined immunodeficiency using histoincompatible parental marrow fractionated by soybean agglutinin and sheep red blood cells: Experience in six consecutive cases. *Transplant. Proc.*, **15**, 1431–1435.
31. Copenhagen Study Group of Immunodeficiencies (1973) Bone marrow transplantation from an HLA non-identical but mixed lymphocyte culture identical donor. *Lancet*, **ii**, 1146–1149.
32. Greenbaum, B.H. (1991) Transfusion-associated graft-versus-host disease: Historical perspectives, incidence, and current use of irradiated blood products. *J. Clin. Oncol.*, **9**, 1889–1902.
33. Hathaway, W.E., Filginiti, V.A., Pierce, C.W., Githens, J.H., Pearlman, D.S., Muschenheim, F. and Klempe, H. (1967) Graft-vs-host reaction following a single blood transfusion. *JAMA*, **201**, 1015–1020.
34. Thaler, M., Shamiss, A., Orgad, S., Huszar, M., Nussinovitch, N., Meisel, S., Gazit, E., Lavee, J. and Smolinsky, A. (1989) The role of blood from HLA-homozygous donors in fatal transfusion-associated graft-versus-host disease after open-heart surgery. *N. Engl. J. Med.*, **321**, 25–33.

Chapter 19

Interleukin 2 Deficiency in Primary Immunodeficiency: Exploration of Recombinant Interleukin 2 as a Potential *In Vivo* Treatment

CHARLOTTE CUNNINGHAM-RUNDLES

Departments of Medicine and Pediatrics, Mount Sinai Medical Center, New York, USA

Defects in the production of interleukin 2 (IL-2) or defective responsiveness to IL-2 have been described in a few animal model systems. In these cases, IL-2 administration can correct the resulting immunological defects *in vitro* and *in vivo*. Deficient IL-2 production has also been described in human systems. In this chapter, the evidence for IL-2 deficiency in congenital immunodeficiency disease is examined, and the potential role of recombinant IL-2 (r-IL-2) or a new compound, polyethylene glycol conjugated r-IL-2 (PEG–IL-2), in the treatment of these diseases is explored.

IL-2 BIOLOGICAL ACTIVITIES

IL-2, first described by Morgan and Ruscetti in 1976 (1), is a glycoprotein produced by activated helper T lymphocytes. The process of T cell activation can be accomplished by a variety of agents, including mitogens, antigens, IL-1 or antibodies to the T cell receptor. *In vitro*, IL-2 is capable of maintaining long-term the growth of T cells (giving rise to its first name, T cell growth factor). IL-2 mediates a large number of immunological functions, both *in vitro*

New Concepts in Immunodeficiency Diseases. Edited by S. Gupta and C. Griscelli
© 1993 John Wiley & Sons Ltd

and *in vivo*, and is understood as essential in the generation of immune responses. The molecular events leading to the production of IL-2 by activated T cells have become more clear in the past few years. T cell activation triggers a cascade of biochemical reactions, including an increase in intracellular calcium concentrations, inositol triphosphate, and the activation of protein kinase C; these events initiate transcription of IL-2 and IL-2 receptor genes. Stimulated T cells become altered in cell surface morphology, and functional receptors for IL-2 appear on the surface of activated T cells; these cells can divide, proliferate, and secrete IL-2. Secreted IL-2 binds to IL-2 receptors, and by still unknown biochemical processes results in the transduction of a proliferative signal. Peak IL-2 concentrations occur about 16 hours after stimulation and subsequently decline, presumably due to consumption of IL-2 by proliferating cells; additionally the increasing development of T suppressor cells after 24 hours inhibits further IL-2 production (1–4).

IL-2 was first described as promoting growth and differentiation of helper/inducer T cells (3, 4), suppressor/cytotoxic T cells (5), natural killer (NK) cells (6), and lymphokine-activated killer cells (7). However, a number of studies have documented that IL-2 can act directly on activated B cells (8–11). For example, IL-2 can up-regulate B cell CD23, an early cell surface marker of B cell activation (12), and can induce B cell responsiveness to IL-6 (13). The essential role of IL-2 in immunoglobulin (Ig) secretion is also revealed by the fact that monoclonal antibodies to either the IL-2 receptor (14) or IL-2 itself (15) can inhibit the generation of Ig-secreting cells. Antibody responses to influenza virus by T cell-depleted human B cells can be completely restored by the addition of exogenous human r-IL-2 (16). Furthermore, in the absence of IL-2, *Streptococcus aureus* Cowan I strain (SAC)-activated B cells do not differentiate into Ig-secreting cells, even if other lymphokines are present (17). The general conclusion has been that IL-2 acts upon activated B cells in the absence of T cells, probably by binding to IL-2 receptors present on B cells (18, 19). However, there is also evidence that IL-2 can initiate B cell differentiation even in the absence of *in vitro* preactivation, an activity which would be unrelated to IL-2 receptors (20). In support of this, Ralph *et al.* have demonstrated that IL-2 induces IgM secretion in a human lymphoblastoid cell line (SKW-6-4) which lacks IL-2 receptors (21).

In addition to these direct actions on B cells, IL-2 causes T cells to secrete additional factors which influence B cell growth and differentiation at crucial steps in the maturational process. For example, IL-2-stimulated T cells produce cytokines which support B cell growth and proliferation such as IL-4, tumor necrosis factor α (TNFα), and high and low-molecular-weight B cell growth factors (BCGF). IL-2-stimulated T cells also produce interferon γ (IFNγ), IL-4, IL-5, IL-6, and B cell differentiation factors (BCDF)—cytokines which support Ig secretion (22–26). These cytokines have differential effects upon activated B cells; for example, IL-6 has minimal effects on human B cell proliferation, but enhances Ig secretion (26), while IL-2 supports both pro-liferation and differentiation (8–10). Cytokines also play an important role in directing the isotype and IgG subclass of the secreted Ig. IL-4, for example, promotes IgE secretion by enhancing the accessibility of the ε switch region to the common recombinase (27), while IFNγ serves as an antagonist to IgE synthesis (28).

RECOMBINANT IL-2 IN CLINICAL TRIALS

In the early 1980s, the purification of IL-2 and subsequent cloning of the IL-2 gene resulted in the availability of large amounts of r-IL-2 for both laboratory and clinical studies (29–32). Important for both kinds of research, the develop-ment of bioassays for IL-2 permitted precise quantitation of IL-2 in biological fluids (32, 33). In clinical medicine the therapeutic potentials of IL-2 have been most extensively investigated in treatment of neoplasms, where the major intent has been to boost cytotoxicity to tumor cells. Significant responses have been seen in renal cell carcinoma and melanoma. Although large doses of IL-2 given intravenously result in high serum levels of IL-2, the initial half-life ($t_{1/2}$ α) is 7–13 minutes and the terminal half-life ($t_{1/2}$ β) is 70–85 minutes, largely due to renal clearance (34–37). Partly as a result of the short half-life, high doses and frequent intravenous treatments for several weeks appear to be needed to produce tumor regression (34–37). Of uncertain biological import-ance is the fact that patients who have been treated with r-IL-2 may develop serum antibodies to this lymphokine. The immunogenicity of IL-2 is believed to be due to the differences between the *Escherichia coli*-produced r-IL-2 and the native form of IL-2. Native IL-2 is glycosylated and readily water soluble; since the recombinant form is not glycosylated and dissolves less well in aqueous solutions, it is possible that the resulting aggregates of r-IL-2 serve to immunize the recipient. Antibodies to IL-2 could conceivably interfere with the effectiveness of treatment (37). When IL-2 is administered either sub-cutaneously, intramuscularly, or intraperitoneally, extended half-lives can be achieved, but r-IL-2 given by these routes appears to be even more capable of serving as an immunogen (38, 39).

Recently, a PEG-conjugated form of IL-2 has been developed (40–42). PEG-conjugated r-IL-2 has an increased molecular weight due to the attach-ment of PEG molecules of defined molecular sizes. The PEG moieties are bound covalently by a succinic anhydride reaction involving one or more lysine residues on the r-IL-2 molecule (Figure 19.1) (40). The "pegylation" procedure increases the effective molecular weight, reduces renal clearance and extends the biological half-life of the r-IL-2 molecule. For example, if two molecules of PEG-5000 are bonded to r-IL-2, the effective molecular size is increased to 75 000 Da and the half-life is extended from 3 to 61 minutes (Table 19.1) (41). As has been shown for other PEG-conjugated pharmacological agents (adenosine deaminase (43), asparaginase (44) and urease (45)), the PEG conjugation procedure extends the half-life of the parent molecule at least 20-fold, and yet generally preserves the spectrum of bio-activities of the native form. For example, PEG–IL-2 has the same ability as r-IL-2 to support the growth of the IL-2-dependent murine cytotoxic T cell line CTLL (Figure 19.2). PEG–IL-2 and IL-2 can similarly induce lysis of the erythroblast target K562 in NK cell assays (Table 19.2a) and induce the function of lymphokine-activated killer cells (Table 19.2b). Since PEG–IL-2 has an extended half-life as compared to r-IL-2, daily administration may not be needed; in some studies, patients have been treated once or twice a week, avoiding the need for an indwelling catheter. PEG–IL-2 has been well tolerated in phase I trials at doses under 4 million IU/m^2 given intra-muscularly once a week (46). In this study, 66 patients with cancer were given escalating doses (0.18×10^6 to 23.1×10^6 IU/m^2 each week). At the high-er doses, the pattern of toxicity was found to be quite similar to that of r-IL-2; however, the half-life of PEG–IL-2 was 10 to 20-fold longer. The clearance of PEG–IL-2 from serum was described as bi-exponential, with a fast compo-nent half-life ($t_{1/2} \alpha$) of 220 minutes and a slow component half-life ($t_{1/2} \beta$) of 942 minutes (46).

Covalent attachment of PEG to r-IL-2 provides an additional advant-ageous feature; r-IL-2 becomes quite soluble in aqueous solutions and does not aggregate. Perhaps for this reason it is rendered very much less immunogenic than native r-IL-2 (42). For example, none of the 66 patients in

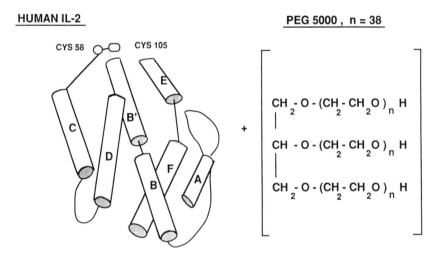

Figure 19.1. Polyethylene glycol conjugated human IL-2 has a molecular structure including seven regions of helical structure and an important cystine bridge (Cys 58–Cys 105). Molecules of polyethylene glycol are covalently bound to r-IL-2, with attachment at available lysine residues on this lymphokine

Table 19.1 PEG modification of r-IL-2: pharmacological changes

r-IL-2 species	No. PEG/ r-IL-2	Half-life α (min)	β	C1[b] (ml/min)	V[c] (ml/kg)	Effective size of PEG-IL-2 (kDa)
r-IL-2	0	3	44	1.15	100	19.5
PEG (350)	5	6	57	0.97	89	21
PEG (4 000)	1	5	44	0.60	93	40
PEG (4 000)	2	14	162	0.23	95	66
PEG (5 000)	2	21	238	0.14	88	72
PEG (10 000)	1	12	263	0.12	80	103
PEG (4 000)	3	32	292	0.12	86	104
PEG (5 000)	4–5	61	370	0.05	60	208
PEG (20 000)	2	32	256	0.11	91	326

[a]Data from Knauf *et al.* (41).
[b]Systemic clearance.
[c]Volume of distribution at steady state.

the phase I trial described above developed detectable IgG antibodies to PEG–IL-2. Currently PEG–IL-2 is being tested in a few clinical trials in adults with HIV infection as a means to restore skin test reactivity (as previously found for subcutaneously delivered r-IL-2) (47, 48) and in congenital immunodeficiency diseases in which IL-2 deficiency has been established.

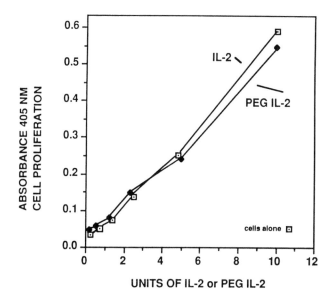

Figure 19.2. The biological effects of r-IL-2 or PEG–IL-2 are compared by their ability to support growth of the murine T cell line, CTLL, using an ELISA assay to measure growth (115)

Table 19.2   Comparisons of r-IL-2 and PEG–IL-2

(a) Activation of cytotoxic cells after 1-day incubation of peripheral blood lymphocytes with r-IL-2 or PEG–r-IL-2[a]

Ratio of effector cells to target cells (K562)	Specific lysis (%)[b]				
		r-IL-2		PEG–r-IL-2[c]	
	0 U/ml	800 U/ml	80 U/ml	800 U/ml	80 U/ml
50:1	0	29.4 ± 1.7	22.8 ± 0.8	25.9 ± 2.6	15.0 ± 0.9
17:1	0	16.7 ± 1.0	13.2 ± 0.4	13.3 ± 0.8	6.7 ± 0.6
6:1	0	0	0	0	0

(b) Lymphokine-activated killer cells after 5-day incubation of peripheral blood lymphocytes with r-IL-2 or PEG–r-IL-2[a,b]

Ratio of effector cells to target cells (Hs695T)	Specific lysis (%)[b]		
		r-IL-2	PEG–r-IL-2
	0 U/ml	100 U/ml	100 U/ml[c]
50:1	0	35.1 ± 3.4	38.4 ± 3.8
17:1	0	23.1 ± 2.9	28.3 ± 5.4
6:1	0	9.7 ± 5.1	13.3 ± 1.8

[a]Data are from Katre *et al.* (40).
[b]Results are mean ± SEM.
[c]Ten moles of PEG ester per mole of r-IL-2 in reaction mixture (36).

DEFICIENT LYMPHOKINE SECRETION IN PRIMARY IMMUNODEFICIENCY

Severe Combined Immunodeficiency

Severe combined immunodeficiency (SCID) is actually a spectrum of syndromes including X-linked and autosomal forms, which has as its main
features failure to thrive, chronic diarrhea, and recurrent, severe bacterial,
viral, and fungal infections (49). In spite of this clinical uniformity, the underlying molecular defects are quite heterogeneous, and the nature of the
specific defects varies from patient to patient. About 40–50% who have the
autosomal recessive form of SCID have a deficiency of adenosine deaminase, or more rarely, a deficiency of nucleoside phosphorylase (50, 51).
In other forms, still uncharacterized at the molecular level, various kinds of
severe T cell deficiency exist, including failure of maturation, activation and
functional differentiation of T cells (52–59). Some infants with SCID appear
to have more normal T cell precursors, but these cells are arrested at various
stages of maturation. Others have phenotypically mature normal T cells, but

lack responses to IL-1, or have abnormal signal transduction, or genetic defects in the expression of class I or II histocompatibility antigens (58–60).

In a few cases of SCID, deficient IL-2 mRNA and resulting deficient secretion of IL-2, or IL-2 unresponsiveness have been documented (53, 54, 61–65). In some of these cases, the addition of IL-2 *in vitro* (and as described below, *in vivo*) was found to rectify the T cell deficiency state, and permit *in vitro* lymphocyte proliferation to mitogens and other stimulators. Partial reconstitution *in vitro* by r-IL-2 has also been described; Rijkers *et al.* studied an 8-year-old child who had severe T cell defects and an oligoclonal expansion of CD8-bearing cells (62). In this case IL-2 *in vitro* could normalize the phorbol-myristate acetate (PMA)/ionomycin proliferative response but not the proliferative response to concanavalin A (Con A). Since PMA and ionomycin bypass T cell receptor-mediated transmembrane signaling, the sustained proliferative abnormality in response to Con A was interpreted as a T cell receptor signaling defect.

Because of the *in vitro* evidence that r-IL-2 could restore T cell immunity in some cases of SCID, at least six patients with a SCID phenotype have been treated parenterally with r-IL-2 in the past 3 years (61, 63–66). In five of six cases, the response of lymphocytes to mitogen activation was improved; in a sixth patient, there was a normalization of T cell numbers. These patients had experienced multiple episodes of bacterial or fungal infections requiring hospitalization; these ailments had been accompanied by weight loss or low weight gain requiring total parenteral nutrition. During IL-2 therapy, many of the infections resolved, parenteral feeding could be stopped, and weight gain was observed. In one well-studied case, a female infant of age 1 was maintained for some months on 30 000 units of r-IL-2 per kilogram body weight per day given intravenously 3 days a week. Clinical improvement occurred and her percentage of peripheral T cells and proliferative responses to mitogens increased to normal (63). In a second case, daily r-IL-2 (40 000 units/kg) was given to an infant with T cell lymphocytosis, impaired proliferative responses to mitogens and antigens, failure of IL-2 production, low NK cell number and function and profound hypogammaglobulinemia. After 1 month severe pyoderma gangrenosum resolved, and after 2 months lymphocyte proliferation responses normalized (63).

The PEG-IL-2 form of r-IL-2 has also been given to several patients with unclassified severe T cell defects. A 6-year-old girl with systemic herpes zoster who had low T cell numbers and no T cell proliferation to mitogens or herpes zoster was given PEG–IL-2 at a dose of 250 000 U/m^2 per week. Previously r-IL-2 had been found to correct the proliferative defect *in vitro*. The child was treated intravenously for some months with PEG–IL-2, with restoration of T cell proliferation and clinical improvement (65).

While T cell responses have been clearly improved in infants and children with SCID treated with IL-2, the effects of this lymphokine on the B cells in these cases have been little studied. Whether or not *de novo* antibody production can be stimulated by IL-2 treatment is unclear.

Nezelof's Syndrome

A second congenital immunodeficiency disease in which there may be IL-2 deficiency due to abnormal T cell maturation, is Nezelof's syndrome. This syndrome, which is similar to SCID, represents a collection of severe T cell defects which may be coupled with abnormal B cell function (67, 68). The first report defined the syndrome as a T cell deficiency disease with little or no abnormality of γ-globulin levels (67). However, despite normal or even increased levels of Igs, antibody synthesis is impaired. In contrast to SCID, Nezelof's syndrome is a somewhat less severe immune defect, which may be compatible with a later presentation and potentially better survival. Nonetheless, probably the best treatment for Nezelof's syndrome is bone marrow transplantation.

Several patients with Nezelof's syndrome have been studied from the point of view of lymphokine deficiency (69, 70). Two males were described in one study who had reduced numbers of circulating T cells, minimal to absent lymphocyte proliferation, and poor antibody production (69). In both cases, deficient IL-2 production was documented, with improved *in vitro* proliferation with additions of exogenous IL-2. One child was treated very briefly with small doses of subcutaneously administered IL-2 but he died of extensive pulmonary aspergillosis (subsequently the possibility that this child had undiagnosed HIV infection was raised) (69). While the other child also had deficient IL-2 production *in vitro*, *in vivo* IL-2 was not given, since a bone marrow transplantation was performed. In a second report, IL-2 was given subcutaneously to a 17-month-old male with Nezelof's syndrome, in a dose of 1600 U/ml every 3–4 days for 50 days. T cell numbers and lymphocyte responsiveness to mitogens improved, but specific antibody production did not change during IL-2 treatment (70).

Hyper IgM Syndrome

A third immunodeficiency in which IL-2 deficiency has been demonstrated is hyper IgM syndrome. The hyper IgM syndrome is a still poorly defined congenital immunodeficiency disease in which IgG and IgA levels are low and serum IgM levels are elevated (71, 72). In this immunodeficiency, peripheral blood B cells bearing IgG and IgA are not found; B cells bear IgM or IgM/IgD only (72). X-linked autosomal recessive or dominant inheritance patterns, as well as acquired forms, have been described. In individual cases it may be difficult to make a clear distinction between hyper IgM syndrome and common variable immunodeficiency with elevated IgM (71, 72).

The cause of hyper IgM syndrome is unknown, although intrinsic B cell defects, or lack of T cell factor(s) needed for an appropriate switch from IgM to IgG production, have been proposed (71, 72). Mayer *et al.* (73) showed that, contrary to previous reports which described intrinsic abnormalities in *in vitro* B cell secretion of IgG and IgA (74), B cells from these immunodeficiency patients were capable of "switching" to IgG and IgA production following incubation with "switch" T cells, but not with culture supernatants of these cells. The nature of the T cell signal needed to initiate such a switch has not been defined, but in several thoroughly investigated cases of hyper IgM, IL-2 secretion by stimulated lymphocytes has been shown to be profoundly deficient or undetectable (75, 76). Since in one group of such patients the production of other lymphokines (IL-1, BCDF, BCGF and IFNγ) was not so depressed, specific functional defects related to IL-2 deficiency were proposed as a plausible explanation for some proportion of the T cell dysfunction observed (77).

Despite the clear lack of various lymphokines in the hyper IgM syndrome, the addition of IL-2 *in vitro* does not seem to enhance proliferation (75), or even when added with IL-6, to induce hyper IgM B cells to switch from IgM-secreting cells to IgG- and IgA-secreting cells (77). However, these *in vitro* experiments do not prove that the administration of IL-2 given *in vivo* would be without effect, since IL-2 *in vivo* encounters cell populations not readily accessible in peripheral blood. Indeed, in one unusual case of hyper IgM syndrome, peripheral blood contained few helper T cells while lymph nodes contained normal numbers of such T cells (76). Nonetheless, the nature of the switch signal has yet to be elucidated in this syndrome, and as far as we are aware no *in vivo* attempts at reconstitution using IL-2 have been performed.

Other Syndromes

Recombinant IL-2 has also been given *in vivo* in another congenital immunodeficiency syndrome: a patient with ataxia telangiectasia (78). The rationale of this treatment was that this 16-year-old male had no IL-2 production *in vitro*, and had recurrent serious infections; 1000–2000 units/kg per day of r-IL-2 were given intravenously for 6 weeks with little change in clinical condition. Interestingly, the production of IgM *in vitro* increased to normal, and the level of serum IgM increased; additionally, lymphocyte proliferation to mitogens improved substantially (78).

Since abnormal T cell development is an essential feature of the DiGeorge syndrome (79), deficiencies of T cell lymphokines in general are likely to be present in such infants. However, specific data are available only for a few cases. In one, a documented IL-2 deficiency was corrected by bone marrow transplantation within 3 months (80). In a second case, IL-2 was found to restore immune functions but no *in vivo* treatment with IL-2 was given (81).

In a third case, an infant with complete DiGeorge syndrome had no detectable peripheral blood lymphocytes bearing the CD3 α/β complex. After 2 months of IL-2 (40 000 units/kg, given intravenously daily) she developed phenotypically normal T lymphocytes (63).

Common Variable Immunodeficiency

Lymphokine Deficiency

Common variable immunodeficiency (CVI) represents another immunodeficiency disease in which lymphokine deficiency has been well described. CVI is a relatively common immunological disorder which affects children or adults of any age (82). Patients with CVI are characterized by abnormally low levels of at least two of the three predominant serum Ig isotypes (IgG, IgA, and IgM). Numerous studies have been performed in the past two decades which point to the probability that the hypogammaglobulinemia in CVI is probably due to a heterogeneous set of immunological defects involving both B and T cell development (83–88). Even though the total number of B cells in CVI is usually normal (82, 83, 89–91), an increased proportion of phenotypically immature B cells may be present. For example, in contrast to normal B cells, CVI B cells (a) display little CD23, (b) have few activation markers (OKT10, TAC 4F2) (90, 91), and (c) show very little (if any) binding of mAb Leu 8 (91). Also suggestive of immaturity, CVI B cells *in vitro* produce an impaired IgG (but often not IgM) response to the T cell-independent B cell activator, Epstein–Barr virus (EBV) (89).

While many abnormalities of B cell development have been documented in CVI, patients vary amongst themselves in the specific defects which are present. However, three main categories of B cell deficiency can be delineated: (a) normal activation and proliferation but poor differentiation; (b) abnormal proliferation and/or differentiation; and (c) no response to activation or proliferation signals (88).

For reasons such as these, CVI has thus often been viewed as a B cell deficiency state; however, numerous T cell defects have been described. For example, poor lymphocyte proliferation is present in about 30–50% of (especially adult) cases (87); loss of T cell help (86), and an excess of T cell suppression (84) have both been documented. Stimulation of autologous T lymphocytes of patients with CVI by phytohemagglutinin (PHA) or monoclonal antibodies to the CD3 complex, OKT3 or PanT2, shows a reduced mitogenic response in 30–50% of patients (92). Perhaps a more frequent abnormality in CVI is a deficiency of various T cell lymphokines. The first deficiency of this kind to be documented was the deficient secretion of IL-2 by CVI T cells activated by mitogens or by monoclonal antibodies to the T cell receptor (84–88) (Figure 19.3). We and others have also shown that IL-2 secretion can be

CVI B CELLS AND CVI T CELLS

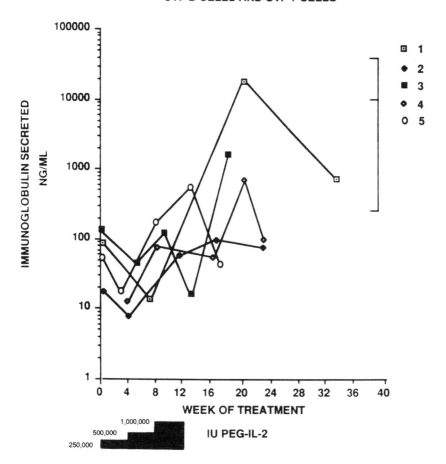

Figure 19.3. Immunoglobulin secreted by CVI B cells with CVT T cells during and after PEG–IL-2 treatment *in vivo*. Prior to, during, and after treatment with PEG–IL-2, B cells of CVI patients were cultured with autologous T cells and PWM (0.1 μg/ml) as a T cell-dependent stimulator. The amount of Ig secreted by the cultured B cells (ng/ml) at the time intervals shown was determined by ELISA. The data for cultures to which PWM (1.0 μg/ml) were added were similar. Data for 38 normal controls are given for comparison, including the mean and the range in the inset in the upper right-hand corner. The doses of PEG–IL-2 are shown, but patient 1 stopped treatment after week 8, and case 4 had only one infusion of 1 000 000 IU/m² of PEG–IL-2 and continued until week 14 on 500 000 IU PEG–IL-2 given weekly. Mean immunoglobulin secretions for patients' B cells (without stimulation) for the dates tested were between 10 and 300 ng/ml, and for normal controls 100 and 400 ng/ml

deficient in CVI T cell cultures which have normal proliferative responses, implying that IL-2 deficiency is an important intrinsic defect in CVI (92–97).

The reason for deficient IL-2 production is unknown; Sneller and Strober have found that PHA-activated, CVI T cells have reduced expression of mRNA for IL-2, as well as mRNA for IL-4, IL-5 and IFNγ (97). These defects could occur as a direct consequence of defects in signal transduction, or as a result of abnormalities in signal reception arising from aberrant T cell receptor/major histocompatibility complex interactions.

Although the production of various lymphokines by CVI T cells may be deficient, the poor proliferative responses displayed by T cells of some patients can be significantly improved by the addition of exogenous IL-2 (92, 93), or overcome by the addition of protein kinase C activators to the cultures (93). For example, a proportion of patients with hypogammaglobulinemia and T cell defects have a normalization of proliferative responses to phytohemagglutinin and OKT3 after incubation with IL-2 (Table 19.3) (92). Here, patients in group A had a full restoration of response, those in group B had a partial restoration, while in group C no response was observed. Patients with CVI may also have defects in the expression of IL-2 receptor; six of seven patients in one study had a profound deficiency (93). However, on the level of RNA, the genes for the IL-2 receptor in these cases were expressed after OKT3 stimulation; after exposure to phorbol ester, there was a normalization of the expression of the receptor itself (94). In another study (97), however, IL-2 receptor expression of PHA-activated peripheral mononuclear cells from four patients was not found depressed, supporting the thesis that considerable heterogeneity in this population is likely.

In addition to deficiencies of IL-2, IL-4, IL-5 and IFNγ, patients with CVI have deficient secretion of BCDF (98–104), although the B cells of many patients respond quite normally *in vitro* when certain BCDFs are supplied (98–104). However, B cells of only some proportion of CVI patients are capable of proliferating normally in the presence of various BCGFs, such as IL-2, IL-4 and low-molecular-weight BCGF (102–105). In addition, it is not known exactly how "normal" these proliferating or differentiated CVI B cells are. In general, patients with CVI may lack the ability to form memory B cells (91, 105). It is possible that CVI B cells may respond poorly (if at all) to BCGFs responsible for developing such memory populations (possibly the high-molecular-weight BCGFs) (105).

An additional perturbation in CVI is the observation that most patients have increased levels of IL-6 in their serum (106), and secrete excess amounts of IL-6 in various cell cultures. These results demonstrate that some elements of immune activation are present; indeed other evidence of intense lymphoid activation is also present in CVI, including increased serum levels of soluble CD8, CD25, and β_2-microglobulin (107).

Table 19.3 IL-2 production and proliferative response by subgroup in CVI patients and controls[a]

	PHA			OKT3		
		Prolif. resp.[c]			Prolif. resp.[c]	
	IL-2 prod.[a]	−IL-2	+IL-2	IL-2 prod.[b]	−IL-2	+IL-2
Controls						
Median	2.0	80.0	99.9	2.0	60.6	82.4
Range	(0.7–6.8)	(565–103.2)	(52–125)	(0.8–16)	(37.6–83.4)	(50.5–127.0)
Group A[d]						
Median	0.6	53.0	108.0	0.7	55.5	100.9
2	0.6	54.3	117.5	0.7	88.1	217.2
3	0.5	53.3	104.8	0.6	13.9	62.3
4	ND	50.0	108.6	ND	55.5	100.9
Group B[d]						
Median	1.7	36.3	55.1	2.0	35.3	53.4
15	0.5	58.6	55.1	0.5	29.2	43.8
9	1.7	29.6	46	2.0	52.4	68.4
5	ND	37.4	38.9	ND	35.3	53.4
Group C[d]						
Median	0.7	14.4	18.2	0.5		16.8
1	0.7	16.7	23.0	1.3	19.2	19.9
16	0.3	7.8	12.5	0.5	7.6	7.6
10	0.6	12.0	13.4	0.5	13.1	13.6
12	7.3	51.4	58.0	0.3	53.3	65.4
13	0.7	48.7	52.4	0.4	38.3	39.4
11	1.2	9.2	2.6	0.6	14.8	7.4

[a]Data are from Kruger *et al.* (92).
[b]Units of IL-2 per milliliter.
[c]Each value listed represents the mean of triplicate values of proliferation of PBL cultures on day 3 with the addition of mitogens or IL-2 as stated in counts per minute in thousands (cpm $\times 10^{-3}$).
[d]Group A patients with full restoration of response with IL-2 addition (numbers are case numbers).
Group B patients with partial restoration of response with IL-2 addition (numbers are case numbers).
Group C patients with no significant response with IL-2 addition (numbers are case numbers).

In Vitro Attempts to Improve Ig Secretion in CVI

Although normal B cell numbers coupled with "intrinsic" B cell defects have been described in CVI, it is not actually known which B cell subset(s) in normals is capable of responding to various T cell-derived signals. It is entirely possible that the pool of these potentially responsive cells is deficient in CVI. This functional B cell immaturity could be caused by defects in T cell maturation alone or superimposed upon intrinsic B cell defects. This hypothesis becomes more tempting considering the fact that CVI has occasionally been found to be reversible when a "T cell" intervention has occurred. For example, cimetidine treatment can normalize antibody secretion in some patients with CVI (108). Normalization of serum Ig levels and restoration of antigen-specific antibody responses have now been reported in a few CVI patients following infection with HIV and concomitant development of impaired *in vitro* T cell-mediated function (109). Perhaps HIV infection in these individuals alters (possibly inhibits?) some pre-existing T cell-mediated suppression of underlying normal humoral immune responses.

Not only can hypogammaglobulinemia be relieved by certain T cell-mediated mechanisms; transient hypogammaglobulinemia can also appear after certain therapies such as hydantoin (110) or gold therapy have been given (111). The observations reinforce the view that there may be reversible B cell defects in CVI.

To investigate if the addition of still-undefined T cell factors could alleviate the B cell deficiency state in CVI *in vitro*, we tested if anti-CD3-stimulated T cells of normal donors and CVI patients could produce factors capable of stimulating Ig secretion by CVI B cells. The use of monoclonal antibodies to the CD3 complex was found to greatly enhance both plaque cell formation and *in vitro* secretion of IgG and IgM for many patients with CVI (103). B cells from many CVI patients were found to differentiate and secrete IgG and IgM in response to either autologous or allogeneic T cell factors. In these experiments CVI B cells appear to mature normally on a percentage basis into Ig-secreting cells (IgSC) but secrete less IgM and especially IgG than do their normal counterparts. Several of the BCDFs which have these capacities have been purified; from anti-CD3 446 stimulated cultures, a 32 000 Da factor with an isoelectric point distinct from IL-6 has been purified (112).

In Vivo PEG–IL-2 in CVI

To assess the potential role of IL-2 in immune reconstitution, we tested 12 CVI patients who had profound T cell helper defects *in vitro* to determine if lymphocyte proliferation occurred after the addition of PEG–IL-2. Five CVI patients who had 0–10% of normal T helper activity were ultimately chosen for PEG–IL-2 treatment *in vivo* (113). Each had an 8–15.1-fold increase in incorporation of [^{3}H]thymidine into cells cultured for 5 days when PEG–IL-2 was added at 10 000 IU/ml, with different degrees of incorporation at lower PEG–IL-2 concentrations (Table 19.4). Ten normal controls had 2.4–32.3-fold increases in uptake of radioisotope (average, 10.3); thus we judged these five CVI patients to be responsive to IL-2 *in vitro*, and thus potentially *in vivo*. These five patients were then treated with PEG–IL-2 for 12 weeks. In this protocol, patients were given weekly intravenous infusions of PEG–IL-2, at a dose of 250 000 units/m^2 body surface area for weeks 0–4, 500 000 units for weeks 4–8, and 1 000 000 units for weeks 8–12. Various immunological analyses were performed to determine the effects of these infusions in the immune system of these patients.

Table 19.4   *In vitro* lymphocyte proliferation response to PEG–IL-2[a]

PEG–IL-2 (IU/ml)	Patient number					Normal controls	
	1	2	3	4	5	(Mean)	(Range)
1	1.5	1.1	1.05	2.3	1.1	2.3	(0–5.9)
10	1.6	1.9	0	2.67	2.3	2.7	(0.7–6.4)
100	1.8	3.2	2.0	4.16	4.8	4.8	(1.5–11.2)
1 000	3.4	4.3	5.9	3.3	6.9	6.9	(2.07–13.2)
10 000	8.0	12.8	15.1	10.8	8.4	10.3	(2.4–32.9)

[a]Data for cultures maintained for 5 days are given. Ten normals had the average and range of values shown. These data are given as a stimulation index, which is the cpm for test cultures ÷ cpm for cultures to which no PEG–IL-2 had been added. Data for additional cultures, harvested at different intervals, are not shown.

After treatment with PEG–IL-2 *in vivo*, no overall changes in peripheral T or B cell numbers, subsets, NK cells or activated T cells occurred, although three patients had increased numbers of IL-2 receptor-bearing cells on several occasions. All patients had somewhat reduced responses to mitogens, phorbol-myristate acetate (PMA), Con A, and pokeweed mitogen (PWM), although these responses remained within the range of control samples tested in our laboratory. Before and after PEG–IL-2 was infused, patients' T cells were tested for their ability to proliferate in response to the soluble recall antigens, tetanus toxoid and *Candida*. Only one patient demonstrated a borderline normal response at the beginning of the trial; the others were negative. Lymphocyte proliferative responses to these antigens were significantly increased for three patients after treatment, although these changes were variable (cases 2, 3, and 5) (Table 19.5).

Although the restoration of antigen-specific T cell proliferative responses in some cases was encouraging, the most dramatic findings occurred in B cell cultures. Profound enhancement of Ig secretion by CVI B cells *in vitro*

Table 19.5   Lymphocyte proliferation to tetanus toxoid and *Candida* antigen

Patient number:	1		2		3		4		5	
Antigen:	Tet.	Can.	Tet.	Can.	Tet.	Can.	Tet.	Can.	Tet.	Can.
Week[a] 0	2.13	2.4	1.68	1.48	1.18	1.1	1.4	1.2	4.78	1.3
4	2.6	2.0	1.33	1.23	84	19.7	1.4	1.2	3.75	1.6
8	ND	ND	ND	1.15	98	1.08	0.9	1.1	1.47	1.12
12	0.9	1.7	7.2	2.23	2.09	1.03	0.86	1.56	0.82	2.55
16	ND	ND	1.9	1.5	48	37	0.57	1.4	3.68	6.8
20	1.0	1.5	1.8	1.67	1.5	4.46	1.1	1.8	1.84	6.68

[a]Data given as stimulation index: cpm for cultures stimulated by Tetanus or *Candida* ÷ cpm non-stimulated cultures. Normal range of immunized individuals is 4.0 or greater; positive responses are underlined. ND = not done.

was observed for all patients (Figures 19.3–19.5) to T-dependent stimuli. B cells of treated patients cultured with autologous T cells demonstrated enhanced Ig secretion in PWM-stimulated cultures by 8 weeks of therapy (Figure 19.3). There was an even greater response when allogenic T cells were used to stimulate CVI B cells (Figure 19.4), such that by 8 weeks all patients demonstrated marked increases in Ig secretion, and by 20 weeks (8 weeks after cessation of therapy) B cells from 3/5 patients were at the mean for normal PWM response (10 µg/ml). Improvement continued well beyond

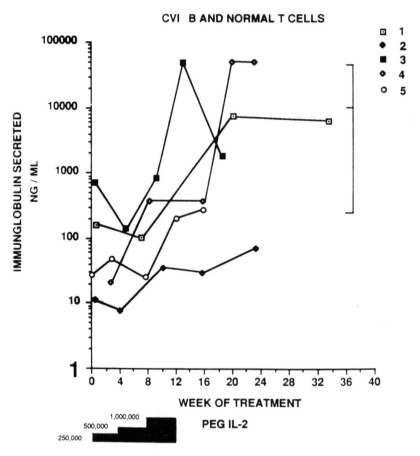

Figure 19.4. Immunoglobulin secreted by CVI B cells with normal T cells during and after PEG–IL-2 treatment *in vivo*. Similar to Figure 19.3, the B cells of CVI patients were cultured with normal T cells at various intervals before, during, and after PEG–IL-2 treatment to assess the amount of secreted Ig that was produced with PWM (0.1 µg/ml) stimulation. Data for cultures to which 1.0 µg/ml of PWM was added were similar. Baseline (unstimulated) secretion by B cells was the same as in the legend to Figure 19.2

cessation of therapy, with values still falling within the normal range 36–40 weeks after treatment.

To determine if these effects were related to activation of B or T cell compartments *in vivo*, T cells of treated CVI patients were incubated with B cells isolated from the blood of normal donors. The results showed that the T cells of CVI patients were also increasingly capable of supporting Ig secretion by normal B cells, normalizing the very defect for which the patients had been selected. As shown in Figure 19.5, normal B cells could secrete up to 10 000-fold more Ig when cultured with T cells of IL-2-treated CVI

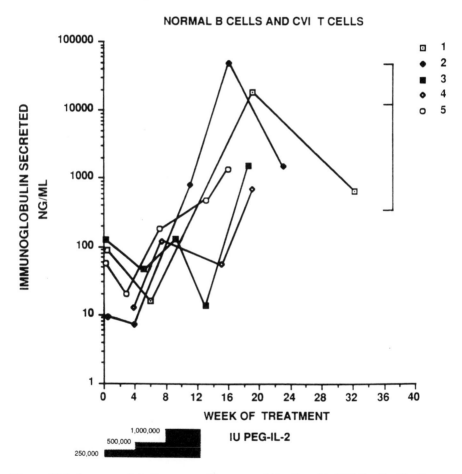

Figure 19.5. Immunoglobulin secreted by normal B cells with CVI T cells. Similar to Figures 19.3 and 19.4 at various time intervals before, during, and after PEG–IL-2 treatment, the amount of immunoglobulin secreted *in vitro* was quantified when normal B cells were incubated with T cells of treated CVI patients in the presence of PWM (0.1 µg/ml)

patients, as compared to cultures to which the T cells of the same patients were added before treatment. In separate assays, the Ig isotype for CVI patients was IgM predominantly, as for all the normal donors tested under these conditions.

All patients were maintained on intravenous Ig, and no increase in serum IgG, IgA or IgM were found during the study. However, for three of the four patients (2, 4 and 5), significant amounts of IgG (but not IgM) anti-tetanus antibody were found in supernatants of CVI B cell cultures stimulated with PWM and cultures stimulated with the T-independent antigens SAC, SAC + IL-2 or BCDF.

Conclusions

Our data show that *in vivo* administration of PEG–IL-2 to patients with severe *in vitro* T cell helper defects, but widely differing manifestations of CVI, can lead to greatly enhanced B cell production of Ig, and specific antibody *in vitro*. Further studies are underway to determine if *de novo* antibody can be detected after r-IL-2 treatment, or if these changes are primarily confined to *in vitro* cell cultures.

OUTLOOK TO THE FUTURE

At the present time, most of the described effects of IL-2 have been on T cell development and the induction of cytotoxicity. As discussed above, there are a group of primary immunodeficiency diseases for which T cell defects and deficient IL-2 production form an integral component. IL-2 could play a clinical role in the treatment of these diseases. At one end of the spectrum, IL-2 deficiency may be a pivotal abnormality, which when corrected may allow for normal T cell proliferation and functional development. In contrast, in other cases, the deficit of IL-2 production may be more an accessory abnormality, for which reconstitution of IL-2 would be a potential adjunctive maneuver. Possibly in the first group would be infants with a SCID phenotype due to an abnormality in translation of the IL-2 gene. Although the infusion of IL-2 could replace the deficient lymphokine, bone marrow transplantation would provide more definitive treatment, perhaps a cure. Much the same view might apply to patients with Nezelof's syndrome. However, in both situations IL-2 could have a role in treatment while preparations for a suitable bone marrow transplantation were being made, or if no donor were available.

Recombinant IL-2 may also find a role in treatment of primary immune deficiency diseases for which bone marrow transplantation is not medically desirable. Into this category could potentially fall patients of common variable immune deficiency, or other syndromes involving T cell deficiency.

Patients with these immunodeficiencies could be treated with r-IL-2 or, as an attractive alternative, PEG–IL-2, since using this form of r-IL-2, infusions or subcutaneous injections appear to be needed at only weekly or bi-weekly intervals. The use of r-IL-2 or PEG–IL-2 in the doses required in primary immunodeficiency is accompanied by few side effects, making long-term administration practical. Such therapy would primarily be expected to boost T cell function, but as we have discussed here positive effects on B cells may well occur.

REFERENCES

1. Morgan, D.A., Ruscetti, F.W. and Gallo, R.C. (1976) Selective *in vitro* growth of T lymphocytes from normal bone marrows. *Science*, **193**, 1007–1008.
2. Welte, K. and Mertelsmann, R. (1985) Human interleukin 2: Biochemistry, physiology, and possible pathogenetic role in immunodeficiency syndromes. *Cancer Invest.*, **3**, 35–49.
3. Robb, R.J. (1981) Interleukin 2: The molecule and its function. *Immunol. Today*, **5**, 203.
4. Smith, R.A., Wang, H.M. and Cantrell, D.A. (1983) The variables regulating T cell growth. In Yamamura, V.Y. and Tada, T. (eds) *Progress in Immunity*. Academic Press, New York, pp. 269–280.
5. Henney, C.S., Kern, D.E. and Gillis, S. (1982) Cytotoxic responses: The regulatory influence of interleukin-2. *Transplant. Proc.*, **14**, 565–569.
6. Lotze, M.T., Grimm, E.A., Mazumder, A., Strausser, J.L. and Rosenberg, S.A. *et al.* (1981) *In vitro* growth of cytotoxic human lymphocytes. *Cancer Res.*, **41**, 4420–4425.
7. Grimm, E.A., Mazumder, A. and Rosenberg, S.A. (1982) Lymphokine activated killer cell phenomenon. *J. Exp. Med.*, **155**, 1823–1841.
8. Ralph, P., Jeong, G., Nakoinz, I., Saiki, O. and Cunningham-Rundles, C. (1985) Rescue of IgM, IgG, and IgA production in common varied immunodeficiency by T cell independent stimulation with Epstein–Barr virus. *J. Clin. Immunol.*, **5**, 122–129.
9. Nakagawa, N., Nakagawa, T., Volkman, D.J., Ambrus, J.L., Jr and Fauci, A.S. (1987) The role of interleukin 2 in inducing Ig production in a pokeweed mitogen-stimulated mononuclear cell system. *J. Immunol.*, **138**, 795–801.
10. Romagnani, S., Prete, G.L., Giudizi, M.G., Biagiotti, G.R., Arimerigogna, F., Tiri, A., Alessi, A., Mazzetti, M. and Ricci, M. (1986) Direct induction of human B cell differentiation by recombinant interleukin-2. *Immunology*, **58**, 31–35.
11. Callard, R.E., Smith, S.H., Shields, J.G. and Levinsky, R.J. (1986) T cell help in human antigen-specific antibody responses can be replaced by interleukin 2. *Eur. J. Immunol.*, **16**, 1037–1042.
12. Hivroz, C., Vallé, A., Brouet, J.C., Banchereau, J. and Guillot-Courvalin (1989) Regulation by IL-2 of CD23 expression of leukemic and normal B cells; comparison with IL-4. *Eur. J. Immunol*, **19**, 1025–1030.
13. Xing, X., Hern-Ku, L., Clark, S.C. and Choi, Y.S. (1989) Recombinant interleukin (IL)2-induced human B cell differentiation is mediated by autocrine IL-6. *Eur. J. Immunol.*, **19**, 2275–2281.

14. Lipsky, P.E., Hirchata, S., Jelinek, D.F., McAnally, L. and Splawski, J.B. (1988) Regulation of human B cell lymphocyte responsiveness. *Scand. J. Rheumatol.*, **76**, 229–235.
15. Mittler, R., Rao, P., Olini, G., Westberg, E., Newman, W., Hoffman, M. and Goldstein, G. (1985) Activated human B cells display a functional IL-2 receptor. *J. Immunol.*, **34**, 2393–2399.
16. Smith, S.H., Shields, J.G. and Callard, R.E. (1989) Human T cell-replacing factor(s): A comparison of recombinant and purified human B cell growth and differentiation factors. *Eur. J. Immunol.*, **19**, 2045–2049.
17. Splawski, J.B., McAnally, L.M. and Lipsky, P.E. (1990) IL-2 dependence of the promotion of human B cell differentiation by IL-6 (BSF-2). *J. Immunol.*, **144**, 562–569.
18. Mingari, M.C., Gerrosa, F., Carra, G., Accola, R.S., Moretta, A., Zubler, R.H., Waldmann, T.A. and Moretta, L. (1984) Human interleukin-2 promotes proliferation of activated B cells via surface receptors similar to those of activated T cells. *Nature*, **312**, 641–643.
19. Muraguchi, A., Kehrl, J.H., Longo, D.L., Volkman, D.J. *et al.* (1985) Interleukin 2 receptors on human B cells: Implications for the role of interleukin 2 in human B cell function. *J. Exp. Med.*, **161**, 181–197.
20. Bich-Thuy, Le thi and Fauci, A.S. (1985) Direct effect of interleukin 2 on the differentiation of human B cells which have not been preactivated *in vitro. Eur. J. Immunol.*, **15**, 1075–9.
21. Ralph, P., Jeong, G., Welte, K., Merteslmann, R., Rabin, H., Henderson, L.E., Souza, L.M., Boone, T.C. and Robb, R.J. (1989) Stimulation of immunoglobulin secretion in human B lymphocytes as a direct effect on high concentrations of IL-2. *J. Immunol.*, **133**, 2442–2445.
22. Defrance, T., Vanbervliet, B., Pène, J. and Banchereau, J. (1988) Human recombinant IL-4 induces activated B lymphocytes to produce IgG and IgM. *J. Immunol.*, **141**, 2000–2005.
23. Jelinek, D.F. and Lipsky, P.E. (1987) Enhancement of human B cell proliferation and differentiation by tumor necrosis factor-α and interleukin 1. *J. Immunol.*, **139**, 2970.
24. Sidman, C.L., Marshall, J.D., Shultz, W., Gray, P.W. and Johnson, H.M. (1984) Gamma interferon is one of several direct B cell modulating cytokines. *Nature*, **309**, 801–804.
25. Harriman, G.R., Kunimoto, D.Y., Elliott, J.F., Paetkau, V. and Strober, W. (1988) The role of IL-5 in IgA B cell differentiation *J. Immunol.*, **140**, 3033–3039.
26. Muraguchi, A.T., Hirano, B., Tang, T., Matsuda, Y., Horii, K., Nakajima, K. and Kishimoto, T. (1988) The essential role of B cell stimulatory factor 2(BSF-2/IL-6) for the terminal differentiation of B cells. *J. Exp. Med.*, **167**, 332.
27. Rothman, P., Lutzker, S., Cook, W., Coffman, R. and Alt, F.W. (1988) Mitogen plus interleukin 4 induction of C epsilon transcripts in B lymphoid cells. *J. Exp. Med.*, **168**, 2385–9.
28. Pène, J.F., Roussett, F., Briere, I., Christian, X., Paliard, J., Banchereau, H., Spits, H. and deVries, J.E. (1988) IgE production by normal human B cells induced by alloreactive T cell clones is mediated by IL-4 and suppressed by IFN-gamma. *J. Immunol.*, **141**, 1218.
29. Devos, R., Plaetinek, G., Cheroutre, H., Simons, G., Degrave, W., Tavernier, J., Remaut, E. and Fiers, W. (1983) Molecular cloning of human interleukin-2 cDNA and its expression in *E. coli. Nucleic Acids Res.*, **11**, 4307–4323.

30. Taniguchi, T., Matsui, H., Fujita, T. *et al.* (1983) Structure and expression of a cloned cDNA for human interleukin-2. *Nature*, **302**, 305–310.

31. Okado, M., Yoshimura, N., Kaieda, T. *et al.* (1981) Establishment and characterization of human T hybrid cells secreting immunoregulatory molecules. *Proc. Nat. Acad. Sci. USA*, **78**, 7717–7721.

32. Frank, M.B., Watson, J. and Gillis, S. (1981) Biochemical and biologic characterization of lymphocyte regulatory molecules. VIII. Purification of interleukin 2 from a human T cell leukemia. *J. Immunol.*, **127**, 2361–2365.

33. Gillis, S., Ferm, M., Ou, W. and Smith, K.A. (1978) T cell growth factor: Parameters of production and a quantitative microassay for activity. *J. Immunol.*, **120**, 2027–2032.

34. Rosenberg, S.A., Lotze, M.T., Muul, L.M., Leitman, S., Chang, A.E., Ettinghausen, S.E., Matory, Y.L., Skibber, J.M., Shiloni, E., Velto, J.T., Seipp, C.A., Simpson, C. and Reichert, C.M. (1985) Observations on the systemic administration of autologous lymphokine activated killer cells and recombinant IL-2 to patients with metastatic cancer. *N. Engl. J. Med.*, **313**, 1485–1492.

35. Lotze, M.L., Matory, Y.L., Ragner, A.A., Ettinghausen, S.E., Vetto, J.T., Slipp, C.A. *et al.* (1986) Clinical effects and toxicity of IL-2 in patients with cancer. *Cancer*, **58**, 2764–2772.

36. Lotze, M.T., Chang, A.E., Seipp, C.A., Simpson, G., Velto, J.T. and Rosenberg, S.A. (1986) High dose interleukin 2 in treatment of patients with disseminated cancer. *JAMA*, **256**, 3117.

37. Thompson, J.A., Lee, D.J., Lindgreen, G.G., Benz, L.A., Collins, C., Shuman, W.P., Levitt, D. and Fefer, A. (1989) Influence of schedule of interleukin 2 administration on therapy with interleukin 2 and lymphokine activated killer cells. *Cancer Res.*, **49**, 235–240.

38. Stein, R.C., Malkovska, V., Morgan, S., Galazka, A. *et al.* (1991) The clinical effects of prolonged treatment of patients with advanced cancer with low-dose subcutaneous interleukin. *Br. J. Cancer*, **63**, 275–278.

39. Okaneya, T. and Ogawa, A. (1991) Induction of cytotoxicity of the renal hilar lymph nodes by pedal subcutaneous administration of interleukin-2 in patients with renal cancer. *Cancer*, **67**, 1332–1337.

40. Katre, N.V., Knauf, M.J. and Laird, W.J. (1987) Chemical modification of recombinant interleukin-2 by polyethylene glycol increases its potency in the murine meth A sarcoma model. *Proc. Nat. Acad. Sci. USA*, **84**, 1487–1491.

41. Knauf, M.J., Bell, D.P., Hirtzer, P., Lou, Z.-P., Young, J.D. and Katre, N.V. (1988) Relationship of effective molecular size to systemic clearance in rats of r-IL-2 chemically modified with water soluble polymers. *J. Biol. Chem.*, **263**, 15064–15070.

42. Katre, N.V. (1990) Immunogenicity of recombinant IL-2 modified by complement attachment of polyethylene glycol. *J. Immunol.*, **144**, 209–213.

43. Hershfield, M.S., Buckley, R.H., Greenberg, M.L., Milton, A.L., Schiff, R., Hatem, C., Kurtzberg, J., Markert, L.M., Kobayashi, R.H., Kobayashi, A.L. and Abuchowski, A. (1987) Treatment of adenosine deaminase deficiency with polyethylene glycol-modified adenosine deaminase. *N. Engl. J. Med.*, **316**, 589–596.

44. Abuchowski, A., Davis, F. and Davis, S. (1981) Immunosuppressive properties and circulating life of *Acromobacter* glutaminase-asparinase covalently attached to PEG in man. *Cancer Treatment Rep.*, **65**, 1077–1081.

45. Chua, C.C., Greenberg, M.L., Viau, A.T., Nucci M., Brenckman, W.D. and Hershfield, M.S. (1988) Use of polyethylene glycol-modified uricase (PEG-

uricase) to treat hyperuricemia in a patient with non-hodgkin lymphoma. *Ann. Intern. Med.*, **109**, 114–116.

46. Meyers, F.J., Paradise, C., Scudder, S.A., Goodman, G. and Konrad, M. (1991) A phase I study including pharmacokinetics of polyethylene glycol conjugated interleukin 2. *Clin. Pharmacol. Ther.*, **49**, 307–313.

47. McElrath, M.J., Kaplan, G., Burkhardt, R.A. and Cohn, Z.A. (1990) Cutaneous response to recombinant interleukin 2 in human immunodeficiency virus 1-seropositive individuals. *Proc. Nat. Acad. Sci. USA*, **87**, 5783–5787.

48. Converse, P., Ottenhoff, T.H., Work Teklemariam, S., Hancock, G.E. *et al.* (1990) Intradermal recombinant interleukin 2 enhances peripheral blood T-cell responses to mitogen and antigens in patients with lepromatous leprosy. *Scand. J. Immunol.*, **32**, 83–91.

49. Durandy, A. and Griscelli, C. (1983) Prenatal diagnosis of severe combined immunodeficiency and X-linked agammaglobulinemia. *Birth Defects*, **19**, 125–7.

50. Gelfand, E.W. and Dosch, H.M. (1983) Diagnosis and classification of severe combined immunodeficiency disease. *Birth Defects*, **19**, 65–72.

51. Hirschhorn, R. (1983) Genetic deficiencies of adenosine deaminase and purine nucleoside phosphorylase: Overview, genetic heterogeneity and therapy. *Birth Defects*, **19**, 73–81.

52. Alarcon, B., Reguerio, J.R., Amaiz-Villena, A. and Terhorst, C. (1988) Familial defect in the surface expression of the T-cell receptor–CD3 complex. *N. Engl. J. Med.*, **319**, 1203–1208.

53. Pagenelli, R., Aiuti, F., Beverly, P.C. and Levinsky, R.J. (1983) Impaired production of interleukins in patients with cell-mediated immunodeficiency. *J. Clin. Exp. Immunol.*, **51**, 338–344.

54. Jung, L.K.L., Fu, S.M., Hara, T., Kapoor, N. and Good, R.A. (1986) Defective expression of T cell associated glycoprotein in SCID. *J. Clin. Invest.*, **77**, 940–946.

55. Chu, E.T., Rosenwasser, L.J., Dinarello, C.A., Rosen, F.S. and Geha, R.S. (1984) Immunodeficiency with defective T cell response to interleukin I. *Proc. Nat. Acad. Sci. USA*, **81**, 4945–4949.

56. Doi, S., Saiki, O., Tanaka, T., Ha-Kawa, K., Igarashi, T., Fujita, T., Taniguchi, T. and Kishimoto, S. (1988) Cellular and genetic analyses of IL-2 production and IL-2 receptor expression in a patient with familial T cell dominant immunodeficiency. *Clin. Immunol. Immunopathol.*, **46**, 24–36.

57. Chatila, T., Wong, R., Young, M., Miller, R., Terhorst, C. and Geha, R.F. (1989) An immunodeficiency characterized by defective signal transduction in T lymphocytes. *N. Engl. J. Med.*, **320**, 696–702.

58. Reith, W., Satola, S., Sanchez, C.H. *et al.* (1988) Congenital immunodeficiency with a regulatory defect in MHC class II gene expression lacks a specific HLA-DR promoter binding protein, RF-X. *Cell*, **53**, 987–1006.

59. Hume, C.R. and Lee, J.S. (1989) Congenital immunodeficiencies associated with absence of HLA class II antigens on lymphocytes result from distinct mutations in trans-acting factors. *Hum. Immun.*, **26**, 288–309.

60. Benichou, B. and Strominger, J.L. (1991) Class II-antigen-negative patient and mutant B cell lines represent at least three, and probably four, distinct genetic defects defined by complementation analysis. *Proc. Nat. Acad. Sci.*, **88**, 4285–4288.

61. Pahwa, R., Paradise, C., Pahwa, S., Chatila, T., Day, N.K., Geha, R., Schwartz, S.A., Slade, H., Oyaizu, N. and Good, R.A. (1989) Recombinant IL-2 therapy in severe combined immunodeficiency disease. *Proc. Nat. Acad. Sci. USA*, **86**, 5069–5073.

62. Rijkers, G.T., Scharenberg, G.M., Van Dongess, J.M., Neijens, H.J. and Zegers, B.J.M. (1991) Abnormal signal transduction in a patient with SCID. *Pediatr. Res.*, **29**, 306–309.
63. Buckley, R., Schiff, S., Markert, L., Gerber, P. and Paradise, C. (1989) Recombinant human interleukin-2 (rIL-2) therapy in primary immunodeficiency. *J. Allergy Clin. Immunol.*, **83**, 296.
64. Weinberg, K. and Parkman, R. (1990) Severe combined immunodeficiency due to a specific defect in the production of interleukin-2. *N. Engl. J. Med.*, **322**, 1718–1723.
65. Weinberg, K., Paradise, C., Annett, G., Kohn, D.B., Sender, C., Lenarsky, C. and Parkman, R. (1990) Polyethylene glycol IL-2 (PEG-IL-2) treatment of T cell immunodeficiency. *Pediatr. Res.* [Abstract], **27**, 163A.
66. Chiron Corp. (data on file).
67. Allibone, E.C., Goldie, W. and Marmion, B.P. (1964) *Pneumocystis carinii* pneumonia and progressive vaccinia in siblings. *Arch. Dis. Child.*, **39**, 26–34.
68. Nezelof, C. (1968) Thymic dysplasia with normal immunoglobulins and immunology deficiency: Pure alymphocytosis. In Good, R.A. (ed.) *Immunologic Deficiency Diseases.* National Foundation, New York, pp. 104–115.
69. Flomemberg, N., Welte, K., Mertelsmann, R., Kernan, N., Ciobanu, N., Venuta, S., Feldman, S., Kruger, A., Kirkpatrick, D., Dupont, B. and O'Reilly, R. (1983) Immunologic effects of interleukin 2 in primary immunodeficiency diseases. *J. Immunol.*, **130**, 2644–2650.
70. Dopfer, R., Niethammer, D., Peter, H.H., Kniep, E.-M., Monner, D.A. and Mühlradt, P.F. (1984) *In vitro* effects of IL-2 or lymphocyte subpopulation in a child with combined immunodeficiency. *Immunobiology*, **167**, 452–461.
71. Rosen, F.S. and Janeway, C.A. (1966) The gammaglobulins III. The antibody deficiency syndromes. *N. Engl. J. Med.*, **275**, 709–715.
72. Geha, R.S., Hyslop, N., Alami, S., Farah, F., Schneeberger, E.E. and Rosen, F.S. (1979) Hyper immunoglobulin immunodeficiency (dysgammaglobulinemia): Presence of immunoglobulin in secretory phasmacytoid cells in peripheral blood and failure of immunoglobulin M–immunoglobulin G switch in B cell differentiation. *J. Clin. Invest.*, **64**, 385–391.
73. Mayer, L., Kwan, S.P., Thompson, C., Ko, H.S., Chiorazzi, N., Waldmann, T. and Rosen, F. (1986) Evidence for a defect in "switch" T cells in patients with immunodeficiency and hyper immunoglobulinemia M. *J. Exp. Med.*, **314**, 409–413.
74. Levitt, D., Harber, P., Rich, K. and Cooper, M.D. (1983) Hyper IgM immunodeficiency: A primary dysfunction of B lymphocyte isotype switching. *J. Clin. Invest.*, **72**, 1650–1656.
75. Ohno, T., Fujii, H., Kanoh, T., Uchino, H., Kuribayachi, K. *et al.* (1987) Selective deficiency of IL-2 production and refractoriness to extrinsic IL-2 in immunodeficiency with hyper IgM. *Clin. Immunol. Immunopathol.*, **45**, 471–480.
76. Fiorilli, M., Russo, G., Paganelli, R., Papetti, G., Larbonari, M., Crescenzi, M., Calvani, M., Quinti, I. and Aiuti, F. (1986) Hypogammaglobulinemia with hyper IgM, severe T cell defect, and abnormal recirculation of OKT4 lymphocytes in a girl with chronic lymphadenopathy. *Clin. Immunol. Immunopathol.*, **38**, 256–264.
77. Gougeon, M.-L., Morelet, L., Doussau, M., Theze, J., Griscelli, G. and Fisher, A. (1992) Hyper-IgM immunodeficiency syndrome: influence of lymphokines in *in vitro* maturation of peripheral B cells. *J. Clin. Immunol.*, **12**, 92–99.
78. Doi, S., Saiki, O., Hara, T., Sugita, T., Ha-Kawa, K., Tanaker, T., Hara, H., Negoro, S., Yabuuchi, H. and Kishimoto, S. (1989) Administration of recombi-

nant IL-2 augments the level of serum IgM in an IL-2 deficient patient. *Eur. J. Pediatr.*, **148**, 630–633.

79. Ammann, A.J. and Hong, R. (1989) Disorders of the T cell system. In Stiehm, E.R. (ed.) *Immunologic Disorders in Infants and Children* (3rd edn). Saunders, Philadelphia, pp. 2257–2313.

80. Borzy, M.S., Ridgway, D., Noya, F. and Shearer, W.T. (1989) Successful bone marrow transplant with split lymphoid chimerism in DiGeorge syndrome. *J. Clin. Immunol.*, **9**, 386–392.

81. Businco, L., Rubaltelli, F.F., Paganelli, R., Galli, E., Ensoli, B., Betti, P. and Aiuti, F. (1986) Results in two infants with DiGeorge syndrome: Effects of long term TP5. *Clin. Immunol. Immunopathol.*, **39**, 222–230.

82. WHO (1989) Primary immunodeficiency diseases: Immunodeficiency reviews. *Immunopathology*, **1**, 173–205.

83. Cunningham-Rundles, C. (1989) Clinical and immunologic analyses of 103 patients with common variable immunodeficiency. *J. Clin. Immunol.*, **9**, 22–33.

84. Waldmann, T.A., Broder, S., Blaese, R.M., Durm, M., Blackman, M. and Strober, W. (1974) Role of suppressor cells in pathogenesis of common variable hypogammaglobulinemia. *Lancet*, **ii**, 609–613.

85. Reinherz, E.L., Cooper, M.D., Schlossman, S.F. and Rosen, F.S. (1981) Abnormalities of T cell maturation and regulation in human beings with immunodeficiency disorders. *J. Clin. Invest.*, **68**, 699–705.

86. Pandolfi, F., Corte, G., Quinti, I., Fiorilli, M., Frieligsdorf, A., Bargellesi, A. and Aiuti, F. (1983) Defect of T helper lymphocytes, as defined by the 5/9 monoclonal antibody, in patients with common variable hypogammaglobulinemia. *Clin. Exp. Immunol.*, **51**, 470–474.

87. Cunningham-Rundles, S., Cunningham-Rundles, C., Ma, D.I., Siegal, F.P., Kosloff, C. and Good, R.A. (1981) Impaired proliferative response to B lymphocyte activators in common variable immunodeficiency. *J. Clin. Immunol.*, **1**, 65–71.

88. Saiki, O., Ralph, P., Cunningham-Rundles, C. and Good, R.A. (1982) Three distinct stages of B cell defects in common varied immunodeficiency. *Proc. Nat. Acad. Sci. USA*, **79**, 6008–6012.

89. Ralph, P., Jeong, G., Nakuinz, I., Saiki, O. and Cunningham-Rundles, C. (1985) Rescue of IgM, IgG, and IgA production in common varied immunodeficiency by T cell independent stimulation with Epstein–Barr virus. *J. Clin. Immunol.*, **5**, 122–129.

90. Fiorilli, M., Crescenzi, M., Carbonari, M., Tedesco, L., Russo, G., Gaetano, C. and Aiuti, F. (1986) Phenotypically immature IgG bearing B cells in patients with hypogammaglobulinemia. *J. Clin. Immunol.*, **6**, 21–25.

91. Saxon, A., Giorgi, J.V., Sherr, E.H. and Kagan, J.M. (1989) Failure of B cells in CVI to transit from proliferation to differentiation is associated with altered B cell surface molecule display. *J. Allergy Clin. Immunol.*, **84**, 44–54.

92. Kruger, G., Welte, K., Ciobanu, N., Cunningham-Rundles, C., Ralph, P., Venuta, S., Feldman, S., Koziner, B., Wang, C.Y., Moore, M.A.S. and Mertelsmann, R. (1984) Interleukin-2 correction of defective *in vitro* T cell mitogenisis in patients with common varied immunodeficiency. *J. Clin. Immunol.*, **4**, 295–303.

93. Fielder, W., Sykora, K.W., Welte, K., Kolitz, J.E., Cunningham-Rundles, C., Holloway, K., Miller, G.A., Souza, L. and Mertelsmann, R. (1987) Defective T cell activation in common variable immunodeficiency is restored by phorbol myristatic acetate (PMA) or allogenic macrophages. *Clin. Immunol. Immunopathol.*, **44**, 206–218.

94. Lopez-Botet, M., Fontan, G., Garcia Rodriguez, M.C. and de Landazuri, M.O. (1982) Relationship between IL-2 synthesis and the proliferative response to PHK in different primary immunodeficiencies. *J. Immunol.*, **128**, 679–683.
95. Spickett, G.P. and Farrant, (1989) The role of lymphokines in common variable hypogammaglobulinemia. *Immunol. Today*, **10**, 192–194.
96. Pastorelli, G., Roncarolo, M.G., Touraine, J.L., Peronne, G., Tovo, P.A. and Devries, J.E. (1989) Peripheral blood lymphocytes of patients with common variable immunodeficiency produce reduced levels of IL-4, IL-2, interferon gamma, but proliferate normally upon activation by mitogens. *Clin. Exp. Immunol.*, **78**, 334–340.
97. Sneller, M.C. and Strober, W. (1990) Abnormalities of lymphokine gene expression in patients with common variable immunodeficiency. *J. Immunol.*, **144**, 3762–3769.
98. Rump, J.A., Schesier, M., Brugger, W., Drager, R., Metchers, I., Adresen, R. and Peter, H.H. (1991) Possible role of IL-2 deficiency for hypogammaglobulinemia in CVI. In Chapel, H.M., Levinsky, R.J. and Webster, A.B.D. (eds) *Progress in Immunodeficiency III*. International Congress and Symposium Series, Royal Society of Medicine Services, London, p. 77.
99. Mayer, L., Fu, S.M., Cunningham-Rundles, C. and Kunkel, H.G. (1984) Polyclonal immunoglobulin secretion in patients with common variable immunodeficiency using monoclonal B cell differentiation factors. *J. Clin. Invest.*, **74**, 2115–2120.
100. Perri, R.T. and Weisdorf, D.J. (1985) Impaired responsiveness to B cell growth factor in a patient with common variable hypogammaglobulinemia. *Blood*, **66**, 345.
101. Matheson, D.S. and Green, B.J. (1987) Defect in production of B cell differentiation factor-like activity by mononuclear cells from a boy with hypogammaglobulinemia. *J. Immunol.*, **138**, 2469.
102. Callard, R.E., Shields, J.G., Smith, S.M., Lau, Y.L. and Levinsky, R.J. (1986) Measurement of human B cell responses to growth and differentiation factors: Relevance for immunodeficiency disease. *Lymphokine Res.*, **5**, 5151.
103. Stohl, W., Cunningham-Rundles, C. and Mayer, L. (1988) *In vitro* induction of T cell dependent B cell differentiation in patients with common varied immunodeficiency. *Clin. Immunol. Immunopathol.*, **49**, 273.
104. Farrant, J., Bryant, A., Almandoz, F., Spickett, G., Evans, S.W. and Webster, A.B.D. (1989) B cell function in acquired "common-variable" hypogammaglobulinemia: Proliferative responses to lymphokines. *Clin. Immunol. Immunopathol.*, **51**, 196–204.
105. Ambrus, J.L. Jr and Fauci, A.S. (1985) Current studies examining regulation of the human B cell cycle. In Webb, D., Pierce, C. and Cohen, S. (eds) *Molecular Basis of Lymphokine Action*. Humana Press, Clifton, NJ, pp. 137–148.
106. Adelman, D.C., Matsuda, T., Hirano, T., Kishimoto, T. and Saxon, A. (1990) Elevated serum IL-6 associated with a failure in B cell differentiation in common variable immunodeficiency. *J. Allerg. Clin. Immunol.*, **86**, 512–520.
107. North, M.E., Spickett, G.P., Webster, A.D.B. and Farrant, J. (1991) Raised serum levels of CD8, CD25, and β2 microglobulin in common variable immunodeficiency. *Clin. Exp. Immunol.*, **86**, 252–255.
108. White, W.B. and Ballow, M. (1985) Modulation of suppressor T cell activity by cimetidine in patients with common variable hypogammaglobulinemia. *N. Engl. J. Med.*, **312**, 198–202.

109. Wright, J.J., Birx, D.L., Wagner, D.K., Waldmann, T.A., Blaese, R.M. and Fleisher, T.A. (1987) Normalization of antibody responsiveness in a patient with common variable hypogammaglobulinemia and HIV infection. *N. Engl. J. Med.*, **317**, 1516–1520.
110. Britigan, B.E. (1991) Diphenylhydantoin-induced hypogammaglobulinemia in a patient infected with HIV. *JAMA*, **90**, 524–526.
111. Dosch, H.M., Jason, J. and Gelfand, E.W. (1982) Transient antibody deficiency and abnormal T suppressor cells induced by phenytoin. *N. Engl. J. Med.*, **306**, 406–409.
112. Sherris, D., Stohl, W. and Mayer, L. (1989) Characteristics of lymphokines mediating B cell growth and differentiation from monoclonal anti-CD3 antibody stimulated T cells. *J. Immunol.*, **142**, 2343–2351.
113. Cunningham-Rundles, C., Mayer, L., Sapira, E.S. and Mendelsohn, L. (1992) Restoration of immunoglobulin secretion in common variable immunodeficiency by *in vitro* treatment with polyethylene glycol conjugated human recombinant interleukin-2. *Clin. Immunol. Immunopathol.*, **64**, 46–56.
114. Weyard, C.M., Goronzy, J., Dallman, M.J., Fathman, G.G. (1986) Administration of recombinant interleukin 2 *in vivo* induces a polyclonal IgM response. *J. Exp. Med.*, **163**, 1607–1612.
115. Tada, H., Shiho, O., Kuroshima, K., Koyama, M. and Tuskamoto, K. (1986) An improved colorimetric assay for interleukin 2. *J. Immunol. Methods*, **93**, 157–165.

Chapter 20

The Role of Polyethylene Glycol–Adenosine Deaminase in the Evolution of Therapy for Adenosine Deaminase Deficiency

MICHAEL S. HERSHFIELD

Division of Rheumatology and Immunology, Duke University Medical Center, Durham, North Carolina, USA

The evolution of therapy for inherited deficiency of adenosine deaminase (ADA) reflects its dual status as an inborn error of metabolism and a primary immunodeficiency syndrome. Following its discovery in 1972 (1) the only treatment was transplantation of HLA-identical bone marrow, just as for other forms of severe combined immunodeficiency disease (SCID) (2). Appreciation of the pathogenic role of deoxyadenosine (dAdo) (3) prompted attempts over the next decade to correct the underlying metabolic defect of patients who lacked a matched marrow donor. Partial exchange transfusion, a form of enzyme replacement, benefited some patients with milder immunodeficiency, but most did not respond (4, 5). A second approach, infusion of deoxycytidine, which can block dAdo phosphorylation and relieve dATP-induced inhibition of ribonucleotide reductase, was of no benefit, even when high deoxycytidine levels were maintained by continuous infusion or by inhibition of its catabolism (6–8). Failure may reflect the inability of deoxycytidine to prevent inactivation of S-adenosylhomocysteine hydrolase (SAHase), another toxic effect of dAdo that occurs in all ADA-deficient patients (9).

New Concepts in Immunodeficiency Diseases. Edited by S. Gupta and C. Griscelli
© 1993 John Wiley & Sons Ltd

Interest in treatment based on the pathogenesis of immune dysfunction waned with the advent of T cell-depleted, haploidentical marrow transplantation (10). Although potentially curative, it soon became apparent that this procedure was neither as benign, nor as likely to produce stable T cell engraftment and recovery of B lymphocyte function, as HLA-matched marrow transplantation (11, 12). By the mid-1980s, cloning of ADA cDNA and the development of retrovirus-based vectors made stem cell gene therapy feasible. However, achieving stable, high-level expression of ADA in lymphoid cells of animals by infusing gene-transfected marrow proved difficult (13). It was unclear when this technique would be attempted in humans. This situation left room for other approaches to therapy and led to a trial of a novel form of enzyme replacement.

Abuchowski and Davis had shown that covalent attachment of polyethylene glycol (PEG) of average molecular weight 5000, an inert, flexible and hydrophilic polymer, could prolong the circulating life and reduce the immunogenicity of enzymes and other proteins (14, 15). PEG-derivatized bovine ADA (PEG–ADA) (16) was produced to test the therapeutic potential of this technology, and as a response to the Orphan Drug Law of 1983, which encouraged the development of therapies for rare disorders. There was initially little interest in PEG–ADA, partly due to the inherent problem of allocating suitable patients with a rare and fatal disease to alternative experimental therapies. Various procedures aimed at improving haploidentical marrow transplantation were under study, and trials of stem cell gene therapy were thought to be imminent (a premature expectation as it turned out). There were also doubts that PEG–ADA would be any more effective in restoring immune function than transfusion therapy, and concerns that it would be too immunogenic or too toxic for chronic therapy.

Several factors led to a trial of PEG–ADA at Duke University in April, 1986. (a) The rationale for enzyme replacement appeared to be sound, provided that higher levels of circulating ADA could be maintained than was possible with erythrocyte transfusion. On a volume basis PEG–ADA possessed ~1800 times the ADA activity of erythrocytes. (b) We felt that key metabolic parameters could be used objectively to establish a minimal effective dose, should effects on immune function be delayed. (c) PEG–ADA was non-toxic in preclinical studies, and available literature indicated that PEG-5000 was harmless and efficiently cleared by the kidney. (d) Finally, the risk of a closely monitored trial seemed justified by the critical and deteriorating condition of the patient under consideration, who had twice failed haploidentical marrow transplantation and had not responded to transfusion therapy. Treatment of this patient and a second child, who had received red cell transfusions monthly for over 8 years, showed that weekly intramuscular injection of PEG–ADA could correct metabolic abnormalities and result in an increase in lymphocyte counts and *in vitro* function (17).

In the past 6 years, 30 patients in North America, Europe, Australia and Japan have been treated with PEG–ADA, which was approved by the US Food and Drug Administration in March 1990. We have acted as a central laboratory for monitoring ADA levels, the metabolic effects of treatment, and the development of anti-ADA antibodies, in collaboration with the physicians and immunologists who have followed clinical status and immune functions. The clinical response of several patients (17–21) and the IgG antibody response to PEG–ADA in 17 patients (22) have been published. We have summarized recommendations for the use of PEG–ADA based on the overall experience through early 1992 (21). The present chapter considers the basis for the effectiveness and limitations of PEG–ADA, and the role of enzyme replacement at a time when therapy for ADA deficiency continues to evolve.

PEG–ADA THERAPY: RATIONALE AND EFFICACY

The long half-life of PEG–ADA in plasma (from 3 to >6 days) is partly achieved at the expense of cellular uptake. Since ADA in plasma is normally much lower than in cells, PEG–ADA is a form of "ectopic" enzyme therapy. However, production of dAdo in viable lymphoid cells is very limited, which is why ADA inhibitors are not toxic to cultured B and T cells in the absence of exogenous ADA substrate (3). Most dAdo is secreted from macrophages that degrade the DNA of senescent cells, red cell progenitors, and presumably other cells undergoing apoptosis (23, 24). If extracellular dAdo is kept low enough (by ADA in plasma), any dAdo arising within lymphocytes should preferentially be exported rather than converted to dATP. This is because the facilitated diffusion transporter that mediates rapid equilibration of intracellular and extracellular nucleoside concentrations has a greater affinity and capacity for dAdo than the cellular kinases capable of phosphorylating dAdo (3, 25, 26). The aim of PEG–ADA therapy is to eliminate circulating dAdo effectively enough to prevent its toxicity to ADA-deficient lymphoid progeny of patient stem cells, enabling them to survive, differentiate, and provide adequate protective immunity.

Immature lymphoid cells are not suitable for biochemical monitoring, but plasma and red cells provide convenient guides for assessing metabolic efficacy, which has been essential in developing replacement therapy. The level of dAXP (total dAdo nucleotides) in ADA-deficient erythrocytes is an index of residual total body ADA activity and an excellent correlate of the severity of immune dysfunction in untreated patients (3, 27, 28). Immunologically normal individuals with "partial ADA deficiency" (undetectable in red cells but 5–70% of normal in nucleated cells) have only slightly elevated red cell dAXP, up to ~20 nmol/ml packed cells (normal, <1–2 nmol/ml). ADA-deficient patients with "delayed onset" of clinical immune deficiency beyond the first year of life generally have levels in the range of 150–300 nmol/ml, compared with 400–1800 nmol/ml in those with typical early-onset SCID. PEG–ADA given once or twice a week (15–60 U/kg per week) maintains plasma ADA activity at ~1.8 to >5 times normal total blood ADA activity. This has reduced red cell dAXP to 3–15 nmol/ml (average ~6 nmol/ml) and normalized SAHase activity in all patients (17–21, and unpublished data), comparable to the metabolic state in "partial ADA deficiency".

In over 80% of patients treated for more than 6 months there is a marked reduction or cessation of opportunistic and life-threatening infections, and in the recurrence and duration of respiratory and gastrointestinal infections. Growth improves and recovery from common childhood infections has been uncomplicated as social interaction is normalized. Clinical improvement is accompanied by recovery of immune function, but aspects of the immune response remain abnormal to some degree in most patients. During the first 2–6 months of therapy a thymic shadow may reappear, and lymphocyte counts and response to mitogens improve to ~30% to >90% of normal (21). In most patients lymphopenia persists and *in vitro* mitogenic responses fluctuate. About half the patients treated for 2 years have discontinued intravenous immunoglobulin (Ig). They have developed specific antibody and antigen-specific *in vitro* proliferative responses after immunization and chicken-pox or other viral infections (21). Discontinuation of intravenous Ig has been based on recovery of functional T helper cells, absence of chronic respiratory insufficiency, and in some cases a normal antibody response to immunization with the bacteriophage φX174 (21a).

About a fifth of patients have shown little improvement in immune function, even when high plasma ADA activity and very low levels of red cell dAXP have been maintained with twice weekly injections of PEG–ADA. While more susceptible to infection than the patients described in the preceding paragraph, during 3 to >5 years of PEG–ADA therapy their clinical course has been relatively good compared with the few long-term responders to chronic erythrocyte transfusion. One child with limited recovery of immune function, now in his fifth year of treatment with PEG–ADA, had two ADA-deficient siblings who died by the age of 2 years, in one case following haploidentical marrow transplantation (A. Rubinstein, unpublished). There have been two deaths in patients receiving PEG–ADA. A respirator-dependent infant who could not be adequately oxygenated died within a week of starting treatment (G. Souillet, unpublished). The second child developed autoimmune hemolytic anemia after a viral infection during the second month of treatment. She did not respond to high-dose intravenous Ig, prednisone, and azathioprine, and died after several weeks from hemolysis and *Candida* sepsis (A. Junker, unpublished).

No allergic or other significant adverse reactions to PEG–ADA have occurred. Antibody to bovine ADA-specific epitopes is detectable by enzyme-linked immunosorbent assay (ELISA) in most patients by 3–8 months of treatment, but these have had little if any effect on enzyme clearance (22). Two patients have developed antibodies that directly inhibit ADA and enhance clearance of PEG–ADA. Tolerance was induced in one, and in the second twice weekly injections of PEG–ADA have compensated for more rapid enzyme elimination; both patients have continued to be treated effectively with PEG–ADA. Based on this experience, we have recommended the monitoring of plasma ADA levels twice monthly during the initial 6–8 months of treatment, then monthly, and testing for anti-ADA antibody if an unexplained fall in enzyme level occurs. We are also investigating the possible use of PEG-modified recombinant human ADA (22).

If the ability to maintain high plasma ADA levels and achieve metabolic detoxification with PEG–ADA is quite uniform, why is immune reconstitution more variable? A growing list of ADA gene mutations, mostly causing amino acid substitutions, have been identified. Although relatively few patients have been studied, thus far there appears to be no overlap of mutations found in patients with SCID and healthy individuals with "partial ADA deficiency" (28–31). Thus genetic differences contribute to clinical heterogeneity among untreated ADA-deficient patients; they may also influence the response to PEG–ADA. We are presently characterizing the mutant ADA alleles of patients receiving PEG–ADA in order to analyze the relationships among genotype, clinical and metabolic severity, and response to enzyme replacement. The relatively large number of patients under treatment, as well as the determination of the three-dimensional structure of ADA (32), provide a strong incentive for undertaking this analysis.

Non-genetic factors also play a role in determining response to PEG–ADA. It is important to appreciate a difference between the group of patients treated prior to approval by the Food and Drugs Administration (FDA), and those who have begun treatment in the last 2 years (21). Most of the former group had been diagnosed before the availability of PEG–ADA; their average age at starting PEG–ADA was 5.0 ± 4.9 years, and only 2 of 13 were less than 1 year of age. This contrasts with an average age of 1.0 ± 1.1 years for the 17 patients who began treatment between April 1990 and March 1992, 14 of whom were ≤ 1 year of age. In addition to cumulative detrimental effects of chronic immunodeficiency on pulmonary function and growth in some older patients, the toxic metabolic effects of prolonged ADA deficiency may have limited the capacity for immune reconstitution. Experience with the first 13 patients ranges from 2 to 6 years (mean, 4.1 years). However, they may not be as representative as the more recent group of 17 patients, who have been under treatment for an average of 10 months, for defining the response to PEG–ADA when it is begun at the time of diagnosis.

THE CURRENT ROLE OF PEG–ADA

Should a new patient with ADA deficiency who has no matched sibling donor be treated by haploidentical marrow transplantation or PEG–ADA as primary therapy? Since this question is not settled, it is worth reviewing how this choice has been made over the past 6 years—a period when experience with PEG–ADA was emerging.

One view is that haploidentical transplantation, which is potentially curative, should always be performed and shown to have failed before enzyme replacement is attempted, as with the first patient to receive PEG–ADA. However, the parents and pediatric immunologists caring for the 29 subsequent patients have carefully considered, but decided against, haploidentical transplantation. It is unlikely that they were uninformed about the potential benefit of transplantation. Many of these physicians had chosen to transplant in previous cases; some had helped to develop haploidentical transplantation procedures. We provided each physician with the names of all investigators following patients under treatment with PEG–ADA so that they might obtain direct information about response to PEG–ADA, as well as any additional recent experience with haploidentical transplantation. We also provided an up-to-date summary of the overall experience with PEG–ADA. Like this chapter, these summaries indicated that while PEG–ADA therapy was safe and could ameliorate the immunodeficiency and clinical course of SCID, it did not restore endogenous immune function to normal, and it might elicit anti-ADA antibodies.

Several factors influenced the choice of therapy. For physicians, these were primarily the age, clinical condition, and residual immune function of the patient, and the morbidity and 25–50% mortality associated with haploidentical transplantation (11, 12). PEG–ADA is currently a very expensive therapy. Although it is available to patients who lack any form of insurance, this has been an obvious concern for parents and physicians. In critically ill patients with active pneumonia, who are at highest risk of dying after transplantation, PEG–ADA was considered a safer therapy (indeed it has been life saving in some severely debilitated patients too ill to undergo transplantation). Conversely, residual immune function of patients with delayed or late-onset disease was considered likely to cause graft rejection; the risk associated with intense cytoablation to promote engraftment in these patients was felt to be unacceptable. For a substantial group of patients the choice of therapy was less clear cut and a matter of judgement, experience, and parental preference. Initially most were transplanted, but the doubling of the number of patients who have begun enzyme replacement in the past 2 years compared to the previous 4 suggests this may be changing. Starting PEG–ADA does not exclude the possibility of other forms of treatment at a later time. If PEG–ADA is discontinued immune function will deteriorate within a few weeks, so that transplantation could then be performed (under appropriate conditions to prevent serious infections from recurring prior to engraftment). This option has not been exercised to date, though it is under consideration in some patients with limited response to PEG–ADA.

PEG–ADA is currently used in conjunction with the form of mature T cell gene therapy under investigation at the National Institutes of Health (NIH), which now involves two patients who are also receiving PEG–ADA (a response to enzyme replacement is necessary to provide the functional mature T cells that are then transfected *in vitro*). One of the patients had a delayed and the other a late onset of immune deficiency; both had responded well to PEG–ADA, with recovery of antigen-specific immune function and gratifying clinical improvement (18, 21). Thus, far, both have continued to receive full doses of PEG–ADA, which provides each week the ADA activity of $\sim 10^{12}$ normal T cells. For these reasons, and others beyond the scope of this discussion, until PEG–ADA is discontinued it will be very difficult to judge the benefit derived from gene therapy alone.

Among the possible reasons offered for targeting ADA cDNA to mature T cells are: (a) that haploidentical marrow transplantation can cure SCID due to ADA deficiency, even though only donor T cells engraft; and (b) that in individuals with "partial ADA deficiency" as little as 5% of normal ADA activity is sufficient to prevent immune dysfunction. The implication that gene-transfected T cells expressing as little as 5% of normal will provide sufficient ADA to treat the underlying enzyme deficiency is not justified by these statements, which require elaboration. After haploidentical transplantation performed without preconditioning, the *only* circulating T cells are donor derived. Recovery of immune function results from the generation of a T cell repertoire from engrafted, not endogenous, stem cells. The simplest explanation for failure of endogenous T cells to reappear is that the engrafted donor cells do not adequately protect the patient's own immature T cells from dAdo toxicity. We have found dAXP in ADA-deficient erythrocytes of six such transplant recipients to be 5–20-fold higher than in red cells of PEG–ADA-treated patients (unpublished data). It has not yet been demonstrated that circulating T cells in the two patients undergoing gene therapy express ADA levels even as high as occur in engrafted T cells after haploidentical transplantation. With regard to the second statement, patients with partial ADA deficiency have substantial residual ADA activity in many tissues, not solely in their T cells. This is clear from the fact they are essentially metabolically, as well as immunologically, normal.

In contrast to mature T cell gene therapy, as little as 5% residual activity expressed in lymphoid progeny of ADA cDNA-transfected patient stem cells might be sufficient to allow immune reconstitution. Success would depend on the efficiency of introducing the gene into stem cells and on the level and stability of ADA expression. As with the response to PEG–ADA, it is also possible that irreversible effects of ADA deficiency may affect the degree of immune reconstitution in some patients. It would be very gratifying one day to see all patients under treatment with PEG–ADA cured by a safe and reliable form of stem cell gene therapy. For the moment, PEG–ADA therapy will continue to play an important role in the treatment of ADA deficiency.

ACKNOWLEDGEMENTS

The author is a consultant to Enzon Inc. We appreciate discussions with the following investigators who have contributed samples and information about the immune function and clinical status of patients under treatment with PEG–ADA: M. Ballow, J. Bastian, M. Berger, C. Bordignon, C. Bory, R. Buckley, S. Chaffee, S. Douglas, J. ElDahr, A. Fischer, D. Girault, B. Hillman, D. Hummell, A. Junker, R. Kobayashi, A. Kobayashi, A. Lawton, G. Marshall, D. Matheson, H. Ochs, M. Okanao, C. Roifman, A. Rubenstein, Y. Sakiyama, R. Schiff, C. Schlossman, R.U. Sorensen, G. Souillet, E.R. Stiehm, D. Umetsu, D. Wara and K. Weinberg.

REFERENCES

1. Giblett, E.R., Anderson, J.E., Cohen, F., Pollara, B. and Meuwissen, H.J. (1972) Adenosine deaminase deficiency in two patients with severely impaired cellular immunity. *Lancet*, **ii**, 1067–1069.

2. Parkman, R., Gelfand, E.W., Rosen, F.S., Sanderson, A. and Hirschhorn, R. (1975) Severe combined immunodeficiency and adenosine deaminase deficiency. *N. Engl. J. Med.*, **292**, 714–719.

3. Kredich, N.M. and Hershfield, M.S. (1989) Immunodeficiency diseases caused by adenosine deaminase deficiency and purine nucleoside phosphorylase deficiency. In Scriver, C.R., Beaudet, A.L., Sly, W.S. and Valle, D. (eds) *The Metabolic Basis of Inherited Disease* (6th edn). McGraw-Hill, New York, pp. 1045–1075.

4. Polmar, S.H., Stern, R.C., Schwartz, A.L., Wetzler, E.M., Chase, P.A. and Hirschhorn, R. (1976) Enzyme replacement therapy for adenosine deaminase deficiency and severe combined immunodeficiency. *N. Engl. J. Med.*, **295**, 1337–1343.

5. Polmar, S.H. (1980) Metabolic aspects of immunodeficiency disease. *Semin. Hematol.*, **17**, 30–43.

6. Davies, E.G., Levinski, R.J., Webster, D.R., Simmonds, H.A. and Perrett, D. (1982) Effect of red cell transfusions, thymic hormone and deoxycytidine in severe combined immunodeficiency due to adenosine deaminase deficiency. *Clin. Exp. Immunol.*, **50**, 303–310.

7. Ammann, A.J., Cowan, M.J., Martin, D.W. and Wara, D. (1983) Dipyridamole and intravenous deoxycytidine therapy in a patient with adenosine deaminase deficiency. In Wedgwood, R.J., Rosen, F.S. and Paul, N.W. (eds) *Primary Immunodeficiency Diseases*. March of Dimes Birth Defects Original Artical Series, Liss, New York, pp. 117–120.

8. Cowan, M.J., Wara, D.W. and Ammann, A.J. (1985) Deoxycytidine therapy in two patients with adenosine deaminase deficiency and severe immunodeficiency diseases. *Clin. Immunol. Immunopathol.*, **37**, 30–36.

9. Hershfield, M.S., Kredich, N.M., Ownby, D.R., Ownby, H. and Buckley, R. (1979) In vivo inactivation of erythrocyte S-adenosylhomocysteine hydrolase by 2'-deoxyadenosine in adenosine deaminase-deficient patients. *J. Clin. Invest.*, **63**, 807–811.
10. Reisner, Y., Kapoor, N., Kirkpatrick, D., Pollack, M.S., Cunningham-Rundles, S., Dupont, B., Hodes, M.Z., Good, R.A. and O'Reilly, R.J. (1983) Transplantation for severe combined immunodeficiency with HLA-A,B,D,DR incompatible parental marrow cells fractionated by soybean agglutinin and sheep red blood-cells. *Blood*, **61**, 341–348.
11. O'Reilly, R.J., Keever, C.A., Small, T.N. and Brochstein, J. (1989) The use of HLA-non-identical T-cell-depleted marrow for transplants for correction of severe combined immunodeficiency diseases. *Immunodef. Rev.*, **1**, 273–309.
12. Fischer, A., Landais, P., Friedrich, W., Morgan, G., Gerritsen, B., Fasth, A., Porta, F., Griscelli, C., Goldman, S.F., Levinsky, R. and Vossen, J. (1990) European experience of bone marrow transplantation for severe combined immunodeficiency. *Lancet*, **336**, 850–854.
13. Belmont, J.W., Henkel, T.J., Wager, S.K., Chang, S.M. and Caskey, C.T. (1986) Towards gene therapy for adenosine deaminase deficiency. *Ann. Clin. Res.*, **18**, 322–326.
14. Abuchowski, A., McCoy, J.R., Palczuk, N.C., van Es, T. and Davis, F.F. (1977) Effect of attachment of polyethylene glycol on immunogenicity and circulating life of bovine liver catalase. *J. Biol. Chem.*, **252**, 3582–3586.
15. Abuchowski, A., van Es, T., Palczuk, N.C. and Davis, F.F. (1977) Alteration of immunological properties of bovine serum albumin by covalent attachment of polyethylene glycol. *J. Biol. Chem.*, **252**, 3578–3581.
16. Davis, S., Abuchowski, A., Park, Y.K. and Davis, F.F. (1981) Alteration of the circulating life and antigenic properties of bovine adenosine deaminase in mice by attachment of polyethylene glycol. *Clin. Exp. Immunol.*, **46**, 649–652.
17. Hershfield, M.S., Buckley, R.H., Greenberg, M.L., Melton, A.L., Schiff, R., Hatem, C., Kurtzberg, J., Markert, M.L., Kobayashi, R.H., Kobayashi, A.L. and Abuchowski, A. (1987) Treatment of adenosine deaminase deficiency with polyethylene glycol-modified adenosine deaminase. *N. Engl. J. Med.*, **316**, 589–596.
18. Levy, Y., Hershfield, M.S., Fernandez-Mejia, C., Polmar, S.H., Scudiery, D., Berger, M. and Sorensen, R.U. (1988) Adenosine deaminase deficiency with late onset of recurrent infections: Response to treatment with polyethylene glycol-modified adenosine deaminase (PEG–ADA). *J. Pediatr.*, **113**, 312–317.
19. Bory, C., Boulieu, R., Souillet, G., Chantin, C., Rolland, M.O., Mathieu, M. and Hershfield, M.S. (1990) Comparison of red cell transfusion and polyethylene glycol-modified adenosine deaminase therapy in an adenosine deaminase-deficient child. *Pediatr. Res.*, **28**, 127–130.
20. Girault, D., Le Deist, F., Debré, M., Pérignon, J.L., Herbelin, C., Griscelli, C., Scudiery, D., Hershfield, M. and Fischer, A. (1992) Traitement du deficit en adenosine desaminase par l'adenosine desaminase couplée au polyethylene glycol (PEG–ADA). *Arch. Fr. Pediatr.*, **49**, 339–343.
21. Hershfield, M.S., Chaffee, S. and Sorensen, R.U. (in press) Enzyme replacement therapy with PEG–ADA in adenosine deaminase deficiency: Overview and case reports of three patients, including two now receiving gene therapy. *Pediatr. Res.*
21a. Ochs, H.D., Buckley, R.M., Kobayashi, R.H., Kobayashi, A.L., Sorensen, R.U., Douglas, S.D., Hamilton, B.L. and Hershfield, M.S. (1992) Antibody responses to bacteriophage ØX174 in patients with adenosine deaminase deficiency. *Blood*, **80**, 1163–1171.

22. Chaffee, S., Mary, A., Stiehm, E.R., Girault, D., Fischer, A. and Hershfield, M.S. (1992) IgG antibody response to polyethylene glycol-modified adenosine deaminase (PEG–ADA) in patients with adenosine deaminase deficiency. *J. Clin. Invest.*, **89**, 1643–1651.
23. Chan, T.-S. (1979) Purine excretion by mouse peritoneal macrophages lacking adenosine deaminase activity. *Proc. Nat. Acad. Sci. USA*, **76**, 925–929.
24. Henderson, J.F. and Smith, C.M. (1981) Mechanisms of deoxycoformycin toxicity in vivo. In Tattersal, M.H.N. and Fox, R.M. (eds) *Nucleosides in Cancer Treatment*. Academic Press, Sydney, pp. 208–217.
25. Jarvis, S.M. (1987) Kinetics and molecular properties of nucleoside transporters in animal cells. In Gerlach, E. and Becker, B.F. (eds) *Topics and Perspectives in Adenosine Research*. Springer, Berlin, pp. 102–117.
26. Hershfield, M.S., Fetter, J.E., Small, W.C., Bagnara, A.S., Williams, S.R., Ullman, B., Martin, D.W.J., Wasson, D.B. and Carson, D.A. (1982) Effects of mutational loss of adenosine kinase and deoxycytidine kinase on deoxyATP accumulation and deoxyadenosine toxicity in cultured CEM cells. *J. Biol. Chem.*, **257**, 6380–6386.
27. Morgan, G., Levinsky, R.J., Hugh, J.K., Fairbanks, L.D., Morris, G.S. and Simmonds, H.A. (1987) Heterogeneity of biochemical, clinical and immunological parameters in severe combined immunodeficiency due to adenosine deaminase deficiency. *Clin. Exp. Immunol.*, **70**, 491–499.
28. Hirschhorn, R. (1990) Adenosine deaminase deficiency. In Rosen, F.S. and Seligmann, M. (eds) *Immunodeficiency Review*. Harwood Academic, New York, pp. 175–198.
29. Hirschhorn, R., Tzall, S. and Ellenbogen, A. (1990) Hot spot mutations in adenosine deaminase deficiency. *Proc. Nat. Acad. Sci. USA*, **87**, 6171–6175.
30. Hirschhorn, R., Chakravarti, V., Puck, J. and Douglas, S.D. (1991) Homozygosity for a newly identified missense mutation in a patient with very severe combined immunodeficiency due to adenosine deaminase deficiency (ADA–SCID). *Am. J. Hum. Genet.*, **49**, 878–885.
31. Akeson, A.L., Wiginton, D.A., Dusing, M.R., States, J.C. and Hutton, J.J. (1988) Mutant human adenosine deaminase alleles and their expression by transfection into fibroblasts. *J. Biol. Chem.*, **263**, 16291–16296.
32. Wilson, D.K., Rudolph, F.B. and Quiocho, F.A. (1991) Atomic structure of adenosine deaminase complexed with a transition-state analog: Understanding catalysis and immunodeficiency mutations. *Science*, **252**, 1278–1284.

Chapter 21

Gene Therapy for Immunodeficiency Disease

KENNETH W. CULVER and R. MICHAEL BLAESE

Cellular Immunology Section, Metabolism Branch, National Cancer Institute,
National Institutes of Health, Bethesda, Maryland, USA

Gene therapy has been traditionally thought of as the ultimate cure for genetic diseases (1). The possibilty of correcting genetic defects at the fundamental level of the gene defect instead of merely treating the associated manifestations is very appealing. In practice, the challenges of this approach have proven to be formidable, but progress in clinical applications are finally being made. However, applications in the non-inherited diseases such as human immunodeficiency virus (HIV)-induced immunodeficiency and cancer will likely have the broadest applications in the next few years.

The development of gene therapy for any genetic disease first requires the identification and cloning of the gene responsible for that condition. Of the more than 20 primary immunodeficiency diseases recognized by the World Health Organization Committee on Primary Immunodeficiency (2), the genes for only four diseases have thus far been cloned (adenosine deaminase deficiency, purine nucleoside phosphorylase deficiency, leukocyte adhesion defect and chronic granulomatous disease). The understanding of the molecular genetics of HIV has made remarkable progress in comparison to the development of a full understanding of the actual mechanism that results in the associated immunodeficiency (3).

New Concepts in Immunodeficiency Diseases. Edited by S. Gupta and C. Griscelli
© 1993 John Wiley & Sons Ltd

OBSTACLES TO THE WIDESPREAD APPLICATION OF GENE THERAPY

Once a gene has been isolated and its function understood, work can begin on developing a gene therapy method. The transfer method must deliver the corrective gene to the proper cells to result in gene expression at a level sufficient to restore normal biochemical functioning. High-efficiency gene transfer may be required to reach this goal in order to prevent residual, defective "non-corrected" cells from interfering with or limiting the effectiveness of the "cured cells". If the corrected cells do not have an intrinsic survival advantage over the defective cells, it may be necessary to use cytoablative therapy (chemotherapy or irradiation) to eliminate the residual defective cells. If the gene defect results in the production of a pathological gene product (e.g. hemoglobin S), a procedure to prevent production of the abnormal gene product must be developed in addition to conferring production of the correct gene product. Gene expression may require tight regulation depending on the cell's position in the cell cycle or to respond rapidly to the concentration of critical intracellular messengers. It might be necessary to coordinate the timing and level of expression of the inserted gene with that of other genes within the cell. Furthermore, the gene delivery procedure should be simple, safe and capable of meeting additional requirements such as avoidance of introducing genes into the patient's germ cells (i.e. spermatozoa).

These requirements pose very significant obstacles to development of gene therapy for many inherited and non-inherited diseases. The current body of scientific knowledge including the isolation of genes, gene transfer methods and ability to regulate gene expression is just not yet sufficiently developed to permit attempts at gene therapy for most of the known 4000 inherited diseases. The primary immunodeficiency diseases appear to be more amenable to gene therapy than many other genetic diseases. Any genetic disease that can be successfully reconstituted by allogeneic bone marrow transplantation should theoretically be treatable by genetic correction of the patient's own bone marrow stem cell population (4). The obstacles to the development of a gene therapy method for the treatment of HIV infection are similar. Ideally, HIV gene therapy would be delivered to all HIV-infected cells to eliminate the HIV-infected cells or permanently block activation of HIV virus production. Methods to target all of the HIV-infected cells *in vivo* have not yet been defined.

IDENTIFICATION AND ISOLATION OF THE DISEASE-CAUSING GENES

The first requirement for application of gene therapy is the identification and cloning of the involved gene. There are an estimated 100 000 or more genes in the human genome. Usually gene isolation follows a sequence, mapping its location to a specific chromosome and then subchromosomal location with the aid of a variety of techniques including linkage analysis of restriction fragment length polymorphisms (RFLP), somatic cell hybrids and reverse genetics (5). The involved gene has been mapped in ten of the primary immunodeficiency disorders, with four of them having been cloned (Table 21.1). In addition to these disorders, several other immunodeficiency diseases have well-characterized defects but the precise molecular genetic basis of the disease has not yet been solved. As an example, class II MHC deficiency syndrome is a severe immunodeficiency disease associated with deficient expression of some or all of the MHC determinants usually expressed on the cell surface. It has been clearly established that the MHC structural genes themselves are not defective in these patients, and evidence has been presented that the defect may lie in the regulatory elements controlling expression of these genes.

Table 21.1 Subchromosomal locations of the gene loci for the primary immunodeficiencies

Disease genes that have been localized and cloned	
Adenosine deaminase deficiency	20q13.4
Purine nucleoside phosphorylase deficiency	14q13.1
Leukocyte adhesion defect (CD18 deficiency)	21q22.3
Chronic granulomatous disease	
gp91-*phox*	Xp21.1
p22-*phox*	16q24
p47-*phox*	7q11.23
p67-*phox*	1q25
Disease genes that have been localized	
Ataxia–telangiectasia	11q22–23
X-linked SCID	Xq1.3
Wiskott–Aldrich syndrome	Xp11–11.3
X-linked agammaglobulinemia	Xp21.33–22
X-linked lymphoproliferative syndrome	Xq26–27
X-linked immunodeficiency with hyper IgM	Xq26–27

Mapping and cloning of the involved gene is just the first step in the process of developing gene therapy. The normal function of that gene and its product must be thoroughly understood before a rational plan can be formulated for genetic correction. For example, genes such as insulin encode for products which are under very close physiological regulation. Therefore, the genetic therapy may require genetic correction of these regulatory elements or gene insertion in conjunction with those regulatory elements. The best initial candidates for gene therapy are diseases that involve a relatively simple "housekeeping" gene that does not require close regulation and whose function is not absolutely critical to the differentiation and development of the affected cell lineage.

GENE TRANSFER TECHNIQUES

A number of methods have been developed for the introduction of genes into living cells (Table 21.2). These include chemical methods (e.g. calcium phosphate precipitation), physical techniques (e.g. electroporation, microinjection, particle bombardment), fusion (e.g. liposomes), receptor-mediated endocytosis (e.g. DNA–protein complexes, viral envelope/capsid-DNA complexes) and recombinant viruses (e.g. herpes simplex, adenovirus, adeno-associated virus (AAV) and Moloney murine leukemia virus (MoMLV)). Each technique has its own theoretical advantages and disadvantages. For example, if a corrective gene is to be inserted into the lympho-hematopoietic stem cell, a process which will give highly efficient stable integration of the inserted gene must be a major feature of the transfer system. Otherwise, as the stem cell proliferates and differentiates, the inserted gene could be progressively diluted out and eventually lost from, or unevenly distributed in, the mature erythroid, myeloid and lymphoid lineages. By contrast, gene insertion into a terminally differentiated non-

Table 21.2 Gene transfer methods

	Transfer efficiency	Integration efficiency
Chemical		
Calcium phosphate precipitation	Low	Low
Physical		
Electroporation	Low	Low
Microinjection[a]	High	High
Particle bombardment	High	Low
Fusion		
Liposomes	High	Low
Receptor-mediated endocytosis		
DNA–protein complexes	Low	Low
Viral envelope/capsid-DNA complexes	Low	Low
Recombinant viruses		
Herpes simplex	High	Low
Adenovirus	High	Low
Adeno-associated virus (AAV)[b]	High	Low
Moloney murine leukemia virus (MoMLV)	High	High
Human immunodeficiency virus (HIV)	High	High

[a]Only a small number of cells can be manipulated.
[b]Potential for site-specific integration.

proliferative tissue such as skeletal muscle or liver might not need integration as a feature of the gene transfer system. Since the immune system involves cells which proliferate actively during differentiation, an integrated gene is probably essential for this population.

MoMLV Vectors

The MoMLV-based retroviral vectors have distinct advantages for gene therapy of proliferating tissues like the lymphoid system (6). Most importantly, these vectors integrate into the chromosomes of the target cell, becoming a stable part of the inheritance of that cell, being passed along to all cell progeny during normal cell division. In addition, retroviral vector systems can be highly efficient for gene transfer, approaching 95% in some cell types *in vitro*. Potential disadvantages of retroviral vectors include the fact that they randomly integrate into the host cell genome. Random integration means that vector-transduced cells may behave differently from one integration site to another (7). This possibility stems from differences in the local environment of the chromosome where neighboring genes may greatly influence the level of gene expression achieved for the vector-carried genes (8). For many functional gene systems, a very wide range of gene expression from cell to cell is not acceptable.

Random integration also provides for the possibility that the integration event could disable a gene which was critical or absolutely required for normal cell function or survival. In such a case, the transduced cell might be killed. With thousands or millions of cells treated, the loss of an occasional cell would probably be of little consequence. A more ominous theoretical problem with random integration would result if vector insertion resulted in the activation of an oncogene or inactivated tumor suppressor gene, potentially contributing to the eventual transformation of that cell to a malignant phenotype (insertional mutagenesis). While this is a theoretical possibility, the use of replication *in*competent retroviral vectors has never been reported to result in malignant transformation in any *in vivo* system (9–11). Finally, retroviral vectors only integrate their genes into cells that are actively proliferating and synthesizing DNA. Totipotent bone marrow stem cells are not generally actively proliferating cells, but are usually in a G0 state. Therefore, before retroviral vectors can be effectively used to insert genes into stem cells, manipulations to induce stem cell proliferation must be applied (12).

HIV Vectors

HIV vectors have been utilized to study selective HIV infectivity and to study their possible use as vehicles for Tat-inducible foreign genes (13–16). Since Tat is normally found only in HIV-infected cells, the use of Tat-inducible promoters may be used to selectively destroy HIV-containing cells. For instance, the diphtheria toxin A chain under control of the Tat and Rev have significantly impaired virus production in Hela cells *in vitro* (17, 18). Since HIV vectors would selectively target gene delivery to CD4+ cells that may harbor the HIV genome, their use warrants intensive study.

HIV vectors can be disabled (19–22). However, there is a substantial risk of HIV recombinatorial events that might lead to new infectious HIV viruses that may render HIV vectors unsuitable for human use. One method to minimize the risk would be the use of an HIV vector containing a "suicide gene" such as herpes simplex thymidine kinase which confers a sensitivity to acyclovir/ganciclovir, a property that allows the destruction of the vector-containing cells when treated with one of the anti-herpes drugs (23–25).

Development of an Injectable, Targetable Vector

The ideal form of gene therapy for the treatment of immunodeficiency diseases would be the direct injection of the gene into the body. In this ideal delivery system, the gene would "home" to the desired tissue, enter the desired cells, cause deletion of the defective gene or irreversibly bind to the target gene in the host cell genome (26, 27). To target specific cell types *in vivo*, one would need to define a specific cell surface receptor (e.g. CD4 for HIV-infected cells or CD34 for stem cells) or a property (e.g. galactose residues found primarily on hepatocytes) that would selectively bind the gene or the vehicle carrying the gene to the specific cell types. The use of the natural specific tropism of different viruses is another strategy for targeting gene delivery (e.g. rabies virus for brain, hepatitis virus for liver). Progress is slow, but many laboratories are working toward the development of some form of injectable targetable vector.

BONE MARROW TRANSPLANTATION FOR IMMUNODEFICIENCY DISEASE

Bone Marrow Transplantation for Primary Immunodeficiency Disorders

Because of the potential wide application of bone marrow gene therapy and the ease of *ex vivo* manipulation, diseases which can be treated by bone marrow transplantation have been the leading candidates for early gene therapy protocols. In 1968, allogeneic bone marrow transplantation was first successfully applied in a child with severe combined immunodeficiency disease (SCID) (28). If a child with SCID has an HLA-matched sibling donor, marrow transplantation usually does not require preparative cytoablation to enhance engraftment (29). This is thought to occur because the engrafted normal bone marrow stem cells have a selective growth advantage *in vivo* over the genetically defective lymphoid cells, allowing the donor cells to predominate. Unfortunately, such a selective growth advantage is not expected in all immunodeficiency diseases (e.g. Wiskott–Aldrich syndrome (WAS)). Autologous stem cell gene therapy for diseases without a selective growth advantage will probably require cytoreduction to allow engraftment of a sufficient number of genetically corrected cells to provide full reconstitution. The need for cytoreduction will increase the morbidity and mortality of the procedure as it does with conventional bone marrow transplantation. However, gene therapy with autologous cells will still have the advantage of a very low risk of graft-versus-host disease.

Bone Marrow Transplantation for HIV Infection

Bone marrow transplantation has been attempted for the treatment of AIDS (30). The administration of HIV-negative syngeneic marrow, syngeneic peripheral blood lymphocytes and zidovudine to identical twins with HIV infection resulted in transient improvement in immune functions without an associated improvement in clinical status. The genetic manipulation to protect non-HIV-infected T cell or stem cells from HIV infection appears to be required for the long-term immunological reconstitution of AIDS patients.

Bone Marrow Versus Peripheral Blood Stem Cells

Stem cells for genetic correction may be obtained by standard bone marrow harvest from the marrow space (BMSC) or from the peripheral blood (PBSC) (31). Infusions of PBSC in humans have engrafted, restoring hematopoiesis following marrow ablation (32, 33). However, it should be noted that it is uncertain if the genetic correction of immunodeficiency diseases using PBSCs will be as effective and durable as correction with BMSCs. The potential advantage of PBSC for gene therapy is the ease with which they could be repeatedly collected if a serial treatment strategy is to be followed.

EXPERIMENTAL MODELS OF BONE MARROW GENE THERAPY

Stem cell gene modification has been under intensive investigation for several years. Initial interest centered on the hemoglobinopathies as candidate diseases for gene therapy with globin gene transfer with retroviral vectors the primary goal (1). In murine systems several genes have been successfully transferred to the hematopoietic stem cells, resulting in long-term expression in transplanted animals. It was found that pretreatment of the bone marrow donor animals with 5-fluorouracil (5-Fu), which killed the proliferating progenitor cells, induced compensatory proliferation of the totipotent stem cells, allowing successful retroviral gene transfer.

Stem Cell Gene Transfer in Large Animals

Unfortunately, attempts to replicate these successes in larger animals were unsuccessful (34). In one model we could readily introduce a corrective adenosine deaminase (ADA) gene into cultural human ADA(–) T cells *in vitro* with the SAX retrovirus vector. We then used the same vector to treat freshly collected bone marrow from rhesus or cynomolgus monkeys. The monkeys were lethally irradiated and then reconstituted by transplantation with the "gene-treated" autologous marrow. In over 20 animals studied in these experiments, some recipients did produce human ADA in their circulating mononuclear cells, but the level of gene expression was low and disappeared within a few weeks to months (35). Although these studies were disappointing in that stable, long-term gene expression was not achieved, they did demonstrate that retroviral vectors could transfer genes into primate cells and that some gene expression could be detected in peripheral cells following bone marrow treatment. In addition, the gene transfer procedure appeared to be safe in that no monkey experienced unexpected consequences following the transplant of gene-modified cells.

There are several factors which probably contribute to the failure of these experiments to result in stable long-term gene expression. Among the most likely is the observation that totipotent stem cells are usually in a non-proliferative (G0) state while the retroviral gene transfer system employed is only effective in introducing its genes into proliferating cells. Thus, genes were probably introduced into a more mature proliferating progenitor population which gave transient expression of the gene before the cells reached senescence, to be replaced by more primitive cells which had not been in cycle earlier and thus had not acquired the gene. Two parallel strategies have been followed in attempts to improve these results: (a) procedures to enrich the stem cells in the population exposed to the retroviral vector, and (b) the use of growth factors to induce the totipotent stem cells to proliferate. While these procedures were being developed, we began a series of studies exploring the use of alternative cellular vehicles for gene therapy, specifically T lymphocytes.

Isolation of Totipotent Stem Cells

Totipotent stem cells are rare relative to the number of more differentiated, progenitor cells in the bone marrow. To improve the efficiency of gene transfer into totipotent stem cells relative to those more mature cells, the PBSCs or BMSCs can be enriched for totipotent stem cells using CD34 monoclonal antibodies (MAb). CD34 is a cell surface glycoprotein found primarily on stem cells. CD34+ cells typically represent 1–4% of mononuclear cells in the bone marrow and 0.02–0.05% of peripheral blood mononuclear cells (36,

37). The percentage of CD34+ mononuclear cells in the peripheral blood increases to 1–2% with injections of certain growth factors (38, 39). Separation of cells with CD34 MAb enriches for totipotent stem cells about 50–150-fold (40, 41). Stem cell gene transfer experiments in man exploiting these new approaches have recently received approval by the Recombinant DNA Advisory Committee of the NIH (RAC) and should be initiated in early 1993.

Introduction of Totipotent Stem Cell Proliferation

The *in vitro* induction of totipotent cell proliferation is a difficult and delicate task because these primitive cells need to remain in the totipotent state. If the induction of proliferation also results in differentiation, then the population of transduced cells may skew to the differentiating lineage(s), possibly diminishing or eliminating the transduction of the essential cell types as well as failing to achieve a truly self-renewing gene-corrected stem cell population. A variety of factors have been tested for their ability to induce proliferation of stem cells (42). These include the colony-stimulating factors (CSF) macrophage-CSF (M-CSF), granulocyte-CSF (G-CSF), granulocyte–macrophage-CSF (GM-CSF) and multi-CSF (interleukin 3, IL-3). Other factors with some effect include IL-1 and IL-6 and stem cell factor (SCF). None of these cytokines alone is sufficient in inducing proliferation to result in retroviral-mediated transduction of more than 1% of primate totipotent cells. However, combinations of these factors (e.g. IL-3 and IL-6) have been quite encouraging as shown by a transduction frequency of 1–5% of human stem cells, measured by G418 resistant colonies *in vitro* and the percentage of gene marked cells in the peripheral blood of transplanted primates (43). The addition of SCF to IL-3 and IL-6 appears to further increase transduction efficiency in murine, primate and human cells without a loss in repopulating ability, as measured in transplanted mice.

GENE THERAPY FOR ADA DEFICIENCY

Genetics

ADA deficiency (EC 3.5.4.4) is inherited as an autosomal recessive disorder with a frequency of less than 1 in 100 000 births. At the molecular and genetic level, ADA deficiency is the most extensively studied of all the congenital immunodeficiency diseases. This was the first of the immunodeficiency diseases in which the molecular defect was identified (44) and the first in which the gene was cloned (1983) (45–47). A defect in the ADA gene may lead to absent or diminished ADA enzyme activity in all tissues of the body but the only consistent clinical consequences affect the immune system, resulting in SCID. Both point mutations and deletions of the gene have been identified (48–52). Most patients studied have point mutations that result in the loss of enzymatic function or an instability of the protein.

Clinical Manifestations

ADA(–) SCID is a heterogeneous disorder with clinical presentations ranging from mild (repeated infections with diagnosis after several years of age) to severe (the development of severe infections within several days of birth) (53). ADA catalyzes the conversion of adenosine and 2'-deoxyadenosine (dAdo) to inosine and 2'-deoxyinosine in the normal pathway of purine catabolism and salvage. In the absence of ADA (dAdo) in particular accumulates to high levels in the tissues and body fluids of these patients. Subsequently the dAdo becomes phosphorylated to deoxy-ATP, which acts to inhibit DNA synthesis and can result in cell death. T cells are the primary site of the toxic effects of ADA deficiency, although B cells may also be severely reduced in number and function (54).

Bone Marrow Transplantation

The current treatment of choice for ADA(–) SCID is an HLA-matched sibling bone marrow transplant. This therapy can be curative for those 20–30% of children fortunate enough to have an HLA-identical sibling donor, with the best results achieved if the transplant can be performed before the child acquires severe opportunistic infections (55). The in-depth understanding of the biochemical and molecular basis of this disease has allowed the development of a number of experimental therapies for children without an HLA identical sibling, including the first use of enzyme replacement therapy and the first trial of gene therapy.

Enzyme Replacement Therapy

In the mid 1970s attempts at enzyme replacement therapy were initiated because of the observation that dAdo was freely diffusible across cell membranes. It was reasoned that it might not be necessary to deliver the enzyme to the substrate in this disease since the freely diffusible substrate could find its way to the enzyme if a concentration gradient was established. Irradiated red blood cell transfusions, as a cellular source of ADA, was administered to a number of children (56). A few patients showed some hopeful signs of early immune reconstitution and evidence that dAdo levels were indeed lowered as a result of the treatment. Unfortunately, the majority of ADA(–) SCID patients experienced only minimal immunological improvement and repeated transfusions risked associated iron overload and infectious transfusion complications. Nevertheless, the concept of enzyme replacement was proved, and in 1985 a new form of enzyme replacement was initiated, with parenteral injections of bovine ADA conjugated to polyethylene glycol (PEG–ADA; Adagen) (57). Children receive this drug as an intramuscular injection once or twice weekly, resulting in a substantial increase in plasma levels of ADA activity and a marked decrease in dAdo levels. The clinical responses to PEG–ADA have generally been better than that achieved with red blood cell transfusions, without the risks associated with transfusions. Most, but not all, children derive some clinical benefit from PEG–ADA, with a few of the children demonstrating near-normalization of immunological functioning. Other patients respond less well to the enzyme replacement even though their levels of dAdo are as effectively decreased as in those patients who experience greater immune reconstitution. The reasons underlying this differential response remain unexplained.

Gene Therapy

For those patients without a matched sibling donor, the ideal curative therapy would seem to be the transfer of a normal ADA gene into the patient's own totipotent stem cells. Expression of the normal ADA gene in the totipotent stem cells and its progeny would then be expected to cure all cell lineages for the duration of that individual's life.

ADA deficiency has a number of characteristics that make it an attractive initial candidate for gene therapy. The gene was isolated independently by three groups in 1983 (45–47), providing almost a decade to gain experience by investigating the gene, its function and regulation. HLA-matched sibling bone marrow transplantation in children with ADA(–) SCID may be curative, even if only the donor T lymphocytes engraft. Thus gene correction of the same autologous population of cells might be expected also to cure the disease. This is a critical feature since it does not make sense to attempt bone marrow gene therapy for a disease in which all of the clinical manifestations cannot be corrected by bone marrow transplantation (e.g. ataxia–telangiectasia, Lesch–Nyhan syndrome). Third, the ADA gene behaves like a "housekeeping" gene that is constitutively expressed in cells and does not appear to require sophisticated regulation of its expression. Therefore an inserted ADA gene should not require the concomitant insertion of regulatory elements. In addition, ADA levels in immunologically normal individuals have been shown to vary over a very broad range. Heterozygote carriers and rare other individuals have been reported with as little as 10% of the normal mean ADA level in their blood cells and yet their immune system function is intact (58). At the other extreme, individuals with 50 times the normal mean ADA concentration have been described with mild hemolytic anemia but no immune abnormality (59). Thus potentially there is a 500-fold range of enzyme concentrations within which we might expect to provide help to these patients' T cells without causing significant unwanted side effects from over-expression of the gene. Since retroviral-mediated gene transfer can result in an extreme variability in gene expression from cell to cell (7), the broad range of expression seen in normals provides a very forgiving system for its clinical application. Also, since dAdo is freely diffusible, ADA produced in one cell might help restore function in a neighboring cell, even though it itself has not acquired the corrective gene. Further, since the experience with allogeneic bone marrow transplantation suggests that ADA-normal cells have a selective growth advantage over the uncorrected ADA(–) cells, gene transfer into only a fraction of the bone marrow stem cell population might be sufficient for the progeny of those cells to completely reconstitute the immune system without the need to eliminate the uncorrected stem cells by ablative treatment.

Preclinical Studies with Bone Marrow Gene Transfer

Based upon the accumulated experience with clinical bone marrow transplantation, there appears to be a growth advantage for ADA-normal lymphoid cells in ADA(–) patients. This conclusion is based on the observation that transplantation with HLA-matched bone marrow would result in stable lymphoid engraftment and immune reconstitution without the need to employ cytoablative preconditioning. This occurred even though the predominant stem cell source in the marrow of the transplanted patients remains ADA(–) host derived cells. Despite this numerical disadvantage, the small number of ADA(+) stem cells were able to produce mature peripheral blood T cells that would reconstitute the patient's immune system (60). Hematopoietic engraftment was less likely to occur without preconditioning, but its lack has apparently not significantly affected the immune reconstitution achieved in these patients.

Although ADA gene transfer into the totipotent bone marrow stem cell was the initial goal of most studies directed at developing gene therapy for this disease, the inability to achieve stable long-term expression of genes transplanted into primate bone marrow with retroviral vectors led us in 1987 to begin to explore the possibility of developing an alternative gene-modified cell population which might be suitable for treatment of this disease. T cells seemed to be a rational choice for this approach for many reasons. Some ADA(–) SCID patients, following allogeneic bone marrow transplantation without cytoreductive conditioning, were found to have engrafted with donor T cells only and yet they were fully immune reconstituted. This suggested that ADA gene-corrected T cells should have a similar growth advantage in these patients and that correction of the T cell defect alone might be sufficient to reconstitute their immune function. We knew that retroviral-mediated gene transfer could completely correct the metabolic defect in ADA(–) T cells because of our earlier work with cultured T cell lines from these patients (7), so that we should be able to deliver the corrective gene to the T cells in culture even if bone marrow gene transfer had not yet been solved. We had also found that the T cells recovered from the blood and bone marrow of ADA(–) SCID patients appeared to be polyclonal since clones prepared from these T cell lines were each found to be utilizing a different T cell receptor β chain gene rearrangement pattern (61). Further, the early experience with transfusion therapy and PEG–ADA treatment had indicated that the T cell lymphopenia in these patients could be substantially reversed by enzyme replacement. The observations on these patients also suggested that these "new" T cells could provide some protective immune function, since the incidence of opportunistic infections and failure to thrive appeared to be significantly reduced following institution of enzyme replacement. This clinical improvement was seen even in some patients who failed to demonstrate objective measures of reconstituted specific immune functions such as antigen-induced T cell proliferation or the development of positive skin tests. Finally, cultured T cells were being employed successfully in the treatment of cancer, so that this new approach to cellular therapy had some precedent.

Preclinical Studies with T lymphocyte Gene Therapy

Our preclinical experiments in mice and monkeys demonstrated prolonged survival of genetically altered T cells with continued expression of the inserted genes *in vivo* (62, 63). These findings further suggested that T cells might be a suitable cellular vehicle for gene therapy in ADA(–) children. Primary ADA(–) T cell cultures were established from five ADA(–) SCID patients. A portion of each culture was genetically corrected following retroviral-mediated transduction with the LASN vector. LASN is a Moloney murine leukemia-based vector constructed by A. Dusty Miller at the Fred Hutchinson Cancer Center (Seattle, Washington) which contains a hADA gene promoted by the 5'-LTR and an internal SV40 early promoter/enhancer-NeoR gene segment, downstream of the hADA gene (64). Parallel growth of these LASN-transduced and non-transduced cultures showed that all of the non-transduced cultures reached senescence and died within a few weeks of the beginning of the culture, while the genetically corrected cells continued to grow for months and continued to express the introduced ADA genes. These observations suggested that production of ADA in an intracellular location provides a survival advantage to the cells even though the cells were not being challenged with exogenous dAdo in this culture situation.

Ferrari and colleagues (65) took these observations one step further by transferring ADA(–) SCID T cells from a child receiving PEG–ADA into immunodeficient BNX mice ± transduction with a hADA gene vector.

Despite the fact that these animals are ADA normal and thus do not have elevated tissue or body fluid levels of dAdo, only the BNX mice receiving ADA gene-corrected cells had evidence of survival of the patient's T cells. In addition, these studies demonstrated that the surviving human T cells were also capable of mediating some T cell effector functions *in vivo*. Taken together, these findings suggested that the insertion of a normal ADA gene into the cell, providing constitutive intracellular ADA production, gives a survival and functional advantage to those cells beyond that which can be obtained by surrounding the cells with ADA enzyme in the extracellular medium or body fluids.

The RAC approved a trial of T cell gene therapy for the treatment of ADA(–) SCID with LASN-transduced T cells in July 1990. Following Food and Drug Administration approval, the first patient was treated on 14 September 1990.

The First Human Gene Therapy Experiment (Figure 21.1)

Two children, 6- and 11-year-old girls, are currently enrolled in the protocol (66). Each had been treated with regular injections of PEG–ADA for at least 2 years and had documented persisting immunodeficiency prior to beginning gene therapy. Every 4–12 weeks, the children undergo apheresis to obtain peripheral blood mononuclear cells (PBMCs). The PBMCs are placed in culture with OKT3 and r-IL-2, which stimulate vigorous T cell proliferation. Twenty-four hours after initiation of culture, the proliferating cells are exposed twice daily to LASN retroviral vector supernatant four to six times. Using this supernate transduction procedure, 1–10% of the cultured ADA(–) T cells acquire and express the human ADA gene. The T cells, which have expanded by 50–100-fold in number, are reinfused intravenously after 9–11 days in culture. This short-term culture process is used to minimize any tendency of the cultured T cells to develop the oligoclonality known to occur with long-term *in vitro* culture. Using mAb analysis of T cell receptor β chain (TCRβ) V region gene usage, we have detected no evidence that oligoclonality has developed in the cell populations infused. No *in vitro* G418 or dAdo selection for gene-expressing cells has been used, since there is a natural selection process *in vitro* and presumably *in vivo* for ADA(+) cells.

In the first child treated, following eight infusions totaling 9×10^{10} T cells, a substantial increase in the number of circulating T cells ($571/\mu l$ pre-gene therapy versus a mean of $2108/\mu l$) has been demonstrated with gene therapy infusions every 6–8 weeks. The ADA activity in peripheral blood T cells regrown from the blood has increased from <1% prior to gene therapy to 25% of normal levels. This is quite significant in light of the fact that her parents have completely normal immune functioning with 50% of normal ADA activity.

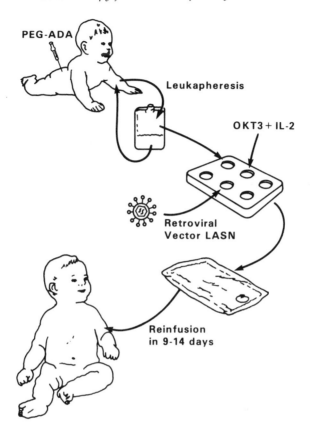

Figure 21.1. Lymphocyte gene therapy schema for ADA(–) SCID protocol. The children must have been maintained on injections of PEG–ADA for at least 9 months without full immunological reconstitution. On a 4–12-week basis, the child undergoes leukapheresis to obtain PBMCs. This procedure generally results in 0.5–2 × 10⁹ PBMCs for genetic manipulation, immune function studies and cryopreservation. The mononuclear cells are then placed in culture in 24 well plates with the monoclonal antibody OKT3 (Ortho) and r-IL-2 (Cetus), which induces vigorous T cell proliferation. Beginning on the second day, the vector LASN is added twice daily for four to six exposures. The cells continue to expand in number and are reinfused after 9–14 days in culture

Persistence of ADA gene-corrected T lymphocytes as measured by polymerase chain reaction (PCR) and vector gene protein expression *in vivo* has been documented in both children even during the discontinuation of T cell infusions for more than 6 months in one child. This suggests that the reinfused ADA gene-corrected T cells may survive for many months and that the survival advantage seen *in vitro, in vivo* in mice and in human bone marrow transplantation is also true for these gene-corrected T cells. Both children have also developed persistent evidence of *in vivo* humoral and cellular immune functions not present while they were being treated with PEG–ADA alone.

In both children, there was no consistent spontaneous production of iso-hemagglutinins prior to gene therapy. However, repeated infusions of gene-corrected T cells has resulted in normal levels of isohemagglutinins and the growth of tonsils in both children. These findings suggest that the gene-corrected T cells can provide the T helper cell function necessary to promote normal spontaneous antibody production. Prior to gene therapy, one child was anergic and the other had only one positive skin test. Now both have positive skin testings to tetanus, *Candida, Streptococcus* and diphtheria. These results suggest that the gene-corrected T cells can perform normal immune functions such as delayed-type hypersensitivity reactions (DTH) and particip-ate in the growth of tonsils. We conclude that: (a) r-IL-2-expanded autologous ADA gene-corrected T lymphocytes will survive and function *in vivo*; and (b) regular infusions of ADA gene-corrected T cells can provide meaningful im-mune reconstitution beyond that achieved with enzyme replacement alone.

Prospects for Peripheral Blood Stem Cell Gene Therapy

The selective growth advantage for ADA gene-corrected T cells *in vivo* has suggested that the genetic correction of a few totipotent stem cells may be sufficient for improvement in the combined immunodeficiency. Until recently, the efficiency of transduction of stem cells has been too low for consideration of a clinical trial for immunodeficiency. However, the growth of totipotent stem cells with combinations of CSFs has resulted in an increased efficiency of transduction from <1% to 10–20% in primate stem cells (67). Transplantation of CSF-driven, vector-transduced CD34-enriched stem cells into irradiated primates has resulted in engraftment of all lineages, with 5–10% of the PBMCs having the vector. Claudio Bordingnon and colleagues in Italy have recently initiated a protocol using the combination of gene-corrected T cells and bone marrow stem cells for two children with ADA deficiency. Our group at NIH will test a similar protocol using G-CSF-mobilized peripheral blood stem cells corrected with an ADA vector different from the one used to insert the correc-tive gene into the T lymphocytes.

OTHER CANDIDATE PRIMARY IMMUNODEFICIENCY DISEASES FOR GENE THERAPY

Purine Nucleoside Phosphorylase (PNP) Deficiency

PNP (EC 2.4.2.1) is also an enzyme in the purine salvage pathway, catalyz-ing the step adjacent to that catabolized by ADA, the conversion of inosine and 2'-deoxyinosine to hypoxanthine. Hypoxanthine may be further metabolized to uric acid and excreted into the urine or rescued to form inosine monophosphate (IMP) through the action of hypoxanthine-guanine phosphoribosyl transferase (HGPRT). PNP deficiency is a rare autosomal recessive disorder with 20 cases described worldwide (68). A deficiency in PNP results in cellular immunodeficiency with susceptibility to viral and fungal agents and variable humoral immune defects. The clinical presentation is heterogeneous, with some children having some residual PNP activity that alters the clinical phenotype.

The PNP gene is located on chromosome 14 and encodes a 289-amino acid polypeptide of 32 kDa. Goddard *et al.* isolated the recombinant PNP cDNA in 1983 (69). Two groups have identified point mutations as the basis for the lack of PNP activity (70, 71). HLA-matched bone marrow transplantation is the treatment of choice for those patients with severe immunodeficiency. The development of gene therapy for PNP deficiency has also been retarded by the lack of success in establishing bone marrow gene therapy. Along with ADA deficiency and for many of the same reasons, PNP deficiency should be an excellent candidate for gene therapy as soon as the problem of bone marrow stem cell gene delivery is solved.

Chronic Granulomatous Disease (CGD)

Four genetic forms of the disease have been identified (Table 21.3) that result in defective phagocyte superoxide-generating production (72–77). The resulting clinical picture is one of repeated and chronic infections with catalase-positive bacteria resulting in granuloma formation. Skin infections are common. Life-threatening infections of the lung, liver or bone may occur. In the 1980s, two groups of investigators noted that interferon γ (IFNγ) increased bactericidal activity of phagocytes from CGD patients (78). The mechanism for this improved function is probably secondary to induction of both oxidative and nonoxidative bactericidal pathways (79). Recently, recombinant human IFNγ (Actimmune) has been administered subcutaneously, with a resulting improvement in the immunological functioning of these children (80–82). This therapy

Table 21.3 Genetic variants of chronic granulomatous disease

	Protein abnormality	Inheritance	Patients (%)
Cytochrome b_{588}	91 kDa chain	X-linked	~60
	22 kDa chain	Autosomal recessive	< 5
Cytosolic proteins	p47*phox*	Autosomal recessive	~33
	47 kDa protein	Autosomal dominant	< 1
	67 kDa protein	Autosomal recessive	~ 5

has been equally effective in all forms of the disease, suggesting IFNγ exerts its effects on myeloid progenitor cells through a common mechanism (83).

The problem of developing gene therapy for CGD is considerably more complex than that posed by ADA deficiency. There are no small animal models of CGD to test the effectiveness of genetic correction *in vivo*. In addition, since granulocytes have such a short survival in culture, it has been difficult to develop a reasonable *in vitro* model to test the effectiveness of gene transfer in these cells. Cobbs *et al.* have expressed a functional p47-*phox* gene in p47-*phox*-deficient B cells (84). However, it has not yet been demonstrated that the transfer of the genes involved in any of the forms of this disorder can actually correct the functional defects in these cells. Further, it is not known if precise regulation of expression of the inserted genes will be required for a satisfactory functional correction of these genetic defects.

In CGD, there is even more reason than in ADA deficiency for the therapy to be directed to the bone marrow stem cell since the mature granulocyte is not in a proliferative state and has a life expectancy of only hours or days. Thus gene correction at the level of the mature cells would result in a "cure" lasting only a very brief time. However, even in this disorder it might be possible to follow the strategy of modifying a more differentiated progenitor cell than the totipotent stem cell with the realization that the treatment would have to be repeated periodically when the previously treated cells had reached senescence and the gene correction has been lost. Half of the circulating polymorphonuclear leukocytes (PMNs) in the heterozygous female carriers of X-linked CGD express the enzyme defect and yet these women are phenotypically normal (85). Therefore CGD shares a characteristic with ADA deficiency in that not all of the defective stem cells may need to be corrected in order to achieve a clinically acceptable outcome. The possibility of using gene therapy to deliver IFNγ to the patients might also be considered.

Leukocyte Adhesion Defect (LAD), CD18 Deficiency

LFA-1 (CD11a), Mac-1 (CD11b) and p150,95 (CD11c) are a family of cell surface proteins that are responsible for cell-to-cell adhesion (86–88). A defect in the common β subunit of these proteins (CD18) results in a partial or complete lack of expression of CD11/CD18 dimers. These dimers (CD18 plus CD11a, b or c) are essential for phagocytes to migrate out of the circulation and bind pathogens. Children suffering with this autosomal recessive disorder have high numbers of neutrophils in their peripheral blood, but they are ineffective protection against invading bacteria, especially encapsulated organisms (89). More than 60 children have been identified with defective expression of the β subunit (CD18). These children have been typically treated with bone marrow transplantation if a matched donor is available (90).

The defective production of these leukocyte adhesion proteins can also result in T lymphocyte dysfunction (91). Using retroviral-mediated gene transfer, the genetic and functional abnormalities in human LAD lymphocytes have been corrected *in vitro*. Wilson *et al.* (92) inserted a normal human CD18 cDNA into LAD human lymphocytes. Antibody staining of the cells demonstrated expression of the heterodimer CD18–CD11a only in those cells containing the vector. Function of these CD18 gene-corrected cells was then determined using an LFA-1-mediated aggregation assay. Stimulation of the lymphocytes with phorbol-myristate acetate (PMA) induced LFA-1-mediated aggregation only in the cells expressing the CD18–CD11a heterodimer. These findings suggest that the ability to insert the CD18 cDNA into a sufficient number of bone marrow stem cells may result in a genetic cure of this disease. The need for precise regulation of gene expression is not completely understood but may not be a limiting condition to the application of retroviral-mediated gene transfer for this disorder. Like the possibility of gene therapy for CGD, the initiation of clinical trials is dependent upon optimization of bone marrow stem cell transduction.

PROSPECTS FOR GENE THERAPY OF OTHER IMMUNODEFICIENCY DISEASES

The development of gene therapy approaches for the other primary immunodeficiency diseases awaits cloning of the involved genes and definition of the role of those genes in the disease process.

Combined Immunodeficiencies

X-linked SCID

The gene defect in this disorder has been mapped to Xq11–13 (93). Bone marrow transplantation has been particularly successful without cytoablation for this disorder if the child has an HLA-matched donor and the transplant is administered before the development of chronic infections. Bone marrow gene therapy could be the mechanism of application if the appropriate progenitor cells are present.

Wiskott–Aldrich Syndrome (WAS)

These children suffer from an X-linked immunodeficiency characterized by eczema, thrombocytopenia and immunodeficiency. The gene has been mapped to Xp11–11.3 (94, 95). The gene has not been isolated and the specific defect resulting in the immunodeficiency has not been characterized. It is cured by allogeneic bone marrow transplantation with cytoreduction, so that again bone marrow gene therapy may be the eventual process used, but cytoreductive conditioning may be required.

Ataxia Telangiectasia (AT)

AT is an autosomal recessive disorder associated with progressive cerebellar dysfunction, variable immunodeficiency and a markedly increased risk of developing cancer. The gene has been localized to chromosome 11q22–q23 (96). It is unlikely that bone marrow gene therapy will correct both the immune and neurological problems.

B Cell Disorders

B cell disorders are quite common and the molecular basis for these diseases is beginning to be defined. Again, until we have the precise gene defect defined it is impossible to predict the strategy which will be required to correct them by gene therapy. The development of efficient methods for homologous recombination may be very valuable for some of these diseases because the corrected gene would then be under the influence of the normal cellular control mechanisms.

Isolated IgA deficiency

Selective IgA is the most common primary immunodeficiency. Autosomal recessive and dominant inheritance patterns have been identified. Other Ig isotypes are normal. The genetic defect(s) may involve chromosomes 6, 14 and/or 18 (97). Some linkage of IgA deficiency with genes encoded within the MHC have been reported but the exact gene defects have not been described (98). No clear strategy for gene therapy has been developed pending definition of the molecular defect.

X-linked Agammaglobulinemia

The gene has been mapped to Xq21.33–22 (99, 100). This genetic defect results in the lack of mature B lymphocytes and a deficiency of all Ig isotypes. These patients develop recurrent pyogenic infections primarily in the respiratory tract. Gene therapy for this disease will also probably involve treatment of autologous bone marrow stem cells.

Immunodeficiency with Hyper IgM

Hyper IgM immunodeficiency is an X-linked disorder that is associated with B lymphocytes expressing only cell surface IgM and/or IgD (101–103). Mayer *et al.* (104) has reported that the Ig defect can be reconstituted with soluble factors for T lymphocytes. Again bone marrow gene therapy is the likely mode of treatment.

Abnormalities in TCR/CD3 Complex and MHC Cell Surface Proteins

The T cell receptor (TCR) is a transmembrane complex of at least seven polypeptide chains. Two chains form a heterodimer that determines antigen specificity (α/β, γ/δ). The CD3 components are involved in signal transduction (γ, δ, ϵ, η, ζ). Defects in both portions of the TCR complex have been described and can result in impaired T cell activation (105–108). Not enough is yet known about the fundamental genetic defect to permit prediction of the ultimate strategy for gene therapy. The occurrence, in the same family, of normal children and children with SCID, each manifesting the defective cell membrane phenotype, suggests a more complicated deficiency than merely the lack of a gene encoding one of the polypeptide chains of the receptor complex.

The lack of HLA class I expression may or may not result in a combined immunodeficiency disorder. HLA class I deficiency was first described by Touraine *et al.* as the "bare lymphocyte syndrome" (109). The lack of HLA class II expression does result in a typical SCID picture with combined cellular and humoral immunodeficiency of specific antigen responses (110). Molecular analysis has shown these cells to lack HLA class II mRNA possibly secondary to an abnormality in the RF-X protein, a specific protein that binds to HLA class II promoter regulatory regions (111). Therefore, HLA class II deficiency may represent a defect involving a regulatory DNA-binding protein (112).

Gene therapy of these primary cell membrane disorders may require complex regulation and assembly of the normal chain components from the endogenous genes and the vector-inserted genes. Krauss *et al.* have shown that insertion of a human CD18 gene into murine cells using retroviral-mediated gene transfer results in expression of human CD18/murine CD11a dimers on the cell surface (113). These dimers are present on the cells that normally express the murine dimers. However, this does not address the possibility that the defective gene may need to be switched off to allow for sufficient expression of functional TCR on the cell surface. There is currently no available methodology to down-regulate expression of abnormal proteins for clinical studies. Correction of defects in constitutive DNA-binding proteins such as RF-X may or may not lend themselves to correction with current gene transfer techniques, depending again on whether complex regulation or coordinated gene expression or assembly of multi-chain proteins will be required.

PROSPECTS FOR GENE THERAPY OF HIV INFECTION

HIV poses a different set of problems compared to many of the primary immunodeficiency diseases where replacement of the defective gene will likely be sufficient for correction of the primary defect and the associated clinical manifestations. In the case of HIV, the HIV genome needs to be eliminated from or genetically blocked from ever expressing its essential genes in all cells. If any cell is left unprotected, there is a risk of development of AIDS.

For individuals that have HIV infection without AIDS, the strategy must be to eliminate the ability of the viral genome to produce infectious virus and prevent spread of HIV to uninfected cells. This might be accomplished by several methods. The first method would be to prevent binding of HIV to uninfected cells such as through the use of CD4 decoys (114). A second method would involve techniques to genetically block the HIV virus from expressing essential genes. This would include using DNA triplexing genes that would irreversibly bind to HIV DNA (27), anti-HIV RNA therapy using ribozymes that would selectively destroy the HIV RNA (115, 116) or anti-sense RNAs that would compete for essential HIV activation sites such as the Tar region, which is required for Tat binding and activation of the HIV LTR (117, 118). In this circumstance, the treatment would be aimed at elimination of the possibility of HIV spread and prevention of AIDS and other consequences of active HIV infection. A third method would be the destruction of HIV-infected cells. This might be accomplished by the genetic alteration of stem cells that would be triggered to self-destruct if infected with the HIV virus, such as might be accomplished with Tat-inducible suicide genes. The possible use of therapies such as these are in early development and are not ready for clinical trials. The development of an injectable, targetable vector, perhaps even using a disabled HIV vector, would be a major advance toward the goal of genetically eliminating the reservoir of HIV within the body.

For patients with AIDS, the strategy would first be the restoration of immune system functioning. The T lymphocyte gene therapy protocol for ADA(–) SCID has demonstrated that the genetic correction of poorly functioning ADA(–) T cells can result in immunocompetent T cells that survive for months *in vivo*. With this knowledge, it might then be reasonable to genetically alter T cells or marrow stem cells from AIDS patients with genes that would prevent their destruction as a consequence of the HIV infection. Infusions of healthy non-genetically altered T cells have recently been shown to be useful in the treatment of human CMV infections (119). However, one would not expect a lasting result in patients with AIDS unless the T cells were genetically protected from HIV infection. Gilboa and colleagues at Sloan-Kettering have developed a retroviral vector containing a Tar decoy that competitively inhibits HIV Tat gene activation and the production of infectious HIV virus (120). We expect that the use of this type of T cell protection strategy may well begin clinical trials in AIDS patients in the next year.

If the use of genetically altered peripheral blood stem cells for the treatment of ADA(–) SCID proves successful, then several therapeutic possibilities become more realistic. First, there is the possibility for long-term T cell protection from the development of the immunodeficiency associated with HIV. Second, there is the possibility that the introduction of a protective gene or a suicide gene that is triggered by HIV infection may be inserted into marrow. Since the marrow stem cells are the source of the CD4+ T cells, monocytes and the dendritic cells—the cells that are the source of the persistent viral infection—it might be possible to replace the infected cells with genetically protected cells over time. While all of these ideas have potential, it is unrealistic to think that any one modality is likely to be curative. Most likely, there will need to be a combination of the methods in order to eliminate the chances for development of AIDS.

CONCLUSIONS

Novel therapies for the treatment of primary immunodeficiency diseases have had a significant impact upon medicine and science. Allogeneic bone marrow transplantation was successfully introduced into clinical practice as a treatment for SCID. Enzyme replacement was also first successfully employed in the treatment of SCID. Similarly, ADA(–) SCID has provided the clinical setting for the first application of human gene therapy. Now, as a result of the new information generated from the T lymphocyte gene therapy experiment for ADA(–) SCID, there may be a first application of gene therapy for the treatment of HIV infection. Even more encouraging is the hope that the upcoming stem cell gene therapy experiment for ADA(–) SCID will prove successful in genetically modifying the totipotent stem cell. If such a protocol is successful, applications to many genetic diseases, autoimmune diseases, cancer and infectious diseases will be ready for human study. As our understanding of the molecular basis of the immunodeficiency diseases accumulate along with parallel progress in basic cell biology and gene transfer modalities, prospects are that gene therapy can be applied successfully to an ever-enlarging number of these often life-threatening diseases.

REFERENCES

1. Anderson, W.F. (1984) Prospects for human gene therapy. *Science*, **226**, 401–409.
2. Report of WHO sponsored meeting (1989) Primary immunodeficiency disease. *Immunodef. Rev.*, **1**, 173–205.
3. Meyaard, L., Otto, S.A., Jonker, R.R. *et al.* (1992) Programmed death of T cells in HIV-1 infection. *Science*, **257**, 217–219.
4. Parkman, R. (1986) The application of bone marrow transplantation to the treatment of genetic diseases. *Science*, **232**, 1373–1378.

5. Schook, L.B., Lewin, H.A. and McLaren, D.G. (eds) (1991) *Gene-mapping Techniques and Applications*. Decker, New York.
6. Miller, A.D. (1992) Human gene therapy comes of age. *Nature*, **357**, 455–460.
7. Kantoff, P.W., Kohn, D.B., Mitsuya, H., *et al.* (1986) Correction of adenosine deaminase deficiency in cultured human T and B cells by retrovirus-mediated gene transfer. *Proc. Nat. Acad. Sci. USA*, **83**, 6563–6567.
8. Blaese, R.M. and Culver, K.W. (1992) Gene therapy for primary immunodeficiency disease. *Immunodef. Rev.*, **3**, 329–349.
9. Cornetta, K., Moen, R.C., Culver, K. *et al.* (1990) Amphotropic murine leukemia virus is not an acute pathogen for primates. *Hum. Gene Ther.*, **1**, 15–30.
10. Rosenberg, S.A., Aebersold, P., Cornetta, K. *et al.* (1990) Gene transfer into humans: Immunotherapy of patients with advanced melanoma, using tumor-infiltrating lymphocytes modified by retroviral gene transduction. *N. Engl. J. Med.*, **323**, 570–578.
11. Anderson, W.F. (1992) Human gene therapy. *Science*, **256**, 808–813.
12. Kohn, D.B., Anderson, W.F. and Blaese, R.M. (1989) Gene therapy for genetic diseases. *Cancer Invest.*, **7**, 179–192.
13. Page, K.A., Landau, N.R. and Littman, D.R. (1990) Construction and use of a human immunodeficiency virus vector for analysis of virus infectivity. *J. Virol.*, **64**, 5270–5276.
14. Poznansky, M., Lever, A., Bergeron, L., Haseltine, W. and Sodroski, J. (1991) Gene transfer into human lymphocytes by a defective human immunodeficiency virus type 1 vector. *J. Virol.*, **65**, 532–536.
15. Shimada, T., Fujii, H., Mitsuya, H. and Nienhuis, A.W. (1991) Targeted and highly efficient gene transfer into CD4+ cells by a recombinant human immunodeficiency virus retroviral vector. *J. Clin. Invest.*, **88**, 1043–1047.
16. Buchschacher, G.L. and Panganiban, A.T. (1992) Human immunodeficiency virus vectors for inducible expression of foreign genes. *J. Virol.*, **66**, 2731–2739.
17. Harrison, G.S., Maxwell, F., Long, C.J. *et al.* (1991) Activation of a diphtheria toxin A gene by expression of human immunodeficiency virus-1 tat and rev proteins in transfected cells. *Hum. Gene Ther.*, **2**, 53–60.
18. Harrison, G.S., Long, C.J., Maxwell, F. *et al.* (1992) Inhibition of HIV production in cells containing an integrated, HIV-regulated diphtheria toxin A chain gene. *AIDS Res. Hum. Retrovirus*, **8**, 39–45.
19. Green, M., Ishino, M. and Loewenstein, P.M. (1989) Mutational analysis of HIV-1 tat minimal domain peptides: Identification of trans-domain mutants suppress HIV-LTR-driven gene expression. *Cell*, **58**, 215–223.
20. Malim, M.H., Bohnlein, S., Hauber, J. and Cullen, B.R. (1989) Functional dissection of the HIV-rev trans activator: derivation of a trans-dominant repressor of rev function. *Cell*, **58**, 205–214.
21. Truono, D., Feinberg, M.B. and Baltimore, D. (1989) HIV-1 gag mutants can dominantly interfere with the replication of the wild-type virus. *Cell*, **59**, 113–120.
22. Freed, E.O., Delwart, E.L., Buchschacher, G.L. and Panganiban, A.T. (1992) A mutation in the human immunodeficiency virus type 1 transmembrane glycoprotein 41 dominantly interferes with fusion and infectivity. *Proc. Nat. Acad. Sci. USA*, **89**, 70–74.
23. Venkatesh, L.K., Arens, M.Q., Subramanian, T. and Chinnaduari, G. (1990) Selective induction of toxicity to human cells expressing human immunodeficiency virus type 1 tat by a conditionally cytotoxic adenovirus vector. *Proc. Nat. Acad. Sci. USA*, **87**, 8746–8750.

24. Caruso, M. and Klatzmann, D. (1992) Selective killing of CD4+ cells harboring a human immunodeficiency virus-inducible suicide gene prevents viral spread in an infected population. *Proc. Nat. Acad. Sci. USA*, **89**, 182–186.

25. Culver, K.W., Ram, Z., Walbridge, S. *et al.* (1992) *In vivo* gene transfer with retroviral vector producer cells for treatment of experimental brain tumors. *Science*, **256**, 1550–1552.

26. Blaese, R.M. (1991) Progress toward gene therapy. *J. Clin. Immunol. Immunopathol.*, **61**, S47–S55.

27. Moffatt, A.S. (1991) Triplexing DNA finally comes of age. *Science*, **252**, 1374–1375.

28. Gatti, R.A., Menwissen, H., Allen, H., Hong, R. and Good, R.A. (1968) Immunologic reconstitution of sex-linked lymphopenic immunological deficiency. *Lancet*, **ii**, 1366–1369.

29. Wijnaendts, L., Le Deist, F., Griscelli, C. and Fischer, A. (1989) Development of immunologic functions after bone marrow transplantation in 33 patients with severe combined immunodeficiency. *Blood*, **74**, 2212–2219.

30. Lane, H.C., Zunich, K.M., Wilson, W. *et al.* (1990) Syngeneic bone marrow transplantation and adoptive transfer of peripheral blood lymphocytes combined with zidovudine in human immunodeficiency virus (HIV) infection. *Ann. Int. Med.*, **113**, 512–519.

31. McCredie, K.B., Hersh, E.M. and Freireich, E.J. (1971) Cells capable of colony formation in the peripheral blood of man. *Science*, **71**, 293–294.

32. Kessinger, A., Armitage, J.O., Landmark, J.D., Smith, D.M. and Weisenberger, D.D. (1988) Autologus peripheral hematopoietic stem cell transplantation restores hematopoietic function following marrow ablative therapy. *Blood*, **71**, 723–727.

33. Kessinger, A. (1990) Autologous transplantation with peripheral blood stem cells: A review of clinical results. *J. Clin. Apheresis*, **5**, 97–99.

34. Williams, D.A. (1990) Expression of introduced genetic sequences in hematopoietic cells following retroviral-mediated gene transfer. *Hum. Gene Ther.*, **1**, 229–239.

35. Kantoff, P.W., Gillio, A.P., McLachlin, J.R. *et al.* (1987) Expression of human adenosine deaminase in nonhuman primates after retrovirus-mediated gene transfer. *J. Exp. Med.*, **166**, 219–234.

36. Serke, S., Sauberlich, S., Abe, Y. and Huhn, D. (1991) Analysis of CD34-positive hemopoietic progenitor cells from normal human adult peripheral blood: Flowcytometrical studies and in-vitro colony (CFU-GM, BFU-E) assays. *Ann. Hematol.*, **62**, 45–53.

37. Heimfeld, S., Andrews, R., Bensinger, W. *et al.* (1991) Peripheral blood stem cell mobilization: Rapid enrichment of progenitor cells using a unique biotin–avidin immunoaffinity column. *Blood*, **78** (suppl. 1), 16a.

38. Siena, S., Bregni, M., Brando, B. *et al.* (1991) Flow cytometry for clinical estimation of circulating hematopoietic progenitors for autologous transplantation in cancer patients. *Blood*, **77**, 400–409.

39. Ravagnani, F., Siena, S., Bregni, M. *et al.* (1991) Methodologies to estimate circulating hematopoietic progenitors for autologous transplantation in cancer patients. *Haematologica*, **76** (Suppl. 1), 46–49.

40. Berenson, R.J., Bensinger, W.I., Hill, R.S. *et al.* (1991) Engraftment after infusion of CD34+ marrow cells in patients with breast cancer or neuroblastoma. *Blood*, **77**, 1717–1722.

41. Bensinger, W.I. and Berenson, R.J. (1990) Peripheral blood and positive selection of marrow as a source of stem cells for transplantation. *Prog. Clin. Biol. Res.*, **337**, 93–98.

42. McNiece, I.K. (1992) Synergism of hematopoietic colony-stimulating factors. *Am. J. Pediatr. Hematol. Oncol.*, **14**, 31–38.

43. Nienhuis, A.W., McDonagh, K.T. and Bodine, D.M. (1991) Gene transfer into hematopoietic stem cells. *Cancer*, **67** (Suppl.) 2700–2704.

44. Giblett, E.R., Anderson, J.E., Cohen, F. *et al.* (1972) Adenosine deaminase deficiency in two patients with severely impaired cellular immunity. *Lancet*, **ii**, 1067–1069.

45. Orkin, S.H., Daddona, P.E., Shewach, D.S. *et al.* (1983) Molecular cloning of human adenosine deaminase gene sequences. *J. Biol. Chem.*, **158**, 12753–12756.

46. Valerio, D., Duyvesteyn, M.G.C., Meera Khan, P. *et al.* (1983) Isolation of cDNA clones for human adenosine deaminase. *Gene*, **25**, 231–240.

47. Wiginton, D.A., Adrian, G.S., Friedman, R.L. *et al.* (1983) Cloning of cDNA sequences of human adenosine deaminase. *Proc. Nat. Acad. Sci. USA*, **80**, 7481–7485.

48. Akeson, A.L., Wiginton, D.A. and Hutton, J.J. (1989) Normal and mutant adenosine deaminase genes. *J. Cell Biochem.*, **39**, 218–228.

49. Bonthron, D.T., Markham, A.F., Ginsburg, D. *et al.* (1985) Identification of a point mutation in the adenosine deaminase gene responsible for immunodeficiency. *J. Clin. Invest.*, **76**, 894–897.

50. Daddona, P.E., Shewach, D.S., Kelley, W.N. *et al.* (1984) Human adenosine deaminase: cDNA and complete primary amino acid sequence. *J. Biol. Chem.*, **259**, 12101–12106.

51. Marker, M.L., Hutton, J.J., Wiginton, D.A. *et al.* (1988) Adenosine deaminase (ADA) deficiency due to deletion of the ADA gene promoter and first exon by homologous recombination between two Alu elements. *J. Clin. Invest.*, **81**, 1323–1327.

52. Valerio, D., Dekker, B.M.M., Duyvesteyn, M.G.C. *et al.* (1986) One adenosine deaminase allele in a patient with severe combined immunodeficiency disease contains a point mutation abolishing enzyme activity. *EMBO J.*, **5**, 113–119.

53. Hirschhorn, R. (1983) Genetic deficiencies of adenosine deaminase and purine nucleoside phosphorylase: Overview, genetic heterogeneity and therapy. *Birth Defect*, **19**, 73–81.

54. Ammann, A.J. and Hong, R. (1989) Disorders of the T cell system. In Steihm, E.R. (ed.) *Immunologic Disorders of Infants and Children*. Saunders, Philadelphia, pp. 257–315.

55. O'Reilly, R.J., Keever, C.A., Small, T.N. and Brochstein, J. (1989) The use of HLA-non-identical T-cell-depleted marrow transplants for the correction of severe combined immunodeficiency disease. *Immunodef. Rev.*, **1**, 273–309.

56 Polmar, S.H., Stern, R.C., Schwartz, A.L. *et al.* (1976) Enzyme replacement therapy for adenosine deaminase deficiency and severe combined immunodeficiency. *N. Engl. J. Med.*, **295**, 1337–1343.

57. Hershfield, M.S., Buckley, R.H., Greenberg, M.L. *et al.* (1987) Treatment of adenosine deaminase deficiency with polyethylene glycol-modified adenosine deaminase. *N. Engl. J. Med.*, **16**, 589–596.

58. Daddona, P.E., Mitchell, B.S., Meuwissen, H.J. *et al.* (1983) Adenosine deaminase deficiency with normal immune function. *J. Clin. Invest.*, **72**, 483–492.

59. Valentine, W.N., Paglia, D.E., Tartaglia, A.P. and Gilsanz, F. (1977) Hereditary hemolytic anemia with increased adenosine deaminase (45–70 fold) and decreased adenosine triphosphates. *Science*, **195**, 783.

60. Vossen, J.M. (1987) Bone marrow transplantation in the treatment of primary immunodeficiencies. *Ann. Clin. Res.*, **19**, 285–292.

61. Kohn, D.B., Mitsuya, H., Ballow, M. *et al.* (1989) Establishment and characterization of adenosine deaminase deficient human T-cell lines. *J. Immunol.*, **142**, 3971–3977.

62. Culver, K., Cornetta, K., Morgan, R. *et al.* (1991) Lymphocytes as cellular vehicles for gene therapy in mouse and man. *Proc. Nat. Acad. Sci. USA*, **88**, 3155–3159.

63. Culver, K.W., Anderson, W.F. and Blaese, R.M. (1991) Lymphocyte gene therapy. *Hum. Gene Ther.*, **2**, 107–109.

64. Osborne, W.R.A., Hock, R.A., Kaleko, M. and Miller, A.D. (1990) Long-term expression of human adenosine deaminase in mice after transplantation of bone marrow infected with amphotropic retroviral vectors. *Hum. Gene Ther.*, **1**, 31–41.

65. Ferrari, G., Rossini, S., Giavazzi, R. *et al.* (1991) An in vivo model of somatic cell gene therapy for human severe combined immunodeficiency. *Science*, **251**, 1363–1366.

66. Culver, K.W., Berger, M., Miller, A.D., Anderson, W.F. and Blaese, R.M. (1992) Lymphocyte gene therapy for adenosine deaminase deficiency. *Pediatr. Res.*, **31**, 149A.

67. Dunbar, C. and Nienhuis, A., personal communication.

68. Carson, D.A. and Carrera, C.J. (1990) Immunodeficiency secondary to adenosine deaminase deficiency and purine nucleoside phosphorylation deficiency. *Semin. Hematol.*, **27**, 260–269.

69. Goddard, J.M., Caput, D., Williams, S.R. and Martin, D.W. (1983) Cloning of human purine-nucleoside phosphorylase cDNA sequences by complementation in *Escherichia coli. Proc. Nat. Acad. Sci. USA*, **80**, 4281–4285.

70. Williams, S.R., Gekeler, V., McIvor, R.S. *et al.* (1987) A human purine nucleoside phosphorylase deficiency carried by a single base change. *J. Biol. Chem.*, **262**, 2332–2338.

71. Andrews, L.G. and Markert, M.L. (1992) Exon skipping in purine nucleoside phosphorylase mRNA processing leading to severe immunodeficiency. *J. Biol. Chem.*, **267**, 7834–7838.

72. Segal, A.W., Cross, A.R. and Garcia, R.C. (1983) Absence of cytochrome b-245 in chronic granulomatous disease: A multicenter European evaluation of its incidence and relevance. *N. Engl. J. Med.*, **308**, 245–251.

73. Royer-Pokora, B., Kunkel, L.M., Monaco, A.P. *et al.* (1986) Cloning the gene for an inherited human disorder—chronic granulomatous disease—on the basis of its chromosomal location. *Nature*, **322**, 32–38.

74. Clark, R.A., Malech, H.L., Gallin, J.I. *et al.* (1989) Genetic variants of chronic granulomatous disease: Prevalence of deficiencies of two cytosolic components of the NADPH oxidase system. *N. Engl. J. Med.*, **321**, 647–652.

75. Lomax, K.J., Leto, T.L., Nunoi, H. *et al.* (1989) Recombinant 47-kD cytosol factor restores NADPH oxidase in chronic granulomatous disease. *Science*, **245**, 409–412 (erratum, **246**: 987).

76. Leto, T.L., Lomax, K.J., Volpp, B.D. *et al.* (1989) Neutrophil oxidase components share homology with the regulatory domains of the src related tyrosine kinase family. *J. Cell Biol.*, **109**, 49a.

77. Dinauer, M.C. and Orkin, S.H. (1992) Chronic granulomatous disease. *Annu. Rev. Med.*, **43**, 117–124.

78. Nathan, C.F., Murray, H.W., Wiebe, M.E. *et al.* (1983) Identification of interferon as the lymphokine that activates human macrophage oxidative metabolism and antimicrobial activity. *J. Exp. Med.*, **158**, 670–689.

79. Gallin, J.I. and Malech, H.L. (1990) Update on chronic granulomatous diseases of childhood. *JAMA*, **263**, 1533–1537.

80. Ezekowitz, R.A.B., Dinauer, M.C., Jaffe, H.S. *et al.* (1988) Partial correction of the phagocyte defects in patients with X-linked chronic granulomatous disease by subcutaneous interferon gamma. *N. Engl. J. Med.*, **319**, 146–151.

81. Newberger, E., Ezekowitz, R.A.B., Whitney, C., Wright, J. and Orkin, S.H. (1988) Induction of phagocyte cytochrome b heavy chain gene expression by interferon γ. *Proc. Nat. Acad. Sci. USA*, **85**, 5215–5219.

82. Ezekowitz, R.A.B., Sieff, C.A., Dinauer, M.C. *et al.* (1990) Restoration of phagocyte function by interferon-γ in X-linked chronic granulomatous disease occurs at the level of a progenitor cell. *Blood*, **76**, 2443–2448.

83. International Collaborative Study Group to assess the efficacy of rIFN-γ in CGD: Clinical recombinant human interferon-gamma (rIFN-γ) in chronic granulomatous disease (1990). *Clin. Res.*, **38**, 465A.

84. Cobbs, C.S., Malech, H.L., Leto, T.L. *et al* (1992) Retroviral expression of recombinant p47^{phox} protein by Epstein–Barr virus-transformed B lymphocytes from a patient with autosomal chronic granulomatous disease. *Blood*, **79**, 1829–1835.

85. Orkin, S. (1989) Molecular genetics of chronic granulomatous disease. *Annu. Rev. Immunol.*, **7**, 277–307.

86. Sanchez-Madrid, F., Nagy, J., Robbins, E., Simon, P. and Springer, T.A. (1983) A human leukocyte differentiation antigen family with distinct alpha subunits and a common beta subunit: The lymphocyte function-associated antigen (LFA-1), the C3bi complement receptor (OKM 1/Mac 1), and the p150,95 molecule. *J. Exp. Med.*, **158**, 1785–1803.

87. Kishimoto, T.K., Hollander, N., Roberts, T.M., Anderson, D.C. and Springer, T.A. (1987) Heterogeneous mutations in the beta subunit common to the LFA 1, Mac 1 and p 150,95 glycoproteins cause leukocyte adhesion deficiency. *Cell*, **50**, 193–202.

88. Todd, R.F. and Freyer, D.R. (1988) The CD11/CD18 leukocyte glycoprotein deficiency. *Hematol. Oncol. Clin. North Am.*, **2**, 13–31.

89. Anderson, D.C. and Springer, T.A. (1987) Leukocyte adhesion deficiency: An inherited defect in the Mac-1, LFA-1, and p150,95 glycoproteins. *Annu. Rev. Med.*, **38**, 175–194.

90. Le Deist, F., Blanche, S., Keable, H. *et al.* (1989) Successful HLA nonidentical bone marrow transplantation in three patients with the leukocyte adhesion deficiency. *Blood*, **74**, 512–516.

91. Van Noesel, C., Miedema, F., Brouwer, M. *et al.* (1988) Regulatory properties of LFA-1 alpha and beta chains in human T-lymphocyte activation. *Nature*, **333**, 850–852.

92. Wilson, J.M., Ping, A.J., Krauss, J.D. *et al.* (1990) Correction of CD18 deficient lymphocytes by retrovirus mediated gene transfer. *Science*, **248**, 1413–1416.

93. de Saint Basile, G., Arveiller, B., Orberle, I. *et al.* (1987) Close linkage of the locus for X chromosome-linked severe combined immunodeficiency to polymorphic DNA markers in Xq11–q13. *Proc. Nat. Acad. Sci. USA*, **84**, 7576–7579.

94. Kwan, S.P., Sandkuyl, L., Blaese, M. *et al.* (1988) Genetic mapping of the Wiskott–Aldrich syndrome with two highly linked polymorphic DNA markers. *Genomics*, **3**, 39–43.

95. de Saint-Basile, G., Fraser, N., Craig, I. *et al.* (1989) Close linkage of hypervariable marker DXS255 to disease locus of Wiskott–Aldrich syndrome. *Lancet*, **ii**, 1319–1320.

96. Gatti, R.A., Berkel, I., Boder, E. *et al.* (1988) Localization of an ataxia–telangiectasia gene to chromosome 11q22–23. *Nature*, **336**, 577–580.

97. Cunningham-Rundles, C. (1990) Genetic aspects of immunoglobulin A deficiency *Adv. Hum. Genet.*, **19**, 235–266.

98. Schaffer, F.M., Palermos, J., Zhu, Z.B. *et al.* (1989) Individuals with IgA deficiency and common variable immunodeficiency share polymorphisms of major histocompatibility complex class III genes. *Proc. Nat. Acad. Sci. USA*, **86**, 8015–8019.

99. Schwartz, M., Yang, H.M., Neibuhr, E., Rosenberg, T. and Page, D.C. (1988) Regional localization of polymorphic DNA loc on the proximal long arm of the X chromosome using deletions associated with chroideremia. *Hum. Genet.*, **78**, 156–160.

100. Kwan, S.P., Kunkel, L., Burns, G., Wedgwood, R.J., Latt, S. and Rosen, F.S. (1986) Mapping of the X-linked agammaglobulinemia locus by use of restriction fragment-length polymorphism. *J. Clin. Invest.*, **77**, 649–652.

101. Rosen, F., Kevy, S., Merler, E., Janeway, C. and Gitlin, D. (1961) Recurrent bacterial infections and dysgammaglobulinemia: Deficiency of 7S gammaglobulins in the presence of elevated 19S gammaglobulins. *Pediatrics*, **28**, 182–195.

102. Geha, R., Hyslop, S., Alami, F. *et al.* (1979) Hyperimmunoglobulin M immunodeficiency (dysgammaglobulinemia): Presence of immunoglobulin M secreting plasmacytoid cells in peripheral blood and failure of immunoglobulin M immunoglobulin G switch in B cell differentiation. *J. Clin. Invest.*, **64**, 385–391.

103. Schwaber, J., Lazarus, H. and Rosen, F. (1981) IgM restricted production of immunoglobulin by lymphoid cell lines from patients with immunodeficiency with hyper IgM (dysgammaglobulinemia). *Clin. Immunol. Immunopathol.*, **19**, 91–97.

104. Mayer, L., Kwam, S.P., Thompson, C. *et al.* (1986) Evidence for a defect in switch T-cells in patients with immunodeficiency and hyperimmunoglobulinemia M. *N. Engl. J. Med.*, **314**, 409–413.

105. Alarcon, B., Regueiro, J.R., Arnaiz-Villena, A. and Terhorst, C. (1988) Familial defect in the surface expression of the T-cell receptor–CD3 complex. *N. Engl. J. Med.*, **319**, 1203–1207.

106. Chatila, T., Wong, R., Young, M. *et al.* (1989) An immunodeficiency characterized by defective signal transduction in T lymphocytes. *N. Engl. J. Med.*, **320**, 696–702.

107. Le Deist, F., de Saint Basile, G., Mazerolles, F. *et al.* (1991) Primary membrane T-cell immunodeficiencies. *Clin. Immunol. Immunopathol.*, **61**, S56–60.

108. Alarcon, B. and Terhorst, C. (1990) Congenital T-cell receptor immunodeficiencies in man. *Immunodef. Rev.*, **2**, 1–16.

109. Touraine, J.L., Betuel, H. and Souillet, G. (1978) Combined immunodeficiency disease associated with absence of cell-surface HLA A and B antigens. *J. Pediatr.*, **93**, 47–51.

110. Griscelli, C., Lisowska-Grospierre, B. and Mach, B. (1989) Combined immunodeficiency with defective expression in MHC class II genes. *Immunodef. Rev.*, **1**, 135–154.

111. Reith, W., Satola, S., Sanchez, C.H. *et al.* (1988) Congenital immunodeficiency with a regulatory defect in MHC class II gene expression lacks a specific HLA-DR promoter binding protein ("RF-X"). *Cell*, **53**, 897–900.

112. Griscelli, C. (1991) Combined immunodeficiency with defective expression in major histocompatibility complex class II genes. *Clin. Immunol. Immunopathol.*, **61**, S106–S110.

113. Krauss, J.C., Ping, A.J., Mayo-Bond, L. *et al.* (1990) Expression of retroviral transduced human CD18 in murine cells: An in vitro model of gene therapy for leukocyte adhesion deficiency. *Hum. Gene Ther.*, **2**, 221–228.

114. Morgan, R.A., Looney, D.J., Muenchau, D.D. *et al.* (1990) Retroviral vectors expressing soluble CD4: A potential gene therapy for AIDS. *AIDS Res. Hum. Retroviruses*, **6**, 9–17.

115. Sarver, N., Cantin, E.M., Chang, P.S. *et al.* (1990) Ribozymes as potential anti-HIV-1 therapeutic agents. *Science*, **247**, 1222–1225.

116. Weerasinghe, M., Leim, S.E., Asad, S., Read, S.E. and Joshi, S. (1991) Resistance to human immunodeficiency virus type 1 (HIV-1) infection in human CD4+ lymphocyte derived cell lines conferred by using retroviral vectors expressing an HIV-1 RNA-specific ribozyme. *J. Virol.*, **65**, 5531–5534.

117. Von Ruden, T. and Gilboa, E. (1989) Inhibition of human T-cell leukemia type 1 replication in primary human T cells that express antisense RNA. *J. Virol.*, **63**, 677–682.

118. Sczakiel, G. and Pawlita, M. (1991) Inhibition of human immunodeficiency virus type 1 replication in human T cells stably expressing antisence RNA. *J. Virol.*, **65**, 468–472.

119. Riddell, S.R., Watanabe, K.S., Goodrich, J.M. *et al.* (1992) Restoration of viral immunity in immunodeficient humans by the adoptive transfer of T cell clones. *Science*, **257**, 238–241.

120. Sullenger, B.A., Gallardo, H.F., Ungers, G.E. and Gilboa, E. (1990) Overexpression of Tar sequences renders cells resistant to human immunodeficiency virus replication. *Cell*, **63**, 601–608.

Chapter 22

Intravenous Immunoglobulin: Current Concepts and Application

John Radcliffe Hospital, Headington, Oxford, UK

HISTORY

The use of immunoglobulin (Ig) replacement therapy for all patients with antibody deficiency syndromes has been indisputable since Bruton treated the first hypogammaglobulinaemic patient with replacement Ig in 1952 (1). Originally the use of Ig, prepared by selective precipitation from serum by cold ethanol fractionation (2), was restricted to the intramuscular route since serious systemic reactions were associated with its use intravenously. The need to give higher doses of Ig, whilst ensuring patient compliance and a reduction of adverse events, led to exploration of additional purification steps to remove aggregates of IgG and other phlogistic contaminants (3).

Preparations of polyclonal Ig, which can be given safely by the intravenous route, have been available for over 10 years. This type of therapy has supplanted intramuscular Ig as the treatment of choice for replacement therapy in most patients with humoral immune deficiencies (4). Several manufacturing processes are used, resulting in products differing in the degree of purity of monomeric IgG, concentration of IgA and the distribution of IgG subclasses. Preparations also differ in the size and source of the original donor pool and may therefore contain different quantities of specific antibodies, both to extrinsic pathogens and to idiotypic determinants. These differences mean that the products are not necessarily interchangeable for therapy, in either immune-deficient patients or those with autoimmune diseases.

New Concepts in Immunodeficiency Diseases. Edited by S. Gupta and C. Griscelli
© 1993 John Wiley & Sons Ltd

INDICATIONS

The indications for the use of intravenous (i.v.) Ig are of two types: immunodeficiency (primary or secondary) and autoimmune disease. In either situation, it is most important that the efficacy and safety of this treatment are proven by randomized trials, double blind and placebo controlled where possible. In immunodeficiency (Table 22.1) i.v. Ig is given as replacement therapy for missing antibodies, and the aim of treatment is to maintain a serum IgG level within the normal range to prevent infections. In contrast, three- to fivefold higher doses are given in autoimmune diseases to modulate inflammation (5–7).

Table 22.1 Indications for prophylactic i.v. Ig therapy in immunodeficient states

Primary
1. Hypogammaglobulinaemia
   - CVI[a]
   - X-linked agammaglobulinaemia[a]
   - X-linked agammaglobulinaemia with hyper IgM[a]
2. IgG subclass(es) deficiency with infections (including Wiskott–Aldrich syndrome)[a]
3. IgA and IgG subclass(es) deficiencies[a]
4. SCID prior to bone marrow transplantation[a]
5. Failure of humoral reconstitution after bone marrow transplantation for SCID[a]

Secondary
1. Infants and children with HIV infection
2. Very low birth weight babies (<1750 g) at risk of late onset (5 days of age) infections
3. Hypogammaglobulinaemia secondary to intestinal lymphangiectasia
4. Adults with secondary hypogammaglobulinaemia due to lymphoproliferative disease[a]
5. Following bone marrow transplantation for non-immune conditions

[a]These groups of patients have suboptimal IgG responses to test immunizations with either protein or carbohydrate (or both) antigens.

All patients presenting with infections who are frankly hypogammaglobulinaemic, i.e. have serum IgA and IgG concentrations significantly below the lower limits of normal for their age, require Ig replacement therapy. Only patients with mild hypogammaglobulinaemia are treated with intramuscular Ig (after loading with i.v. Ig), since limited doses can be given by the intramuscular route. Patients must also be compliant with the weekly regimen of uncomfortable injections; failure of adequate therapy can lead to gradual deterioration in lung function (8). Most patients with primary hypogammaglobulinaemia, whether due to common variable immunodeficiency, X-linked agammaglobulinaemia or failure of B cell reconstitution after bone marrow transplantation for severe combined immunodeficiency disease (SCID) (Table 22.1), have fewer breakthrough infections (acute and chronic) with the larger doses of Ig provided by the i.v. route.

Children with SCID are also given i.v. Ig prior to bone marrow transplantation to prevent lung infections which reduce the chances of a successful outcome for the transplant (9). Once transplanted, these children's bone marrow may not fully reconstitute (10), particularly if an HLA non-identical donor is used (11). Although the infection risk from fungal and viral infections is corrected, such children may require continued i.v. Ig for persistent antibody failure.

The clinical significance of deficiencies in one or more of the IgG subclasses is unclear (12). Some healthy individuals with isolated or several IgG subclass deficiencies have been noted and heavy chain gene deletions leading to IgG subclass deficiencies in asymptomatic individuals is well documented. However, a substantial number of patients with IgG subclass deficiencies do suffer repeated infections. Amongst such patients with low-normal levels of total serum IgG, IgG subclass deficiencies have been found in association with failure to respond to test immunizations. A reduction of the infection rate by Ig therapy would be good evidence of the clinical significance of IgG subclass deficiency. In a double-blind, 2-year cross-over study involving 31 infection-prone adult patients with levels of IgG subclasses below the 3rd percentiles, replacement Ig significantly reduced the number of days of infection ($p<0.035$). This was despite the low doses given (25 mg/kg per week); there was also a significant reduction in days with asthma (12). Preliminary reports of higher doses (50 mg/kg per week) suggest that i.v. Ig would be substantially better in these patients. (Hanson, personal communication). It is our practice to immunize those patients who have low IgG subclass levels in association with bacterial infections and give replacement therapy to those with poor antibody responses to either proteins (tetanus and diphtheria toxoids) (13) or carbohydrates (pneumococcal or *Haemophilus* polysaccharides) (14) or both. This includes patients with Wiskott–Aldrich syndrome who fail to make antibodies to carbohydrate antigens.

Those patients with recurrent infections in association with IgA deficiency may also have an underlying IgG subclass or specific antibody deficiency (12). Infections usually involve the respiratory and gastrointestinal tracts, are often long standing and may be severe, with an overall clinical picture resembling that of common variable immunodeficiency (CVI) (15). A controlled study of Ig prophylaxis is urgently needed, since uncontrolled reports and general clinical experience have shown i.v. Ig to be as efficacious in this situation as in CVI. We test immunize all such IgA-deficient patients, and if suboptimal immunization responses are seen it is our practice to give replacement Ig therapy on a year's trial and to monitor infections carefully during this time.

There are a few patients with histories typical of classical immunodeficiency in whom serum Ig, IgG subclass levels and antibody responses are normal at the time of initial investigation. Such patients should be followed carefully and their serum antibody levels checked at regular intervals, since there have been anecdotal reports of patients who gradually developed hypogammaglobulinaemia over a number of years. Such patients often present with immune complex diseases; presumably low-affinity antibodies are produced, initially resulting in immune complexes which are difficult to clear, and leading to glomerulonephritis, skin damage or thrombocytopenia. Once antibody production has ceased altogether, infection risk is increased and typical hypogammaglobulinaemia becomes apparent. Such patients need replacement therapy several years after initial investigation.

Primary antibody deficiency states in which Ig replacement therapy is still controversial include transient hypogammaglobulinaemia of infancy. In this rare condition infants are able to make specific antibodies on immunization although their total serum levels of IgG and IgA are low for their age. This ability to respond to extrinsic antigens may explain why the infants are not at continued risk of serious infection (16). Occasional children with severe infections in this transient phase may require temporary replacement therapy but this is unusual. Test immunization with killed vaccines is used to distinguish between transient and persistent hypogammaglobulinaemia in infants presenting with recurrent infections.

Situations in which i.v. Ig is used as prophylaxis against infection in secondary antibody deficiencies (Table 22.1) include those in association with prematurity, HIV infection in infants, lymphoproliferative diseases and following bone marrow transplantation for malignancies and lethal, non-malignant conditions such as metabolic disorders (i.e. other than SCID). These and the use of i.v. Ig in autoimmune diseases are discussed later.

EFFICACY

The efficacy of replacement Ig in hypogammaglobulinaemia was originally shown by the Medical Research Council trial, when intramuscular Ig was first used on a wide scale (17). Intravenous Ig was initially shown to be as good as intramuscular (18); later trials (19–21) demonstrated increased efficacy of Ig with higher doses of i.v. Ig. Furthermore Roifman *et al.* (22) were able to show an improvement of FEV_1 and vital capacity after 6 months of high-dose Ig infusions in patients with chronic lung disease.

The more persistent complications of hypogammaglobulinaemia, such as those due to granulomata or atrophic gastritis, are not usually reversed by Ig therapy, though nodular lymphoid hyperplasia may disappear in children (24). The increased risk of cancer (13%), particularly lymphoma or gastric carcinoma, is unlikely to be changed by i.v. Ig, though this will not be known for another decade (24).

DOSE

The dose of Ig used for replacement in humoral immunodeficiencies has gradually increased over the years, as it has become apparent that larger doses were safe and more efficacious. Initial trials with 200 mg/kg per month intravenously versus 100 mg/kg per month intramuscularly showed some improvement in infection prophylaxis, though there were still a considerable number of breakthrough infections. Roifman *et al.* (22) showed that much larger doses could be used safely in a cross-over study of 600 mg/kg per month versus 200 mg/kg per month. Doses up to a 1g/kg per month (in divided weekly doses) have now been given satisfactorily, with further reduction in chronic infections and few adverse reactions. However, very few patients need such doses and most patients receive approximately 400 mg/kg per month, usually in two doses, 2 weeks apart.

The dose of i.v. Ig required by a given patient is initially determined by the severity and frequency of infections as well as the starting level of serum IgG concentration. Initially i.v. Ig infusions may be given weekly or 2-weekly, in order to provide protection against infection rapidly; concurrent infection should be treated vigorously with antibiotics prior to the first infusion to reduce the risk of an adverse reaction (see later). Once stabilized, the dose of i.v. Ig is adjusted according to the clinical state of the patient, by changing the infusion interval as well as the amount of material infused at any one time.

HALF-LIFE

An alternative method of raising the serum IgG concentration is to shorten the interval between infusions as this reduces the differences between the peak (post-infusion) and trough (pre-infusion) levels. Initially infusions were given at 3-weekly intervals as studies of IgG half-life in volunteers, using radiolabelled myeloma IgG proteins, suggested a half-life of 21–28 days (25). More recently this has been confirmed using polyclonal Ig and a variety of statistical methods. An infusion of 10–20 g of i.v. Ig raises the plasma (and extravascular) concentration sharply, and since the rate of metabolism of infused IgG depends on the IgG concentration at the time (26–28), stability of IgG levels (and thus protection) is best achieved by frequent (weekly or 2-weekly) infusions of 5–15 g of i.v. Ig. The advent of home therapy (self-infusion at home) enables patients to have weekly i.v. Ig infusions easily. The increased frequency of infusions provides more stable levels of Ig and fewer breakthrough infections. Some patients with interstitial lung disease or intestinal lymphangiectasia require weekly infusions as they have demonstrably shortened serum IgG half-lives.

MONITORING

The dose and interval of i.v. Ig replacement therapy is titrated primarily against the clinical state of the patient; all patients should be warned that the benefit of i.v. Ig therapy may not be clinically apparent for several months. The trough serum IgG levels are measured to ensure that reasonable levels are reached within a few months. Once the steady state is reached, serum IgG is checked to ensure that IgG is not lost secondarily via the kidney, gastrointestinal tract or into inflamed tissues.

The level at which the IgG is maintained in order for the patient to stay infection free varies between patients; a general aim is to keep the IgG concentration within the normal range. Liver function tests must be measured regularly (every 2 months or so) to exclude subclinical, passively transmitted hepatitis (see below). Regular lung function tests (on a yearly basis) ensure that there is no subclinical deterioration due to insufficient replacement (8, 29).

ADMINISTRATION

Most adverse reactions experienced by immunodeficient patients occur during the first few infusions of i.v. Ig. This is probably due to a high antigenic load of pathogen-derived material which reacts rapidly with the infused Ig; the resultant increase in circulating immune complexes can lead to local and systematic complement activation. In order to avoid this, the first few infusions should be given slowly with antihistamine and hydrocortisone cover (30). Intensive antibiotic therapy for 2 weeks prior to the first infusion should be given, if appropriate, to reduce the bacterial load.

Most adverse reactions are related to the infusion rate (31) and are therefore avoidable, provided that the maximum rate (4 mg/kg per minute) is not exceeded. There has been a suggestion recently that very rapid infusion may be possible in selected patients who tolerate i.v. Ig preparations well, though the incidence of rate-related, moderate reactions is higher (12%) than that seen with more conservative rates (<2% of infusions) (32).

ADVERSE REACTIONS: IMMEDIATE

Adverse reactions may be mild, moderate or severe (Table 22.2). Mild reactions include headache, flushing, chills, low back pain, muscle pain, nausea and fatigue. Children too young to describe symptoms may scream or hold their head or abdomen to indicate an adverse reaction. It is interesting that in recent double-blind, controlled trials of i.v. Ig against placebo in patients with secondary hypogammaglobulinaemia, those receiving infusions of 0.3% albumin (placebo) also suffered these types of reaction, though at a lower frequency than those receiving Ig (33). Such reactions do not require the infusion to be stopped, but the rate should be slowed until the symptoms have subsided.

Table 22.2   Adverse reactions of i.v. Ig (in order of severity and frequency)

Mild
Headache
Fatigue/sleepiness
Flushing
Chills
Low back pain
Muscle pain
Nausea
Abdominal pain

Moderate
Persistence of mild symptoms despite slowing infusion rate
Worsening of mild symptoms
Wheezing—mild
Chest tightness
Vomiting
Unexplained anxiety

Severe
Chest pain
Stridor with acute shortness of breath ⎫
Hypotension   ⎭ Anaphylaxis

Moderate reactions, such as chest tightness, mild wheezing or vomiting, may require the infusion to be discontinued. Antihistamines, aspirin or hydrocortisone may be used both as treatment and prophylaxis for such adverse reactions (30). Adrenaline should always be available, even at home, in case an anaphylactoid reaction (hypotension and bronchospasm) should occur, though this is extremely uncommon with the present generation of i.v. Ig products.

Some patients get delayed symptoms within 24 hours following an infusion. These are usually mild (such as migraines), do not persist and respond to aspirin or paracetamol.

The cause of reactions remains unknown. It has been suggested that rapidly formed immune complexes between microbial antigens in the infected host and the infused antibodies activate complement, and subsequently provoke mast cells and leucocytes to release inflammatory mediators (34). Such a mechanism was also proposed to explain the increased incidence of reactions with older i.v. Ig products, known to contain complement-activating aggregates of IgG. To avoid such reactions, patients with active infection are treated with antibiotics for 24 hours before an infusion, which is then given slowly. The World Health Organization (WHO) standards require that the present i.v. Ig preparations are free of vasoactive substances.

Rare patients with CVI and complete absence of IgA may develop anti-IgA antibodies after infusion of blood, plasma or Ig containing IgA. The precise significance of such antibodies is unknown but three patients with very high and rising titres of anti-IgA antibodies have been reported in whom life-threatening, anaphylactic reactions occurred after only a few millilitres of IgA were infused (35). IgA-free material should be used for patients with high-titre anti-IgA antibodies and the titre of these antibodies monitored regularly in all patients without detectable IgA.

HOME THERAPY

The low incidence of adverse reactions with current i.v. Ig preparations and the ability to take avoidance measures to prevent such reactions have enabled self-infusion at home to be undertaken safely. Such programmes are available both in the UK (36) and in North America (37). Selection of patients is obviously important and they must have received several months of the i.v. Ig preparation used without adverse effects. Patients must be well motivated and be able to recognize and treat any reactions. They should be technically competent to take blood samples for monitoring of Ig levels and liver function tests, to solubilize the Ig powder (the liquid preparations are an advantage) as well as to perform the infusions. All patients are carefully followed up in the outpatient clinic in order to diagnose any complications of hypogammaglobulinaemia, as well as to check the adequacy of i.v. Ig therapy.

The advantages of self-infusion at home include vastly greater convenience for the patient, who avoids travel to and from the hospital. Patients also have a greater involvement in their therapy and disease, giving increased self-esteem and confidence. It has been shown to be a less expensive option than hospital-based infusions (36, 38) and enables infusion intervals to be reduced to optimize replacement therapy (37). Compliance is monitored with infusion logs and return of blood samples for serum IgG measurements. A register of home-based i.v. Ig infusion patients in the UK has shown how rapidly patients are recruited to this type of programme (39).

In Sweden, home therapy is provided using the subcutaneous route for rapid infusion of Ig replacement (40). A trial is planned in the UK to investigate the efficacy of this method for those patients in whom i.v. infusions at home are not considered feasible. The use of intramuscular preparations which do not contain either mercury compounds or high concentrations of sugars enables this route to be used without serious local reactions or sterile abscesses.

METHODS OF PREPARATION

There are over 17 preparations of i.v. Ig available in the world. Some countries are self-sufficient in Ig production, and manufacture only enough i.v. Ig for internal use (Scotland, France, Australia). Others produce more i.v. Ig than is required within the country and the excess is exported (Netherlands). Much i.v. Ig is made commercially from plasma obtained in several different countries and often from paid donors. This widens the risk of transmission of infection, and stringent standards have been established by the WHO to reduce this risk (41), since most countries depend on these commercial products.

All preparative methods involve an initial cold ethanol precipitation step (2); further purification of the Cohn fraction II paste to provide a preparation containing 90% intact monomeric IgG molecules free of fragments and aggregates is done in different ways, resulting in products with differing characteristics. WHO requirements include normal opsonic activity and complement binding of IgG antibodies and normal distribution of IgG subclasses, as well as absence of kinins, plasmin and prekallikrein activators (41).

The different methods of manufacture (see Table 22.3) result in preparations with varying amounts of IgA. Preparations which employ ion-exchange chromatography are very low in IgA content. These products are recommended for those few patients with selective IgA deficiency who have high-titre anti-IgA antibodies, in order to avoid potential systemic reactions (35, 42). The use of i.v. Ig containing low concentrations of IgA in those patients without anti-IgA antibodies (but capable of an IgG subclass response) in order to prevent sensitization to IgA (which might provoke a future blood transfusion reaction) is still controversial. Other methods for purification of IgG include the use of low pH, polyethylene glycol or low concentration of enzyme(s). The use of large amounts of cleavage enzymes to remove the Fc portion of IgG (in order to prevent complement activation) has been discarded, as the resulting preparations were less effective against pathogenic organisms.

Most immunologists are able to select a product for a particular patient since many countries have a choice of products. In practice this is not essential other than in patients with anti-IgA antibodies (see above). The liquid preparations are particularly suitable in clinical situations requiring ease of handling (e.g. self-infusion) or rapid availability for infusion, such as in

Table 22.3

Method of manufacture	IgA content (mg/l)
Acid pH 4.0 and trace of pepsin	720
Acid pH 4.2 and low salt	270
Ethanol fractionation	≥ 20
Polyethylene glycol	24
Polyethylene glycol and trace of trypsin	≤ 10
Ion-exchange chromatography	≤ 2

acute Guillain–Barré syndrome or life-threatening haemorrhage in a patient with idiopathic thrombocytopenic purpura (see later). Intravenous Ig products should not be used interchangeably; not only is the IgA content widely different but there remains the risk of transmission of blood-borne agents, albeit low. Indiscriminate use of more than one product in a given patient will prevent identification of the source of such infection if this occurs. If one particular method is more prone to viral transmission than others, this would be obscured (43).

SAFETY

The common starting material, Cohn fraction II, is obtained from cold ethanol precipitation of plasma; this is the method used for manufacturing intramuscular Ig. It is probably due to Cohn fractionation that no Ig preparation has been found to transmit retroviral infection, since cold ethanol appears to destroy this group of viruses (44). However, several preparations have been associated with outbreaks of non-A non-B hepatitis (45, 46). The associations of these transmissions with particular batches of i.v. Ig suggest that Cohn fractionation does not affect this group of viruses, and the deciding factor for transmission of non-A, non-B (including hepatitis C) viruses will depend on the size of the inoculum (46). To prevent contaminated donations being used, most manufacturers previously tested for liver enzyme abnormalities all the 6–15 000 units of blood used prior to pooling the plasma; those units with abnormal liver enzymes were discarded. Recently this has been superseded by screening all units for hepatitis C antibodies. A fourth generation of i.v. Ig products are just becoming available in which heat inactivation or the addition of a detergent solvent to specifically inactivate viruses is included in the manufacturing process.

The extension of the use of i.v. Ig to conditions other than hypogammaglobulinaemia has led to its use in patients with compromised renal function. Replacement doses (0.4–0.6 g/kg per month) do not appear to have a deleterious effect on renal function, even in patients with amyloidosis or renal tubular dysfunction secondary to multiple myeloma. Transient increases of serum creatinine have been reported following large doses (0.4 g/kg daily for 5 days) in patients with pre-existing nephrotic syndrome but these changes were short lived (47). High doses of i.v. Ig have also been associated occasionally with aseptic meningitis, and rarely with vascular haemolysis (48).

However, a 44-year-old woman with a mixed IgM/IgG cryoglobulinaemia due to an IgM paraprotein with rheumatoid activity suffered from acute renal failure when infused with 15 g of i.v. Ig; the patient's paraprotein, along with polyclonal IgG, was found in the renal deposits (49). Cryoglobulinaemia with rheumatoid factor should be considered a contraindication for i.v. Ig therapy. Recently small increases in plasma viscosity have been demonstrated in patients receiving high doses of i.v. Ig (0.4 g/kg daily × 5). These changes did not result in symptoms nor were the levels of plasma viscosity associated with the hyperviscosity syndrome reached. However, care should be taken in elderly patients with evidence of pre-existing ischaemia (50).

USES OF i.v. Ig IN SECONDARY IMMUNE DEFICIENCY

Intravenous Ig is also used in several situations in which bacterial infections are common as a result of a secondary immune deficiency state. These are new indications for i.v. Ig replacement therapy, and each clinical condition has undergone a randomized, placebo-controlled study. Since intramuscular Ig was not used previously in these conditions, these trials could use an i.v. placebo (often 0.3% albumin) in a double-blind manner.

Bacterial infections are known to be a problem in children infected with HIV, although these children in general do not have demonstrable hypogammaglobulinaemia and very often have raised levels of serum IgG. The recent double-blind, placebo-controlled study of HIV-infected children showed that i.v. Ig therapy increased the length of time free of serious bacterial infections for those children who have early disease (with a circulating CD4 lymphocyte count of $>200 \times 10^9$ per litre) (51). Similarly those children with intestinal lymphangiectasia with acquired secondary lymphocyte and humoral immune deficiencies appear to do well on i.v. Ig replacement, though the levels of IgG detectable in the serum remain low, due to the decreased half-life of IgG.

Pre-term infants, especially those of low birth weight, are hypogammaglobulinaemic due to inadequate placental transport of IgG (52) which takes place after 32 weeks of gestational age. Children born before this often suffer from late-onset sepsis since they have no maternal antibody for protection. Furthermore, neonates are unable to produce antibodies to polysaccharide antigens, whilst antibodies to protein antigens are restricted to the IgM isotype and are of low affinity (53). Several early studies suggested that i.v. Ig was protective against late-onset sepsis, although varying protocols

very high doses of i.v. Ig in several autoimmune (Table 22.4) and other diseases (Table 22.5) has raised the possibility of mechanisms other than simple replacement for the mode of action of i.v. Ig in both immunodeficient and autoimmune states. In immunodeficiency it has been assumed that the provision of antibodies with wide-ranging multiple specificities to invading organisms provides protection against most pathogens encountered in the environment. Whether or not the anti-inflammatory actions of i.v. Ig (at replacement doses) are also involved in preventing complications of hypogammaglobulinaemia, particularly those of chronic lung disease and granulomata, remains unproven. The other mechanisms by which high-dose i.v. Ig cause immune modulation (see Table 22.6), such as the reduction of B cell synthesis of autoantibodies or anti-idiotypic antibodies, in addition to Fc blockade, may not be applicable in immune deficiencies, since at least a fivefold lower dose is used for replacement therapy; overwhelming sepsis which might result from Fc blockade is not seen with the doses of i.v. Ig used for replacement therapy (33, 58).

Table 22.5   Other diseases[a]

Asthma	Several encouraging open studies in children
Recurrent seizures	Treatment-resistant seizures in children with/without IgG2 deficiency
Chronic fatigue syndrome	Conflicting reports of placebo-controlled studies using different patient selection criteria and doses of i.v. Ig

[a]These are unproven indications where blinded, placebo-controlled studies on well-defined homogeneous patient groups are urgently needed.

Table 22.6   Possible mechanisms of action of i.v. Ig when used in very high doses[a]

1. Blockade of Fc receptors for IgG
2. Regulation of idiotypic network and neutralization of existing autoantibodies
3. Direct action to reduce autoantibody synthesis by B cells
4. Decreased cytokine production by macrophages
5. Changes of proportions of and inhibition of functional activity in circulating T cells
6. Alteration of complement activation and complement-mediated clearance

[a]These are not mutually exclusive and several/all may act together.

INFECTIONS

Specific Ig with high-titre antibodies to particular organisms are used following exposure to viral infections (measles and chicken-pox) of cell-mediated immunodeficient subjects (such as children with acute leukaemia undergoing cytotoxic therapy). Likewise intramuscular Ig has been used for prophylaxis for hepatitis A and hepatitis B in normal subjects, as there are high titres of antibodies to these viruses in polyclonal Ig. The use of i.v. Ig for CMV prophylaxis in CMV-positive individuals having bone marrow transplantation is now established (57), but the use of high-titre CMV Ig to treat established CMV infections (either primary or reactivation) remains unclear. Similarly i.v. Ig has been used to treat X-linked antibody-deficient patients who have established enteroviral encephalitis; i.v. Ig has been used intraventricularly as well as intravenously, though not always with success (61).

The use of Ig to treat infection in otherwise immunocompetent individuals is doubtful. To date the only successful antibody treatment for severe bacterial disease has been with IgM mouse monoclonal antibodies (62); this may indicate that very high doses of multivalent opsonizing antibodies are required if antibody enhancement is to help in recovery. The anti-inflammatory action of human polyclonal IgG may be insufficient or even inappropriate in this situation.

CONCLUSION

The ability to give much larger doses of Ig intravenously, the widespread availability of i.v. Ig and its apparent safety have led to a rapid increase in the clinical indications for its use. Not only has the range of immunodeficient states widened, for both primary and secondary immune deficiencies, but i.v. Ig is used extensively in autoimmune diseases (5–7).

Intravenous Ig is an expensive form of therapy, whose efficacy needs to be proved in double-blind, placebo-controlled trials before widespread adoption in any disease. The use of anecdotal cases and open trials to justify the use of this expensive material is not sufficient. This is particularly important where the immune mechanisms by which i.v. Ig results in improvement remain largely speculative. Appropriate, placebo-controlled, double-blind trials are obligatory, before i.v. Ig is adopted as an efficacious mode of treatment.

ACKNOWLEDGEMENTS

I am grateful to Mrs Lynda Beckley and Mrs Vanessa Johnson for their patient and careful processing of the manuscript, and Dr Siraj Misbah for critical evaluation of the text.

REFERENCES

1. Bruton, O. (1952) Agammaglobulinaemia. *Paediatrics*, **9**, 722–728.
2. Cohn, E.J., Oncley, J.L., Strong, L.E. *et al.* (1944) Chemical, clinical and immunological studies of the products of human plasma fractionation: Characterisation of the protein fractions of human plasma. *J. Clin. Invest.*, **23**, 417–432.
3. Barandun, S. and Isliker, H. (1986) Development of immunoglobulin preparation for intravenous use. *Vox Sang.*, **51**, 157–160.

40. Gardulf, A., Hammarstrom, L. and Smith, C.I.E. (1991) Home treatment of hypogammaglobulinaemia with subcutaneous gammaglobulin by rapid infusion. *Lancet*, **338**, 162–166.
41. IUIS/WHO (1983) Appropriate use of human immunoglobulin in clinical practice. *Clin. Exp. Immunol.*, **52**, 417–422.
42. Bjorkander, J., Hammarstrom, L., Smith, C.I.E. *et al.* (1987) Immunoglobulin prophylaxis in patients with antibody deficiency states and anti IgA antibodies. *J. Clin. Immunol.*, **7**, 8–15.
43. Dorey, J., Collinge, D., Chapel, H.M. and Dolton, R. (1990) Intravenous Immunoglobulin Preparations. *Pharm. J.*, **245**, 775.
44. Hamamoto, Y., Harada, H., Yamamoto, M. *et al.* (1987) Elimination of viruses from an IVIg preparation. *Vox Sang.*, **53**, 65–69.
45. Bjorkander, J., Cunningham-Rundles, C., Lundin, P., Olsson, R., Soderstrom, R. and Hanson, L.A. (1988) Intravenous immunoglobulin prophylaxis causing liver damage in 16 of 77 patients with hypogammaglobulinemia or IgG subclass deficiency. *Am. J. Med.*, **84**, 107–111.
46. Williams, P.E., Yap, P.-L., Gillon, J. *et al.* (1989) Transmission of non-A non-B hepatitis by pH4 treated intravenous immunoglobulin. *Vox Sang.*, **57**, 15–18.
47. Schifferli, J., Favere, H., Nydegger, U. *et al.* (1991) High dose IVIg treatment and renal function. *Lancet*, **337**, 457–458.
48. Chapel, H.M. and Misbah, S.A. (1993) Adverse effects of immunoglobulin therapy. *Drug Safety* (in press).
49. Barton, J., Herrera, G.A., Galla, J.H., Bertoli, L.F., Work, J. and Koopman, W.J. (1987) Acute cryoglobulinaemic renal failure after intravenous infusion of gammaglobulin. *Am. J. Med.*, **82**, 624–629.
50. Reinhart, W.H. and Berchtold, P.E. (1992) Effect of high-dose intravenous immunoglobulin therapy on blood rheology. *Lancet*, **339**, 662–664.
51. National Institute of Child Health and Human Development (1991) Intravenous immunoglobulin study group: IVIg for prevention of bacterial infections in children with symptomatic human immunodeficiency virus infection. *N. Engl. J. Med.*, **325**, 73–80.
52. Ugazio, A.G., Chirico, G., Duse, M., Plebani, A., Notarangelo, L.D., Rondini, G. and Burgio, G.R. (1991) Immunoglobulin treatment and prophylaxis in the neonate. In Imbach, P. (ed.) *Immunotherapy with Intravenous Immunoglobulins*. Academic Press, New York, pp. 75–92.
53. Butler, J.L., Suzuki, T., Kubagawa, H. and Cooper, M.D. (1986) Humoral immunity in the human neonate. In Burgio, G.R., Hanson, L.A. and Ugazio, A.G. (eds) *Immunology of the Neonate*. Springer Verlag, Berlin, pp. 27–36.
54. Clapp, D.W., Kliegman, R.M., Baley, J.E., Shenker, N., Kyllonen, K., Fanaroff, A.A. and Berger, M. (1989) Use of intravenously administered immune globulin to prevent nosocomial sepsis in low birth weight infants: A pilot study. *J. Pediatr.*, **115**, 973–978.
55. Eibl, M.M., Wolf, H.M., Furnkranz, H. and Rosenkranz, A. (1988) Prevention of necrotising enterocolitis in low birth weight infants by IgA–IgG feeding. *N. Engl. J. Med.*, **319**, 1–7.
56. Lum, L.G. (1987) The kinetics of immune reconstitution after human marrow transplantation. *Blood*, **69**, 369–380.
57. Sullivan, K.M., Kopecky, K.J., Jocom, J. *et al.* (1990) Immunomodulating and antimicrobial efficacy of intravenous immunoglobulin in bone marrow transplantation. *N. Engl. J. Med.*, **323**, 705–712.

58. Griffiths, H., Brennan, V., Lea, J., Bunch, C., Lee, M. and Chapel, H. (1989) Crossover study of immunoglobulin replacement therapy in patients with low grade B cell tumours. *Blood*, **73**, 366–368.
59. Weeks, J.C., Tierney, M.R. and Weinstein, M.C. (1991) Cost effectiveness of prophylactic IVIg in chronic lymphocytic leukaemia. *N. Engl. J. Med.*, **325**, 81–86.
60. Besa, E.C. and Klumpe, D. (1992) Prophylactic immunoglobulinin chronic lymphocytic leukaemia. *N. Engl. J. Med.*, **326**, 139.
61. Misbah, S.A., Spickett, G.P., Hockaday, J.M., Kroll, J.S., Kurtz, J.B., Moxon, E.R. and Chapel, H.M. (1992) Chronic enteroviral meningoencephalitis in agammaglobulinaemia: Case report and literature review. *J. Clin. Immunol.*, **12**, 266–270.
62. Ziegler, E.J., Fisher, C.J., Sprung, C.L. *et al.* (1991) Treatment of gram-negative bacteraemia and septic shock with HA-1A human monocloncal antibody against endotoxin: A randomized, double-blind, placebo-controlled trial. *N. Engl. J. Med.*, **324**, 429–436.
63. Newland, A.C., Macey, M.G. and Keys, P.A. (1991) IVIg: Mechanisms of action and their clinical application. In Imbach, P. (ed.) *Immunotherapy with Intravenous Immunoglobulins*. Academic Press, London, pp. 15–26.
64. Newburger, J.W., Takahashi, M., Beiser, A.S. *et al.* (1991) A single intravenous infusion of gamma globulin as compared with four infusions in the treatment of acute Kawasaki syndrome. *N. Engl. J. Med.*, **234**, 1633–1639.
65. Van der Merché, F.G.A. and Schumitz, P.I.M. for the Dutch Guillain–Barré Study Group (1992) High dose intravenous immunoglobulin versus plasma exchange in Guillain–Barré Syndrome. *N. Engl. J. Med.*, **326**, 1123–1129.
66. Van Doorn, P.A., Brand, A., Strengers, P.F.W. *et al.* (1990) High dose IVIg in chronic inflammatory demyelinating polyneuropathy: A double blind placebo controlled, cross over study. *Neurology*, **40**, 209–212.

Index

Index compiled by Jill Halliday